CONTENTS

CAROLYN JARVIS, PhD, APN, CNP

Professor of Nursing
School of Nursing
Illinois Wesleyan University
Bloomington, Illinois
and
Family Nurse Practitioner
Bloomington, Illinois

Physical Examination & Health Assessment

Seventh Edition

Original Illustrations by Pat Thomas, CMI, FAMI
East Troy, Wisconsin

Assessment Photographs by Kevin Strandberg
Professor of Art
Illinois Wesleyan University
Bloomington, Illinois

ELSEVIER

ELSEVIER

3251 Riverport Lane
St. Louis, Missouri 63043

Notices

Knowledge and best practice in this field are constantly changing. As new research and experience broaden
our understanding, changes in research methods, professional practices, or medical treatment may become
necessary.

Practitioners and researchers must always rely on their own experience and knowledge in evaluating and
using any information, methods, compounds, or experiments described herein. In using such information
or methods they should be mindful of their own safety and the safety of others, including parties for
whom they have a professional responsibility.

With respect to any drug or pharmaceutical products identified, readers are advised to check the most
current information provided (i) on procedures featured or (ii) by the manufacturer of each product to be
administered, to verify the recommended dose or formula, the method and duration of administration,
and contraindications. It is the responsibility of practitioners, relying on their own experience and
knowledge of their patients, to make diagnoses, to determine dosages and the best treatment for each
individual patient, and to take all appropriate safety precautions.

To the fullest extent of the law, neither the Publisher nor the authors, contributors, or editors, assume
any liability for any injury and/or damage to persons or property as a matter of products liability,
negligence or otherwise, or from any use or operation of any methods, products, instructions, or ideas
contained in the material herein.

International Standard Book Number: 978-1-4557-2810-7

Executive Content Strategist: Lee Henderson
Content Development Manager: Laurie Gower
Senior Content Development Specialist: Heather Bays
Publishing Services Manager: Deborah L. Vogel
Senior Project Manager: Jodi M. Willard
Design Direction: Julia Dummitt

Printed in Canada

Last digit is the print number: 9 8 7 6 5 4 3 2

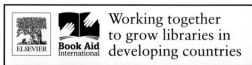

To Paul, who read every word, with love and thanks

Carolyn Jarvis received her BSN cum laude from the University of Iowa, her MSN from Loyola University (Chicago), and her PhD from the University of Illinois at Chicago, with a research interest in the physiologic effect of alcohol on the cardiovascular system. She has taught physical assessment and critical care nursing at Rush University (Chicago), the University of Missouri (Columbia), and the University of Illinois (Urbana), and she has taught physical assessment, pharmacology, and pathophysiology at Illinois Wesleyan University (Bloomington).

Dr. Jarvis is a recipient of the University of Missouri's Superior Teaching Award; has taught physical assessment to thousands of baccalaureate students, graduate students, and nursing professionals; has held 150 continuing education seminars; and is the author of numerous articles and textbook contributions.

Dr. Jarvis has maintained a clinical practice in advanced practice roles—first as a cardiovascular clinical specialist in various critical care settings and as a certified family nurse practitioner in primary care. She is currently a Professor at Illinois Wesleyan University; is a nurse practitioner in Bloomington, Illinois; and is licensed as an advanced practice nurse in the state of Illinois. During the last 8 years, her enthusiasm has focused on using Spanish language skills to provide health care in rural Guatemala and at the Community Health Care Clinic in Bloomington. Dr. Jarvis has been instrumental in developing a synchronous teaching program for Illinois Wesleyan students both in Barcelona, Spain, and at the home campus.

CONTRIBUTORS

Susan Caplan, PhD, MSN, APRN-BC
The contributor for Chapter 2, Cultural Competence, and the culture content in Chapter 7, Domestic and Family Violence Assessments, is an Assistant Professor and Family Nurse Practitioner Specialty Director at Rutgers University. Dr. Caplan completed her PhD in Nursing at Yale University. She has published and lectured extensively about cultural competency in the health care professions.

Martha Driessnack, PhD, PNP-BC
The contributor for the Health Promotion boxes is an Associate Professor in the School of Nursing at Oregon Health & Science University. She received her PhD from Oregon Health & Science University and completed a postdoctoral research fellowship in clinical genetics. Her primary focus is as an advocate for including the voices of children in health-related decisions that affect them.

Ann Eckhardt, PhD, RN
The co-contributor for Chapter 1, Evidence-Based Assessment; Chapter 3, The Interview; Chapter 9, General Survey, Measurement, Vital Signs; the new adult case studies; and the electronic health recording content in Chapter 29 is an assistant professor in the School of Nursing at Illinois Wesleyan University. She received her PhD from the University of Illinois at Chicago and has over a decade of clinical experience in critical care and nursing leadership. Her research focus is symptomatology in heart disease.

Carla Graf, PhD, RN, CNS-BC
The co-contributor for Chapter 31, Functional Assessment of the Older Adult, is a board-certified Geriatric Clinical Nurse Specialist and is an Assistant Clinical Professor at the University of California San Francisco School of Nursing. She is currently the Manager for Innovations in Transitions of Care at UCSF Medical Center.

Amanda F. Hopkins, PhD, RN
Dr. Hopkins contributed the pediatric case studies within each of the body systems chapters. She is an Assistant Professor in the School of Nursing at Illinois Wesleyan University. She specializes in pediatric health care and cross-cultural awareness.

Sarah Jarvis, BSN, RN, DNPc
The co-contributor for Chapter 10, Pain Assessment: The Fifth Vital Sign, is a hematology and oncology nurse at the University of Michigan Health System in Ann Arbor, Michigan. She has 7 years of experience working with cancer-related pain management. She is also a doctoral student at Wayne State University in Detroit, Michigan.

Joyce K. Keithley, DNSc, RN, FAAN
The contributor for Chapter 11, Nutritional Assessment, is a Professor at Rush University College of Nursing and Rush University Medical Center in Chicago. Because she has worked in both clinical and instructional settings, she is an experienced and well-known practitioner, teacher, researcher, and author in the area of clinical nutrition.

Kelsey Merl, MSN, MPH, PNP-C
The co-contributor for Chapter 7, Domestic and Family Violence Assessments, is a Pediatric Nurse Practitioner on the surgical trauma team at the UCSF Benioff Children's Hospital Oakland. She is on the hospital's forensic center for child protection team, serving children who have endured possible abuse and neglect. She conducts domestic violence research to help keep women and college students safe in their relationships.

Shawna S. Mudd, DNP, PNP-BC, CPNP-AC
Dr. Mudd is a co-contributor for Chapter 7, Domestic and Family Violence Assessments. She is an Assistant Professor at The Johns Hopkins University School of Nursing and senior pediatric nurse practitioner in the pediatric emergency department at The Johns Hopkins Hospital.

Daniel J. Sheridan, PhD, RN, FAAN
The co-contributor for Chapter 7, Domestic and Family Violence Assessments, is a Professor at the Goldfarb School of Nursing Graduate Studies Department at Barnes-Jewish College. Dr. Sheridan is also an adjunct Associate Professor at the Flinders University School of Nursing and Midwifery in Adelaide, South Australia. Dr. Sheridan has 30 years of research and experience working with survivors of family abuse and sexual assault.

INSTRUCTOR AND STUDENT ANCILLARIES

Key Point Summaries

Joanna Cain, BSN, BA, RN
Auctorial Pursuits, Inc.
President and Founder
Austin, Texas

NCLEX® Review Questions and PowerPoint Presentations

Daryle Wane, PhD, ARNP-BC
Professor of Nursing
Pasco-Hernando Community College
New Port Richey, Florida

TEACH for Nurses

Melanie Cole, MA
Freelance Editor
Community Treatment, Inc.
University of Missouri–St. Louis
St. Louis, Missouri

Test Bank

Christine Kessel, PhD, MSN, RN, CNE
Professor
Trinity College of Nursing and Health Sciences
Rock Island, Illinois

REVIEWERS

Jennifer Taylor Alderman, MSN, RNC-OB, CNL
Clinical Assistant Professor/Academic Counselor
School of Nursing
The University of North Carolina at Chapel Hill
Chapel Hill, North Carolina

Susan Caplan, PhD, MSN, FNP-BC
Assistant Professor
Rutgers University
Newark, New Jersey

Elizabeth Day, RN, MSN, CHPN
Nursing Faculty
Fresno City College;
Academic Faculty
University of Phoenix
Fresno, California

Debra B. Gordon, RN-BC, MS, DNP, ACNS-BC, FAAN
Teaching Associate
Department of Anesthesiology & Pain Medicine
University of Washington
Seattle, Washington

Christine Kessel, PhD, MSN, RN, CNE
Professor
Trinity College of Nursing and Health Sciences
Rock Island, Illinois

Karen Klosinski, PhD(c), MSN/Ed, RN
Assistant Professor of Nursing
Purdue University North Central
Westville, Indiana

Mary Lashley, PhD, RN, APHN, BC
Professor
Community Health Nursing
Towson University
Towson, Maryland

Phillip J. Moore, MSN, RN, FNP-BC
Clinical Instructor
University of Tennessee, College of Nursing
Knoxville, Tennessee

Kathryn Schartz, MSN, RN, PPCPNP-BC
Assistant Professor
School of Nursing
Baker University
Topeka, Kansas

Gwen Sherwood, PhD, RN, FAAN
Professor and Associate Dean for Academic Affairs
University of North Carolina at Chapel Hill
Chapel Hill, North Carolina

Constance Sinclair, CNM, MSN
Chief Nurse-Midwife
Kaiser Santa Rosa Medical Center
Santa Rosa, California

Tammy Spencer, RN, MS, CNE, ACNS-BC, CCNS
Senior Instructor
University of Colorado
College of Nursing
Aurora, Colorado

Troy Spicer, MS, FNP-BC
Dean and Associate Professor
School of Nursing and Health Sciences
Abraham Baldwin Agricultural College
Tifton, Georgia

Mary Charles Sutphin, MSN, CNM
Certified Nurse Midwife
Clinical Instructor
University of North Carolina School of Nursing
Chapel Hill, North Carolina

Christina Tomkins, RN, MSN, CEN, CCRN, CRNP, PHRN
Assistant Professor
Misericordia University
Dallas, Pennsylvania

Jo A. Voss, PhD, RN, CNS
Associate Professor
South Dakota State University
West River Department of Nursing
Rapid City, South Dakota

INSTRUCTOR AND STUDENT ANCILLARIES

Christine Kessel, PhD, MSN, RN, CNE
Professor
Trinity College of Nursing and Health Sciences
Rock Island, Illinois

Kathryn Schartz, MSN, RN, PPCPNP-BC
Assistant Professor
School of Nursing
Baker University
Topeka, Kansas

This book is for those who still carefully examine their patients and for those of you who wish to learn how to do so. You develop and practice, and then learn to trust, your health history and physical examination skills. In this book, I give you the tools to do that. Learn to listen to the patient—most often he or she will tell you what is wrong (and right) and what you can do to meet his or her health care needs. Then learn to inspect, examine, and listen to the person's body. The data are all there and are accessible to you by using just a few extra tools. High-tech machinery is a smart and sophisticated adjunct, but it cannot replace your own bedside assessment of your patient. Whether you are a beginning examiner or an advanced-practice student, this book holds the content you need to develop and refine your clinical skills.

NEW TO THE SEVENTH EDITION

The 7th edition retains the strengths of the first six editions: a clear, approachable writing style; an attractive and user-friendly format; integrated developmental variations across the life span with age-specific content on the infant, child, adolescent, pregnant woman, and older adult; cultural competencies in both a separate chapter and throughout the book; hundreds of meticulously prepared full-color illustrations; sample documentation of normal and abnormal findings and 60 clinical case studies; integration of the complete health assessment in 2 photo essays at the end of the book where all key steps of a complete head-to-toe examination of the adult, infant, and child are summarized; and a photo essay highlighting a condensed head-to-toe assessment for each daily shift of nursing care.

The 7th edition has a new chapter section and several new content features. A new **Electronic Health Recording** section in Chapter 29 discusses the documenting of assessment findings with the new technology. Chapter 28 is a new photo essay on the complete physical assessment of the Infant, Child, and Adolescent. There are 45 new **clinical case studies** and 15 revised studies of frequently encountered situations that show the application of assessment techniques to patients of varying ages and clinical situations. These case histories, in SOAP format ending in diagnosis, use the actual language of recording. Diagnoses are derived from assessment data and show the relationship between medical and nursing diagnoses. I encourage professors and students to use these as critical thinking exercises to discuss and develop a Plan for each one.

My focus throughout is evidence-based practice. Chapter 1, **Evidence-Based Assessment,** is reoriented to conducting the most effective, accurate exams based on data showing their usefulness in patient assessment. Throughout the text, examination techniques are explained and included depending on current clinical **evidence.**

Pat Thomas has designed 32 new art pieces in beautiful detail. We have worked together to design new teaching tables for students; note Table 13-4, Thyroid Hormone Disorders; Fig. 19-12; Jugular venous pulsations; Table 21-2, Clinical Portrait of Intestinal Obstruction; Fig. 23-59 The Glascow Coma Scale; Table 23-6, Ischemic and Hemorrhagic Stroke; and many others. Kevin Strandberg and I have had many new photo shoots, replacing exam photos in Chapter 18, Thorax and Lungs, and many others.

All **Promoting a Healthy Lifestyle** boxes have been rewritten to respond to current health-related concerns. These boxes describe an important teaching topic related to the body system discussed in each chapter—a teaching topic you can use to enhance patient health. Also, new content on **obesity** is added to numerous chapters to address the important role we health care providers have in assessing and addressing obesity in adults and children.

The **Abnormal Findings** tables located at the end of the chapters are revised and updated with many new clinical photos. These are still divided into two sections. The Abnormal Findings tables present frequently encountered conditions that every clinician should recognize, and the Abnormal Findings for Advanced Practice tables isolate the detailed illustrated atlas of conditions encountered in advanced practice roles.

All chapters are **revised and updated,** with accurate coverage in anatomy and physiology, physical examination, and assessment tools. **Developmental Competence** sections provide updated growth and development information, and the Examination section of each body system chapter details **exam techniques and clinical findings for infants, children, adolescents, and aging adults.**

Culture and Genetics data have been revised and updated in each chapter. Together with a revised Chapter 2 on cultural competence, these data highlight the importance of diversity and cultural awareness.

Chapter bibliographies are up-to-date and are meant to be used. They include the best of clinical practice readings as well as basic science research and nursing research, with an emphasis on scholarship from the last 5 years.

DUAL FOCUS AS TEXT AND REFERENCE

Physical Examination & Health Assessment is a **text for beginning students** of physical examination as well as a **text and reference for advanced practitioners.** The chapter progression and format permit this scope without sacrificing one use for the other.

Chapters 1 through 7 focus on **health assessment of the whole person,** including health promotion for all age-groups, cultural environment and assessment, interviewing and complete health history gathering, the social environment of mental status, and the changes to the whole person on the occasions of substance use or domestic violence.

Chapters 8 through 11 begin the approach to the **clinical care setting,** describing physical data-gathering techniques, how to set up the examination site, body measurement and vital signs, pain assessment, and nutritional assessment.

Chapters 12 through 26 focus on the **physical examination and related health history** in a body systems approach. This is the most efficient method of performing the examination and is the most logical method for student learning and retrieval of data. Both the novice and the advanced practitioner can review anatomy and physiology; learn the skills, expected findings, and common variations for generally healthy people; and study a comprehensive atlas of abnormal findings.

Chapters 27 through 31 **integrate the complete health assessment.** Chapters 27, 28, and 29 present the choreography of the head-to-toe exam for a complete screening examination in various age-groups and for the focused exam in this **unique chapter on a hospitalized adult.** Chapters 30 and 31 present special populations—the health assessment of the pregnant woman and the functional assessment of the older adult, including assessment tools and caregiver and environmental assessment.

This text is valuable to both advanced practice students and experienced clinicians because of its comprehensive approach. *Physical Examination & Health Assessment* can help clinicians learn the skills for advanced practice, refresh their memory, review a specific examination technique when confronted with an unfamiliar clinical situation, compare and label a diagnostic finding, and study the Abnormal Findings for Advanced Practice.

CONCEPTUAL APPROACH

Physical Examination & Health Assessment is committed to:
- **Holism,** the individual as a whole, both in wellness needs and illness needs.
- **Health promotion** in the health history questions that elicit self-care behaviors, the Promoting a Healthy Lifestyle boxes, nutrition information, and the self-examination teaching presented for skin, breast, and testicles.
- Contracting with the person as an **active participant in health care** by discussing what the person currently is doing to promote health and by engaging the person to participate in self-care.
- **Cultural competencies** that take into account this global society in which culturally diverse people seek health care.
- Individuals **across the life cycle,** supporting the belief that a person's state of health must be considered in light of developmental stage. All chapters integrate relevant devel-

opmental content. Developmental anatomy, modifications of examination technique, and expected findings are given for infants and children, adolescents, pregnant females, and aging adults.

FEATURES FROM EARLIER EDITIONS

Physical Examination & Health Assessment is built on the strengths of the previous edition and is designed to engage students and enhance learning:
1. **Method of examination** (Objective Data section) is clear, orderly, and easy to follow. Hundreds of original examination illustrations are placed directly with the text to demonstrate the physical examination in a step-by-step format.
2. **Two-column format** begins in the Subjective Data section, where the running column highlights the rationales for asking history questions. In the Objective Data section, the running column highlights selected abnormal findings to show a clear relationship between normal and abnormal findings.
3. **Abnormal Findings tables** organize and expand on material in the examination section. The atlas format of these extensive collections of pathology and original illustrations helps students recognize, sort, and describe abnormal findings. When applicable, the text under a table entry is presented in a Subjective Data–Objective Data format.
4. **Genetics and racial variations** in disease incidence and response to treatment are cited throughout using current research. The Jarvis text has the richest amount of cultural-racial-genetic content available in any assessment text.
5. **Developmental approach** in each chapter presents a prototype for the adult, then age-specific content for the infant, child, adolescent, pregnant female, and aging adult so students can learn common variations for all age-groups.
6. **Cultural competencies** are extensive throughout and present the expected variations for culturally diverse people. Chapter 2 keynotes the cultural content, including customs to consider when planning the interview, cultural variations to consider when reviewing examination findings, and a Heritage Assessment Guide.
7. **Stunning full-color art** shows detailed human anatomy, physiology, examination techniques, and abnormal findings.
8. **Health history** (Subjective Data) appears in two places: (1) in Chapter 4, The Complete Health History, and (2) in pertinent history questions that are repeated and expanded in each regional examination chapter, including history questions that highlight health promotion and self-care. This presentation helps students understand the relationship between subjective and objective data. Considering the history and examination data together, as you do in the clinical setting, means that each

chapter can stand on its own if a person has a specific problem related to that body system.

Chapter 3, The Interview, has the most complete discussion available on the process of communication, interviewing skills, techniques and traps, and cultural considerations (for example, how nonverbal behavior varies cross-culturally and the use of an interpreter).

9. **Summary checklists** at the end of each chapter provide a quick review of examination steps to help develop a mental checklist.

10. **Sample recordings** of normal and abnormal findings show the written language you should use so that documentation, whether written or electronic, is complete yet succinct.

11. **Integration of the complete health assessment** for the adult, infant, and child is presented as illustrated essays in Chapters 27 and 28. This approach integrates all the steps into a choreographed whole. Included is a complete write-up of a health history and physical examination.

12. **User-friendly design** makes the book easy to use. Frequent subheadings and instructional headings assist in easy retrieval of material.

13. **Spanish-language translations** highlight important phrases for communication during the physical examination and appear on the inside back cover.

SUPPLEMENTS

- The *Pocket Companion for Physical Examination & Health Assessment* continues to be a handy and current clinical reference that provides pertinent material in full color, with over 200 illustrations from the textbook.

- The *Laboratory Manual* with physical examination forms is a workbook, now in full color, that includes for each chapter a student study guide, glossary of key terms, clinical objectives, regional write-up forms, and review questions. The pages are perforated so students can use the regional write-up forms in the skills laboratory or in the clinical setting and turn them in to the instructor. This edition adds review questions to help students prepare for the NCLEX® examination.

- The revised *Health Assessment Online* is an innovative and dynamic teaching and learning tool with more than **8000 electronic assets**, including video clips, anatomic overlays, animations, audio clips, interactive exercises, laboratory/diagnostic tests, review questions, and **electronic charting activities**. Comprehensive **Self-Paced Learning Modules** offer increased flexibility to faculty who wish to provide students with tutorial learning modules and in-depth capstone case studies for each body system chapter in the text. The **Capstone Case Studies** now include **Quality and Safety Challenge** activities. Additional **Advance Practice Case Studies** put the student in the exam room and test history taking and documentation skills. The comprehensive **video clip library** shows exam procedures across the life span, including clips on the pregnant woman. Animations, sounds, images, interactive activities, and video clips are embedded in the learning modules and cases to provide a dynamic, multimodal learning environment for today's learners.

- *Physical Examination & Health Assessment Video Series* is an 18-video package developed in conjunction with this text. There are 12 body system videos and 6 head-to-toe videos, with the latter containing complete examinations of the neonate, child, adult, older adult, pregnant woman, and the bedside examination of a hospitalized adult. This series is available in DVD or streaming online formats. There are over 5 hours of video footage with highlighted Cross-Cultural Care Considerations, Developmental Considerations, and Health Promotion Tips, as well as Instructor Booklets with video overviews, outlines, learning objectives, discussion topics, and questions with answers.

- The companion *EVOLVE Website* (http://evolve.elsevier .com/Jarvis/) contains learning objectives, more than 300 multiple-choice and alternate-format review questions, system-by-system exam summaries, bedside exam summaries, printable key points from the chapter, and a comprehensive physical exam form for the adult. **Case studies**—including a variety of developmental and cultural variables—help students apply health assessment skills and knowledge. These include 25 in-depth case studies with critical thinking questions and answer guidelines, as well as printable health promotion handouts. Also included is a complete Head-to-Toe Video Examination of the Adult that can be viewed in its entirety or by systems, as well as a new printable section on Quick Assessments for Common Conditions.

- *Simulation Learning System.* The new *Simulation Learning System* (SLS) is an online toolkit that incorporates medium- to high-fidelity simulation with scenarios that enhance the clinical decision-making skills of students. The SLS offers a comprehensive package of resources, including leveled patient scenarios, detailed instructions for preparation and implementation of the simulation experience, debriefing questions that encourage critical thinking, and learning resources to reinforce student comprehension.

- For instructors, the Evolve website presents TEACH for Nursing, PowerPoint slides with Audience Response Questions for iClicker and Case Studies, a comprehensive Image Collection, and a Test Bank. **TEACH for Nurses** provides annotated learning objectives, key terms, teaching strategies for the classroom in a revised section with strategies for both clinical and simulation lab use and a focus on QSEN competencies, critical thinking exercises, websites, and performance checklists. The **PowerPoint** slides include 2000 slides with integrated images. **Audience Response Questions** provide 90 questions for in-class student participation. A separate 1200-illustration **Image Collection** is featured and, finally, the ExamView **Test Bank** has over 1000 multiple-choice and alternate-format questions with coded answers and rationales.

IN CONCLUSION

Throughout all stages of manuscript preparation and production, we make every effort to develop a book that is readable, informative, instructive, and vital. Thank you for your enthusiastic response to the earlier editions of *Physical Examination & Health Assessment*. I am grateful for your encouragement and for your suggestions, which are incorporated wherever possible. Your comments and suggestions continue to be welcome for this edition.

Carolyn Jarvis
c/o Education
Elsevier
3251 Riverport Lane
Maryland Heights, MO 63043

ACKNOWLEDGMENTS

I am grateful for the many talented and dedicated colleagues who helped make the revision of the 7th edition of this textbook possible.

Thank you to the bright, hardworking professional team at Elsevier. I am fortunate to have the support of Laurie Gower, Content Development Manager. Laurie is positive and skilled in directing the big picture of the books, as well as the endless details. She has a calm and forthright manner that is so welcome. Also, I am grateful to work daily with Heather Bays, Senior Content Development Specialist. Heather juggled all the deadlines, readied all the manuscript for production, searched out endless photos for abnormal examination findings, kept current with the permissions, and so many other daily details. Her work is pivotal to our success. I feel lucky she joined our team.

I had a wonderful production team and I am most grateful to them. Debbie Vogel, Publishing Services Manager, supervised the schedule for book production. I am especially grateful to Jodi Willard, Senior Project Manager, who has been in daily contact to keep the production organized and moving. She works in so many extra ways to keep production on schedule. I am pleased with the striking colors of the interior design of the 7th edition and the beautiful cover; both are the work of Julia Dummitt, Book Designer. The individual page layout is the wonderful work of Leslie Foster, Illustrator/Designer. Leslie hand-crafted every page, always planning how the page can be made better. Because of her work, I added 45 new case studies and scores of new art and tables, and we still came out with comparable page length for the 7th edition.

I have gifted artistic colleagues, who made this book such a vibrant teaching display. Pat Thomas, Medical Illustrator, is so talented and contributes format ideas as well as brilliant drawings. Kevin Strandberg patiently sets up equipment for all our photo shoots and then captures lovely exam photos of children and adults. Julia Jarvis also photographed our infant photos with patience and clarity.

I am fortunate to have dedicated research assistants. Molly Gray Guenette searched and retrieved countless articles and sources. She was always prompt and accurate. Karolina Sierzputowska just joined as a research assistant and has helped in many ways. I am most grateful to Paul Jarvis, who read and reread endless copies of galley and page proof, finding any errors and making helpful suggestions.

Thank you to the faculty and students who took the time to write letters of suggestions and encouragement—your comments are gratefully received and are very helpful. I am fortunate to have the skilled reviewers who spend time reading the chapter manuscript and making valuable suggestions.

Most important are the members of my wonderful family, growing in number and in support. Their constant encouragement has kept me going throughout this process.

Carolyn Jarvis

CONTENTS

CHAPTER 1

Evidence-Based Assessment

1-1

C.D. is a 23-year-old Caucasian woman who works as a pediatric nurse at a children's hospital. She comes to clinic today for a scheduled physical examination to establish with a new primary care provider (Fig. 1-1). On arrival the examiner collects a health history and performs a complete physical examination. The preliminary list of significant findings looks like this:

- Recent graduate of a BSN program. Strong academic record (A/B). Reports no difficulties in college.

Past medical history:

- Diagnosed with type 1 diabetes at age 12 years. Became stuporous during a family vacation. Rushed home; admitted to ICU with decreased level of consciousness (LOC) and heavy labored breathing; blood sugar 1200 mg/dL. Coma × 3 days; ICU stay for 5 days. Diabetic teaching during hospital stay with follow-up with diabetic educator prn.
- Now uses insulin pump. Reports HbA1c <7%.

- Finger fracture and ankle sprains during childhood (unable to remember exact dates).
- Bronchitis "a lot" as a child.
- Tympanostomy tubes at age 5 because of frequent ear infections. No issues in adulthood.
- Diabetic seizures at ages 16 and 18 caused by hypoglycemia. Family gave glucagon injection. Did not go to ED.
- Denies tobacco use. Reports having 1 glass of red wine approximately 5-6 days in the past month.
- Current medications: Insulin, simvastatin, birth control pills, fish oil, multivitamin, melatonin (for sleep).
- Birth control since age 16 because of elevated blood sugar during menstruation. Gynecologic examinations annually. Last Pap test 6 months ago; told was "negative."
- Family history: Mother and paternal grandfather with hypertension; maternal grandfather transient ischemic attack, died at age 80 from a myocardial infarction; maternal grandmother died at age 49 of cervical and ovarian cancer; paternal grandmother with arthritis in the hands and knees; paternal grandfather with kidney disease at age 76; sister with migraine headaches.
- BP 108/72 mm Hg right arm, sitting. HR 76 beats/min, regular. Resp 14/min unlabored.
- Weight 180 lbs. Height 5ft 6 in. BMI 29 (overweight).
- Health promotion: Reports consistently wearing sunscreen when outside and completing skin self-examination every few months. Consistently monitors blood glucose. Walks 2 miles at least 3 days per week and does strength training exercises 2 days per week. No hypoglycemic episodes during exercise. Reports weekly pedicure and foot check to monitor for skin breakdown. Biannual dental visits. Performs BSE monthly.
- Relationships: Close relationship with family (mother, father, brother, and sister); no significant other. Feels safe in home environment and reports having close female friends.
- Health perception: "Could probably lose some weight," but otherwise reports "good" health. Primarily concerned with blood sugar, which becomes labile with life transitions.
- Expectations of provider: Establish an open and honest relationship. Listen to her needs and facilitate her health goals.

Physical examination:

- Normocephalic. Face symmetric. Denies pain on sinus palpation.
- Vision tested annually. Has worn corrective lenses since 4th grade. PERRLA.
- Scarring bilateral tympanic membranes. Denies hearing problems. Whispered words heard bilaterally.
- Gums pink; no apparent dental caries except for 3 noticeable fillings. Reports no dental pain.
- Compound nevus on left inner elbow; patient reports no recent changes in appearance. No other skin concerns.
- Breath sounds clear and equal bilaterally. Heart S_1S_2, neither accentuated nor diminished. No murmur or extra heart sounds.
- CBE done with annual gynecologic visit.
- Abdomen is rounded. Bowel sounds present. Reports BM daily.
- Extremities warm and = bilat. All pulses present, 2+ and = bilat. No lymphadenopathy. Sensory modalities intact in legs and feet. No lesions.

The examiner analyzed and interpreted all the data; clustered the information, sorting out which data to refer and which to treat; and identified the diagnoses. It is interesting to note how many significant findings are derived from data the examiner collected. Not only physical data but also cognitive, psychosocial, and behavioral data are significant for an analysis of C.D.'s health state. The findings also are interesting when considered from a life-cycle perspective (i.e., she is a young adult who predictably is occupied with the developmental tasks of emancipation from parents, building an independent lifestyle, establishing a vocation, making friends, forming an intimate bond with another, and establishing a social group). C.D. appears to be meeting the appropriate developmental tasks successfully.

A body of clinical **evidence** has validated the use of the particular assessment techniques in C.D.'s case. For example, measuring the BP screens for hypertension and early intervention here wards off heart attack and stroke. Monitoring blood sugar levels and HbA1c facilitates management of her type 1 diabetes. Completing a skin assessment reveals a nevus on her elbow that needs to be watched for any changes. Collecting health promotion data allows the examiner to personalize risk reduction and health promotion information while reinforcing positive behaviors already in place. The physical examination is not just a rote formality. Its parts are determined by the best clinical evidence available and documented in the professional literature.

ASSESSMENT—POINT OF ENTRY IN AN ONGOING PROCESS

Assessment is the collection of data about the individual's health state. Throughout this text you will be studying the techniques of collecting and analyzing **subjective data** (i.e., what the person *says* about himself or herself during history taking) and **objective data** (i.e., what you as the health professional *observe* by inspecting, percussing, palpating, and auscultating during the physical examination). Together with the patient's record and laboratory studies, these elements form the **database**.

From the database you make a clinical judgment or diagnosis about the individual's health state, response to actual or potential health problems, and life processes. Thus the purpose of assessment is to make a judgment or diagnosis.

An organized assessment is the starting point of diagnostic reasoning. Because all health care diagnoses, decisions, and treatments are based on the data you gather during assessment, it is paramount that your assessment be factual and complete.

Diagnostic Reasoning

The step from data collection to diagnosis can be a difficult one. Most novice examiners perform well in gathering the data (given adequate practice) but then treat all the data as being equally important. This makes decision making slow and labored.

Diagnostic reasoning is the process of analyzing health data and drawing conclusions to identify diagnoses. Novice examiners most often use a diagnostic process involving hypothesis forming and deductive reasoning. This hypothetico-deductive process has four major components: (1) attending to initially available cues; (2) formulating diagnostic hypotheses; (3) gathering data relative to the tentative hypotheses; and (4) evaluating each hypothesis with the new data collected, thus arriving at a final diagnosis. A *cue* is a piece of information, a sign or symptom, or a piece of laboratory data. A *hypothesis* is a tentative explanation for a cue or a set of cues that can be used as a basis for further investigation.

Once you complete data collection, develop a preliminary list of significant signs and symptoms for all patient health needs. This is less formal in structure than your final list of diagnoses will be and is in no particular order.

Cluster or group together the assessment data that appear to be causal or associated. For example, with a person in acute pain, associated data are rapid heart rate, increased BP, and anxiety. Organizing the data into meaningful clusters is slow at first; experienced examiners cluster data more rapidly because they recall proven results of earlier patient situations and recognize the same patterns in the new clinical situation.[10]

Validate the data you collect to make sure they are accurate. As you validate your information, look for gaps in data collection. Be sure to find the missing pieces, because identifying missing information is an essential critical-thinking skill. How you validate your data depends on experience. If you are unsure of the BP, validate it by repeating it yourself. Eliminate any extraneous variables that could influence BP results such as recent activity or anxiety over admission. If you have less experience analyzing breath sounds or heart murmurs, ask an expert to listen. Even with years of clinical experience, some signs always require validation (e.g., a breast lump).

Critical Thinking and the Diagnostic Process

The standards of practice in nursing, traditionally termed the **nursing process**, include six phases: assessment, diagnosis, outcome identification, planning, implementation, and evaluation.[3] This is an iterative process allowing practitioners to move back and forth while caring for the needs of complex patients (Fig. 1-2).

Although the nursing process is a problem-solving approach, the way in which we apply the process depends on our level and years of experience. The *novice* has no experience with a specified patient population and uses rules to guide performance. It takes time, perhaps 2 to 3 years in similar clinical situations, to achieve *competency,* in which you see actions in the context of arching goals or daily plans for patients. With more time and experience the *proficient* nurse understands a patient situation as a whole rather than as a list of tasks. At this level you can see long-term goals for the patient. You project that today's interventions apply to the point at which you want the patient to be in the future. Finally it seems that *expert* nurses vault over the steps and arrive at a clinical judgment in one leap. The expert has an intuitive grasp of a clinical situation and zeroes in on the accurate solution.[5]

ASSESSMENT
- Collect data:
  Review of the clinical record
  Health history
  Physical examination
  Functional assessment
  Risk assessment
  Review of the literature
- Use evidence-based assessment techniques
- Document relevant data

EVALUATION
- Progress toward outcomes
- Conduct systematic, ongoing, criterion-based evaluation
- Include patient and significant others
- Use ongoing assessment to revise diagnoses, outcomes, plan
- Disseminate results to patient and family

DIAGNOSIS
- Compare clinical findings with normal and abnormal variation and developmental events
- Interpret data
  Identify clusters of clues
  Make hypotheses
  Test hypotheses
  Derive diagnoses
- Validate diagnoses
- Document diagnoses

IMPLEMENTATION
- Implement in a safe and timely manner
- Use evidence-based interventions
- Collaborate with colleagues
- Use community resources
- Coordinate care delivery
- Provide health teaching and health promotion
- Document implementation and any modification

OUTCOME IDENTIFICATION
- Identify expected outcomes
- Individualize to the person
- Culturally appropriate
- Realistic and measurable
- Include a timeline

PLANNING
- Establish priorities
- Develop outcomes
- Set timelines for outcomes
- Identify interventions
- Integrate evidence-based trends and research
- Document plan of care

THE INDIVIDUAL

1-2

Functioning at the level of expert in clinical judgment includes using intuition (i.e., knowledge received as a whole). Intuition is characterized by immediate recognition of patterns; expert practitioners learn to attend to a pattern of assessment data and act without consciously labeling it. Whereas the beginner operates more from a set of defined, structured rules, the expert practitioner uses intuitive links, has the ability to see salient issues in a patient situation, and knows instant therapeutic responses.[5] The expert has a storehouse of experience concerning which interventions have been successful in the past.

For example, compare the actions of the nonexpert and the expert nurse in the following situation of a young man with *Pneumocystis jiroveci* pneumonia:

> He was banging the side rails, making sounds, and pointing to his endotracheal tube. He was diaphoretic, gasping, and frantic. The nurse put her hand on his arm and tried to ascertain whether he had a sore throat from the tube. While she was away from the bedside retrieving an analgesic, the expert nurse strolled by, hesitated, listened, went to the man's bedside, reinflated the endotracheal cuff, and accepted the patient's look of gratitude because he was able to breathe again. The nonexpert nurse was distressed that she had misread the situation. The expert reviewed the signs of a leaky cuff with the nonexpert and pointed out that banging the side rails and panic help differentiate acute respiratory distress from pain.[15]

The method of moving from novice to becoming an expert practitioner is through the use of critical thinking. We all start as novices, when we need the familiarity of clear-cut rules to guide actions. Critical thinking is the means by which we learn to assess and modify, if indicated, before acting. We may even be beginners more than once during our careers. As we transition to different specialties, we must rebuild our data base of experiences to become experts in new areas of practice.

Critical thinking is required for sound diagnostic reasoning and clinical judgment. During your career you will need to sort through vast amounts of data to make the sound judgments to manage patient care. These data will be dynamic, unpredictable, and ever changing. There will not be any one protocol you can memorize that will apply to every situation.

Critical thinking is recognized as an important component of nursing education at all levels.[2,20] Case studies and simulations frequently are used to encourage critical thinking with students. As a student, be prepared to think outside the box and think critically through patient-care situations. Critical thinking goes beyond knowing the pathophysiology of a disease process and requires you to put important assessment cues together to determine the most likely cause of a clinical problem and develop a solution. Critical thinking is a multidimensional thinking process, not a linear approach to problem solving.

Remember to approach problems in a nonjudgmental way and to avoid making assumptions. Identify which information you are taking for granted or information you may overlook based on natural assumptions. Rates of incorrect diagnoses are estimated to be as high as 10% to 15%, and one of the primary causes of misdiagnosis is the clinician's bias.[12] An overweight young adult comes to your clinic for a scheduled physical examination. Are you making assumptions about her lifestyle and eating habits? Make sure that you double-check the accuracy of your data (subjective and objective), identify normal and abnormal findings, and group like findings together. For example, a man who has heart failure may exhibit shortness of breath, palpitations, ankle edema, and weight gain. Alone each of these may appear unrelated, but together they are signs of an exacerbation of heart failure.

Once you have clustered items that are related, you are ready to identify relevant information and anything that does not fit. In the case of your heart failure patient, his complaints of a headache may be viewed as unrelated to the primary diagnosis, whereas abdominal pain and difficulty buttoning his pants are related (presence of ascites). As you gather clinical cues and complete an assessment, also think about priority setting (Table 1-1).

- **First-level priority problems** are those that are emergent, life threatening, and immediate, such as establishing an airway or supporting breathing.
- **Second-level priority problems** are those that are next in urgency—those requiring your prompt intervention to forestall further deterioration (e.g., mental status change, acute pain, acute urinary elimination problems, untreated medical problems, abnormal laboratory values, risks of infection, or risk to safety or security).
- **Third-level priority problems** are those that are important to the patient's health but can be addressed after more urgent health problems are addressed. Interventions to treat these problems are more long term, and the response to treatment is expected to take more time.
- **Collaborative problems** are those in which the approach to treatment involves multiple disciplines. Collaborative problems are certain physiologic conditions in which nurses have the primary responsibility to diagnose the onset and monitor the changes in status.[8] For example, C.D.'s data regarding diabetes represent a collaborative problem. With this problem the sudden imbalance of insulin and blood sugar has profound implications on the central nervous and gastrointestinal (GI) systems. Her care will be monitored by nurses, doctors, dietitians, and case managers. Or another patient with an alcohol-use disorder presents to the hospital for unrelated surgery and experiences sudden alcohol withdrawal symptoms. This causes rebound effects on the central nervous and cardiovascular systems that must be managed by a team of clinicians.

Once you have determined problems, you must identify expected outcomes and work with the patient to facilitate outcome achievement. Remember, your outcomes need to be measurable. Set small goals that can be accomplished in a given time frame. For your heart failure patient your goal may be to eliminate supplemental oxygen needs before discharge. Include your patient in your outcome identification and his or her input as appropriate.

TABLE 1-1 Identifying Immediate Priorities

Principles of Setting Priorities

1. **Make a complete list of current medications, medical problems, allergies, and reasons for seeking care. Refer to them frequently because they may affect how you set priorities.**
2. **Determine the *relationships* among the problems:** If problem Y causes problem Z, problem Y takes priority over problem Z. **Example:** If pain is causing immobility, *pain management* is a high priority.

Setting priorities is a dynamic, changing process; at times the order of priority changes, depending on the seriousness and relationship of the problems. **Example:** If abnormal laboratory values are at life-threatening levels, they become a higher priority; if the patient is having trouble breathing because of acute rib pain, managing the pain may be a higher priority than dealing with a rapid pulse (first-level priority, listed in the next section).

Steps to Setting Priorities

1. Assign high priority to *first-level* priority problems (immediate priorities): Remember the "ABCs plus V":
   - **A**irway problems
   - **B**reathing problems
   - **C**ardiac/circulation problems
   - **V**ital sign concerns (e.g., high fever)

   Exception: With cardiopulmonary resuscitation (CPR) for cardiac arrest, begin chest compressions immediately. Go to www.americanheart.org for the most current CPR guidelines.
2. Next attend to *second-level* priority problems:
   - Mental status change (e.g., confusion, decreased alertness)
   - Untreated medical problems requiring immediate attention (e.g., a person with diabetes who has not had insulin)
   - Acute pain
   - Acute urinary elimination problems
   - Abnormal laboratory values
   - Risks of infection, safety, or security (for the patient or for others)
3. Address *third-level* priority problems (later priorities):
   - Health problems that do not fit into the previous categories (e.g., problems with lack of knowledge, activity, rest, family coping)

© 2014 Alfaro-LeFevre Workshop Handouts. www. AlfaroTeachSmart.com.

The final steps to the critical-thinking process include evaluation and planning. You must continuously evaluate whether you are on the right track and correct any missteps or misinterpretation of data. If you are not on the right path, reassess, reanalyze, and revise. The final step is the development of a comprehensive plan that is kept up-to-date. Communicate the plan to the multidisciplinary team. Be aware that this is a legal document and that accurate recording is important for evaluation, insurance reimbursement, and research.

EVIDENCE-BASED ASSESSMENT

Does honey help burn wounds heal more quickly? Is St. John's wort effective in relieving the symptoms of major depression? Does male circumcision reduce the risk of transmitting human immunodeficiency virus (HIV) in heterosexual men? Can magnesium sulfate reduce cerebral palsy risk in premature infants? Can infusing hearts with stem cells help heal tissue damage after a heart attack?

Health care is a rapidly changing field. The amount of medical and nursing information available today has skyrocketed. Current efforts of cost containment result in a hospital population composed of people who have a higher acuity but are discharged earlier than in the past. Clinical research studies are continuously pushing health care forward. Keeping up with these advances and translating them into practice are very challenging. Budget cuts, staff shortages, and increasing patient acuity mean that the clinician has little time to grab a lunch break, let alone browse the most recent journal articles for advances in a clinical specialty.

The conviction that all patients deserve to be treated with the most current and best-practice techniques led to the development of **evidence-based practice (EBP)**. In 1972 a British epidemiologist and early proponent of EBP, Archie Cochrane, identified a pressing need for systematic reviews of randomized clinical trials. In a landmark case Dr. Cochrane noted multiple clinical trials published between 1972 and 1981 showing that the use of corticosteroids to treat women in premature labor reduced the incidence of infant mortality. A short course of corticosteroid stimulates fetal lung development, thus preventing respiratory distress syndrome, a serious and common complication of premature birth. Yet these findings had not been implemented into daily practice, and thousands of low-birth-weight premature infants were dying needlessly. Following a systematic review of the evidence in 1989, obstetricians finally accepted the use of corticosteroid treatment as standard practice for women in preterm labor. Corticosteroid treatment has since been shown to reduce the risk of infant mortality by 30% to 50%.[9]

EBP is more than the use of best-practice techniques to treat patients. "EBP is a systematic approach to practice that emphasizes the use of best evidence in combination with the clinician's experience, as well as the patient preferences and values, to make decisions about care and treatment"[16] (Fig. 1-3). This definition is comprehensive and holistic. Note how clinical decision making depends on all four factors: the best evidence from a critical review of research literature; the patient's own preferences; the clinician's own experience and expertise; and finally physical examination and assessment. Assessment skills must be practiced with hands-on experience and refined to a high level.

Although assessment skills are foundational to EBP, it is important to question tradition when no compelling research evidence exists to support it. Some time-honored assessment techniques have been removed from the examination repertoire because clinical evidence indicates that these techniques are not as accurate as once believed. For example, the

1-3

traditional practice of auscultating bowel sounds was found to be a poor indicator of returning GI motility in patients having abdominal surgery.[17] The research team first reviewed earlier studies suggesting that early postoperative bowel sounds probably do *not* represent the return of normal GI motility and therefore listening to the abdomen is not useful in this situation. Research showed the primary markers for returning GI motility after abdominal surgery to be the return of flatus and the first postoperative bowel movement. The Madsen team instituted a new practice protocol and monitored patient outcomes to determine whether discontinuing the auscultation of bowel sounds was detrimental to abdominal surgery patients. Detrimental outcomes did not occur; the new practice guideline was shown to be safe for patients' recovery and a better allocation of staff time.

Evidence shows that other assessment skills *are* effective for patient care. For example, clinicians should measure the ankle brachial index (ABI), as described in Chapter 20 of this text. Evidence is clear about the value of ABI as a screening measure for peripheral artery disease.

Despite the advantages to patients who receive care based on EBP, it often takes up to 17 years for research findings to be implemented into practice.[4] This troubling gap has led researchers to examine closely the barriers to EBP, both as individual practitioners and as organizations. As individuals, nurses lack research skills in evaluating quality of research studies, are isolated from other colleagues knowledgeable in research, and lack confidence to implement change. Other significant barriers are the organizational characteristics of health care settings. Nurses lack time to go to the library to read research; health care institutions have inadequate library research holdings; and organizational support for EBP is lacking when nurses wish to implement changes in patient care.[13]

Fostering a culture of EBP at the undergraduate and graduate levels is one way in which health care educators attempt to make evidence-based care the "gold standard" of practice. Students of medicine and nursing are now taught how to filter through the wealth of scientific data and critique their findings. They are learning to discern which interventions would best serve their individual patients. Facilitating support for EBP at the organizational level includes time to go to the library; teaching staff to conduct electronic searches; journal club meetings; establishing nursing research committees; linking staff with university researchers; and ensuring that adequate research journals and preprocessed evidence resources are available in the library.[13] "*We have come to a time when the credibility of the health professions will be judged by which of its practices are based on the best and latest evidence from sound scientific studies in combination with clinical expertise, astute assessment, and respect for patient values and preferences.*"[18]

COLLECTING FOUR TYPES OF DATA

Every examiner needs to establish four different types of databases, depending on the clinical situation: complete, focused or problem-centered, follow-up, and emergency.

Complete (Total Health) Database

This includes a complete health history and a full physical examination. It describes the current and past health state and forms a baseline against which all future changes can be measured. It yields the first diagnoses.

The complete database often is collected in a primary care setting such as a pediatric or family practice clinic, independent or group private practice, college health service, women's health care agency, visiting nurse agency, or community health agency. When you work in these settings, you are the first health professional to see the patient and have primary responsibility for monitoring the person's health care. Collecting the complete database is an opportunity to build and strengthen your relationship with the patient. For the well person this database must describe the person's health state; perception of health; strengths or assets such as health maintenance behaviors, individual coping patterns, support systems, and current developmental tasks; and any risk factors or lifestyle changes. For the ill person the database also includes a description of the person's health problems, perception of illness, and response to the problems.

For well and ill people, the complete database must screen for pathology and determine the ways people respond to that pathology or to any health problem. You must screen for pathology because you are the first, and often the only, health professional to see the patient. This screening is important to refer the patient to another professional, help the patient make decisions, and perform appropriate treatments. But this database also notes the human responses to health problems. This factor is important because it provides additional information about the person that leads to nursing diagnoses.

In acute hospital care the complete database also is gathered on admission to the hospital. In the hospital, data related specifically to pathology may be collected by the admitting physician. You collect additional information on the patient's perception of illness, functional ability or patterns of living, activities of daily living, health maintenance behaviors, response to health problems, coping patterns, interaction patterns, and health goals.

Focused or Problem-Centered Database

This is for a limited or short-term problem. Here you collect a "mini" database, smaller in scope and more targeted than the complete database. It concerns mainly one problem, one cue complex, or one body system. It is used in all settings—hospital, primary care, or long-term care. For example, 2 days after surgery a hospitalized person suddenly has a congested cough, shortness of breath, and fatigue. The history and examination focus primarily on the respiratory and cardiovascular systems. Or in an outpatient clinic a person presents with a rash. The history follows the direction of this presenting concern such as whether the rash had an acute or chronic onset; was associated with a fever, new food, pet, or medicine; and was localized or generalized. Physical examination must include a clear description of the rash.

Follow-Up Database

The status of any identified problems should be evaluated at regular and appropriate intervals. What change has occurred? Is the problem getting better or worse? Which coping strategies are used? This type of database is used in all settings to follow up both short-term and chronic health problems.

Emergency Database

This is an urgent, rapid collection of crucial information and often is compiled concurrently with lifesaving measures. Diagnosis must be swift and sure. For example, a person is brought into a hospital ED with suspected substance overdose. The first history questions are, "What did you take?" "How much did you take?" and "When?" The person is questioned simultaneously while his or her airway, breathing, circulation, level of consciousness, and disability are being assessed. Clearly the emergency database requires more rapid collection of data than the episodic database. Once the person has been stabilized, a complete database can be compiled.

EXPANDING THE CONCEPT OF HEALTH

Assessment is the collection of data about a person's health state. A clear definition of health is important because this determines which assessment data should be collected. In general the list of data that must be collected has lengthened as our concept of health has broadened.

Consideration of the whole person is the essence of **holistic health.** Holistic health views the mind, body, and spirit as interdependent and functioning as a whole within the environment. Health depends on all these factors working together. The basis of disease is multifaceted, originating from both within the person and from the external environment. Thus the treatment of disease requires the services of numerous providers. Nursing includes many aspects of the holistic model (i.e., the interaction of the mind and body, the oneness and unity of the individual). Both the individual human and the external environment are open systems, dynamic and continually changing and adapting to one another. Each person is responsible for his or her own personal health state and is an active participant in health care. Health promotion and disease prevention form the core of nursing practice.

In a holistic model assessment factors are expanded to include such things as lifestyle behaviors, culture and values, family and social roles, self-care behaviors, job-related stress, developmental tasks, and failures and frustrations of life. All are significant to health.

Health promotion and disease prevention now round out our concept of health. Guidelines to prevention emphasize the link between health and personal behavior. The report of the U.S. Preventive Services Task Force[26] asserts that the great majority of deaths among Americans younger than 65 years are preventable. Prevention can be achieved through counseling from primary care providers designed to change people's unhealthy behaviors related to smoking, alcohol and other drug use, lack of exercise, poor nutrition, injuries, and sexually transmitted infections.[14] Health promotion is a set of positive acts that we can take. In this model the focus of the health professional is on teaching and helping the consumer choose a healthier lifestyle.

The frequency interval of assessment varies with the person's illness and wellness needs. Most ill people seek care because of pain or some abnormal signs and symptoms they have noticed, which prompts an assessment (i.e., gathering a complete, a focused, or an emergency database). In addition, risk assessment and preventive services can be delivered once the presenting concerns are addressed (Fig. 1-4).

But for the well person opinions are inconsistent about assessment intervals. The term *annual checkup* is vague. What does it constitute? Is it necessary or cost-effective? How can primary-care clinicians deliver preventive services to people with no signs and symptoms of illness? Periodic health checkups are an excellent opportunity to deliver preventive services and update the complete database. Although periodic health

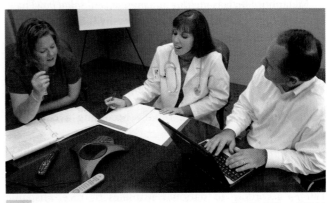

1-4 (Yoder-Wise, 2014.)

checkups could induce unnecessary costs and promote non-recommended services, advocates justify well-person visits because of delivery of some recommended preventive services and reduction of patient worry.[7]

The *Guide to Clinical Preventive Services* is a positive approach to health assessment and risk reduction.[26] The *Guide* is updated annually and is accessible online or in print. It presents evidence-based, gold standard recommendations on screening, counseling, and preventive topics and includes clinical considerations for each topic. These services include screening factors to gather during the history, age-specific items for physical examination and laboratory procedures, counseling topics, and immunizations. This approach moves away from an annual physical ritual and toward a rational and varying periodicity based on factors specific to the patient. Health education and counseling are highlighted as the means to deliver health promotion and disease prevention.

For example, the guide to examination for C.D. (23-year-old female, nonpregnant, not sexually active) would recommend the following services for preventive health care:

1. **Screening history** for dietary intake, physical activity, tobacco/alcohol/drug use, and sexual practices
2. **Physical examination** for height and weight, BP, and screening for cervical cancer and HIV
3. **Counseling** for physical activity and risk prevention (e.g., secondhand smoke, seatbelt use)
4. **Depression** screening
5. **Healthy diet** counseling, including lipid disorder screening and obesity screening
6. **Chemoprophylaxis** to include multivitamin with folic acid (females capable of or planning pregnancy)

C.D. is living successfully with a serious chronic condition. Because she has diabetes, including periodic checks of hemoglobin A1c and a fasting glucose level is important. In addition, you should ask how her pump is functioning and whether she is having any difficulties with blood sugar control.

CULTURE AND GENETICS

In a holistic model of health care, assessment factors must include culture. An introduction to cross-cultural concepts follows in Chapter 2. These concepts are developed throughout the text as they relate to specific chapters.

Metaphors such as *melting pot, mosaic,* and *salad bowl* have been used to describe the cultural diversity that characterizes the United States. According to the U.S. Census Bureau, close to 50% of the population of the United States will consist of people from diverse racial, ethnic, and cultural groups by the year 2050. *Emerging minority* is a term that has been used to classify the populations, including Blacks, Hispanics, and Asian Americans, that are rapidly becoming a combined numeric majority.[22]

The population of the United States surpassed 311 million people in the autumn of 2011; approximately 1 in 3 U.S. residents was part of a group other than single-race non-Hispanic Whites according to national estimates by race, Hispanic origin, and age released by the Census Bureau.

In 2043 the United States is expected to become a majority-minority nation. Although non-Hispanic Whites will remain the largest single group, they will no longer constitute a numeric majority. By 2060 the U.S. Census Bureau projects that minorities will comprise 57% of the population. The Hispanic and Asian populations are projected to more than double by 2060, and all other racial groups are expected to increase as well. By 2060 nearly 33% of the population will be Hispanic, 15% Blacks, 8.2% Asian, and 1.5% American Indians or Alaska Natives. In 2050 the U.S. Census Bureau anticipates that there will be more people over the age of 65 years than under the age of 18 years for the first time in history.[25]

As the United States population is becoming more diverse, the U.S. health care providers go abroad to work in a variety of health care settings in the international community. Medical and nursing teams volunteer to provide free medical and surgical care in developing countries (Fig. 1-5). International interchanges are increasing among health care providers, making attention to the cultural aspects of health and illness an even greater priority.

During your professional career you may be expected to assess short-term foreign visitors who travel for treatments, international university faculty, students from abroad studying in U.S. high schools and universities, family members of foreign diplomats, immigrants, refugees, members of more than 106 different ethnic groups, and American Indians from 510 federally recognized tribes. A serious conceptual problem exists in that nurses and physicians are expected to know, understand, and meet the health needs of people from culturally diverse backgrounds with minimal preparation in cultural competence.

Culture has been included in each chapter of this book. Understanding the basics of a variety of cultures is important in health assessment. People from different cultures may interpret symptoms differently; therefore asking the right questions is imperative for you to gather data that are accurate and meaningful. Members of some cultural groups are demanding culturally relevant health care that incorporates their specific beliefs and practices. An increasing expectation exists among

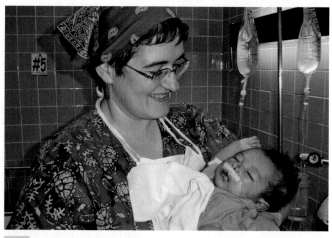

1-5

members of certain cultural groups that health care providers will respect their "cultural health rights," an expectation that may conflict with the unicultural Western biomedical worldview taught in U.S. educational programs that prepare nurses, doctors, and other health care providers.

Given the multicultural composition of the United States and the projected increase in the number of individuals from diverse cultural backgrounds anticipated in the future, a concern for the cultural beliefs and practices of people is increasingly important.

BIBLIOGRAPHY

1. Alfaro-LeFevre, R. (2013). *Critical thinking, clinical reasoning and clinical judgment.* (5th ed.). St. Louis: Saunders.
2. American Association of Colleges of Nursing. (2008). *Essentials of baccalaureate education for professional nursing practice.* Available at https://www.aacn.nche.edu/education-resources/baccessentials08.pdf.
3. American Nurses Association. (2010). *Nursing scope and standards of performance and standards of clinical practice.* Washington, DC: American Nurses Publishing.
4. Balas, E. A., & Boren, S. A. (2000). Managing clinical knowledge for health care improvements. In Bemmel, J., & A. T. McCray (Eds.). *Yearbook of medical informatics 2000.* Stuttgart, Germany: Schattauer.
5. Benner, P., Tanner, C. A., & Chesla, C. A. (1996). *Expertise in nursing practice.* New York: Springer.
6. Benner, P., Tanner, C. A., & Chesla, C. A. (1997). Becoming an expert nurse. *Am J Nurs, 97*(6), 16BBB-16DDD.
7. Boulware, L. E., Marinopoulos, S., & Phillips, K. A. (2007). Systematic review: the value of the periodic health evaluation. *Ann Intern Med, 146*(4), 289-300.
8. Carpenito-Moyet, L. J. (2012). *Nursing diagnosis: application to clinical practice.* (14th ed.). Philadelphia: Lippincott Williams & Wilkins.
9. Cochrane Collaboration. (2013). Available at www.cochrane.org.
10. Coderre, S., Mandin, H., Harasym, P. H., et al. (2003). Diagnostic reasoning strategies and diagnostic success. *Med Educ, 37*(8), 695-703.
11. Crisp, N., & Chen, L. (2014). Global supply of health professionals. *N Engl J Med, 370*(10), 950-957.
12. Croskerry, P. (2013). From mindless to mindful practice—cognitive bias and clinical decision making. *N Engl J Med, 368,* 2445-2450.
13. DiCenso, A., Guyatt, G., & Ciliska, D. (2005). *Evidence-based nursing: a guide to clinical practice.* St. Louis: Mosby.
14. Ezzati, M., & Riboli, E. (2013). Behavioral and dietary risk factors for noncommunicable diseases. *N Engl J Med, 369*(10):954-964.
15. Hanneman, S. K. (1996). Advancing nursing practice with a unit-based clinical expert. *Image, 28*(4), 331-337.
16. Leufer, T. C. (2009). Evidence-based practice: improving patient outcomes. *Nurs Stand, 23*(32), 35-39.
17. Madsen, D., Sebolt, T., Cullen, L., et al. (2005). Listening to bowel sounds: an evidence-based practice project. *Am J Nurs, 105*(12), 40-50.
18. Melnyk, B. M., & Fineout-Overholt, E. (2011). *Evidence-based practice in nursing & healthcare.* (2nd ed.). Philadelphia: Lippincott Williams & Wilkins.
19. Melnyk, B. M., Fineout-Overhold, E., Stillwell, B., et al. (2009). Evidence-based practice step by step: igniting the spirit of inquiry. *Am J Nurs, 109*(11), 49-52. First in a 12-part series.
20. National League for Nursing Accrediting Commission. (2006). *Accreditation manual and interpretive guidelines by program type for postsecondary and higher degree programs in nursing.* New York: Author.
21. Robert, R. R., & Petersen, S. (2013). Critical thinking at the bedside: providing safe passage to patients. *Medsurg Nurs, 22*(2):85-93.
22. Spector, R. E. (2013). *Cultural diversity in health and illness.* (8th ed.). Indianapolis, IN: Pearson.
23. Throckmorton, T., & Windle, P. E. (2009). Evidence-based case management practice. Part 1: the systemic review. *Prof Case Manage, 14*(2), 76-81.
24. U.S. Bureau of the Census. (2014). *Quickfacts.* Washington, DC: U.S. Government Printing Office. www.census.gov.
25. U.S. Census Bureau. (2012). *U.S. Census Bureau projections show a slower growing, older, more diverse nation a half century from now.* Available at https://www.census.gov/newsroom/releases/archives/population/cb12-243.html.
26. U.S. Preventive Services Task Force (USPSTF). (2012). *Guide to clinical preventive services. (2012).* Available at http://www.ahrq.gov/professionals/clinicians-providers/guidelines-recommendations/guide/guide-clinical-preventive-services.pdf.

CHAPTER 2

Cultural Competence

http://evolve.elsevier.com/Jarvis/

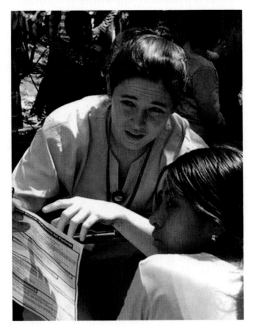

2-1

A health profession role encompasses your relationships with people—your ability to listen to, empathize with, and understand people. How can you fulfill this role to the best of your ability? First be open to people who are different from you, have a curiosity about people, and begin the lifelong journey of becoming culturally competent (Fig. 2-1). The United States is becoming more diverse, not only through globalization and immigration, but also because of a wide range of subcultures and an increasing acceptance of lifestyle choices that may differ from the mainstream. For example, in 2011 approximately 4% of the U.S. adult population (or 9 million people) identified themselves as lesbian, gay, bisexual, or transgender (LGBT), and even larger numbers stated that they had same-sex experiences or were attracted to the same sex without necessarily identifying themselves as LGB.[16]

A key to understanding cultural diversity is self-awareness and knowledge of one's own culture, which may be African American, Euro American, Chinese American, Dominican American, Mexican American, Southeast Asian–American, or any combination of self-identified ethnicities and races. Your cultural identification might include the subculture of nursing or health care professionals. You might identify yourself as a Midwesterner, a college student, an athlete, a member of the Polish community, or a Buddhist. These multiple and often changing cultural and subcultural identifications help define an individual and influence one's beliefs about health and illness, coping mechanisms, and wellness behaviors.

Over the course of your professional education, you will study physical examination and health promotion across the life span and learn to conduct numerous assessments such as a health history, a physical examination, a mental health assessment, a domestic violence assessment, a nutritional assessment, and a pain assessment. However, depending on the cultural and racial background of the person, the data you gather in the assessments may vary. Therefore a cultural assessment must be an integral component of a complete physical and health assessment.

DEMOGRAPHIC PROFILE OF THE UNITED STATES

The estimates of the U.S. population illustrate the increasing diversity in the population and explain the rationale for learning about the cultural aspects of health* and illness† from the point of view of the person seeking health care.[46] The population of the United States exceeded 311 million people in 2011.[44] Approximately 1 in every 6 to 7 people was an immigrant, and greater than one third of U.S. residents were part of a group other than single-race non-Hispanic White.[27,44] The national minority, actually *emerging majority*, population totaled 37% of the total population.[27] Among this emerging majority, the largest ethnic group is Hispanic, who make up 16.7% of the population and are the fastest-growing minority group. The largest racial minority group is African American or Black (12.2%), followed by Asians (4.8%), other races (4.7%), two or more races (2.8%), American Indians and Alaska natives (0.8%), and Native Hawaiians and other Pacific Islanders (0.2%).[44]

There are differences among the emerging majority groups when compared to non-Hispanic Whites. These demographic differences are age, poverty level, and household

---

*Health: "The **balance** of the person, both within one's being (i.e., physical, mental, and/or spiritual) and in the outside world (i.e., natural, communal, and/or metaphysical), is a complex, interrelated phenomenon."[41]

†Illness: "The loss of the person's **balance**, both within one's being (i.e., physical, mental, and/or spiritual) and in the outside world (i.e., natural, communal, and/or metaphysical)."[41]

composition. The median age of the non-Hispanic White population in 2012 was 40.2 years, and one fourth was younger than 18 years. The median age of some racial and ethnic groups was younger than the total population as a whole. Hispanics had the youngest median age (27.7 years), followed by Native Hawaiian/Pacific Islanders (30.4 years), American Indians and Alaska Natives (31.9 years), African Americans, (32.9 years), and Asians (36 years).[44] The family size of some racial and ethnic groups is larger than that of non-Hispanic Whites (3.14 people). Native Hawaiian/Pacific Islanders have the largest average family size (4.16 people), followed by Hispanics, (3.95 people), American Indians and Alaska Natives (3.68 people), Asians (3.61 people), and African Americans (3.47 people).[44] The number of relatives living in the household is higher for all racial and ethnic minorities compared to non-Hispanic Whites, as is the number of multigenerational families. African Americans, American Indians, and Alaska Natives are more likely to have grandparents who are responsible for the care of grandchildren compared with other groups.[44]

All ethnic and racial minority groups have poverty rates exceeding the national average for non-Hispanic Whites of 13%.[44] American Indians and Alaska Natives (29.1%), African Americans, (28.1%), and Hispanics (25.4%) have about twice as many people living in poverty as non-Hispanic Whites.[44] Contributing to the high rates of poverty is low educational attainment. Thirty six percent of Hispanics, 21% of American Indians and Alaska Natives, and 17% of Blacks have less than a high school education compared to 12% of non-Hispanic Whites.[44] Female-headed households with children under 18 years are most likely to be living in poverty. Dominicans, Puerto Ricans, Somalians, and African Americans are 3 times more likely to be in female-headed households with children under 18 compared to non-Hispanic Whites.[46] Ten percent of the population is living with a disability; this rate is higher among African Americans (13.6%) and American Indians and Alaska Natives (16.7%).[44]

Within these groups are subgroup variations (e.g., Cubans in the U.S. have a median age of 39.8 years, whereas Guatemalans have a median age of 27.8 years). In terms of educational attainment: more than half of Guatemalans, Mexicans, and Salvadorans have less than a high school education compared to 9% of Chileans; 36% of Somalis have less than a high school education compared to 4% of Nigerians; 19% of Koreans have a graduate or professional degree compared to 4% of Cambodians.[44] Among Asian ethnic groups, poverty rates are highest for Hmong (27%) and Cambodians (21%) compared to Japanese (8.5%). Among Hispanics, poverty rates are highest for Dominicans and Hondurans (29%), followed by Guatemalans and Mexicans (28%) and Puerto Ricans (27%), compared to Bolivians at 9%.[44]

IMMIGRATION

Immigrants are people who are not U.S. citizens at birth. The United States accepts more immigrants than any other county in the world.[36] Some new immigrants have minimal understanding of health care resources and how to navigate the health care system. They may not speak or understand English, and they may not be literate in the language of their country of origin. Therefore it is imperative that health care address the needs of this growing population.

In 2011 the population in the United States included over 40 million foreign-born people, including legal and undocumented immigrants, representing 13% of the U.S. population and an increase of 9 million people since 2000.[27,44] Although the number of foreign born is the greatest in U.S. history, the foreign born as a percent of the entire population does not reach the high point in American history (i.e., from 1890 to 1920) when immigrants from Southern and Eastern Europe made up 15% of the population.[36] The current wave of immigrants is predominantly from Latin America (50%) and Asia (27%). Mexico has by far the largest number of immigrants to the U.S. at 29% of the foreign-born population, followed by India at 4.6%, the Philippines at 4.5%, China at 4.1%, and Vietnam at 3.1%.[36]

The Immigration and Nationality Act of 1965 abolished quota systems that denied entrance into the United States to Latin Americans, Asians, and Africans, thus opening the way for the current wave of immigration. In 2011 there were also 11.1 million people who were foreign born and living in the United States without legal documents (unauthorized or undocumented immigrants), which decreased from 12 million in 2007. This is the result of a decrease or reversal of net immigration from Mexico, the origin of the largest number of unauthorized immigrants.[34] The new wave of immigration and the numbers of unauthorized immigrants have engendered a great deal of controversy in the United States and have prompted new policy changes. The proposed Immigration Reform Bill would create a mechanism for the 11 million undocumented immigrants to achieve legal citizenship after proving that they can speak English, pass background checks, and pay taxes and a penalty.[7]

DETERMINANTS OF HEALTH AND HEALTH DISPARITIES

An individual's health status is influenced by a constellation of personal, social, economic, and environmental factors, collectively known as the *Determinants of Health*.[45] The determinants of health comprise political action and legislation; health care services; social factors such as poverty, occupational status, the quality of the neighborhood, and environment; lifestyle factors and individual behaviors; and biology and genetics. However, evidenced-based research has consistently shown that **poverty** has the greatest influence on health status.

The purposes of Healthy People 2020 are to address the multiple determinants of health and evaluate interventions that go beyond the traditional health care provider–patient model. For the past two decades the goals of Healthy People have been to eliminate health disparities. Healthy People 2020 defines a health disparity as "a particular type of health difference that is closely linked with social, economic, and/or environmental disadvantage. Health disparities adversely affect groups of people who have systematically experienced greater obstacles to health based on their racial or ethnic group; religion; socioeconomic status; gender; age; mental health; cognitive, sensory, or physical disability; sexual orientation or gender identity; geographic location; or other characteristics historically linked to discrimination or exclusion."[45]

The new framework for health care delivery strives for social and physical environments that promote quality of life free from preventable illness, disability, and premature death. This new framework encourages public health sectors to address the needs for safe and affordable housing; reliable transportation; nutritious food that is accessible to everyone; safe, well-integrated neighborhoods and schools; health care providers that are culturally and linguistically competent; and clean water and air.

Health Care Disparities Among Vulnerable Populations

Health disparities or *unfair and avoidable* health differences affect people who experience social, economic, and/or environmental disadvantage. These people are "vulnerable populations" and include ethnic and racial minorities, people with disabilities, and the LGBT community. Health care disparities can be measured by comparing the percent of difference from one group to the best group rate for a disease. Among African Americans the 7 largest health care disparities include gonorrhea, congenital syphilis, new cases of acquired immunodeficiency syndrome (AIDS), and deaths from AIDS—these reflect over 1000% difference from the group with the lowest indicators (Asians and/or Non-Hispanic Whites).[19] These are followed by nonfatal firearm-related injuries, new cases of tuberculosis, homicides, and drug-induced deaths. For Hispanics the five largest indicators of health disparities were congenital syphilis, new cases of tuberculosis, new cases of AIDS, exposure to environmental contaminants, and cirrhosis deaths. Following these are no source of ongoing care, drug-induced deaths, carbon monoxide poisoning, no completion of high school, and death from poisoning. The American Indian or Alaska Native population also had the same largest disparities as the Black non-Hispanic population, including high rates of gonorrhea, new tuberculosis cases, and drug-induced deaths. Some of its largest disparities were similar to those of the Hispanic population: new cases of tuberculosis, cirrhosis deaths, and deaths from poisoning. The American Indian or Alaska Native population had the highest rates of fetal alcohol syndrome, smoking by pregnant women, alcohol-related motor vehicle deaths, and physical assault.

The Asian population had the largest disparities in congenital syphilis and new tuberculosis cases and also had high rates of exposure to particulate matter, carbon monoxide, and no source of ongoing care. In addition, the Asian population had low rates of Pap testing, greater exposure to ozone, greater lack of knowledge of stroke symptoms, and lower rates of self-monitoring of blood glucose levels among people with diabetes.

Non-Hispanic Whites had the highest rates of all racial and ethnic groups in drug-induced deaths and death from cirrhosis, death by poisoning, smoking in pregnant women, physical assault, chronic obstructive pulmonary disease, binge drinking among high school seniors, firearm-related deaths, steroid use among 10th graders, and prostate cancer deaths.

Few of the differences in health between ethnic and racial groups have a biologic basis but rather pertain to the social determinants of health. Moreover, some differences suggest the benefits of targeted educational strategies such as toward Asians' lack of Pap testing, lower rates of self-monitoring for diabetes or fetal alcohol syndrome, and smoking by pregnant women among Alaska Natives and Pacific Islanders. However, disparities in exposure to environmental contaminants, violence, and substance abuse among some racial and ethnic minorities suggest the need for a major transformation of the neighborhoods and social contexts of people's lives.

Note that information regarding specific health disparities is included in the CULTURE AND GENETICS section of chapters in this text.

National Cultural and Linguistic Standards

The determinants of health most relevant to health care disparities fall under the areas of policy and legislation; health care services; social factors such as poverty, occupational status, and the quality of the neighborhood and environment; lifestyle factors and individual behaviors; and biology and genetics. Many forms of discrimination based on race or national origin frequently limit the opportunities of people to gain equal access to health care services. Many health and social service programs provide information about their services in English only. It is said that "language barriers have a deleterious effect on health care; patients are less likely to have a usual source of health care and have an increased risk of non-adherence to medication regimens."[15]

Because immigration occurs at high levels and immigrants with limited English proficiency (LEP) have particular needs, the Office of Minority Health published the *National Standards for Culturally and Linguistically Appropriate Services in Health Care*. The first and landmark standard states: "Health care organizations should ensure that patients receive from all staff members effective, understandable, and respectful care that is provided in a manner compatible with their cultural health beliefs and practices and preferred language."[29]

- EFFECTIVE CARE results in positive outcomes and satisfaction for the patient.
- RESPECTFUL CARE takes into consideration the values, preferences, and expressed needs of the patient.
- CULTURAL AND LINGUISTIC COMPETENCE is a set of congruent behaviors, attitudes, and policies that come together in a system among professionals that enables work in cross-cultural situations (Fig. 2-2).

Linguistic Competence

Under the provisions of Title VI of the Civil Rights Act of 1964, when people with LEP seek health care in settings such

2-2

as hospitals, nursing homes, clinics, daycare centers, and mental health centers, services cannot be denied to them.

English is the predominant language of the United States. However, among people at least 5 years old living in the United States in 2012, 21% spoke a language other than English at home.[44] Of those, 62% spoke Spanish, and 38% spoke some other language; 40.5% reported that they did not speak English "very well." The most common non-English languages spoken by people older than 5 years at home are Spanish (62%), Chinese (4.8%), Tagalog (2.6%), Vietnamese (2.3%), French (2.1%), Korean (1.9%), German (1.8%), Arabic (1.6%) Russian (1.5%), and African languages (1.5%).[38]

When people with LEP seek health care, they are frequently faced with receptionists, nurses, and physicians who speak English only. These health care professionals may be judgmental of people who do not speak English or become impatient with the added time it takes to provide service to them. The language barrier may result in the denial of medical care or social services, delay in the receipt of care and services, or the provision of care and services based on inaccurate or incomplete information. To prevent serious adverse health outcomes for LEP persons, it is incumbent on health care professionals to communicate effectively.

Chapter 3 describes in more detail how to communicate with people who do not understand English, how to interact with interpreters, and which services are available when no interpreter is available. It is vital that interpreters be present who not only serve to verbally translate the conversation but who can also describe to you the cultural aspects and meanings of the person's situation.

CULTURE AND CULTURE-RELATED CONCEPTS

There is no single definition of culture; often definitions tend to omit salient aspects of culture or are too general to have any real meaning. One definition is that culture is a pattern of shared attitudes, beliefs, self-definitions, norms, roles, and values that can occur among those who speak a particular language or live in a defined geographic region.[43] Culture is a complex whole in which each part is related to every other

part. It is also a web of communication, and much of culture is transmitted nonverbally through socialization or enculturation.[41] *Socialization* or *enculturation* is the process of being raised within a culture and acquiring the norms, values, and behaviors of that group.

In addition, culture has four basic characteristics: (1) *learned* from birth through the processes of language acquisition and socialization; (2) *shared* by all members of the same cultural group; (3) *adapted* to specific conditions related to environmental and technical factors and to the availability of natural resources; and (4) *dynamic* and ever changing.

Culture is a universal phenomenon without which no person exists. Yet the culture that develops in any given society is always specific and distinctive, encompassing all the knowledge, beliefs, customs, and skills acquired by members of that society. However, within cultures some groups of people share different beliefs, values, and attitudes. Differences occur because of ethnicity, religion, education, occupation, age, and gender. When such groups function within a large culture, they are referred to as *subcultural groups*.

Many people think about race and ethnicity as a part of the concept of culture. The concept of **race** reflects self-identification by people according to race or races with which they closely identify. The U.S. Census Data lists 15 racial categories: White, Black (African American or Negro), American Indian or Alaskan native, Asian Indian, Chinese, Filipino, Japanese, Korean, Vietnamese, Native Hawaiian, Guamanian or Chamorro, Samoan, other Pacific Islander, some other race, or more than one race. Some people have a biologic view of race (i.e., that race is characterized by genetic differences or innate, unchangeable physical characteristics that distinguish one group of people from another).[18]

In reality there are no genetic characteristics that distinguish one group of people from another, and today's scientific community asserts that race is not a useful construct when examining disease prevalence. It is more important to think about differences in drug metabolism and/or prevalence of some hereditary disease as the result of genetic variations caused by markers that are defined by geographic origins of ancestry. Although sickle cell anemia is commonly thought of as a disease that affects Blacks, the trait is found in Mediterranean groups as well. Therefore the disease can also be found in Whites who have a Spanish, Italian, or Greek background.[4]

Ethnicity refers to a social group that may possess shared traits such as a common geographic origin, migratory status, religion, language, values, traditions or symbols, and food preferences. The ethnic group may have a loose group identity with few or no cultural traditions in common or a coherent subculture with a shared language and body of tradition. Similarly *ethnic identity* is one's self-identification with a particular ethnic group. This identity may be strongly adherent to one's country of origin or background or weakly identified, depending on one's acculturation strategy.

Acculturation is the process of social and psychological exchanges that take place when there are ongoing encounters between individuals of different cultures, with subsequent

2-3

changes in either or both groups.[37] During the late 1800s and early part of the 1900s when the United States experienced its greatest period of immigration, the expectation was that immigrants would take on the characteristics of the dominant culture, known as *assimilation.* One was discouraged from having a unique ethnic identity in favor of the nationalist identity. The acculturation process during this period of our history became known as the *melting pot*[30] and also as *Americanization.*[13]

The recent wave of immigrants in the latter part of the 20th century has developed different strategies of acculturation. Rather than solely relying on assimilation, new immigrants developed new means of forging identities between the countries of origin and their host country such as "biculturalism" and "integration."[39] Assimilation is a unidirectional and one-dimensional means of acculturation, proceeding in a linear fashion from unacculturated to acculturated. However, biculturalism and integration are bidirectional and bidimensional, inducing reciprocal changes in both cultures and maintaining aspects of the original culture in one's ethnic identity (Fig. 2-3).

Those who emigrate here from non-Western or nonmodern countries may find the process of acculturation, whether in schools or society, to be an extremely difficult and painful process. The losses and changes that occur when adjusting to or integrating a new system of beliefs, routines, and social roles are known as **acculturative stress,** which has important implications for health and illness.[9-11] When caring for patients, please be aware of the factors that contribute to acculturative stress as defined in Table 2-1.[7]

Religion and Spirituality

Other major aspects of culture are **religion and spirituality.** An important distinction needs to be made. **Spirituality** is borne out of each person's unique life experience and his or her personal effort to find purpose and meaning in life.[40] On the other hand, **religion** refers to an organized system of beliefs concerning the cause, nature, and purpose of the universe, especially belief in a divine or superhuman power to be obeyed and worshipped as the creator(s) and ruler(s) of the universe (called by names such as Allah, God, Yahweh, and Jehovah).[1] Religion is a shared experience of spirituality or the values, beliefs, and practices into which people either are born or which they may adopt to meet their personal spiritual needs through communal actions such as religious affiliation; attendance and participation in a religious institution, prayer, or meditation; and religious practices.

The Landscape Survey detailed statistics on religion in America.[35] The study found that religious affiliation in the United States is both diverse and extremely fluid. The number of people who say they are not affiliated with any particular faith is 16.1%. Those reporting religious affiliation with a Christian church number 78.4%. The Christian denominations include Roman Catholic (23.9%); Protestant (51.3%), which includes Mainline Protestant (18.1%), Evangelical churches (26.3%), and historical Black churches (6.9%); Mormon (1.3%); Jehovah's Witness (0.7%); and others. Those belonging to non-Christian and other religions total 4.7% of the U.S. population; of these the largest group is Jewish (1.7%), followed by Buddhist (0.7%), Muslim (0.6%), and Hindu (0.4%). The Landscape Survey also found that, among the foreign-born adult population, Catholics outnumbered Protestants by nearly a 2-to-1 margin (46% Catholic versus 24% Protestant) and that immigrants are also disproportionately represented among several world religions in the United States, including Islam, Hinduism, and Buddhism.[35]

Religious affiliation and practices can support spiritual harmony and health in the following ways:

1. Religious affiliation and attendance at religious functions may promote health through social networks and social support systems that buffer and affect stress and isolation.[23]

TABLE 2-1 **Dimensions of Acculturative Stress**		
INSTRUMENTAL/ENVIRONMENTAL	**SOCIAL/INTERPERSONAL**	**SOCIETAL**
Financial	Loss of social networks	Discrimination/stigma
Language barriers	Loss of social status	Level of acculturation
Lack of access to health care	Family conflict	Political/historical forces
Unemployment	Family separation	Legal status
Lack of education	Intergenerational conflict	
	Changing gender roles	

Modified from Caplan, S. (2007). Latinos, acculturation, and acculturative stress: a dimensional concept analysis. *Policy Politics Nurs Pract, 8*(2), 93-106.

2-4 **A,** The Vietnam Veterans Memorial. **B,** Saint Peregrine. **C,** Thai Spirit House. **D,** Buddhist shrine. (Spector, 2006.)

2. Religious affiliation and membership benefit health by promoting healthy behavior and lifestyles.[29]
3. Regular religious fellowship benefits health by offering social support. Faith benefits health by leading to thoughts of hope, optimism, and positive expectation.[8,31]

In times of crisis such as serious illness and impending death, religion may be a source of consolation for the person and his or her family.[32] Religious dogma and spiritual leaders may exert considerable influence on the person's decision making concerning acceptable medical and surgical treatment such as vaccinations, choice of healer(s), and other aspects of the illness.

There are many examples of how spirituality and religion are apparent in daily life and frequently play a role in one's health. People may take religious pilgrimages to shrines. There are countless shrines, both secular and from a religious tradition, which people visit to remember and/or pray for favors or healing. Fig. 2-4, *A,* is an image of the Vietnam Veterans Memorial in Washington, DC, an example of a secular/spiritual shrine where people go to remember loved ones who died in the Vietnam War. Fig. 2-4, *B,* is a statue of Saint Peregrine, the patron saint of people with cancer, in the Mission San Juan Capistrano in California. Fig. 2-4, *C,* is the Thai Spirit House in Los Angeles, California. The shrine is on a public street and is visited by believers; offerings such as flowers and food are frequently left at the base. Fig. 2-4, *D*, is an example of a sacred Buddhist shrine that can be found in a store or in a home.

In health care settings you frequently encounter people who are searching for a spiritual meaning to help explain their illnesses or disabilities. Some health care providers find spiritual assessment difficult because of the abstract and personal nature of the topic. This aspect of the person may be ignored, and the question "What is your religious preference?" is not asked. This may be to protect against discrimination based on religion. Yet the omission of questions about spiritual and religious practices can raise barriers to holistic care.

Several well-validated questionnaires assess how a person is coping with loss such as a serious illness. Perhaps the most well-known and widely used is the Brief R-COPE, a short 14-item assessment for use in clinical practice (Table 2-2).[33] The Brief R-COPE helps practitioners understand the patient's religious coping to enable them to integrate spirituality in treatment.[33] It examines whether a patient is using positive or negative religious coping. Positive religious coping mechanisms indicate that the person is strongly connected to a divine presence, is spiritually connected with others, and has a benevolent outlook on life, whereas negative religious coping methods reflect a spiritual struggle with one's self or with God. Illness may be attributed to God's punishment, to an act of the Devil, or totally within the hands of God. Just as positive religious coping has been linked to positive health (described previously), negative religious coping is associated with poor health outcomes[33] and provides an opportunity for the nurse to intervene.

In summation we need to understand a patient's cultural and religious beliefs because countless health-related behaviors are promoted by nearly all cultures and religions. Meditating, exercising and maintaining physical fitness, getting enough sleep, being willing to have the body examined, telling the truth about how you feel, maintaining family viability, hoping for recovery, coping with stress, being able to live with a disability, and caring for children are all intricately related to one's core values and beliefs.

HEALTH-RELATED BELIEFS AND PRACTICES

Healing and Culture

HEALTH is defined as the **balance** of the person, both within one's being (physical, mental, or spiritual) and in the outside world (natural, communal, or metaphysical). It is a complex, interrelated phenomenon. Before determining whether cultural practices are helpful, harmful, or neutral, you must first understand the logic of the traditional belief systems coming from a person's culture and then grasp the nature and meaning of the health practice from the person's cultural perspective.

Wide cultural variation exists in the manner in which certain symptoms and disease conditions are perceived, diagnosed, labeled, and treated. You should not assume that the perceived symptoms or complaints of patients are equivalent to the names of recognized diseases or syndromes familiar to nurses, physicians, and other health care professionals.[11] The

---

TABLE 2-2 **Spirituality Assessment: the Brief R-COPE***
The following items deal with how you coped with a significant trauma or negative event in your life. There are many ways to try to deal with problems. These items ask which part religion played in what you did to cope with this negative event. Obviously different people deal with things in different ways, but we are interested in how you tried to deal with it. Each item says something about a particular way of coping. We want to know to what extent you did what the item says: *how much or how frequently*. Don't answer on the basis of what worked or not—just whether or not you did it. Use these response choices.

Try to rate each item separately in your mind. Make your answers as true *for you* as you can.

    1 = Not at all
    2 = Somewhat
    3 = Quite a bit
    4 = A great deal

1. Looked for a stronger connection with God. _____
2. Sought God's love and care. _____
3. Sought help from God in letting go of my anger. _____
4. Tried to put my plans into action together with God. _____
5. Tried to see how God might be trying to strengthen me in this situation. _____
6. Asked forgiveness for my sins. _____
7. Focused on religion to stop worrying about my problems. _____
8. Wondered whether God had abandoned me. _____
9. Felt punished by God for my lack of devotion. _____
10. Wondered what I did for God to punish me. _____
11. Questioned God's love for me. _____
12. Wondered whether my church had abandoned me. _____
13. Decided the devil made this happen. _____
14. Questioned the power of God. _____

From Pargament, K., Feuille, M., & Burdzy, D. (2011). The Brief RCOPE: current psychometric status of a short measure of religious coping. *Religions* 2, 51-76.
*The reproduction of any copyrighted material is prohibited without the express permission of the copyright holder.

---

same disease that is considered grounds for social ostracism in one culture may be reason for increased status in another. For example, epilepsy is seen as contagious and untreatable among Ugandans, as a cause for family shame among Greeks, as a reflection of a physical imbalance among Mexican Americans, as the entry of a "spirit" into the person's body by the Hmong,[14] and as a sign of having gained favor by enduring a trial by God among the Hutterites.

Bodily symptoms are also perceived and reported in a variety of ways. For example, people of Mediterranean descent tend to report common physical symptoms more often than people of Northern European or Asian heritage. Among Chinese, no translation exists for the English word "sadness," yet all people experience the feeling of sadness at some time in life. To express emotion, Chinese patients somatize their symptoms or convert mental experiences or states into bodily symptoms (e.g., complain of cardiac symptoms because the center of emotion in the Chinese culture is the heart). For example, you may collect in-depth data about the cardiovascular system only to learn later that all diagnostic tests are negative. On further assessment you find that the person has experienced a loss and is grieving (e.g., has experienced the death of a close relative or friend or has been divorced or separated). This is a culturally acceptable somatic expression of emotional disharmony.

For patients, symptom labeling and diagnosis depend on the degree of difference between the person's behaviors and those that the group has defined as normal (e.g., beliefs about the causation of illness, level of stigma attached to a particular set of symptoms, prevalence of the pathologic condition, and the meaning of the illness to the person and his or her family).

Beliefs About Causes of Illness

Throughout history people have tried to understand the cause of illness and disease. Theories of causation have been formulated on the basis of ethnic identity, religious beliefs, social class, philosophic perspectives, and level of knowledge.[22] Many people who maintain traditional beliefs would define HEALTH in terms of balance and a loss of this balance. This understanding includes the balance of mind, body, and spirit in the overall definitions of HEALTH and ILLNESS.

Disease causation may be viewed in three major ways: from a biomedical or scientific, a naturalistic or holistic, or a magicoreligious perspective.[21]

Biomedical

The first, called the **biomedical** or **scientific** theory of illness causation, assumes that all events in life have a cause and effect, that the human body functions more or less mechanically (i.e., the functioning of the human body is analogous to the functioning of an automobile), that all life can be reduced or divided into smaller parts (e.g., the reduction of the human person into body, mind, and spirit), and that all of reality can be observed and measured (e.g., intelligence tests and psychometric measures of behavior). Among the biomedical explanations for disease is the germ theory, which holds that microorganisms such as bacteria and viruses cause specific disease conditions. Most educational programs for physicians, nurses, and other health care providers embrace the biomedical or scientific theories that explain the causes of both physical and psychological illnesses.[20]

Naturalistic

The second way in which people explain the cause of illness is from the **naturalistic** or **holistic** perspective, found most frequently among American Indians, Asians, and others who believe that human life is only one aspect of nature and a part of the general order of the cosmos. These people believe that the forces of nature must be kept in natural balance or harmony.

Some Asians believe in the **yin/yang theory,** in which health exists when all aspects of the person are in perfect balance.[26] Rooted in the ancient Chinese philosophy of *Tao,* the yin/yang theory states that all organisms and objects in the universe consist of yin and yang energy forces. The seat of the energy forces is within the autonomic nervous system, where balance between the opposing forces is maintained during health. Yin energy represents the female and negative forces such as emptiness, darkness, and cold, whereas yang forces are male and positive, emitting warmth and fullness. Foods are classified as hot and cold in this theory and are transformed into yin and yang energy when metabolized by the body. Yin foods are cold, and yang foods are hot. Cold foods are eaten with a hot illness, and hot foods are eaten with a cold illness. The yin/yang theory is the basis for *Eastern* or *Chinese* medicine and is commonly embraced by many Asian Americans.

The naturalistic perspective holds that the laws of nature create imbalances, chaos, and disease. People embracing this view use metaphors such as the healing power of nature, and they call the earth "Mother." For example, from the perspective of the Chinese, illness is not seen as an intruding agent but as a part of the rhythmic course of life and an outward sign of disharmony within.

Many Hispanic, Arab, Black, and Asian groups embrace the **hot/cold theory** of health and illness, an explanatory model with origins in the ancient Greek humoral theory. The four humors of the body—blood, phlegm, black bile, and yellow bile—regulate basic bodily functions and are described in terms of temperature, dryness, and moisture. The treatment of disease consists of adding or subtracting cold, heat, dryness, or wetness to restore the balance of the humors.

Beverages, foods, herbs, medicines, and diseases are classified as hot or cold according to their perceived effects on the body, not on their physical characteristics. Illnesses believed to be caused by cold entering the body include earache, chest cramps, paralysis, gastrointestinal discomfort, rheumatism, and tuberculosis. Among illnesses believed to be caused by overheating are abscessed teeth, sore throats, rashes, and kidney disorders.

According to the hot/cold theory, the person is whole, not just a particular ailment. Those who embrace the hot/cold theory maintain that health consists of a positive state of total well-being, including physical, psychological, spiritual, and social aspects of the person. Paradoxically the language used to describe this artificial dissection of the body into parts is itself a reflection of the biomedical/scientific perspective, not a naturalistic or holistic one.

Magicoreligious

The third major way that people explain the causation of ILLNESS is from a **magicoreligious** perspective. The basic premise is that the world is an arena in which supernatural forces dominate.[14] The fate of the world and those in it depends on the action of supernatural forces for good or evil. Examples of magical causes of illness include belief in voodoo or witchcraft among some Blacks and others from circum-Caribbean countries. *Faith healing* is based on religious beliefs and is most prevalent among certain Christian groups, including Christian Scientists, whereas various healing rituals may be found in other religions such as Roman Catholicism and Mormonism.

Traditional Treatments and Folk Healers

All cultures have their own preferred lay or popular healers, recognized symptoms of ill health, acceptable sick role behavior, and treatments. In addition to seeking help from you as a biomedical/scientific health care provider, patients may also seek help from folk or religious healers. Each culture has its own healers, most of whom speak the person's native tongue, make house calls, understand the person's cultural health beliefs, and cost significantly less than practitioners in the biomedical/scientific health care system. Table 2-3 lists examples of traditional HEALTH and ILLNESS beliefs and practices, causes of illness, and examples of traditional healers.

In some religions spiritual healers may be found among the ranks of the ordained and official religious hierarchy and may be known by a variety of names such as *priest, bishop, elder, deacon, rabbi, brother,* and *sister.* In other religions a separate category of healer may be found (e.g., Christian Science "nurses" [not licensed by states] or practitioners). Spirituality is included in the perceptions of health and illness.

Hispanics may rely on *curandero(ra), espiritualista* (spiritualist), *yerbo(ba)* (herbalist), *partera* (lay midwife), or *sabedor* (healer who manipulates bones and muscles). Blacks may mention having received assistance from a *hougan* (a voodoo priest or priestess), *spiritualist,* or *"old lady"* (an older woman who has successfully raised a family and who specializes in child care and folk remedies). American Indians may seek assistance from a *shaman* or *medicine (wo)man.* Asians may mention that they have visited *herbalists, acupuncturists,* or *bone setters.* Among the Amish the term *braucher* refers to folk healers who use herbs and tonics in the home or community context. *Brauche,* a folk healing art, refers to sympathy curing, which is sometimes called *powwowing* in English.

Many cultures believe that the cure is incomplete unless healing of body, mind, and spirit are all carried out. The division of the person into parts is itself a Western concept. For example, a Hispanic person with a respiratory infection may take the antibiotics prescribed by a physician or nurse practitioner and herbal teas recommended by a *curandero* and may say prayers for healing suggested by a Catholic priest.[5] American Indians may frequent sweat lodges or use talking circles and other healing ceremonies such as smudging or ritual purifying with the smoke of sacred herbs.[17] Many people from different faith traditions practice prayer or visit healing shrines, as discussed earlier.

Amulets are objects such as charms that may be worn on a string or chain around the neck, wrist, or waist to protect the wearer from the "evil eye" or the "evil spirits" that could be transmitted from one person to another or that could have supernatural origins. They may also be hung in the home, car, or workplace. Natural folk medicine uses remedies from the natural environment (i.e., herbs, plants, minerals, and animal substances) to treat illnesses. Amulets and remedies have

2-5 The interior of a *botanica.*   (Spector, 2006.)

come to the United States from every corner of the world, the East and the West. They may be purchased in pharmacies, markets, and natural food stores. Fig. 2-5 illustrates the interior of a *botanica,* a store in which a person can purchase amulets and remedies used by people from many Latino ethnicities. Others may be objects or substances used externally. Fig. 2-6 presents samples of traditional amulets.

The variety of healing beliefs and practices used by the many ethnocultural populations found in this country far exceeds the limitations of this chapter. Fig. 2-7 presents samples of traditional remedies used for recovery. In addition to folk practices, many other complementary healing practices exist. In the United States an estimated 38% of adults use some form of complementary therapy to treat an illness, including acupuncture, Ayurveda, biofeedback, chiropractic or osteopathic manipulation, deep-breathing exercises and guided imagery, diet-based therapies, homeopathy, hypnosis, meditation, Tai-Chi and Yoga, and traditional folk healers.[28] Furthermore, U.S. adults spent $33.9 billion out-of-pocket on visits to complementary and alternative medicine practitioners, to traditional healers, and for the purchase of related products.[2]

The availability of over-the-counter medications, the relatively high literacy level of Americans, the growing availability of herbal remedies, and the influence of the Internet and mass media in communicating health-related information to the general population have contributed to the high percentage of cases of self-treatment. Home treatments are attractive for their accessibility, especially compared with the inconvenience associated with traveling to a physician, nurse practitioner, or pharmacist, particularly for people from rural or sparsely populated areas. Furthermore, home treatment may mobilize the person's social support network and provide the sick person with a caring environment in which to convalesce. However, not all home remedies are inexpensive.

TABLE 2-3   **Selected Examples of Traditional HEALTH and ILLNESS Beliefs and Practices**

ORIGIN	HEALTH BELIEFS	ILLNESS BELIEFS	ILLNESS CAUSATION	HEALTH MAINTENANCE	HEALTH PROTECTION	HEALTH RESTORATION	TRADITIONAL HEALERS
Asian Heritages							
China India Japan Korea Philippines Southeast Asia Laos Cambodia Vietnam	Balance of *"yin and yang"*	Imbalance of *"yin and yang"*	Upset in the balance of *"yin and yang"* Overexertion Prolonged sitting Lying in bed	Prevent imbalances of *"yin and yang"* and changes in climate	Wear amulets such as jade Eat correct and compatible foods	Traditional remedies such as ginseng root Acupuncture Moxibustion Cupping	Chinese physicians Herbalists
African Heritages							
Africa— west coast (as slaves) (e.g., Ghana Nigeria) Haiti Jamaica West Indian islands	Harmony with nature	Disharmony with nature	Demons Evil spirits Voodoo Hexes	Prevent disharmony; respect cleanliness Religion Avoid sick people	Wear bangles Faith	*Asafoetida,* herbs and roots	Root worker Spiritualists "Old Lady"
European Heritages							
England France Germany Poland Russia Others	Physical and emotional well-being; feeling okay	Absence of well-being; feeling bad	Evil eye Evil spirits Hexes	Proper nutrition, exercise, cleanliness, and faith in God	Wear amulets Shawls	Home remedies such as swamp root and *Olbas*	Homeopathic physicians Brauchers
American Indian/Alaska Native Heritages							
North American Indians/ Alaska Natives 550+ federally or state recognized nations	Living in harmony with nature Balance of the mind, emotions, body, and spirit	Disharmony with nature	Evil spirits Ghosts Displeasing holy people	Respect nature; avoid evil spirits Masks	Use of amulets and sweet grass	Sand paintings Herbs	Medicine man (shaman)
Iberian, Central and South American Heritages							
Spain and Portugal Brazil Cuba Mexico Puerto Rico Colombia	Reward for good behavior Balance of "hot and cold" humors	Punishment for wrongdoing Imbalance of hot and cold	Evil eye Envy of other people Jealousy	Use proper diet to maintain balance of "hot and cold" Faith	Amulets such as a *mano negro,* soaps, candles	Prayers Promises to saints Herbs, *Anis,* and *Manzanilla*	Folk healers such as the *santro/a, partera,* or *curandero/a*

2-6   A, The glass blue eye from Turkey seen here is an example of an amulet that may be hung in the home. **B,** A seed with a red string may be placed on the crib of a baby of Mexican heritage. **C,** These bangles may be worn for protection by a person of Caribbean heritage. **D,** This small packet is placed on a crib or in the room of a baby of Japanese heritage. (Spector, 2006.)

A wide variety of alternative, complementary, or traditional interventions is gaining the recognition of health care professionals in the biomedical/scientific health care system. Acupuncture, acupressure, therapeutic touch, massage, therapeutic use of music, biofeedback, relaxation techniques, meditation, hypnosis, distraction, imagery, iridology, reflexology, and herbal remedies are examples of interventions that people may use either alone or in combination with other treatments. Many pharmacies and grocery stores routinely carry herbal treatments for a wide variety of common illnesses. The effectiveness of complementary and alternative interventions for specific health problems has been studied extensively (see National Center for Complementary and Alternative Medicine at www.nccam.nih.gov).

❖ DEVELOPMENTAL COMPETENCE

Illness during childhood may pose a difficult clinical situation. Children and adults have spiritual needs that vary according to the child's developmental level and the religious climate that exists in the family. Parental perceptions about the illness of the child may be partially influenced by religious beliefs. For example, some parents may believe that a transgression against a religious law is responsible for a congenital anomaly in their offspring. Other parents may delay seeking medical care because they believe that prayer should be tried first. Certain types of treatment (e.g., administration of blood; medications containing caffeine, pork, or other prohibited substances) and selected procedures may be perceived as *cultural taboos* (i.e., practices to be avoided by both children and adults).

Values held by the dominant U.S. and Canadian cultures such as emphasis on independence, self-reliance, and productivity influence the aging members of society. North Americans define people as old at the chronologic age of 65 years and then limit their work, in contrast to other cultures in which people are first recognized as being unable to work and then identified as being "old." The generation born just before or at the end of World War II (1940-1949) comprises the early range of older adults who are eligible for Social Security and Medicare.

Older persons may develop their own means of coping with illness through self-care, assistance from family members, and support from social groups. Some cultures have attitudes and specific behaviors for older adults that include humanistic care and identification of family members as care providers. The older adults may have special family responsibilities (e.g., providing hospitality to visitors [Amish cultures] and communicating their skills and accrued wisdom to members of younger generations [Filipinos]).

Older immigrants who have made major lifestyle adjustments in their move from their homelands to the United States or from a rural to an urban area (or vice versa) may not be aware of health care alternatives, preventive programs, health care benefits, and screening programs for which they are eligible. These people also may be in various stages of *culture shock* (i.e., the state of disorientation or inability to

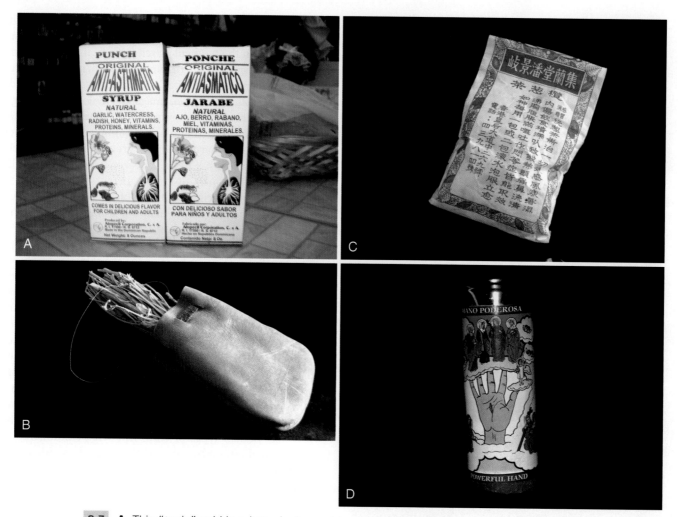

2-7 **A,** This "tonic" sold in a *botanica* is used to treat asthma. **B,** The traditional medicine bag of an American Indian shaman is used to carry necessary medicines. **C,** The leaves in this package may be used by a person of Chinese heritage to treat indigestion. **D,** This candle may be burned for cleansing by a person of Mexican heritage (Spector, 2006).

respond to the behavior of a different cultural group because of its sudden strangeness, unfamiliarity, and incompatibility with the newcomer's perceptions and expectations). For example, to maintain ties with their native heritage, people may purchase food in stores that specialize in selling products from their homelands.

TRANSCULTURAL EXPRESSION OF PAIN

To illustrate how symptom expression may reflect the person's cultural background, let us use an extensively studied symptom—pain. Pain is a universally recognized phenomenon, and it is an important aspect of assessment. It is a private, subjective experience that is greatly influenced by cultural heritage. Expectations, manifestations, and management of pain are all embedded in a cultural context. The definition of pain, like that of health or illness, is culturally determined.

The word *pain* is derived from the Greek word for *penalty*, which helps explain the long association between pain and

punishment in Judeo-Christian thought. The meaning of painful stimuli, the way people define their situations, and the impact of personal experience all help determine the experience of pain.

In addition to expecting variations in pain perception and tolerance, you also should expect variations in the expression of pain. It is well known that people turn to their social environment for validation and comparison. A first important comparison group is the family, which transmits cultural norms to its children.

STEPS TO CULTURAL COMPETENCY

Cultural competency includes the attitudes, knowledge, and skills necessary for providing quality care to diverse populations.[2,6] You must climb several steps on the journey to cultural competency. The integration of this knowledge into day-to-day practice takes time because many practitioners in the health care system hesitate to adopt new ideas. Cultural competency does not come after reading a chapter or several

Spector's Heritage Assessment

The following set of questions can be used by caregivers to begin to determine a person's ethnic, cultural, or religious heritage and its relationship to his or her personal and health care traditions. The stronger the association of these items to a person's identification, the more traditional is his or her heritage.

1. Where were you born? _____
2. Where were your parents/grandparents born?
   a. Mother: _____
   b. Father: _____
   c. Mother's mother: _____
   d. Mother's father: _____
   e. Father's mother: _____
   f. Father's father: _____
3. How many brothers _____ and sisters _____ do you have?
4. What setting did you grow up in? Urban _____ Rural _____ Suburban _____
   Where? _____
5. What country did your parents/grandparents grow up in?
   a. Mother: _____
   b. Father: _____
   c. Mother's mother: _____
   d. Mother's father: _____
   e. Father's mother: _____
   f. Father's father: _____
6. How old were you when you came to the United States? _____
7. How old were your parents/ grandparents when they came to the United States?
   a. Mother: _____
   b. Father: _____
   c. Mother's mother: _____
   d. Mother's father: _____
   e. Father's mother: _____
   f. Father's father: _____
8. When you were growing up, who lived with you? _____
9. Have you maintained contact with:
   a. Aunts, uncles, cousins? _____ Yes _____ No
   b. Brothers and sisters? _____ Yes _____ No
   c. Parents? _____ Yes _____ No
   d. Your own children? _____ Yes _____ No
10. Does most of your family live near you? _____ Describe: _____
11. Approximately how often did you visit your family members who lived outside your home? _____ Daily _____ Weekly _____ Monthly _____ <Once a year _____ Never
12. Was your original family name changed? _____ Yes _____ No
13. What is your religious preference? _____ Catholic _____ Jewish _____ Protestant–Denomination _____ Other _____ None
14. Is your spouse of the same religion? _____ Yes _____ No
    Describe: _____
15. Is your spouse of the same ethnic background as you? _____ Yes _____ No
    Describe: _____
16. What kind of school did you go to? _____ Public _____ Private _____ Parochial
17. As an adult, do you live in a neighborhood where the neighbors are the same religion and ethnic background as yourself? _____ Yes _____ No
18. Do you belong to a religious institution? _____ Yes _____ No
    Describe: _____
19. Would you describe yourself as an active member? _____ Yes _____ No
20. How often do you attend your religious institution? _____ More than once a week _____ Weekly _____ Monthly _____ Special holidays only _____ Never
21. Do you practice your religion or other spiritual practices in your home? _____ Yes _____ No
    If yes, please specify: _____ Praying _____ Bible reading _____ Diet _____ Celebrating religious holidays _____ Meditating _____ Other: describe_____
22. Do you prepare foods of your ethnic background? _____ Yes _____ No
    Describe: _____
23. Do you participate in ethnic activities? _____ Yes _____ No
    If yes, specify: _____ Singing _____ Holiday celebrations _____ Dancing _____ Costumes _____ Festivals _____ Other
    Describe: _____
24. Are your friends from the same religious background? _____ Yes _____ No
25. Are your friends of the same ethnic background as you? _____ Yes _____ No
26. What is your native language? _____
    Do you speak this language? _____ Prefer _____ Occasionally _____ Rarely
27. Do you read in your native language? _____ Prefer _____ Occasionally _____ Rarely

From Spector, R. E. (2013). *Cultural diversity in health and illness* (8th ed.). Upper Saddle River, NJ: Pearson, pp. 376-378.

2-8

chapters or books on this highly specialized area. It is complex and multifaceted, and many facets change over time. The areas of knowledge include sociology, psychology, theology, cultural anthropology, demography, folklore, and immigration history and policies. One must also have an understanding of poverty and environmental health. Cultural competency also involves soul searching about your own culture and health.

One response to the government mandates for cultural competency is the development of cultural care that describes professional health care as culturally sensitive, appropriate, and competent. There is a discrete body of knowledge, and much of the content is introduced in this chapter.

- *Culturally sensitive* implies that caregivers possess some basic knowledge of and constructive attitudes toward the diverse cultural populations found in the setting in which they are practicing.
- *Culturally appropriate* implies that the caregivers apply the underlying background knowledge that must be possessed to provide a given person with the best possible health care.
- *Culturally competent* implies that the caregivers understand and attend to the total context of the individual's situation, including awareness of immigration status, stress factors, other social factors, and cultural similarities and differences.[39]

Cultural care is the provision of health care across cultural boundaries and considers the context both in which the patient lives and the situations in which the patient's health problems arise.[41] Each chapter in this text includes information necessary for delivery of cultural care.

CULTURAL ASSESSMENT

Cultural Formulation Model

The Cultural Formulation Model[24] is a well-recognized tool to use to provide an in-depth exploration of the patient's issues in the context of culture. The model has five categories: cultural identity of the individual, cultural explanation of the individual's illness, cultural factors related to psychosocial environment and levels of functioning, and cultural elements of the relationship between the individual and the clinician. This assessment tool provides an overall cultural assessment to promote culturally competent diagnosis and care.

Heritage Assessment

The following are the factors of heritage consistency that determine the depth to which you and the given patient identify with a traditional heritage (i.e., the cultural beliefs and practices of the family, the extended family, and an ethnoreligious community).

The Heritage Assessment tool (Fig. 2-8), lists all of the questions that may be asked. It is important to ask the questions slowly over time. If the person appears anxious, it is best to postpone asking the questions or to weave them into other parts of the health history. The responses can be scored, and an image arises as to whether the person identifies with his or her traditional heritage or whether he or she is acculturated and assimilated into the mainstream of modern American culture.

In addition to the background information, four short questions may be asked:

1. Do you mostly participate in social activities with members of your family?
2. Do you mostly have friends from a similar cultural background as you?
3. Do you mostly eat the foods of your family's tradition?
4. Do you mostly participate in the religious traditions of your family?

If the person answers two to four of these questions positively, the probability of being more likely to use health practices relevant to their traditional heritage is high.

BIBLIOGRAPHY

1. Abramson, H. J. (1980). Religion. In Thernstrom, S. (Ed.), *Harvard encyclopedia of American ethnic groups.* Cambridge: Harvard University Press.
2. American Association of Colleges of Nursing (2008). *Cultural competency in baccalaureate nursing education.* Available at http://www.aacn.nche.edu/leading-initiatives/education-resources/competency.pdf.
3. Barnes, P. M., Bloom, B., & Nahin, R. CDC National Health Statistics Report #12. (December 2008). *Complementary and alternative medicine use among adults and children: United States, 2007.* Available at https://nccam.nih.gov/sites/nccam.nih.gov/files/news/nhsr12.pdf.
4. Brawley, O. W. (2003). Population categorization and cancer statistics. *Cancer Metastasis Rev, 22*(1)11-19.
5. Cabassa, L. J., Lester, R., & Zayas, L. H. (2007). It's like being in a labyrinth: Hispanic immigrants' perceptions of depression and attitudes toward treatments. *J Immigrant Minor Health, 9*(1), 1-16.
6. Campinha-Bacote, J. (2003). *The process of cultural competence in the delivery of healthcare services,* ed 4. Cincinnati: Transcultural C.A.R.E. Associates.
7. Caplan, S. (2007). Latinos, acculturation, and acculturative stress: a dimensional concept analysis. *Policy Polit Nurs Pract 8*(2):93-106.
8. Clements, A. D., & Ermakova, A. V. (2012). Surrender to God and stress: a possible link between religiosity and health. *Psychol Religion Spirituality, 4*(2), 93-107.
9. Cuellar, I., Bastida, E., & Braccio, S. M. (2004). Residency in the United States, subjective well-being, and depression in an older Mexican-origin sample. *J Aging Health, 16*(4), 447-466.
10. Dalla, R. I., & Christensen, A. (2005). Latino immigrants describe residence in rural Midwestern meatpacking communities. *Hispanic J Behav Sci, 27*(1), 23-41. Available at PsychINFO database.
11. Engstrom, D. W., & Piedra, L. M. (2005). Central American survivors of political violence. Gonzales, G., & Gonzalez, R.,

(Eds.), *Mental health care for new Hispanic immigrants.* Binghamton, NY: Hayworth Press, (pp. 161-189).

12. Erikson, E., & Erik, H. (1959). *Identity and the life cycle.* New York: International Universities Press.

13. Escobar, J. I., & Vega, W. A. (2000). Mental health and immigrations AAAs. *J Nervous Mental Dis, 188*(11), 736-740.

14. Fadiman, A. (1997). *The spirit catches you and you fall down: a Hmong child, her American doctors, and the collision of two cultures.* New York: Farrar, Straus and Giroux.

15. Flores, G. (2006). Language barriers to health care in the United States. *New Engl J Med, 355,* 229-231.

16. Gates, G. J. (April 2011). *How many people are lesbian, gay, bisexual, and transgender?* The Williams Institute, University of California–Los Angeles School of Law.

17. Hamdy, S. L. (2004). *Sexual victimization in Indian country: barriers and resources for native women seeking help.* Harrisburg, PA: VAWnet. Available at http://www.vawnet.org.

18. Haney Lopez, I.F.: *The social construction of race,* 29 Harvard Civil Rights-Civil Liberties Law Review 1-62, 6-7, 11-17, Winter 1994.

19. Keppel, K. G. (2007). Ten largest US racial and ethnic health disparities. *Am J Epidemiol, 166,* 97-103. Available at http://aje.oxfordjournals.org.

20. Kleinman, A. (1978). Concepts and a model for the comparison of medical systems as cultural systems. *Social Sci Med, 12*(2-B), 85-95.

21. Kottak, C. P. (2008.). *Cultural anthropology.* (12th ed.). Boston: McGraw Hill.

22. Landrine, H., & Klonoff, E. A. (1994). Cultural diversity in causal attributions for illness: the role of the supernatural. *J Behav Med 17,* 181-93.

23. Levin, J. (2001). *God, faith and health: exploring the spirituality-healing connection.* New York: John Wiley & Sons.

24. Lewis-Fernandez, R., & Diaz, N. (2002). The cultural formulation: a method for assessing cultural factors affecting the clinical encounter. *Psych Q, 7*(4), 271-295.

25. Maselko, J., Hughes, C., & Cheney, R. (2011). Religious social capital. *Soc Sci Med, 73*(5):759-67.

26. Men, J., & Guo, L. (2010). *A general introduction to traditional Chinese medicine.* Boca Raton, FL: CRC Press.

27. Motel, S., & Patten, E. (January 29, 2013). *Statistical portrait of the foreign-born population in the United States, 2011.* Available at http://www.pewhispanic.org/2013/01/29/statistical-portrait-of-the-foreign-born-population-in-the-united-states-2011/.

28. Nahin, R. L., Barnes, P. M., Stussman, B. J., et al. (2009). *Costs of complementary and alternative medicine (CAM) and frequency of visits to CAM practitioners: United States, 2007. National health statistics reports; no 18.* Hyattsville, MD: National Center for Health Statistics.

29. *National standards for culturally and linguistically appropriate services in health care, final report,* March 2001, Washington, DC: Office of Minority Health, Department of Health and Human Services.

30. Novak, M. (1972). *The rise of the unmeltable ethnics.* New York: Macmillan.

31. Page, R. L., Ellison, C. G., & Lee, J. (2009). Does religiosity affect health risk behaviors in pregnant and postpartum women? *Matern Child Health J, 13,* 621–632.

32. Pargament, K. I. (1997). *The psychology of religion and coping. Introduction,* p. 2. New York: Guilford Press.

33. Pargament, K., Feuille, M., & Burdzy, D. (2011). The Brief RCOPE. *Religions 2,* 51-76.

34. Passel, J. S., & Cohn, D. (December 6, 2012). *Unauthorized immigrants: 11.1 million in 2011.* Washington, DC: Pew Hispanic Center.

35. Pew Forum on Religion and Public Life. (2007). *U.S. Religious Landscape Survey.* Available at http://religions.pewforum.org/pdf/report2religious-landscape-study-key-findings.pdf.

36. Pew Research Center. (January 29, 2013). *A nation of immigrants: a portrait of the 40 million, including 11 million unauthorized.* Available at http://www.pewhispanic.org/files/2013/01/statistical_portrait_final_jan_29.pdf.

37. Redfield, R., Linton, R., & Herskovits, M. J. (1936). Memorandum for the study of acculturation. *Am Anthropol, 38,* 149-152.

38. Ryan, C. (August 2013). ACS-22. *American Community Survey Reports. Language use in the United States: 2011.* Available at http://www.census.gov/prod/2013pubs/acs-22.pdf.

39. Sam, D. L., & Berry, J. W. (2006). Introduction. *The Cambridge handbook of acculturation psychology* (1st ed.). Cambridge, UK: Cambridge University Press, pp. 1-7, 12.

40. Skalla, K. A., & McCoy, J. P. (2006). Spiritual assessment of patients with cancer. *Oncol Nurs Forum, 33,* 752.

41. Spector, R. E. (2013). *Cultural diversity in health and illness* (8th ed.). Upper Saddle River, NJ: Pearson.

42. The White House. (2014). *Creating an immigration system for the 21st century.* Available at http://www.whitehouse.gov/issues/immigration.

43. Triandis, H. C. (1996). The psychological measurement of cultural syndromes, *Am Psychol 51*(4), 407-415.

44. U.S. Census Bureau. (2012). *American FactFinder–Selected social characteristics in the United States: 2012 American community survey 1-year estimates.* Available at http://factfinder2.census.gov/faces/tableservices/jsf/pages/productview.xhtml?pid=ACS_12_1YR_DP02&prodType=table.

45. U.S. Department of Health and Human Services. The Secretary's Advisory Committee on National Health Promotion and Disease Prevention Objectives for 2020. (2008). *Phase I report: recommendations for the framework and format of Healthy People 2020.* Available at http://www.healthypeople.gov/hp2020/advisory/PhaseI/sec4.htm#_Toc211942917.

46. Vespa, J., Lewis, J. M., &. Kreider, R. M. (2013). *America's families and living arrangements: 2012: population characteristics P20-570.* Source: U.S. Census Bureau, American Community Survey, 2011. Available at http://www.census.gov/prod/2013pubs/p20-570.pdf.

The Interview

ℯ http://evolve.elsevier.com/Jarvis/

3-1

The interview is the first point of contact with a client* and the most important part of data collection. During the interview you collect **subjective data** (i.e., what the person says about himself or herself) (Fig. 3-1). Although the purpose of the interview isn't to collect **objective data** (i.e., what you obtain through physical examination), you will collect some objective data as you note the person's posture, physical appearance, ability to carry on a conversation, and overall demeanor. The interview is the best chance a person has to tell you what *he or she* perceives the health state to be. Once people enter the health care system, they relinquish some control. However, at the interview the client is still in charge. The individual knows everything about his or her own health state, and you know nothing. Skilled interviewers are able to glean all necessary information while establishing a rapport with the client. Successful interviews allow you to:

1. Gather complete and accurate data about the person's health state, including the description and chronology of any symptoms of illness.

2. Establish trust so the person feels accepted and thus free to share all relevant data.
3. Teach the person about his or her health state.
4. Build rapport for a continuing therapeutic relationship; this rapport facilitates future diagnoses, planning, and treatment.
5. Discuss health promotion and disease prevention.

Consider the interview a **contract** between you and your client. The contract concerns what the client needs and expects from health care and what you as a clinician have to offer. Your mutual goal is optimal health for the client. The terms of the contract include:

- Time and place of the interview and succeeding physical examination.
- Introduction of yourself and a brief explanation of your role.
- The purpose of the interview.
- How long it will take.
- Expectation of participation for each person.
- Presence of any other people (e.g., family, other health professionals, students).
- Confidentiality and to what extent it may be limited.
- Any costs to the client.

Although the person already may know some of this information through telephone contact with receptionists or the admitting office, the remaining points need to be stated clearly at the outset. Any confusion or unclear expectations can cause mistrust and resentment rather than the openness and trust required to facilitate the interview.

THE PROCESS OF COMMUNICATION

The vehicle that carries you and your client through the interview is communication. Communication is exchanging information so each person clearly understands the other. If you do not understand one another, if you have not *conveyed meaning,* no communication has occurred.

It is challenging to teach the skill of interviewing because initially most people think that it is common sense. They assume that if they can talk and hear, they can communicate. But much more than talking and hearing is necessary. Communication is based on behavior, conscious and unconscious, and *all behavior has meaning.*

---

*The term "client" is being used throughout this chapter to encompass the variety of settings in which you may encounter an individual where they are not considered a patient, including the home setting.

Sending

Likely you are most aware of *verbal* communication—the words you speak, vocalizations, the tone of voice. *Nonverbal* communication is as important as verbal communication. This is your body language—posture, gestures, facial expression, eye contact, foot tapping, touch, even where you place your chair. Because nonverbal communication is under less conscious control than verbal communication, it may be more reflective of true feelings.

Receiving

Being aware of the messages you send is only part of the process. Your words and gestures must be interpreted in a *specific context* to have meaning. You have a specific context in mind when you send your words, but your context may not be understood by the receiver. The receiver uses his or her own interpretations on your words. These interpretations are based on past experiences, culture, and self-concept. Physical and emotional states also play a role in a person's interpretation. Your context and that of the receiver may not coincide, which can cause frustration and conflict. Your message can be sabotaged by the listener's bias or any preconceived notions. It takes mutual understanding by the sender and receiver to have successful communication.

Even greater risk for misunderstanding exists in the health care setting than in a social setting. The client's frame of reference is narrowed and focused on illness. The client usually has a health problem, and this factor emotionally charges your professional relationship. It *intensifies* the communication because the person feels dependent on you to get better.

Communication is one of the most important *basic skills* that can be learned and refined when you are a beginning practitioner. It is a tool, as basic to quality health care as the tools used in physical assessment. To maximize your communication skills, first you need to be aware of internal and external factors and their influence.

Internal Factors

Internal factors are those specific to you, the examiner. As you cultivate your communication skills, you need to focus on the four inner factors of liking others, empathy, the ability to listen, and self-awareness.

Liking Others

One essential factor for an examiner's "goodness of fit" into a helping profession is a genuine liking of other people. This means a generally optimistic view of people—an assumption of their strengths and a tolerance for their weaknesses. An atmosphere of warmth and caring is necessary, and the client must believe that he or she is accepted unconditionally.

The respect for other people extends to respect for their own control over their health. Your goal is *not* to make your clients dependent on you, but to help them to be increasingly responsible for themselves. You wish to promote their growth, and you have the health care resources to offer them in that pursuit. Clients must choose how to apply those resources to their own lives, and you have to respect their choice to follow the guidelines or disregard them.

Empathy

Empathy means viewing the world from the other person's inner frame of reference while remaining you. It is a recognition and acceptance of the other person's feelings without criticism. It is described as "feeling *with* the person rather than feeling *like* the person." Empathy does not mean that you lose yourself in the other person at your own expense. By losing yourself, you cease to be useful. Empathy is the ability to understand with the person and recognize how he or she perceives his or her world.

The Ability to Listen

Listening is not a passive role in the communication process; it is active and demanding. Listening requires complete and focused attention. You are not only hearing the person's words; you are interpreting their meaning, asking follow-up questions, and ensuring a thorough understanding of what the person is telling you. If you are preoccupied with your own needs or those of other clients, you may miss important information. The needs of the person you are interviewing should be your sole concern.

Active listening is the route to understanding. Listen not only to *what* the person says but the way he or she says it. Be aware of nonverbal communication and ask follow-up questions as appropriate. Do not interrupt. The story may not come out in the order you ask it, but it is important to allow the person to speak from his or her outline. As the person speaks, be aware of the way the story is told—did he or she have any difficulty with language? What was the tone of his or her voice? What is the person leaving out?

CLINICAL ILLUSTRATION

S.B., 29 years of age, is seeking care for a variety of medical complaints that appear unrelated. She continually provides conflicting accounts of the information, does not make eye contact, and is fidgeting. During the interview you notice that she sometimes uses inappropriate pronouns when describing symptoms. For example, when asked what makes her headaches better, she responds, "He says that nothing helps." As you continue questioning and delve into social history, you find her evading questions about her children. She continually questions you about what you think is wrong and asks what kind of medication you think she needs. After continued questioning, she finally confides in you that she cannot afford health insurance for her children and is trying to get medication that she can give to her son who is ill. Had you rushed through the interview and taken her account at face value without follow-up questions, you never would have known the true problem. Knowing your client's personal history and listening to what he or she doesn't say can inform you as much as listening to what is actually said.

Self-Awareness

To effectively communicate with others, you must know yourself. Understanding your personal biases, prejudices, and stereotypes is an important part of developing your skills as an interviewer. By knowing your behaviors and responses, you become aware of how some unintentional actions can have a negative impact on your communication. You may have strong feelings about teen pregnancy, sexual orientation, or illicit drug use. By recognizing your biases and values, you can put them aside when dealing with people who may have a very different set of values. Part of your job as an interviewer is to recognize and set aside personal prejudices so you can effectively care for all types of clients. If you recognize that you cannot put aside certain values, you may have to ask a colleague to step in when you are confronted with certain situations. For example, you are a devout Catholic who feels strongly that abortion is wrong. You are preparing to interview a 15-year-old who is 8 weeks' pregnant. You know that she has made the appointment to discuss her options. If you are unable to put aside your stance that abortion is wrong and believe that you cannot counsel the young woman effectively, you may need to ask a colleague to complete the interview so the young woman is presented with all options.

External Factors

Prepare the physical setting. The setting may be in a hospital room, an examination room in an office or clinic, or the person's home (where you have less control). In any location optimal conditions are important to have a smooth interview.

Ensure Privacy

Aim for geographic privacy—a private room in the hospital, clinic, office, or home. This may involve asking an ambulatory roommate to step out or finding an unoccupied room or empty lounge. If geographic privacy is not available, create "psychological privacy" using curtained partitions, but make sure that the person feels comfortable with the privacy provided. Privacy extends to ensuring that the client is comfortable with the people in the room. Consider a teenager being interviewed before an annual physical. You will need to ask questions about risky behaviors, including alcohol, illicit drugs, and sexual behaviors. Do you think the teenager is going to be forthright and honest with a parent or guardian sitting right there? He or she may not be comfortable asking the parent or guardian to leave; however, it is your job to advocate for the teenager, which may include asking a parent or guardian to step out during the interview.

Refuse Interruptions

Most people resent interruptions except in cases of an emergency. Inform any support staff of your interview and ask that they not interrupt you during this time. Discourage other health professionals from interrupting you with *their* need for access to the patient. You need to concentrate and establish rapport. An interruption can destroy in seconds what you have spent many minutes building up. If you anticipate an interruption, let the person know ahead of time.

Physical Environment

- Set the room temperature at a comfortable level.
- Provide sufficient lighting so you can see each other clearly, but avoid strong, direct lighting that may cause squinting.
- Secure a quiet environment. Turn off televisions, radios, and any unnecessary equipment.
- Remove distracting objects or equipment. It is appropriate to leave some professional equipment (otoscope/ophthalmoscope, blood pressure manometer) in view, but avoid clutter; stacks of mail, other files, or your lunch should not be seen. The room should advertise a trained professional.
- Place the distance between you and the client at 4 to 5 feet. Personal space is any space within 4 feet of a person. Encroaching on personal space can cause anxiety, but if you position yourself farther away, you may seem aloof and distant. The personal reaction bubble depends on a variety of factors, including culture, gender, and age. (See Table 3-1 for information on personal space.)
- Arrange **equal-status seating** (Fig. 3-2). Both you and the client should be comfortably seated, at eye level. Placing the chairs at 90 degrees is good because it allows the person

TABLE 3-1	Functional Use of Space
ZONE	**REMARKS**
Intimate zone (0 to 1½ ft)	Visual distortion occurs
	Best for assessing breath and other body odors
Personal distance (1½ to 4 ft)	Perceived as an extension of the self, similar to a bubble
	Voice moderate
	Body odors inapparent
	No visual distortion
	Much of physical assessment occurs at this distance
Social distance (4 to 12 ft)	Used for impersonal business transactions
	Perceptual information much less detailed
	Much of interview occurs at this distance
Public distance (12+ ft)	Interaction with others impersonal
	Speaker's voice must be projected
	Subtle facial expressions imperceptible

From Hall, E. (1963). Proxemics: the study of man's spatial relations. In Galdston, I. (Ed.). *Man's image in medicine and anthropology*. New York: International University Press, pp. 109-120.

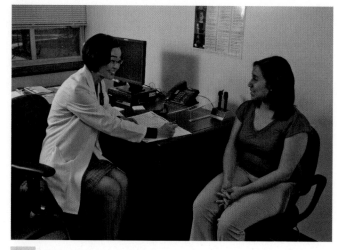

3-2   Equal-status seating.

either to face you or to look straight ahead from time to time. Make sure that you avoid facing a client across a desk because this creates a barrier and, most important, avoid standing. Standing does two things: (1) it communicates your haste, and (2) it assumes superiority. Standing makes you loom over the client as an authority figure. When you are sitting, the person feels some control in the setting.

- When interviewing a hospitalized bedridden person, arrange a face-to-face position, and avoid standing over him or her (Fig. 3-3). The person should not be staring at the ceiling but should have access to eye contact. Without eye contact the person loses the visual message of your communication.

3-3   Avoid this position.   (Potter et al., 2015.)

Dress

- The client should remain in street clothes during the interview except in an emergency. A hospital gown causes a power differential and may make the person feel exposed and uncomfortable. Establish rapport before asking the person to change into a gown.
- Your appearance and clothing should be appropriate to the setting and should meet conventional professional standards: a uniform or lab coat over conservative clothing, a name tag, and neat hair. Avoid extremes.

Note-Taking

Some use of history forms and note-taking may be unavoidable (see Fig. 3-2). For example, when you sit down later to record the interview, you cannot rely completely on memory to furnish details of previous hospitalizations or the review of body systems. But be aware that excessive note-taking during the interview has disadvantages:

- It breaks eye contact too often.
- It shifts your attention away from the person, diminishing his or her sense of importance.
- Trying to record everything a person says may cause you to ask him or her to slow down, or the person may slow his or her tempo to allow for you to take notes. Either way, the client's natural mode of expression is lost.
- It impedes your observation of the client's nonverbal behavior.
- It is threatening to the client during the discussion of sensitive issues (e.g., amount of alcohol and drug use, number of sexual partners, or incidence of physical abuse).

Keep note-taking to a minimum and try to focus your attention on the person. Any recording you do should be secondary to the dialogue and should not interfere with the person's spontaneity. With experience you will not rely on note-taking as much. The use of standardized forms can help decrease it by providing quick check boxes for some of the information.

Electronic Health Record (EHR)

Direct computer recording of the health record has moved into many outpatient offices and hospital rooms in the 21st century. This eliminates handwritten clinical data and provides access to online health education materials. Although computer entry facilitates data retrieval from numerous locations, this new technology poses problems for the provider-client relationship. In the worst-case scenario the person sits idly by while the examiner interacts silently with the computer.[35]

If this technology is used in your setting, do not let the computer screen become a barrier between you and the client. Begin the interview as you usually would by greeting the person, establishing rapport, and collecting his or her narrative story in a direct face-to-face manner. Explain the computerized charting, and position the monitor so the client can see it. Typing directly into the computer may ease entry of some sections of history such as past health occurrences, family history, and review of systems (see Chapter 4). Be aware that the client narrative, emotional issues, and complex health problems can only be addressed by the reciprocal communication techniques and client-centered interviewing presented in this chapter.

TECHNIQUES OF COMMUNICATION

Introducing the Interview

You may be nervous at the beginning of the interview. Keep in mind that the client likely is nervous as well. Keep the introduction short and formal. Address the person using his or her surname and shake hands if appropriate. Unless the client directs you otherwise, avoid using the first name during the interview. Automatic use of the first name is too familiar for most adults and lessens dignity. The exception is with children and adolescents. You can also ask the person about his or her preference.

Introduce yourself and state your role in the agency (if you are a student, say so). If you are gathering a complete history, give the reason for this interview:

> *"Mrs. Sanchez, I would like to talk about your illness that caused you to come to the hospital."*
> *"Mr. Craig, I want to ask you some questions about your previous medical history, family history, and any current complaints before we complete your physical examination."*

If the person is in the hospital, more than one health team member may be collecting a history. This repetition can be disconcerting because some people think that multiple clinicians asking the same questions indicates incompetence or a refusal to take the time to review the chart. Making sure that you indicate the reason for the interview can help lessen this exasperation.

After this brief introduction, ask an open-ended question (see the following section) and then let the person proceed. You do not need much friendly small talk to build rapport. This is not a social visit; the person wants to talk about some concern and wants to get on with it. You build rapport best by letting him or her discuss the concern early.

The Working Phase

The working phase is the data-gathering phase. Verbal skills for this phase include your ability to form questions appropriately and your responses to the answers given by the client. You will likely use a combination of open-ended and closed questions during the interview.

Open-Ended Questions

The **open-ended** question asks for narrative information. It states the topic to be discussed but only in **general** terms. Use it to begin the interview, to introduce a new section of questions, and whenever the person introduces a new topic.

> *"Tell me how I can help you."*
> *"What brings you to the hospital?"*
> *"You mentioned shortness of breath. Tell me more about that."*
> *"How have you been feeling since your last appointment?"*

The open-ended question is unbiased; it leaves the person free to answer in any way. This question encourages the person to respond in paragraphs and give a spontaneous account in any order chosen. It lets the person express himself or herself fully.

As the person answers, make eye contact and *listen*. Typically he or she will provide a short answer, pause, and then look at you for direction on whether to continue. How you respond to this nonverbal question is key. If you pose new questions on other topics, you may lose much of the initial story. Instead lean forward slightly toward the client and make eye contact, looking interested. With your posture indicating interest, the person will likely continue his or her story. If not, you can respond to his or her statement with, "Tell me about it," or "Anything else?"

Closed or Direct Questions

Closed or **direct** questions ask for specific information. They elicit a short, one- or two-word answer, a "yes" or "no," or a forced choice. Whereas the open-ended question allows the client to have free rein, the direct question limits his or her answer (Table 3-2).

Direct questions help you elicit specific information and are useful to fill in any details that were initially left out after the person's opening narrative. Direct questions are also useful when you need specific facts such as past medical history or during the review of systems. You need direct questions to speed up the interview. Asking all open-ended questions would be unwieldy and extend the interview for hours, but be careful not to overuse closed questions. Follow these guidelines:

1. Ask only one direct question at a time. Avoid bombarding the person with long lists: "Have you ever had pain, double vision, watering, or redness in the eyes?" Avoid double-barreled questions such as, "Do you exercise

TABLE 3-2 Comparison of Open-Ended and Closed Questions

OPEN-ENDED	DIRECT, CLOSED
Used for narrative information	Used for specific information
Calls for long paragraph answers	Calls for short one- to two-word answers
Elicits feelings, opinions, ideas	Elicits cold facts
Builds and enhances rapport	Limits rapport and leaves interaction neutral
Tell me all about your headaches.	*Are your headaches on one side or both?*

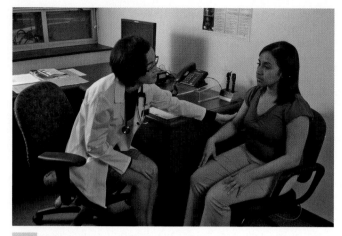

3-4 Showing empathy.

and follow a diet for your weight?" The person will not know which question to answer. And if the person answers "yes," you will not know which question the person has answered.

2. Choose language the person understands. You may need to use regional phrases or colloquial expressions. For example, "running off" means running away in standard English, but it means diarrhea to Appalachian mountain people.

Verbal Responses—Assisting the Narrative

You have asked the first open-ended question, and the client answers. As the person talks, your role is to encourage free expression while keeping the person focused at the same time. Your responses help the teller amplify the story.

Some people seek health care for short-term or relatively simple needs. Their history is direct and uncomplicated; for these people you may require only a subset of your full communication arsenal. Other people have a complex story, a long history of a chronic condition, or accompanying emotions that will require you to pull out all the stops during your interaction. There are nine types of verbal responses. The first five responses (facilitation, silence, reflection, empathy, clarification) involve your *reactions* to the facts or feelings that the person has communicated (Fig. 3-4). Your response focuses on the client's frame of reference. Your own frame of reference does not enter into the response. In the last four responses (confrontation, interpretation, explanation, summary), you start to express your *own* thoughts and feelings. In the first five responses the client leads; in the last four responses you lead. Study the array of possible responses in Table 3-3.

Ten Traps of Interviewing

The verbal responses presented in Table 3-3 are productive and enhance the interview. Now we will consider *traps*, which

are nonproductive verbal and nonverbal messages. Because you want to help your client, it is easy to fall into the traps and send negative verbal messages that may do the opposite of what you intended by cutting off communication. These traps restrict the person's response and create obstacles as you attempt to establish rapport. Be aware of the following traps and work to avoid them as you establish your communication style.

1. Providing False Assurance or Reassurance

A pregnant woman says, "I've been spotting on and off all day, and I haven't felt the baby kick. I just know I'm going to miscarry." Your automatic response may be to provide reassurance, "Don't worry. I'm sure you and the baby will be fine." Although this helps relieve your anxiety and gives you the sense that you have provided comfort, it actually trivializes the woman's anxiety and closes off communication. You have also just promised something that may not be true, which can diminish rapport. Consider these responses:

> *"You're really worried about your baby, aren't you?"*
> *"It must be hard to wait for the doctor. Is there anything I can get you or anything that you'd like to talk about?"*

These responses acknowledge the feeling and open the door for more communication.

A genuine, valid form of reassurance does exist. You *can* reassure clients that you are listening to them, that you understand them, that you have hope for them, and that you will take good care of them.

> *Client:* "I feel so lost here since they transferred me to the medical center. My family lives too far away to visit, and no one here knows me or cares."
> *Response:* "I care what happens to you. I will be here all day today and for the next 3 days. Please call if you need anything."

This type of reassurance makes a commitment to the client, and it can have a powerful impact.

2. Giving Unwanted Advice

It is important as a health care provider to recognize when giving advice is warranted and when it should be avoided. People often seek health care because they want professional advice. A parent may ask how to care for a child with chickenpox, or an older man may ask if it is appropriate to receive a pneumonia vaccine. These are straightforward requests for information, and you respond by providing the appropriate information.

But if advice is based on a hunch or feeling or is your personal opinion, then it is likely inappropriate. Consider a young woman who has just met with her physician about her infertility issues: "Dr. Compton just told me I have to have surgery and that, if I don't, I won't be able to get pregnant. I'm just not sure. What would you do?" If you provide an

TABLE 3-3 Examiner's Verbal Responses

RESPONSE	REASON FOR USE	EXAMPLE(S)
Client's Perspective		
Facilitation, general leads, minimal cues	• Encourages client to say more • Shows person you are interested	• *mm-hmmm, go on, uh-huh* • Maintaining eye contact, shifting forward • Nodding *yes*
Silence	• Communicates that client has time to think • Silence can be uncomfortable for novice examiner, but interruption can make client lose his or her train of thought • Provides you with chance to observe client and note nonverbal cues	• Waiting for response without interruption • Sitting quietly; **don't fidget** • Counting silently 1 to 10
Reflection	• Echoes client's words by repeating part of what person has just said • Can help express feelings behind words • Mirroring client's words can help person elaborate on problem	• Client: *It's so hard having to stay in bed during my pregnancy. I have kids at home I'm worried about.* • Response: *You feel worried and anxious about your children?*
Empathy	• Names a feeling and allows its expression • Allows person to feel accepted and strengthens rapport • Useful in instances when client hasn't identified the feeling or isn't ready to discuss it	• Client (sarcastically): *This is just great! I own a business, direct my employees; now I can't even go to the bathroom without help.* • Response: *It must be hard—one day having so much control and now feeling dependent on someone else.* • Other responses include: *This must be very hard for you* or just placing hand on person's arm (see Fig. 3-4)
Clarification	• Useful when person's word choice is ambiguous or confusing • Summarize person's words, simplify the statement, and ensure that you are on the right track	• Response: *The heaviness in your chest occurs with walking up 1 flight of stairs or more than 1 block, but it stops when you rest. Is that correct?* • Client: *Yes, that's it.*
Examiner's Perspective		
Confrontation	• Clarifying inconsistent information • Focusing client's attention on an observed behavior, action, or feeling	• *You look sad,* or *You sound angry.* • *Earlier you said that you didn't drink, but just now you said you go out every night after work for 1-2 beers.* • *When I press here you grimace, but you said it doesn't hurt.*
Interpretation	• Links events, makes associations, and implies cause • Not based on direct observations but instead on inference or conclusion • Your interpretation may be incorrect but helps prompt further discussion	• *It seems that every time you feel the stomach pain, you have some type of stress in your life.* • Client: *I don't want any more treatment, but I can't seem to tell the doctor I'm ready to stop.* • Response: *Could it be that you're afraid of her reaction?*
Explanation	• Informing person • Sharing factual and objective information	• *You order your dinner from the menu provided, and it takes approximately 30 minutes to arrive.* • *You may not eat or drink for 12 hours before your blood test because the food may change the results.*
Summary	• Condenses facts and validates what was discussed during the interview • Signals that termination of interview is imminent • Both client and examiner should be active participants	• Review pertinent facts • Allow client time to make corrections

answer, especially if the answer begins with "If I were you …" you would be falling into a trap. You are not your client and therefore cannot make decisions for her. Providing an answer shifts accountability to you instead of the client. The woman must work out her own decision. So what do you do?

> Response: *What are your concerns about the recommendation?*
> Woman: *I'm terrified of being put to sleep. What if I don't wake up?*

Now you know her *real* concern and can help her deal with it. She will have grown in the process and may be better equipped to make her decision.

When asked for advice, other preferred responses are:

> "*What are the pros and cons of _____ [this choice] for you?*"
> "*What is holding you back?*"

Although it is quicker just to give advice, take the time to involve the patient in a problem-solving process. When a person participates, he or she is more likely to learn and to change behavior.

3. Using Authority

"Your doctor/nurse knows best" is a response that promotes dependency and inferiority. You effectively diminish the client's concerns with one short sentence, and you cut off communication. Using authority should be avoided. Although you may have more professional knowledge than the client, you both have equally important roles since the client must make the final decision about his or her health.

4. Using Avoidance Language

People use euphemisms instead of discussing unpleasant topics. For example, people use "passed on" or "has gone to a better place" to avoid the reality of dying. Using euphemisms promotes avoidance of reality and allows people to hide their feelings. Not talking about uncomfortable topics doesn't make them go away but instead makes them even more frightening. The best way to deal with frightening or uncomfortable topics is by using direct language.

5. Distancing

Distancing is the use of impersonal speech to put space between a threat and the self: "There is a lump in *the* left breast." By using "the" instead of "your," you are allowing the woman to deny any association with her diseased breast and protect herself from it. Health professionals use distancing to soften reality, but in actuality it may communicate that you are afraid of the procedure or disease. Clients use distancing to avoid admitting that they have a problem: "My doctor told me that the prostate was enlarged." Using blunt specific terms is actually preferable to defuse anxiety. Using specific language and blunt terms indicates that you are not fearful of

the disease or procedure and may help the person cope with the reality of the situation.

6. Using Professional Jargon

The medical profession is fraught with jargon that sounds exclusionary and paternalistic. It is important that you can adjust your vocabulary to ensure understanding without sounding condescending. Just because your client uses medical jargon, don't assume that he or she understands the correct meaning. Some people think "hypertensive" means tense. This misunderstanding may cause them to take their medication only when they are feeling tense and stressed instead of taking it all the time. Misinformation must be corrected immediately to ensure compliance. However, mispronunciations do not need to be corrected every time (e.g., when a client says "prostrate" for prostate gland).

7. Using Leading or Biased Questions

Asking a client, "You don't smoke, do you?" or "You don't ever have unprotected sex, correct?" implies that one answer is "better" than another. If the client wants to please you, he or she will either answer in a way corresponding to your values or feel guilty when he or she must admit the other answer. The client feels that he or she risks your disapproval by not answering the question "correctly." If the client feels dependent on you for care, he or she won't want to alienate you and may not answer truthfully. Make sure that your questions are unbiased and do not lead clients to a certain "correct" answer. Better questions are: "Do you smoke?" or "When you have sexual intercourse, do you use any type of protection?"

8. Talking Too Much

Some examiners positively associate helpfulness with verbal productivity. If the air has been thick with their oratory and advice, these examiners leave thinking that they have met the client's needs. Just the opposite is true. Eager to please the examiner, the client lets the professional talk at the expense of his or her need to express himself or herself. A good rule for every interviewer is to *listen more than you talk*.

9. Interrupting

When you think you know what the client is going to say next, it is easy to cut him or her off and finish the statement. Unfortunately you are not proving that you are clever, but you are signaling impatience or boredom. Related to interruption is preoccupation with yourself. As the client speaks, you may be thinking about what to say next. If you are focused on your next statement instead of his or her statements, you are unable to fully understand what the person is saying. You become so preoccupied with being a good interviewer that you forget to be a good listener. The goal of the interview is to include two people listening and two people speaking. Leave at least a second of space between the end of the client speaking and your next statement. This ensures that the person is finished.

10. Using "Why" Questions

Children ask why questions constantly. Why is the sky blue? Why can't I have a cookie for dinner? Their motive is an innocent search for information. The adult's use of "why" questions usually implies blame and condemnation; it puts the person on the defensive. Consider your use of "why" questions in the health care setting. "Why did you take so much medication?" Or "Why did you wait so long before coming to the hospital if you were having chest pain?" The only possible answer to a "why" question is "because …" and the person may not know the answer. The use of a why question makes the interviewer sound accusatory and judgmental. By using a why question, the client must produce an excuse to rationalize his or her behavior. To avoid this trap, say, "I see you started to have chest pains early in the day. What was happening between the time the pains started and the time you came to the emergency department?"

Nonverbal Skills

As a novice interviewer you may be focused on what the client says, but listening with your eyes is just as important as listening with your ears. Nonverbal modes of communication include physical appearance, posture, gestures, facial expression, eye contact, voice, and touch. They are important in establishing rapport and conveying information. They provide clues to understanding feelings. When nonverbal and verbal messages are congruent, the verbal is reinforced. When they are incongruent, the nonverbal message tends to be the true one because it is under less conscious control.

Physical Appearance

In his classic work *The Stress of Life,* Hans Selye reports that his interest in the total response of his body to stress began when he was a student.[29] He noted that some people just "looked sick," even though they did not exhibit the specific signs that would lead to a precise medical diagnosis. The same view can work for you. Inattention to dressing or grooming suggests that the person is too sick to maintain self-care or has an emotional dysfunction such as depression. Choice of clothing also sends a message, projecting such varied images as role (student, worker, or professional) or attitude (casual, suggestive, or rebellious).

You are concerned with the client's image, and he or she is just as concerned with yours. Your appearance sends a message to the client. Professional dress varies among agencies and settings. Professional uniforms can create a positive (expertise or ease of identification) or a negative (distance or formality) image. Whatever your personal choice in clothing or grooming is, the aim should be to convey a competent, professional image and should follow agency guidelines.

Posture

On beginning the interview, note the client's position. An open position with extension of large muscle groups shows relaxation, physical comfort, and a willingness to share information. A closed position with arms and legs crossed looks defensive and anxious. Changes in posture during the interview can also suggest a different comfort level with new topics. For example, if your client began the interview in an open posture but immediately assumes a closed posture when asked about his or her sexuality, he or she may be uncomfortable with the new topic.

Make sure that you are aware of your own posture. Assuming a calm, relaxed posture conveys interest. On the other hand, standing and hastily filling out forms while peeking at your watch communicates that you are busy with many more important things than interviewing this person. Even when your time is limited, it is important to appear unhurried. Sit down, even if it is only for a few minutes, and look as if nothing else matters except this person. If you are aware of a possible emergency that will require interruption, let the client know when you enter the room. "I'm on call today and may be interrupted during our time together. That doesn't mean that your appointment isn't important to me. If I do need to step out for a minute, rest assured that I will return promptly so we can finish without rushing."

Gestures

Gestures send messages; therefore make sure that you are aware of your own gestures while also noting those of the client. Nodding the head or openly turning out the hand shows acceptance, attention, or agreement; whereas wringing the hands or picking the nails often indicates anxiety. Hand gestures can also reinforce descriptions of pain. When describing crushing substernal chest pain, the person often holds a fisted hand in front of the sternum. Sharply localized pain is often indicated by using one finger—"It hurts right here." Along with gestures, be aware of fidgeting. We have all spoken with people who constantly bounce a leg, click a pen, play with hair, or drum fingers on the table. These movements can distract the client and cause him or her to lose focus. Make sure that you know if you tend to fidget, and work on controlling that urge during interviews.

Facial Expression

Typically the face and facial expression are some of the first things we notice when we meet someone. The face reflects our emotions and conditions. Physical conditions such as pain are often reflected by expressions such as a frown or grimace. As an interviewer it is important to note your client's facial expression. Does it match what he or she is saying or is it incongruous?

As you pay attention to the client's expression, it is equally important that you are aware of your own facial expression. Your expression should reflect a person who is attentive, sincere, and interested. Avoid expressions that may be construed as boredom, disgust, distraction, criticism, or disbelief. A negative facial expression can severely damage your rapport with the client and may lead to the person ceasing communication.

Eye Contact

Lack of eye contact suggests that the person is shy, withdrawn, confused, bored, intimidated, apathetic, or depressed. This applies to examiners too. You should aim to maintain eye contact, but do not "stare down" the person. Do not have a fixed, penetrating look but rather an easy gaze toward the person's eyes, with occasional glances away. One exception to this is when you are interviewing someone from a culture that avoids direct eye contact.

Voice

Although spoken words have meaning, it is important that you are keenly aware of the tone of your voice and that of the client. Meaning comes not only from the words spoken, but from the tone of voice, the intensity and rate of speech, the pitch, and any pauses. The tone of voice may show sarcasm, disbelief, sympathy, or hostility. People who are anxious often speak louder and faster than normal. A soft voice may indicate shyness or fear, whereas a loud voice may indicate that the person is hearing impaired.

Even the use of pauses conveys meaning. When your question is easy and straightforward, a client's long, unexpected pause indicates that the person is taking time to think of an answer. This raises some doubt as to the honesty of the answer

or whether the client heard the question. When unusually frequent and long pauses are combined with speech that is slow and monotonous and a weak, breathy voice, it indicates depression.

Touch

The meaning of physical touch is influenced by the person's age, gender, cultural background, past experience, and current setting. The meaning of touch is easily misinterpreted. In most Western cultures physical touch is reserved for expressions of love and affection or for rigidly defined acts of greeting. Do not use touch during the interview unless you know the person well and are sure how it will be interpreted.

In summation, an examiner's nonverbal messages that show attentiveness and unconditional acceptance are productive and help build rapport. Defeating, nonproductive nonverbal behaviors are those of inattentiveness, authority, and superiority (Table 3-4).

Closing the Interview

The session should end gracefully. An abrupt or awkward closing can destroy rapport and leave the person with a negative impression of the interaction. To ease into the closing, ask the person:

> *"Is there anything else you would like to mention?"*
> *"Are there any questions you would like to ask?"*
> *"We've covered a number of concerns today. What would you most like to accomplish?"*

This gives the person the final opportunity for self-expression. Once this opportunity has been offered, you will need to make a closing statement that indicates that the end of the interview is imminent, such as, "Our interview is just about over." At this point no new topics should be introduced, and no unexpected questions should be asked. This is a good time to give your **summary** or a recapitulation of what you have learned during the interview. The summary is a final statement of what you and the client agree the health state to be. It should include positive health aspects, any health problems that have been identified, any plans for action, and an explanation of the following physical examination. As you part from clients, thank them for the time spent and for their cooperation.

❖ DEVELOPMENTAL COMPETENCE

Interviewing the Parent or Caregiver

When your client is a child, you must build rapport with two people—the child and the accompanying caregiver. Greet both by name, but with a younger child (1 to 6 years old) focus more on the caregiver. Ignoring the child temporarily allows him or her to size you up from a safe distance. The

TABLE 3-4 **Nonverbal Behaviors of the Interviewer**	
POSITIVE	**NEGATIVE**
Appropriate professional appearance	Appearance objectionable to client
Equal-status seating	Standing
Close proximity to client	Sitting behind desk, far away, turned away
Relaxed, open posture	Tense posture
Leaning slightly toward person	Slouched in chair
Occasional facilitating gestures	Critical or distracting gestures: pointing finger, clenched fist, finger-tapping, foot-swinging, looking at watch
Facial animation, interest	Bland expression, yawning, tight mouth
Appropriate smiling	Frowning, lip biting
Appropriate eye contact	Shifty, avoiding eye contact, focusing on notes
Moderate tone of voice	Strident, high-pitched tone
Moderate rate of speech	Rate too slow or too fast
Appropriate touch	Too frequent or inappropriate touch

3-5

child can use this time to observe your interaction with the caregiver. If the child sees that the caregiver accepts and likes you, he or she will begin to relax (Fig. 3-5).

Begin by interviewing the caregiver and child together. If any sensitive topics arise (e.g., the parents' troubled relationship or the child's problems at school or with peers), explore them later when the caregiver is alone. Provide toys to occupy a young child as you and the caregiver talk. This frees the caregiver to concentrate on the history and gives you information about the child's level of attention span and ability for independent play. Throughout the interview observe the caregiver-child interaction.

For younger children, the parent or caregiver will provide all or most of the history. Thus you are collecting the child's health data from the caregiver's frame of reference, which typically is considered reliable. Most caregivers have the child's well-being in mind and will cooperate with you to enhance it. Bias can occur when caregivers are asked to describe the child's achievements or when their ability to provide proper care seems called into question. For example, if you say "His fever was 103, and you didn't bring him in?" you are implying a lack of skills, which puts the caregiver on the defensive and increases anxiety. Instead use open-ended questions that increase description and defuse threat such as, "What happened when the fever went up?"

A parent with more than one child has more than one set of data to remember. Be patient as the parent sorts through his or her memory to pull out facts of developmental milestones or past history. A comprehensive history may be lacking if the child is accompanied by a family friend or daycare provider instead of the primary caregiver.

When asking about developmental milestones, avoid judgmental behavior or inferring that the behavior occurred late.

Parents are understandably proud of their child's achievements and are sensitive to insinuations that these milestones occurred late. "So he didn't say any words until he was 15 months old? Did you take him to speech therapy?" Instead consider saying, "I see that Jon began speaking when he was 15 months old. How is his speech progressing now that he is 2 years old?"

Always refer to the child by name and ensure that he or she is included in the interview as appropriate. Refer to the parent by his or her proper surname instead of "Mom" or "Dad." Remember not to make any assumptions. The person accompanying the child may not be the biologic mother or father. Don't assume that a couple bringing in a child is mom and dad or that two women bringing a child in are mom and aunt; they may be the child's two mothers. Instead of assuming, ask who is accompanying the child.

Most of your communication is with the caregiver of a younger child, but make sure that you don't ignore the child completely. Allow him or her to size you up but engage him or her in conversation as well. Contact made during the nonthreatening interview can ease the physical examination. Ask the child about the toy with which he or she is playing or about the special toy brought from home. Make sure that you stoop to meet the child at his or her eye level. Your size can seem overwhelming to young children, and standing at your full height may emphasize his or her smallness.

Nonverbal communication is even more important to children than it is to adults. Children are quick to pick up feelings, anxiety, or comfort from nonverbal cues. Keep your physical appearance neat and clean, and avoid formal uniforms that distance you. Keep your gestures slow, deliberate, and close to your body. Children are frightened by quick or grandiose gestures. Do not try to maintain constant eye contact; this feels threatening to a small child. Use a quiet, measured voice and choose simple words in your speech. Considering the child's level of language development is valuable in planning your communication.

Stages of Cognitive Development

A child's thought process, perception of the world, and emotional responses to situations are very different from those of an adult. As an interviewer it is important that you consider the stage of development as you approach the child and converse with him or her. Piaget's cognitive-developmental theory can help you understand the child's current level and construct your approach to the interview (Table 3-5). Piaget observed children moving through sequential stages of development. Although this provides a guide, keep in mind that the ages are approximated and will differ slightly based on the maturity level of the child. Also keep in mind that you may be approaching children who are in crisis as a result of illness. Regression is a common response during times of acute stress; therefore a child may regress in his or her ability to communicate at this time.

TABLE 3-5	Stages of Cognitive Development		
AGE	**PIAGET'S STAGE**	**CHARACTERISTICS**	**LANGUAGE DEVELOPMENT**
Birth to 2 years	**Sensorimotor**	Infant learns by manipulating objects At birth reflexive communication, then moves through six stages to reach actual thinking	**Presymbolic** Communication largely nonverbal Vocabulary of more than 4 words by 12 months, increase to >200 words, and use of short sentences before age 2 years
2-6 years	**Preoperational**	Beginning use of symbolic thinking Imaginative play Masters reversibility	**Symbolic** Actual use of structured grammar and language to communicate Uses pronouns Average vocabulary > 10,000 words by age 6 years
7-11 years	**Concrete operations**	Logical thinking Masters use of numbers and other concrete ideas such as classification and conservation	Mastery of passive tense by age 7 years and complex grammatical skills by age 10 years
12+ years	**Formal operations**	Abstract thinking. Futuristic; takes broader, more theoretical perspective	Near adult-like skills

Adapted from Piaget J. (1972). *The child's conception of the world*, Savage, MD: Littlefield, Adams. In Arnold, E. C., & Boggs, K. U. (2011). *Interpersonal relationships: professional communication skills for nurses* (ed. 6). Philadelphia: Saunders.

COMMUNICATING WITH DIFFERENT AGES

The Infant (Birth to 12 months)

Infants use coos, gurgles, facial expressions, and cries to identify their needs. Although you will not "interview" an infant, it is important to establish a rapport. Nonverbal communication is the primary method of communicating with infants. When their needs are met, most infants will be calm and relaxed. When they are frightened, hungry, tired, or uncomfortable, they will cry or be difficult to console. Respond quickly to changes in infant communication. If a baby begins to cry, respond to the communication. Use gentle handling and a quiet, calm voice. Face infants directly. They are fascinated by adult faces and enjoy looking at them, but remember that eyesight does not develop right away; thus you will need to hold them close. As infants get older, they may begin to exhibit stranger anxiety and will be more cooperative when the caregiver is kept in view or allowed to hold the infant during the examination.

The Toddler (12 to 36 months)

At this stage the child is beginning to develop communication skills. At first they communicate with one- or two-word sentences and a limited vocabulary, which may include grunts and pointing intertwined with words. Language progresses from a vocabulary of about two words at 1 year to a spurt of about 200 words by 2 years. Then the 2-year-old begins to combine words into simple two-word phrases—"all gone," "me up," "baby crying." This is **telegraphic speech,** which is usually a combination of a noun and a verb and includes only words that have concrete meaning. Interest in language is high during the second year, and a 2-year-old seems to understand all that is said to him or her.

Older toddlers want to know why; therefore it is important that you provide a simple explanation of what you want. You can help them communicate by labeling their emotions and expanding on their one- or two-word sentences. Give toddlers one direction at a time, keeping it simple, and provide warnings before transitions when possible. Toddlers also struggle for control and autonomy; therefore provide simple choices when possible.

The Preschooler (3 to 6 years)

A 3- to 6-year-old is egocentric. He or she sees the world mostly from his or her own point of view. Everything revolves around him or her. Only the child's own experience is relevant; thus telling what someone else is doing will not have any meaning.

A 3-year-old uses more complex sentences with more parts of speech. Between 3 and 4 years of age the child uses three- to four-word **telegraphic** sentences containing only essential words. By 5 to 6 years, the sentences are six to eight words long, and grammar is well developed.

Preschoolers' communication is direct, concrete, literal, and set in the present. Avoid expressions such as "climbing the walls," because they are easily misinterpreted by young children. Use short, simple sentences with a concrete explanation. Take time to give a short, simple explanation for any unfamiliar equipment that will be used on the child. Preschoolers can have *animistic* thinking about unfamiliar objects. They may imagine that unfamiliar inanimate objects can come alive and have human characteristics (e.g., that a blood-pressure cuff can wake up and bite or pinch). Preschoolers have active imaginations, and that can work to your benefit. Education and explanations can be provided with play (e.g., puppet shows, dress-up, drawings).

The School-Age Child (7 to 12 years)

A child 7 to 12 years old can tolerate and understand others' viewpoints. This child is more objective and realistic. He or she wants to know functional aspects—how things work and why things are done. At this age children are beginning to recognize that things they do can affect others. It is very important that you are nonjudgmental.

The school-age child can read. By using printed symbols for objects and events, the child can process a significant amount of information. At this age thinking is more stable and logical. School-age children can **decenter** and consider all sides of a situation to form a conclusion. They are able to reason, but this reasoning capacity still is limited because they cannot yet deal with abstract ideas.

Children of this age-group have the verbal ability to add important data to the history. Interview the caregiver and child together; but, when a presenting symptom or sign exists, ask the child about it first and then gather data from the caregiver. For the well child seeking a checkup, pose questions about school, friends, or activities directly to the child.

The Adolescent

Adolescence begins with puberty. Puberty is a time of dramatic physiologic change. It includes a growth spurt—rapid growth in height, weight, and muscular development; development of primary and secondary sex characteristics; and maturation of the reproductive organs. A changing body affects a teen's self-concept.

Adolescents want to be adults, but they do not have the cognitive ability yet to achieve their goal. They are between two stages. Sometimes they are capable of mature actions, and other times they fall back on childhood response patterns, especially in times of stress. You cannot treat adolescents as children; yet you cannot overcompensate and assume that their communication style, learning ability, and motivation are consistently at an adult level.

Adolescents value their peers. They crave acceptance and sameness with their peers. Adolescents think that no adult can understand them. Because of this, some act with aloof contempt, answering only in monosyllables. Others make eye contact and tell you what they think you want to hear, but inside they are thinking, "You'll never know the full story about me." This knowledge about adolescents is apt to paralyze you in communicating with them. However, successful communication is possible and rewarding. The guidelines are simple.

The first consideration is your attitude, which must be one of respect. Respect is the most important thing you can communicate to the adolescent. The adolescent needs to feel validated as a person.

Second, your communication must be totally honest. The adolescent's intuition is highly tuned and can detect when information is withheld. Always give them the truth. Play it straight or you will lose them. Providing rationale for your questions will increase cooperation.

Stay in character. Avoid using language that is absurd for your age or professional role. It is helpful to understand some of the jargon used by adolescents, but you cannot use those words yourself to bond with the adolescent. You are not part of the adolescent's peer group, and he or she will not accept you as a peer.

Focus first on the adolescent, not on the problem. Although an adult wants to talk about the health concern immediately, the adolescent wants to talk about himself or herself as a person. Show an interest in the adolescent (Fig. 3-6). Ask open, friendly questions about school, activities, hobbies, and friends. "*How are things at school?*" "*Are you in any sports? Any activities?*" "*Do you have any pets at home?*" Refrain from asking questions about parents and family for now—these topics can be emotionally charged during adolescence.

Do not assume that adolescents know *anything* about a health interview or a physical examination. Explain every step and give the rationale. They need direction. They will cooperate when they know the reason for the questions or actions. Encourage their questions. Adolescents are afraid that they will sound "dumb" if they ask a question to which they assume everybody else knows the answer.

Keep your questions short and simple. "Why are you here?" sounds brazen to you, but it is effective with the adolescent. Be prepared for the adolescent who does *not* know why he or she is there. Some adolescents are pushed into coming to the examination by a caregiver.

The communication responses described for the adult need to be reconsidered when talking with the adolescent. Silent periods usually are best avoided. Giving adolescents a

3-6

little time to collect their thoughts is acceptable, but silence for other reasons is threatening. Also avoid reflection. If you use reflection, the adolescent is likely to answer, "What?" They just do not have the cognitive skills to respond to that indirect mode of questioning. Adolescents are also more sensitive to nonverbal communication than are adults. Be aware of your expressions and gestures. Adolescents are struggling to develop their self-identity and may withdraw from you if you make a comment that they take as a criticism. It is important that you are cognizant of how the person may misinterpret your questions or comments.

Later in the interview, after you have developed rapport with the adolescent, you can address the topics that are emotionally charged, including smoking, alcohol and drug use, sexual behaviors, suicidal thoughts, and depression. Adolescents undertake risky behaviors that may yield serious consequences.

Adolescents will assume that health professionals have similar values and standards of behavior as most of the other authority figures in their lives, and they may be reluctant to share this information. You can assure them that your questions are not intended to be curious or intrusive but cover topics that are important for most teens and on which you have relevant health information to share. You will want to ensure privacy during these questions. Adolescents may be more willing to share this information without a caregiver in the room, but they may feel uncomfortable asking the caregiver for privacy. As the health professional, you can ask the caregiver to step out during the interview, explaining that privacy is important.

If confidential material is uncovered during the interview, consider what can remain confidential and what you believe you must share for the well-being of the adolescent. State laws vary about confidentiality with minors, and in some states caregivers are not notified about some health treatments such as birth control prescriptions or treatment for sexually transmitted infections (STIs). However, if the adolescent talks about an abusive home situation or risk of imminent physical harm, state that you must share this information with other health professionals for his or her own protection. Ask the adolescent, *"Do you have a problem with that?"* and then talk it through. Tell the adolescent, *"You will have to trust that I will handle this information professionally and in your best interest."*

Finally, take every opportunity for positive reinforcement. Praise every action regarding healthy lifestyle choices: *"That's great that you don't smoke. It will save you lots of money that you can use on other things, you won't smell like smoke, and your skin won't be so wrinkled when you get older."*

For lifestyle choices that are risky, this is a premium opportunity for discussion and early intervention. *"Have you ever tried to quit smoking?" "I'm concerned about your extra weight for someone so young. What kind of exercise do you like?" "What do you like to drink when you're at a party with your friends?" "Did you use a condom the last time you had sex?"* Providing information alone is not enough. Listen to their stories in an open, nonjudgmental way. Give them a small, achievable goal, and encourage another visit in a few weeks for follow-up on the behaviors of concern.

The Older Adult

The aging adult has the developmental task of finding the purpose of his or her own existence and adjusting to the inevitability of death. Some people have developed comfortable and satisfying answers and greet you with a calm demeanor and self-assurance, but be alert for the person who sounds hopeless and despairing about life and his or her future. Symptoms of illness and worries over finances are even more frightening when they mean physical limitation or threaten independence.

Always address the person by his or her proper surname, and avoid using the first name. Some older adults resent being called by their first name by younger people and think that it demonstrates a lack of respect. Above all, avoid "elderspeak,"[36] which consists of (1) diminutives (honey, sweetie, dearie); (2) inappropriate plural pronouns ("Are we ready for our interview?"); (3) tag questions ("You would rather sit in this nice, soft chair, wouldn't you?"); and (4) shortened sentences, slow speech rate, and simple vocabulary that sounds like baby talk.

Older adults have a longer story to tell; therefore plan accordingly. The interview will likely take longer, and you don't want to appear rushed. Depending on the person's physical condition, you may need to break the interview into more than one session, making sure to cover the most important data during the first interview. You can also gather certain portions of the data such as past history or the review of systems on a form that is filled out at home, as long as the person's vision and handwriting are adequate. Take time to review any forms completed at home during the interview.

It is important to adjust the pace of the interview to the aging person (Fig. 3-7). The older person has a great amount of background material through which to sort, and this takes some time. Allow appropriate periods of silence during these times. Some aging people also need a greater amount of

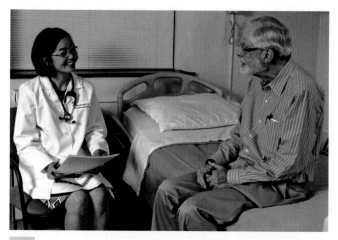

3-7

response time to interpret the question and process the answer. Avoid hurrying them because this only affirms their stereotype of younger people in general and health care providers in particular; that is, people who are interested merely in numbers of clients and filling out forms. You will lose valuable data and not meet their needs if you urge them to go through information quickly or appear rushed.

Consider physical limitations when planning the interview. Make sure that you face the person with impaired hearing directly so your mouth and face are fully visible. Do not shout; it does not help and actually distorts speech. For a person in a wheelchair, make sure you move the chairs so an appropriate position is available for the client.

Touch is a nonverbal skill that is very important to older persons. Their other senses may be diminished, and touch grounds you in reality. In addition, a hand on the arm or shoulder is an empathic message that communicates that you want to understand his or her problem.

INTERVIEWING PEOPLE WITH SPECIAL NEEDS

Hearing-Impaired People

As the population ages, you will encounter more people who are deaf or hard of hearing. They see themselves as a linguistic minority, not as disabled.[15] People who are hearing impaired may feel marginalized by professionals and think that their intelligence is questioned because they cannot always understand what is being asked of them. Although some people will tell you in advance that they have a hearing impairment, others will not readily divulge the information. In the latter case you must use cues to recognize potential hearing loss, such as the client staring at your mouth, not answering unless looking at you, speaking in an unusually loud voice, or frequently requesting that you repeat a question. Full communication is important with every client. People with a hearing impairment may feel isolated and anxious because they cannot understand everything that is happening. Ask the person his or her preferred way to communicate—by signing, lip reading, or writing. If the person has hearing aids, make sure that he or she is using them properly. If you notice a hearing impairment but no hearing aids are in use, consider a referral for a hearing test and follow-up.

A complete health history of someone who is deaf requires a sign language interpreter. Because most health care professionals are not proficient in signing, try to find an interpreter through a social service agency or the person's own social network. You may use family members, but be aware that they sometimes edit for the person. Use the same guidelines as for the bilingual interpreter (see p. 45).

If the person prefers lip reading, be sure to face him or her squarely and have good lighting on your face. Examiners with a beard, mustache, or foreign accents are less effective. Do not exaggerate your lip movements because this distorts your words. Similarly, shouting distorts the reception of a hearing aid. Speak slowly and supplement your voice with appropriate hand gestures or pantomime. Nonverbal cues are important adjuncts because the lip reader understands at best only 50% of your speech when relying solely on vision. Be sure that the person understands your questions. Many hearing-impaired people nod "yes" just to be friendly and cooperative but really do not understand.

Written communication is efficient in sections such as past health history or review of systems when forms can easily be used. For the present history of illness, writing is very time consuming and laborious. The syntax of the person's written words will read like English if the hearing impairment occurred after speech patterns developed. If the deafness occurred before speech patterns developed, the grammar and written syntax may follow that of sign language, which is different from that of English.

Acutely Ill People

Emergent situations require combining the interview with the physical examination. In this case focus the interview on pertinent information only, including history of present illness, medications, allergies, last meal, and basic health state. Subjective information is a crucial component of providing care; therefore it is important that you try to interview as much as possible while performing lifesaving actions. Abbreviate your questioning. Identify the main area of distress and inquire about that. Family or friends often can provide important data.

A hospitalized person with a critical or severe illness is usually too weak, too short of breath, or in too much pain to talk. Focus on making him or her comfortable first and then ask priority questions about the history. Explore the first concern the person mentions. You will find that you ask closed, direct questions earlier in the interview to decrease response burden. Finally make sure that you are clear in your statements. When a person is very sick, even the simplest sentence can be misconstrued. The person will react according to preconceived ideas about what a serious illness means; thus anything you say should be direct and precise.

People Under the Influence of Street Drugs or Alcohol

It is common for people under the influence of alcohol or other mood-altering drugs to be admitted to a hospital; all of these drugs affect the central nervous system (CNS), increasing risk for overdose, accidents, and injuries. Also, chronic alcohol or drug use creates complex medical problems that require more care.

Many substance abusers are poly-drug abusers. The client's behavior depends on which drugs were consumed. Alcohol, benzodiazepines, and the opioids (heroin, methadone, morphine, oxycodone) are CNS depressants that slow brain activity and impair judgment, memory, intellectual performance, and motor coordination. Stimulants of the central nervous system (cocaine, amphetamine) can cause an intense high, agitation, and paranoid behavior. Hallucinogens (LSD, ketamine, PCP) cause bizarre, inappropriate, sometimes even violent behavior accompanied by superhuman strength and insensitivity to pain.

When interviewing a person currently under the influence of alcohol or illicit drugs, ask simple and direct questions. Take care to make your manner and questions nonthreatening. Avoid confrontation while the person is under the influence and avoid displaying any scolding or disgust since this may make the person belligerent.

The top priority is to find out the time of the person's last drink or drug, how much he or she took, and the name and amount of each drug that was taken. This information will help assess any withdrawal patterns. (A full discussion of substance use assessment is presented in Chapter 6.) For your own protection, be aware of hospital security or other personnel who could be called on for assistance. Avoid turning your back, and make sure that you are aware of your surroundings.

Once a hospitalized substance abuser has been detoxified and is sober, he or she should be assessed for the extent of the problem and its meaning for the person and family. Initially you will encounter denial and increased defensiveness; special interview techniques are needed (see Chapter 6).

Personal Questions

Occasionally people will ask you questions about *your* personal life or opinions such as, "Are you married?" "Do you have children?" or "Do you smoke?" You do not need to answer every question, but you may supply information that you think is appropriate. Beware that there may be an ulterior motive to the questions such as anxiety or loneliness. Try directing your response back to the person's frame of reference. You might say something like, *"No, I don't have children; I wonder if your question is related to how I can help you care for little Jamie?"*

Sexually Aggressive People

On some occasions personal questions extend to flirtatious compliments, seductive innuendo, or sexual advances. Some people see illness as a threat to their self-esteem and sexual adequacy; this feeling creates anxiety that makes them act out in sexually aggressive ways.

Your response must make it clear that you are a health professional who can best care for the person by maintaining a professional relationship. It is important to communicate that you cannot tolerate sexual advances, but you should also communicate that you accept the person and understand his or her need to be self-assertive. This may be difficult, considering that the person's words or gestures may have left you shocked, embarrassed, or angry. Your feelings are normal. You need to set appropriate verbal boundaries by saying, *"I am uncomfortable when you talk to me that way; please don't."* A further response that would open communication is, *"I wonder if the way you're feeling now relates to your illness or to being in the hospital?"* If the behavior continues, you may need to remove yourself from the situation.

Crying

A beginning examiner usually feels horrified when the client starts to cry, but crying is a big relief to a person. Health problems come with powerful emotions, and it takes a good deal of energy to keep worries about illness, death, or loss bottled up. When you say something that "makes the person cry," do not think you have hurt the person. You have just broached a topic that is important. Do not go on to a new topic. It is important that you allow the person to cry and express his or her feelings fully before you move on. Have tissues available and wait until the crying subsides to talk. Reassure the crying client that he or she does not need to be embarrassed and that you are there to listen.

Sometimes your client looks as if he or she is on the verge of tears but is trying hard to suppress them. Again, instead of moving on to something new, acknowledge the expression by saying, "You look sad." Don't worry that you will open an uncontrollable floodgate." The person may cry but will be relieved, and you will have gained insight to a serious concern. Use of appropriate therapeutic touch can help show empathy while a person is crying.

CLINICAL ILLUSTRATION

M.P., a 49-year-old White male, is at the clinic today for a physical examination. He hasn't been seen in over 5 years and readily admits a dislike of doctors' offices.

M.P.: I haven't been seen in quite a while, but I thought I should come in soon.

Response: What made you decide to come see the doctor?

M.P.: (appears uncomfortable) My father died of a heart attack when he was 47 years old, so I figure I'm living on borrowed time (lip folds in; tears in eyes).

Response: You look sad. (places hand on forearm)

M.P.: (crying now) It's just that I have kids and a wife, and I worry about what's going to happen if I die. When my father died, my mother struggled so much to raise us. I don't want to leave my wife with that burden.

Response: I understand how worried you are, and I'm glad you came in for a checkup today. We'll take this one step at a time and work together to minimize your risk of having a heart attack.

Anger

Occasionally you will try to interview a person who is already angry. Don't take the anger personally; it typically doesn't relate to you. The person is showing aggression as a response to his or her own feelings of anxiety or helplessness. Do ask about the anger and hear the person out. Deal with the angry feelings before you ask anything else. An angry person cannot be an effective participant in a health interview.

Threats of Violence

The health care setting is not immune to violent behavior, and an individual may act in such a way that you believe that your personal safety is being threatened. Red-flag behaviors of a potentially disruptive person include fist clenching, pacing back and forth, a vacant stare, confusion, statements out of touch with reality or that do not make sense, a history of recent drug use, or perhaps a recent history of intense bereavement (loss of partner, loss of job). If you sense any suspicious or threatening behavior, act immediately to defuse the situation or obtain additional support from other staff or security. Make sure that you leave the door to the examination room open, and never turn your back to a potentially aggressive person. You also want to make sure to position yourself between the person and door so you can easily leave the room. Make sure that you know the hospital policies and which resources are available. Do not raise your own voice or try to argue with the threatening person. Act calm and talk to the person in a soft voice. Act interested in what the person is saying, and behave in an unhurried way. Your most important goal is safety; avoid taking any risks.

Anxiety

Finally take it for granted that nearly all sick people have some anxiety. This is a normal response to being sick. It makes some people aggressive and others dependent. Appearing unhurried and taking the time to listen to all of the client's concerns can help diffuse some anxiety. Avoiding the traps to interviews and using therapeutic responses are other ways to help diffuse anxiety.

CULTURE AND GENETICS

Cultural Considerations on Gender

Violating cultural norms related to appropriate male-female relationships may jeopardize a professional relationship. Among some Arab Americans an adult male is never alone with a female (except his wife) and is generally accompanied by at least one other male when interacting with females. This behavior is culturally very significant; a lone male could be accused of sexual impropriety. Ask the person about culturally relevant aspects of male-female relationships at the beginning of the interview. When gender differences are important to the patient, try strategies such as offering to have a third person present. If a family member or friend has accompanied the patient, inquire whether the patient would like that person to be in the examination room during the history and/or physical examination. It is not unusual for a female to refuse to be examined by a male and vice versa. Modesty is another issue. It is imperative to ensure that the patient is carefully draped at all times, curtains are closed, and, when possible, doors are closed. Do not enter a room without knocking first and announcing yourself.

Cultural Considerations on Sexual Orientation

Lesbian, gay, bisexual, and transgender (LGBT) individuals are aware of heterosexist biases and the communication of these biases during the interview and physical examination. *Heterosexism* refers to the belief that heterosexuality is the only natural choice and assumes that everyone is or should be heterosexual. Heterosexism is a form of homophobia and leads to discrimination. Most admitting and health history forms are heterosexist. The form asks for marital status and does not include an option for a long-term committed relationship or partner. Many same-sex couples are in monogamous, committed relationships, but there is seldom a category that acknowledges this relationship on the form. Although technically and legally the person may be single, this trivializes the relationship with his or her significant other. If this type of form is in use, the interviewer may not realize that the person is in a relationship and may make inappropriate comments based on incorrect assumptions.

Simple, basic changes in your communication and nursing practice can help avoid heterosexism.

- Instead of asking marital status or referring to a spouse, husband, or wife, use the term partner, and make sure that all forms have this as an option.
- Do not marginalize a homosexual relationship. Ask the same questions of a homosexual couple that you would of a heterosexual couple as long as the questions are applicable.
- Know your state laws. Every state differs; therefore it is important that you know applicable laws in your state. For example, some states allow both same-sex parents to be listed on the birth certificate, whereas others do not.
- Use appropriate health teaching materials, including those that depict same-sex couples.
- Do not make assumptions about a person's sex based on his or her appearance.
- Avoid heterosexist assumptions. Make sure that you ask all appropriate questions while avoiding assumptions that heterosexism is the norm. For example, ask a sexually active woman, "Have you ever used birth control?" instead of, "Which type of birth control measures have you used?" The latter question assumes that the woman has had the need for birth control, which assumes that she has engaged in relations with a man.
- Make sure that registration and admitting forms allow for identification of a same-sex partner by using terms such as "partner" or "significant other" while avoiding terms such as "marital status."
- Be nonjudgmental, and make sure that your workplace has adopted policies to avoid discrimination.

Most important, be aware of your personal bias and baggage. Being familiar with considerations for treatment of the LGBT community is the first step in providing culturally competent care.

Working With (and Without) an Interpreter

Over 60.5 million people in the United States speak a language other than English at home.[33] One of the greatest challenges in cross-cultural communication occurs when you and the client speak different languages (Fig. 3-8). After assessing the language skills of non–English-speaking people, you may find yourself in one of two situations: trying to communicate

3-8

effectively through an interpreter or trying to communicate effectively when there is no interpreter. Either way, it is important that you consider not only the meaning of the spoken language, but also nonverbal communication. See Chapter 2 for culturally competent care.

Clients with language barriers experience many negative health outcomes, especially if an interpreter is not used. Non–English-speaking clients have longer hospital stays, receive fewer preventive services, and are less satisfied. Clients who need but do not receive an interpreter undergo more unnecessary testing, are at greater risk of being discharged from the emergency department without a follow-up appointment, and are more likely to be admitted to the hospital.[3,18] The use of trained interpreters has been linked to lower admission rates and increased use of preventive services. Trained interpreters can improve overall health outcomes, improve use of primary care, and increase client satisfaction. Their use may also result in a cost savings and reduced rate of complications.[18]

Interviewing the non–English-speaking person requires a bilingual interpreter for full communication. Even clients who seem to have a basic command of English as a second language may need an interpreter when faced with the anxiety-provoking situation of entering a hospital, describing a strange symptom, or discussing sensitive topics such as those related to reproductive or urologic concerns.

It is tempting to ask an "ad hoc" interpreter (e.g., a relative, friend, or even another client) to interpret because this person is readily available. Although convenient, it is disadvantageous for a number of reasons to ask an untrained interpreter to translate. The client's confidentiality is violated by asking for an "ad hoc" interpreter because the client may not want his or her information shared. Furthermore, the friend or relative, although fluent in ordinary language usage, is unlikely to be familiar with medical terminology, hospital or clinic procedures, and medical ethics. Having a relative interpret adds stress to an already stressful situation and may disrupt family relationships. In some cultures talk about death or cancer is taboo, and a family interpreter may edit out this language.[11]

Whenever possible, work with a bilingual team member or a trained medical interpreter. This person knows interpreting techniques, has a health care background, and understands clients' rights. A trained interpreter is also knowledgeable about cultural beliefs and health practices. This "cultural broker" can help you bridge the cultural gap and advise you concerning the cultural appropriateness of your recommendations.

Many clients with limited English proficiency do not have access to interpreters. It is your responsibility to ensure that the provisions of Title VI as discussed in Chapter 2 are met. It is well known that few clinicians are receiving the necessary preparation to practice with interpreters; only 23% of teaching hospitals in the United States provide this training.[9] As a first preference, language services should include the availability of a bilingual staff or on-site medical interpreters who can communicate directly with clients in their preferred language and dialect. When a trained interpreter isn't available, telephone translation services such as the AT&T Language Line (www.languageline.com) can be used 24 hours a day.

Although interpreters are trained to remain neutral, they can influence both the content of information exchanged and the nature of the interaction. Many trained medical interpreters are members of the linguistic community they serve. Although this is largely beneficial, it has limitations. For example, interpreters may know clients and details of their circumstances before the interview begins. Although acceptance of a code of ethics governing confidentiality and conflicts of interest is part of the training that interpreters receive, discord may arise if an interpreter relates information that the client has not volunteered to the examiner.

Note that being bilingual does not always mean that the interpreter is culturally aware. For example, the Latino culture is so diverse that a Spanish speaking interpreter from one country, class, race, and gender does not necessarily understand the cultural background of a Spanish-speaking person from another country and different circumstances. Even trained interpreters, who are often from urban areas and represent a higher socioeconomic class than the clients whom they interpret, may be unaware of or embarrassed by rural attitudes and practices. Summarized in Table 3-6 are suggestions for the selection and use of an interpreter.

Although you will be in charge of the focus and flow of the interview, view yourself and the interpreter as a team. Ask the interpreter to meet the client beforehand to establish rapport and to determine the client's age, occupation, educational level, and attitude toward health care. This enables the interpreter to communicate on the client's level. Place the interpreter next to the client, but speak directly to the client. Although it can be difficult, focus on the client and address your questions to him or her. For example, do not say to the interpreter, "Ask him if he has pain," but rather ask the client directly, "Do you have pain?"

Although a trained interpreter is your best choice, you may find yourself in a situation in which the client insists on using a friend or family member or when you may have no other choice. In either of these situations, make sure to document who was used as the interpreter and whether it was the client's choice. Unless there is an emergency, never use a minor as an interpreter. Keep in mind that friends and family members may edit, add, or change the message. Make sure that you assess the "ad hoc" interpreter's ability to translate complex medical terminology. You may have to change your phrasing and terminology with an untrained interpreter. Keep your questioning in mind as well. If you are going to ask about sensitive topics such as domestic violence, sexually transmitted infections, illicit drugs, end-of-life care, or other controversial topics, the client may not be as forthcoming with a friend or family member as the translator.

You will need to allow more time for the interview. Having a third person repeat everything will take considerably longer than your interview with English-speaking clients. If you have limited time, focus on priority data.

There are two styles of interpreting: line-by-line and summarizing. Translating line-by-line takes more time, but it ensures accuracy. Use this style for most of the interview. Both you and the client should speak only a sentence or two and then allow the interpreter some time. Use simple language yourself, not medical jargon that the interpreter must simplify before it can be translated. Summary translation progresses faster and is useful for teaching relatively simple health techniques with which the interpreter is already familiar. Be alert for nonverbal cues as the client talks. These cues can give valuable data. A good interpreter also notes nonverbal messages and passes them on to you.

TABLE 3-6   Use of an Interpreter

Choosing an Interpreter
- Before locating an interpreter, identify the language the person speaks at home. Be aware that it may differ from the language spoken publicly (e.g., French is sometimes spoken by well-educated and upper-class members of certain Asian, African, or Middle Eastern cultures, but it is not the language spoken in the home).
- Whenever possible, use a *trained* interpreter, preferably one who knows medical terminology.
- Avoid interpreters from a rival tribe, state, region, or nation (e.g., a Palestinian who knows Hebrew may not be the best interpreter for a Jewish person).
- Be aware of gender differences between interpreter and client. In general the same gender is preferred.
- Be aware of age differences between interpreter and client. In general an older, more mature interpreter is preferred to a younger, less experienced one.
- Be aware of socioeconomic differences between interpreter and client.

Strategies for Effective Use of an Interpreter
- Plan what you want to say ahead of time. Meet privately with the interpreter before the interview. Avoid confusing the interpreter by backing up, hesitating, or inserting a proviso.
- Ask the interpreter to provide a line-by-line verbatim account of the conversation. Ask for a detailed interpretation when provided with brief summaries of longer exchanges between interpreter and client.
- Be patient. When using an interpreter, interviews often take 2 to 3 times longer.
- Longer-than-expected explanatory exchanges are often required to convey the meaning of words such as *stress, depression, allergy, preventive medicine,* and *physical therapy* because there may not be comparable terms in the language that the client understands.
- When discussing diagnostic tests such as mammograms, magnetic resonance imaging (MRI), computed tomography (CT) scans, or those involving body fluids such as blood, urine, stool, spinal fluid, or saliva, be sure to clarify the nature of the test to the interpreter. Indicate the purpose of the test, exactly what will happen to the client, approximately how long the test will take, whether the procedure is invasive or noninvasive, and which part(s) of the body will be tested.
- Be aware that the interpreter may modify or edit some aspects of the conversation, especially if he or she thinks you might not understand the cultural context of the client's response (e.g., traditional or folk beliefs and practices related to healing).
- Avoid ambiguous statements and questions. Refrain from using conditional or indefinite phrasing such as "if," "would," and "could," especially for target languages such as Khmer (Cambodia) that lack nuances of conditionality or distinctions of time other than simple past and present. Conditional statements may be mistaken for actual agreement or approval of a course of action.
- Avoid abstract expressions, idioms, similes, metaphors, and medical jargon.
- To ensure confidentiality and privacy, avoid using as interpreters children or strangers who may be visiting other clients.
- Be aware that an interpreter who is a nonrelative may seek compensation for services rendered. Be sure to negotiate fees ahead of time.

Recommendations for Institutions
- Maintain a current, computerized list of interpreters who may be contacted as needed.
- Network with area hospitals, colleges, universities, and other organizations that may serve as resources.
- Use over-the-telephone interpretation services provided by telephone companies. For example, since 1989 AT&T has operated the Language Line Services, which provides interpretation in more than 140 languages. Services are available around the clock every day of the year. Call (800) 628-8486 or visit www.languageline.com for further information on services and charges.

Although use of an interpreter is the ideal, you may find yourself in a situation with a non–English-speaking client when no interpreter is available. Table 3-7 summarizes some suggestions for overcoming language barriers when no interpreter is present. Communicating with these clients may require that you combine verbal and nonverbal communication.

TABLE 3-7   What to Do When No Language Interpreter Is Available

1. Be polite and formal.
2. Pronounce name correctly. Use proper titles of respect such as "Mr.," "Mrs.," "Ms.," "Dr." Greet the person using the last or complete name.
   Gesture to yourself and say your name.
   Offer a handshake or nod. Smile.
3. Proceed in an unhurried manner. Pay attention to any effort by the client or family to communicate.
4. Speak in a low, moderate voice. Avoid talking loudly. Remember that there is a tendency to raise the volume and pitch of your voice when the listener appears not to understand. The listener may perceive that you are shouting and/or angry.
5. Use any words that you might know in the person's language. This indicates that you are aware of and respect his or her culture.
6. Use simple words such as "pain" instead of "discomfort." Avoid medical jargon, idioms, and slang. Avoid using contractions (e.g., don't, can't, won't). Use nouns repeatedly instead of pronouns.
   Do not say: "He has been taking his medicine, hasn't he?"
   Do say: "Does Juan take medicine?"
7. Pantomime words and simple actions while you verbalize them.
8. Give instructions in the proper sequence.
   Do not say: "Before you rinse the bottle, sterilize it."
   Do say: "First wash the bottle. Second, rinse the bottle."
9. Discuss one topic at a time. Avoid using conjunctions.
   Do not say: "Are you cold and in pain?"
   Do say: "Are you cold (while pantomiming)? Are you in pain?"
10. Validate whether person understands by having him or her repeat instructions, demonstrate the procedure, or act out the meaning.
11. Write out several short sentences in English and determine the person's ability to read them.
12. Try a third language. Many Indochinese speak French. Europeans often know two or more languages. Try Latin words or phrases.
13. Ask who among the person's family and friends could serve as an interpreter.
14. Obtain phrase books from a library or bookstore, make or purchase flash cards, contact hospitals for a list of interpreters, and use both formal and informal networks to locate a suitable interpreter.

Health Literacy: Ensuring We Are understood

You might have perfected the communication techniques described and feel fully prepared to interview the most challenging client, but are you sure that he or she understands everything you say? Several decades ago the concept of **health literacy** was introduced because it was clear that people did not always understand the health information provided.[7] Literacy is the ability to read and write; however, health literacy refers to the ability to understand instructions, navigate the health care system, and communicate concerns with the health care provider.[16] A person can have adequate literacy and not have health literacy. In 2006 the U.S. Department of Education released the National Assessment of Adult Literacy, which estimated that only 12% of people have proficient health literacy. Said another way, nearly 9 out of 10 people that you encounter do not have adequate health literacy to navigate the health care system and understand health instructions.[21]

Health literacy encompasses a variety of factors beyond basic reading, including the ability to use quantitative (numeric) information and to understand and remember verbal instructions. People with low health literacy struggle to navigate the health care system and may be noncompliant because of a misunderstanding. Low health literacy has been associated with low medication compliance, more emergency department visits, increased readmission rates, inability to recall information after a clinic visit, and an inability to effectively manage chronic illness.[7] Low health literacy leads to increased cost of care and poor outcomes for this population.

Tools for Determining Literacy

As a clinician you are on the front line in the battle for adequate health literacy for your clients. A wide variety of tools to measure health literacy exist—some more challenging than others. Table 3-8 presents three commonly used screening tools.

Each of the tools can be used in the clinical setting. A Single-Item Literacy Screener has been suggested, but with only marginal effectiveness. Some clinics simply ask standardized questions such as, "Do you have any limitations in learning?" or "What is the last grade level completed?" instead of requiring a specific assessment tool.

What Can You Do?
Oral Teaching

As a clinician there are steps you can take to ensure that your clients understand the information you are providing. Although completing a health literacy screener gives you objective data and can help you determine the appropriate level of information, most clients (regardless of literacy level) want to be provided with simple, easy-to-understand instructions; therefore the practice of giving all clients simple instructions at a lower reading level is acceptable. When discussing medical information with clients, keep it simple, use short sentences and words containing no more than two syllables (when possible), limit the number of messages you are

TABLE 3-8 **Tools for Assessing Health Literacy**		
TOOL	**DESCRIPTION**	**EXAMPLE QUESTIONS**
Test of Functional Health Literacy (TOFHLA)	• Designed for use in research • Measures reading comprehension and numeracy • Uses actual client instructions and forms • Takes approximately 22 minutes	Do not eat _____ a. appointment b. walk-in c. breakfast d. clinic
Rapid Estimate of Adult Literacy in Medicine (REALM)	• Designed for use in clinical setting • Person reads 66 medical terms aloud • Score based on number of words read and pronounced correctly • Takes 2-3 minutes to administer	Words include: flu, smear, stress, gallbladder, inflammatory, diagnosis, potassium
Newest Vital Sign (NVS)	• Assesses numeracy and comprehension • Uses nutrition label that clients must read and interpret • Total of six questions related to label provided • Takes approximately 3 minutes	Give client the nutrition label and ask: • If you eat the entire container, how many calories will you eat? • If you usually eat 2,500 calories in a day, what percentage of your daily value of calories will you be eating if you eat one serving?

giving the client, be sure to tell the person what they will gain by following your instructions, present only needed information, focus on the client, use the active voice, and avoid jargon. Although you may think using complex terms and sentences makes you sound more professional or smarter, it can confuse the client. You are better off speaking to them as you would to a friend, using a conversational structure that includes time for them to ask questions. A few examples follow:

Say: Feel for lumps about the size of a pea.
Don't say: Feel for lumps about 5 to 6 millimeters.
Say: Birth control
Don't say: Contraception
Say: Mad cow disease
Don't say: Bovine spongiform encephalitis
Say: Place your hand palm up.
Don't say: Supinate your hand.
Say: Cook chicken until it is no longer pink.
Don't say: Cook chicken to an internal temperature of 165° F.

Written Materials

When preparing or using written materials, make sure to assess the appropriateness of the materials. Most client education materials are created at a reading level that is not suitable for the majority of clients. Written materials should be at the 5th-grade reading level or below. Reading level can be determined with a variety of formulas that use number of syllables per word and complexity of sentences to determine reading level. Materials should be at least 12-point font. Also avoid all capital letters, use headings and subheadings, use bullet points, and limit medical jargon. Pictures are often used in written materials, but you must be careful to select appropriate graphics. See Fig. 3-9 for examples of appropriate pictures.

Choosing Appropriate Pictures for Low-Literacy Patients

Instead of this...	Use this...	Because
		Poor readers may not understand the "night cap" reference and the yawning moon to indicate bedtime.
		Giving inanimate objects human characteristics is very confusing to poor readers; in this case, to indicate daytime use simply the sun.
		Poor readers might not understand the concept of a "brown bag" referring to lunch and might focus only on the apple.
		Poor readers might see the three pills in the illustration on the left and think it means their dose is three pills.
		Poor readers might be confused by the clock-as-plate metaphor for the midday meal, as ideal as it may seem to the practitioner with high-level literacy.
		Poor readers have no frame of reference with the free-floating lungs: many people think this picture looks more like kidneys.

3-9

(Carroll, 2007.)

Teach Back

Although ensuring appropriate verbal and written communication is important, one of the easiest things you can do when teaching a client is to use the teach-back approach. Teach back is simple and free. It allows you to assess whether the person understands and to immediately correct misconceptions. Many health care professionals ask, "Do you understand?" or "Do you have any questions?" throughout the teaching sessions. Just because your client has no questions and indicates understanding with a nod doesn't mean that he or she actually understands the information. Using teach back encourages the client to repeat in his or her own words what you have just said. This verbal discussion allows you to assess the understanding and may open the door for the client to ask questions.

BIBLIOGRAPHY

1. Reference deleted in proofs.
2. Arnold, E., & Boggs, K. (2011). *Interpersonal relationships: professional communication skills for nurses* (6th ed.). Philadelphia: Saunders.
3. Association of American Medical Colleges. (2013). *Guidelines for use of medical interpreter services.* Available at www.aamc.org.
4. Centers for Disease Control and Prevention. (2009). *Simply put: a guide for creating easy-to-understand materials* http://www.cdc.gov/healthliteracy/learn/index.html..
5. Centers for Medicare and Medicaid Services: http://www.cms.gov/Outreach-and-Education/Outreach/WrittenMaterialsToolkit/index.html?redirect=/WrittenMaterialsToolkit/.
6. Deering, C. G., & Cody, D. J. (2002). Communicating with children and adolescents. *Am J Nurs, 103*(3), 34-42.
7. Dickens, C., & Piano, M. R. (2013). Health literacy and nursing: an update. *Am J Nurs, 113*(6), 52-58.
8. Diversity Rx website: www.diversityrx.org.
9. Flores, G. (2006). Language barriers to health care in the United States. *N Engl J Med, 355*(3), 229-231.
10. Flores, G., Abreu, M., Barone, C. P., et al. (2012). Errors of medical interpretation and their potential clinical consequences: a comparison of professional versus ad hoc versus no interpreters. *Ann Emerg Med 60*(5), 515-553. doi: 10.1016/j.annemergmed.2012.01.025.
11. Ho, A. (2008). Using family members as interpreters in the clinical setting. *J Clin Ethics, 19*(3), 223-231.
12. Reference deleted in proofs.
13. HSTAT: National Library of Medicine website: http://nlm.gov/outreach/consumer/healthlit.html.
14. Reference deleted in proofs.
15. Iezzoni, L. I., O'Day, B. L., Killeen, M., et al. (2004). Communicating about health care: observations from persons who are deaf or hard of hearing. *Ann Intern Med, 140*(5), 356-362.
16. Institute of Medicine. Health literacy: a prescription to end confusion. In Nielsen-Bohlman, L., Panzer, A., Kindig, D. A., (Eds.). (2004). Washington, DC: National Academies Press.
17. Interactive Patient website: http://healthweb.org.
18. Interpreting Stakeholder Group. (2009). *How to work effectively with interpreters.* Available at www.umtia.org.
19. Jacobs, E. A., Sadowski, L. S., & Rathouz, R. J. (2007). The impact of an enhanced interpreter service intervention on hospital costs and patient satisfaction. *J Gen Intern Med, 22*(Suppl 2), 306-311, 2007.
20. Jolly, K., Weiss, J. A., & Liehr, P. (2007). Understanding adolescent voice as a guide for nursing practice and research. *Issues Compr Pediatr Nurs, 30*(1-2), 3-13.
21. Kutner, M., et al. The health literacy of America's adults. (2006). Washington, DC: National Center for Education Statistics, U.S. Department of Education; Sep. NCES 2006-483. http://nces.ed.gov/pubs2006/2006483.pdf.
22. Lange, N., & Tigges, B. B. (2005). Influence positive change with motivational interviewing. *Nurse Pract, 30*(3), 44-53.
23. Levensky, E. R., Forcehimes, A., O'Donohue, W. T., et al. (2007). Motivational interviewing. *Am J Nurs, 107*(10), 50-59.
24. Martindell, D. (2012). Violence prevention training for ED staff. *Am J Nurs, 112*(9), 65-68.
25. Microsoft Office Support: *Test your document's readability.* Available at http://office.microsoft.com/en-us/word-help/test-your-document-s-readability-HP010148506.aspx.
26. National Cancer Institute. *Clear and simple: developing effective print materials for low-literate readers.* Available at http://www.cancer.gov/cancertopics/cancerlibrary/clear-and-simple/page1/AllPages.
27. Richardson, K. J. (2014). Deaf culture: competencies and best practices. *Nurse Pract, 39*(5), 21-28.
28. Rollnick, S., Miller, W. R., & Butler, C. C. (2008). *Motivational interviewing in health care: helping patients change behavior.* New York: Guilford Publications.
29. Selye, H. (1956). *The stress of life.* New York: McGraw-Hill.
30. Reference deleted in proofs.
31. Taylor, J. L. (2010). Workplace violence. *Am J Nurs, 110*(3), 11.
32. The Joint Commission. (2011). *Advancing effective communication, cultural competence, and patient- and family-centered care for the lesbian, gay, bisexual and transgender (LGBT) community: a field guide.* Available at www.jointcommission.org.
33. U.S. Bureau of the Census. *2011 American community survey.* Available at www.factfinder.census.gov.
34. U.S. Department of Health and Human Services. *The Health Insurance Portability and Accountability Act of 1996 (HIPAA) privacy rule.* Website: www.hhs.gov/ocr/privacy/index.html.
35. Ventres, W., Kooienga, S., Vuckovic, N., et al. (2006). Physicians, patients, and the electronic health record: an ethnographic analysis. *Ann Fam Med, 4*(2), 124-131.
36. Williams, K., Kemper, S., & Vockevic, N. (2005). Enhancing communication with older adults: overcoming elderspeak. *J Psychosoc Nurs, 43*(5), 12-16.

CHAPTER 4

The Complete Health History

The purpose of the health history is to collect **subjective data**—what the person says about himself or herself. This is different from **objective data**—what you observe through measurement, inspection, palpation, percussion, and auscultation. The history is combined with the objective data from the physical examination and laboratory studies to form the database. The database is used to make a judgment or a diagnosis about the health status of the individual (Fig. 4-1).

The following health history provides a complete picture of the person's past and present health. It describes the individual as a whole and how the person interacts with the environment. It records health strengths and coping skills. The history should recognize and affirm what the person is *doing right:* what he or she is doing to help stay well. For the well person, the history is used to assess his or her lifestyle, including such factors as exercise, healthy diet, substance use, risk reduction, and health promotion behaviors.

For the ill person, the health history includes a detailed and chronologic record of the health problem. For everyone the health history is a screening tool for abnormal symptoms, health problems, and concerns; and it records ways of responding to the health problems.

In many settings the patient fills out a printed or electronic history form or checklist. This allows the person ample time to recall and consider such items as dates of health landmarks and relevant family history. You then review and validate the written data and collect more data on lifestyle management and current health problems.

Although history forms vary, most contain information in the sequence of categories listed to the right. This health history format presents a generic database for all practitioners. Those in primary care settings may use all of it, whereas those in a hospital may focus primarily on the history of present illness and the functional, or patterns of living, data.

4-1

Health History Sequence
1. Biographic data
2. Reason for seeking care
3. Present health or history of present illness
4. Past history
5. Medication reconciliation
6. Family history
7. Review of systems
8. Functional assessment or activities of daily living (ADLs)

THE HEALTH HISTORY—THE ADULT

Record the date and time of day of the interview.

Biographic Data

Biographic data include name, address, and phone number; age and birth date; birthplace; gender; marital partner status; race; ethnic origin; and occupation (both usual and present; an illness or disability may have prompted a change in occupation). Record the person's primary language. Try to find a language-concordant provider to collect the history or a medical interpreter fluent in the patient's language. Evidence supports that language-concordance providers increase accuracy of communication and patient satisfaction.[18]

Source of History

1. Record who furnishes the information—usually the person himself or herself, although the source may be an interpreter or caseworker. Less reliable is a relative or friend.
2. Judge how reliable the informant seems and how willing he or she is to communicate. What is reliable? A reliable person always gives the same answers, even when questions are rephrased or repeated later in the interview.
3. Note if the person appears well or ill; a sick patient may communicate poorly.
See sample recordings at right.

Sample Statements:
Patient herself, who seems reliable
Patient's son, John Ramirez, who seems reliable
Mrs. R. Fuentes, interpreter for Theresa Castillo, who does not speak English

Reason for Seeking Care*

This is a brief, spontaneous statement in the person's own words that describes the reason for the visit. Think of it as the "title" for the story to follow. It states one (possibly two) symptoms or signs and their duration. A **symptom** is a subjective sensation that the person feels from the disorder. A **sign** is an objective abnormality that you as the examiner could detect on physical examination or in laboratory reports. Try to record whatever the person *says* is the reason for seeking care, enclose it in quotation marks to indicate the person's exact words, and record a time frame. See examples at right.

The reason for seeking care is not a diagnostic statement. Avoid translating it into the terms of a medical diagnosis. For example, Mr. J.S. enters with shortness of breath, and you ponder writing "emphysema." Even if he is known to have emphysema from previous visits, it is not the chronic emphysema that prompted *this visit* but, rather, the "increasing shortness of breath" for 4 hours.

Some people try to self-diagnose based on similar signs and symptoms in their relatives or friends or on conditions they know they have. Rather than record a woman's statement that she has "strep throat," ask her what symptoms she has that make her think this is present, and record those symptoms.

Occasionally a person may have *many* reasons for seeking care. After the first reason, ask, "Is there anything else we should take care of today?" The most important reason to the person may not necessarily be the one stated first. Try to focus on which is the most pressing concern by asking the person which one prompted him or her to seek help *now*.

Sample Statements:
"Chest pain for 2 hours"
"Sore throat for 3 days now and just getting worse"
"Earache and fussy all night"
"Need annual physical for work"
"Want to start jogging and need checkup"

Present Health or History of Present Illness

For the well person, this is a short statement about the general state of health: *"I feel healthy right now." "I am healthy and active."*

For the ill person, this section is a chronologic record of the reason for seeking care, from the time the symptom first started until now. Isolate each reason for care identified by the person and say, for example, "Please tell me all about your headache, from the time it started until the time you came to the hospital" (Fig. 4-2). If the concern started months or years ago, record what occurred during that time and find out why the person is seeking care *now*.

As the person talks, do not jump to conclusions and bias the story by adding your opinion. Collect *all* the data first. Although you want the person to respond in a narrative format without interruption from you, your final summary of any symptom the person has should include these *eight critical characteristics:*

1. **Location.** Be specific; ask the person to point to the location. If the problem is pain, note the precise site. "Head pain" is vague, whereas descriptions such as "pain behind the eyes," "jaw pain," and "occipital pain" are more precise and diagnostically significant. Is the pain localized to this site or radiating? Is the pain superficial or deep?
2. **Character** or **Quality.** This calls for specific descriptive terms such as burning, sharp, dull, aching, gnawing, throbbing, shooting, viselike. Use similes: Does blood in the stool look like sticky tar? Does blood in vomitus look like coffee grounds?
3. **Quantity** or **Severity.** Attempt to quantify the sign or symptom such as "profuse menstrual flow soaking five pads per hour." Quantify the symptom of pain using the scale shown on the right. With pain, avoid adjectives, and ask how it affects daily activities. Then record if the person says, "I was so sick I was doubled up and couldn't move" or "I was able to go to work, but then I came home and went to bed."
4. **Timing** (Onset, Duration, Frequency). When did the symptom first appear? Give the specific date and time or state specifically how long ago the symptom started prior to arrival (PTA). "The pain started yesterday" will not mean much when you return to read the record in the future. The report must include answers to questions such as, "How long did the symptom last (duration)? Was it steady (constant) or did it come and go during that time (intermittent)? Did it resolve completely and reappear days or weeks later (cycle of remission and exacerbation)?"

4-2

Pain Scale
Quantify the symptom of pain by asking: *"On a 10-point scale, with 10 being the most pain you can possibly imagine and 1 being mild pain you barely notice, tell me how your pain feels right now."* (See Chapter 10 for a full description.)

---

*In the past, this statement was called the *chief complaint (CC)*. Avoid this title because it labels the person a "complainer" and, more important, does not include wellness needs.

5. **Setting.** Where was the person or what was the person doing when the symptom started? What brings it on? For example, "Did you notice the chest pain after shoveling snow, or did the pain start by itself?"

6. **Aggravating** or **Relieving Factors.** What makes the pain worse? Is it aggravated by weather, activity, food, medication, standing bent over, fatigue, time of day, or season? What relieves it (e.g., rest, medication, or ice pack)? What is the effect of any treatment? Ask, "What have you tried?" or "What seems to help?"

7. **Associated Factors.** Is this primary symptom associated with any others (e.g., urinary frequency and burning associated with fever and chills)? Review the body system related to this symptom now rather than waiting for the Review of Systems section later. Many clinicians review the person's medication regimen now (including alcohol and tobacco use) because the presenting symptom may be a side effect or toxic effect of a chemical.

8. **Patient's Perception.** Find out the meaning of the symptom by asking how it affects daily activities (Fig. 4-3). "How has this affected you? Is there anything you can't do now that you could do before?" Also ask directly, "What do you think it means?" This is crucial because it alerts you to potential anxiety if the person thinks the symptom may be ominous.

You may find it helpful to organize this same question sequence into the mnemonic **PQRSTU** to help remember all the points. Note that you still need to address the patient's perception of the problem.

P: Provocative or Palliative. What brings it on? What were you doing when you first noticed it? What makes it better? Worse?

Q: Quality or Quantity. How does it look, feel, sound? How intense/severe is it?

R: Region or Radiation. Where is it? Does it spread anywhere?

S: Severity Scale. How bad is it (on a scale of 1 to 10)? Is it getting better, worse, staying the same?

T: Timing. Onset—Exactly when did it first occur? Duration—How long did it last? Frequency—How often does it occur?

U: Understand Patient's Perception of the problem. What do you think it means?

4-3

Past Health

Past health events are important because they may have residual effects on the current health state. The previous experience with illness may also give clues about how the person responds to illness and the significance of illness for him or her.

Childhood Illnesses. Measles, mumps, rubella, chickenpox, pertussis, and strep throat. Avoid recording "usual childhood illnesses," because an illness common in the person's childhood (e.g., mumps) may be unusual today. Ask about serious illnesses that may have sequelae for the person in later years (e.g., rheumatic fever, scarlet fever, poliomyelitis).

Accidents or Injuries. Auto accidents, fractures, penetrating wounds, head injuries (especially if associated with unconsciousness), and burns.

Serious or Chronic Illnesses. Asthma, depression, diabetes, hypertension, heart disease, human immunodeficiency virus (HIV) infection, hepatitis, sickle-cell anemia, cancer, and seizure disorder.

Hospitalizations. Cause, name of hospital, how the condition was treated, how long the person was hospitalized, and name of the physician.

Operations. Type of surgery, date, name of the surgeon, name of the hospital, and how the person recovered.

Obstetric History. Number of pregnancies (gravidity), number of deliveries in which the fetus reached full term (term), number of preterm pregnancies (preterm), number of incomplete pregnancies (miscarriages or abortions), and number of children living (living). For each complete pregnancy, note the course of pregnancy; labor and delivery; sex, weight, and condition of each infant; and postpartum course.

Recorded as:
Grav 3
Term 2
Preterm 1
Ab 0
Living 3

Immunizations. Routinely assess vaccination history and urge the recommended vaccines. Your strong recommendation increases compliance.[1] Use the current Centers for Disease Control (CDC) recommendations for adults, but be aware of primary contraindications and precautions as well as the person's lifestyle, occupation, and travel.[1] The 2013 recommendations for adults include: influenza (annually), tetanus-diphtheria-pertussis (Td/Tdap) (once and boost every 10 years), varicella, human papilloma virus (HPV) for female and male (3 doses ages 9 to 26 years), zoster (after 60 years), measles-mumps-rubella (1 or 2 doses), pneumococcal (once and boost after 65 years), meningococcal, and hepatitis A and B. Recommendations for Tdap now include routine vaccination for those over 65 years and for repeat Tdap with each pregnancy during 27 to 36 weeks' gestation.

You can find a printable color-coded table of the 2013 adult immunization schedule at http://www.cdc.gov/vaccines/schedules/hcp/adult.html.

Advise gay and bisexual men to receive HPV, hepatitis A, and hepatitis B vaccinations. If they are not in a long-term monogamous relationship, they should have annual testing for HIV, syphilis, gonorrhea, and chlamydia.[2a]

Last Examination Date. Physical, dental, vision, hearing, electrocardiogram (ECG), chest x-ray film, mammogram, Pap test, stool occult blood, serum cholesterol.

Allergies. Note both the allergen (medication, food, or contact agent such as fabric or environmental agent) and the reaction (rash, itching, runny nose, watery eyes, or more serious difficulty breathing). With a drug this symptom should not be a side effect but a true allergic reaction.

Current Medications. **Medication reconciliation** is a comparison of a list of current medications with a previous list, which is done at every hospitalization and every clinic visit. The purpose is to reduce errors and promote patient safety. For all currently prescribed medications, note the name (generic or trade), dose, and schedule, and ask: "How often do you take it each day? What is it for? How long have you been taking it? Do you have any side effects?" and if not taking it, "What is the reason you stopped taking it?"

A person could take furosemide from one bottle and Lasix from another prescriber and not know that it is the same medication.

Ask about nonprescription and over-the-counter (OTC) drugs. The average U.S. home medicine cabinet holds 24 OTC medications, and 40% of Americans take at least one OTC medicine every 2 days.[12b] Specifically ask about aspirin (because many people do not consider it a medication even though they take it every day) and other medications: vitamins, birth control pills, antacids, cold remedies, acetaminophen. Be aware that acetaminophen is a component in many OTC pain and cold medications. It has close to 25 trade names, including Tylenol. Serious liver damage may ensue if a person unknowingly doubles or triples the maximum daily acetaminophen intake. For any pain reliever (e.g., acetaminophen, ibuprofen [Advil, Motrin]) ask how many milligrams the person takes.

Ask about herbal medications. Although not regulated by the Food and Drug Administration (FDA), they are popular because consumer advertising promises weight loss, improved memory, or relief from insomnia or depression. Many are considered safe, but some interact with prescribed medications. For example, St. John's wort is often taken for depression, but because it enters the CYP 450 enzyme metabolism, it has many herb-drug interactions.[12]

Inquire about substances (alcohol, tobacco, street drugs) here or later in Personal Habits (see p. 57).

Family History

In the age of genomics an accurate family history highlights diseases and conditions for which a particular patient may be at increased risk. A person who learns that he or she may be vulnerable for a certain condition may seek early screening and periodic surveillance. A person with significant coronary heart disease history (e.g., a cardiac event in a first-degree male relative < 55 years or female relative < 65 years) may be influenced to adopt a healthy lifestyle when possible to mitigate that risk.

The most fruitful way to compile a complete family history is to send home a detailed questionnaire before the health care/hospital encounter because the information takes time to compile and often comes from multiple family members. Then you can use the health visit to complete the pedigree. A **pedigree** or **genogram** is a graphic family tree that uses symbols to depict the gender, relationship, and age of immediate blood relatives in at least three generations such as parents, grandparents, and siblings (Fig. 4-4). The health of close

Family History Tools in Electronic and Print Format
U.S. Surgeon General (My Family Health Portrait): www.hhs.gov/familyhistory/
Utah Health Family Tree: www.health.utah.gov/genomics
American Medical Association: www.ama-assn.org/ama/pub/category/2380.html

Drawing Your Family Tree:
- Make a list of all of your family members.
- Use this sample family tree as a guide to draw your own family tree.
- Write your name at the top of your paper and the date your drew your family tree.
- In place of the words *father*, *mother*, etc., write the names of your family members.

- When possible, draw your brothers and sisters and your parents' brothers and sisters starting from oldest to the youngest, going from left to right across the paper.
- If dates of birth or ages are not known, then estimate or guess ("50s," "late 60s").

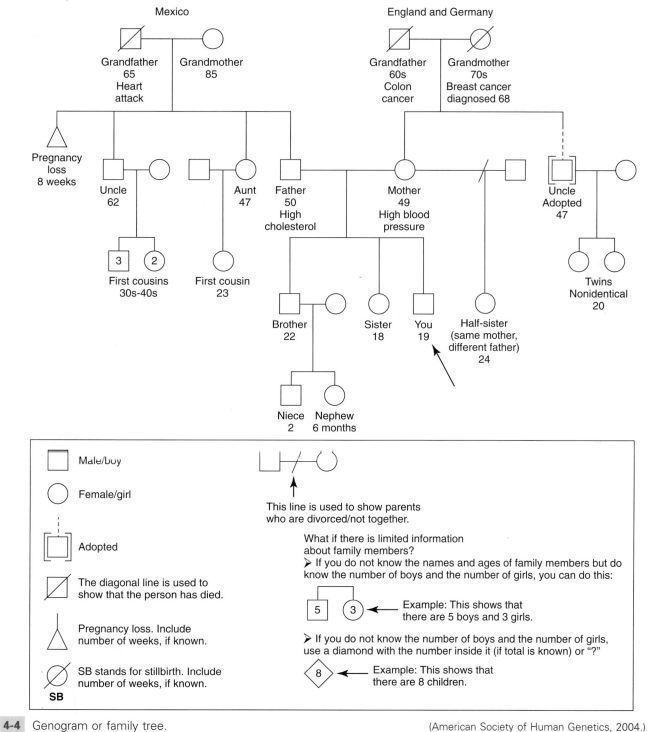

4-4   Genogram or family tree.   (American Society of Human Genetics, 2004.)

family members such as spouse or partner and children is equally important to highlight the patient's prolonged contact with any communicable disease or environmental hazard such as tobacco smoke, or to flag the effect of a family member's illness on this person.

Record the medical condition of each relative and other significant health data such as age and cause of death, twinning, tobacco use, and heavy alcohol use. When reviewing the family history data, ask specifically about coronary heart disease, high blood pressure, stroke, diabetes, obesity, blood disorders, breast/ovarian cancer, colon cancer, sickle-cell anemia, arthritis, allergies, alcohol or drug addiction, mental illness, suicide, seizure disorder, kidney disease, and tuberculosis (TB).

CULTURE AND GENETICS

Add several questions to the complete health history when the person is a new immigrant:
- Biographical data—When did the person enter the United States and from what country. If a refugee, under which conditions did he or she come? Was there harrassment or torture?
  - The older adult may have come to this country after World War II and may be a Holocaust survivor—Questions regarding family and past history may evoke painful memories and must be asked carefully.
- Spiritual resources/religion—Assess whether certain procedures, such as administering blood to a Jehovah's Witness or drawing large amounts of blood from a Chinese patient, are prohibited.
- Past health—Which immunizations were given in the homeland (e.g., was the person given *Bacillus Calmette-Guérin* [BCG])? This vaccine is used in many countries to prevent TB; it is not administered in the United States. If the person has had BCG, he or she will have a positive tuberculin test; further diagnostic procedures must be done, including a sputum test and chest x-ray film.
- Health perception—How does the person describe health and illness, and what does he or she see as the problem that he or she is now experiencing?
- Nutritional—Which foods and food combinations are taboo?

Many immigrants have significant health care needs (e.g., diabetes, accidents on the job, muscle pain) but are in the country without documentation. Unless your facility ensures anonymity, they are reluctant to furnish biographic data for fear of deportation.

Review of Systems

The purposes of this section are (1) to evaluate the past and present health state of each body system, (2) to double-check in case any significant data were omitted in the Present Illness section, and (3) to evaluate health promotion practices. The order of the examination of body systems is roughly head to toe. The items within each system are not inclusive, and only the most common symptoms are listed (Fig. 4-5). If the Present Illness section covered a body system, you do not need to repeat all the data here. For example, if the reason for seeking care is earache, the Present Illness section describes most of the symptoms listed for the auditory system. Just ask now what was not asked in the Present Illness section.

4-5

Medical terms are listed here, but they need to be translated for the patient. (Note that symptoms and health promotion activities are merely listed here. These terms are repeated and expanded in each related physical examination chapter, along with suggested ways to pose questions and a rationale for each question.)

When recording information, avoid writing "negative" after the system heading. You need to record the *presence* or *absence* of all symptoms; otherwise the reader does not know about which factors you asked.

A common mistake made by beginning practitioners is to record some physical finding or objective data here such as "skin warm and dry." Remember that the history should be limited to patient statements or subjective data—factors that the person *says* were or were not present.

General Overall Health State. Present weight (gain or loss, over what period of time, by diet or other factors), fatigue, weakness or malaise, fever, chills, sweats or night sweats.

Skin. History of skin disease (eczema, psoriasis, hives), pigment or color change, change in mole, excessive dryness or moisture, pruritus, excessive bruising, rash or lesion.

Hair. Recent loss, change in texture. Nails: change in shape, color, or brittleness.
Health Promotion. Amount of sun exposure; method of self-care for skin and hair.

Head. Any unusually frequent or severe headache; any head injury, dizziness (syncope), or vertigo.

Eyes. Difficulty with vision (decreased acuity, blurring, blind spots), eye pain, diplopia (double vision), redness or swelling, watering or discharge, glaucoma or cataracts.

Health Promotion. Wear glasses or contacts; last vision check or glaucoma test; how coping with loss of vision if any.

Ears. Earaches, infections, discharge and its characteristics, tinnitus or vertigo.

Health Promotion. Hearing loss, hearing aid use, how loss affects daily life, any exposure to environmental noise, and method of cleaning ears.

Nose and Sinuses. Discharge and its characteristics, any unusually frequent or severe colds, sinus pain, nasal obstruction, nosebleeds, allergies or hay fever, or change in sense of smell.

Mouth and Throat. Mouth pain, frequent sore throat, bleeding gums, toothache, lesion in mouth or tongue, dysphagia, hoarseness or voice change, tonsillectomy, altered taste.

Health Promotion. Pattern of daily dental care, use of dentures, bridge, and last dental checkup.

Neck. Pain, limitation of motion, lumps or swelling, enlarged or tender nodes, goiter.

Breast. Pain, lump, nipple discharge, rash, history of breast disease, any surgery on breasts.

Health Promotion. Performs breast self-examination, including its frequency and method used; last mammogram.

Axilla. Tenderness, lump or swelling, rash.

Respiratory System. History of lung diseases (asthma, emphysema, bronchitis, pneumonia, TB), chest pain with breathing, wheezing or noisy breathing, shortness of breath, how much activity produces shortness of breath, cough, sputum (color, amount), hemoptysis, toxin or pollution exposure.

Health Promotion. Last chest x-ray study, TB skin test.

Cardiovascular. Chest pain, pressure, tightness or fullness, palpitation, cyanosis, dyspnea on exertion (specify amount of exertion [e.g., walking one flight of stairs, walking from chair to bath, or just talking]), orthopnea, paroxysmal nocturnal dyspnea, nocturia, edema, history of heart murmur, hypertension, coronary heart disease, anemia.

Health Promotion. Date of last ECG or other heart tests, cholesterol screening.

Vigorously pursue all vague chest pain similarities. Consider a woman with fatigue or vague indigestion as a cardiac patient until proven otherwise.

Peripheral Vascular. Coldness, numbness and tingling, swelling of legs (time of day, activity), discoloration in hands or feet (bluish red, pallor, mottling, associated with position, especially around feet and ankles), varicose veins or complications, intermittent claudication, thrombophlebitis, ulcers.

Health Promotion. Does the work involve long-term sitting or standing? Avoid crossing legs at the knees. Wear support hose?

Gastrointestinal. Appetite, food intolerance, dysphagia, heartburn, indigestion, pain (associated with eating), other abdominal pain, pyrosis (esophageal and stomach burning sensation with sour eructation), nausea and vomiting (character), vomiting blood, history of abdominal disease (liver or gallbladder, ulcer, jaundice, appendicitis, colitis), flatulence, frequency of bowel movement, any recent change, stool characteristics, constipation or diarrhea, black stools, rectal bleeding, rectal conditions (hemorrhoids, fistula).

Health Promotion. Use of antacids or laxatives. (Alternatively, diet history and substance habits can be placed here.)

Urinary System. Frequency, urgency, nocturia (the number of times the person awakens at night to urinate, recent change); dysuria; polyuria or oliguria; hesitancy or straining, narrowed stream; urine color (cloudy or presence of hematuria); incontinence; history of urinary disease (kidney disease, kidney stones, urinary tract infections, prostate); pain in flank, groin, suprapubic region, or low back.

Health Promotion. Measures to avoid or treat urinary tract infections, use of Kegel exercises after childbirth.

Male Genital System. Penis or testicular pain, sores or lesions, penile discharge, lumps, hernia.

Health Promotion. Perform testicular self-examination? How frequently?

Female Genital System. Menstrual history (age at menarche, last menstrual period, cycle and duration, any amenorrhea or menorrhagia, premenstrual pain or dysmenorrhea, intermenstrual spotting), vaginal itching, discharge and its characteristics, age at menopause, menopausal signs or symptoms, postmenopausal bleeding.

Health Promotion. Last gynecologic checkup and last Pap test.

Sexual Health. Begin with: "I usually ask all patients about their sexual health." Then ask: "Are you presently in a relationship involving intercourse? Are the aspects of sex satisfactory to you and your partner? Are condoms used routinely? Is there any dyspareunia (for female) or are there any changes in erection or ejaculation (for male)? Are contraceptives used? Is the contraceptive method satisfactory? Are you aware of contact with a partner who has any sexually transmitted infection (gonorrhea, herpes, chlamydia, venereal warts, HIV/acquired immunodeficiency syndrome (AIDS), or syphilis)?"

Musculoskeletal System. History of arthritis or gout. In the joints: Pain stiffness, swelling (location, migratory nature), deformity, limitation of motion, noise with joint motion? In the muscles: Any muscle pain, cramps, weakness, gait problems, or problems with coordinated activities? In the back: Any pain (location and radiation to extremities), stiffness, limitation of motion, or history of back pain or disk disease?

Health Promotion. How much walking per day? What is the effect of limited range of motion on ADLs such as grooming, feeding, toileting, dressing? Are any mobility aids used?

Neurologic System. History of seizure disorder, stroke, fainting, blackouts. Motor function: Weakness, tic or tremor, paralysis, or coordination problems? Sensory function: Numbness, tingling (paresthesia)? Cognitive function: Memory disorder (recent or distant, disorientation)? Mental status: Any nervousness, mood change, depression, or history of mental health dysfunction or hallucinations?

Health Promotion. Alternatively, data about interpersonal relationships and coping patterns are placed here.

Hematologic System. Bleeding tendency of skin or mucous membranes, excessive bruising, lymph node swelling, exposure to toxic agents or radiation, blood transfusion and reactions.

Endocrine System. History of diabetes or diabetic symptoms (polyuria, polydipsia, polyphagia), history of thyroid disease, intolerance to heat and cold, change in skin pigmentation or texture, excessive sweating, relationship between appetite and weight, abnormal hair distribution, nervousness, tremors, and need for hormone therapy.

Functional Assessment (Including Activities of Daily Living)

Functional assessment measures a person's self-care ability in the areas of general physical health or absence of illness; ADLs such as bathing, dressing, toileting, eating, walking; instrumental ADLs (IADLs) or those needed for independent living such as housekeeping, shopping, cooking, doing laundry, using the telephone, managing finances; nutrition; social relationships and resources; self-concept and coping; and home environment.

Functional assessment may mean organizing the entire assessment around functional "pattern areas."[11] Instruments that emphasize functional categories may help to lead to a nursing diagnosis.

Functional assessment may also mean the use of a standardized instrument that objectively measures a person's present functional status and monitors any changes over time (see Chapter 31 for more information).

Functional assessment questions listed here provide data on the lifestyle and type of living environment to which the person is accustomed. Because the person may consider these questions "private," they are best asked at this later point in the interview after you have had time to establish rapport.

Self-Esteem, Self-Concept. Education (last grade completed, other significant training), financial status (income adequate for lifestyle and/or health concerns), value-belief system (religious practices and perception of personal strengths).

Activity/Exercise. A daily profile reflecting usual daily activities. Ask, "Tell me how you spend a typical day." Note ability to perform ADLs: independent or needs assistance with feeding, bathing, hygiene, dressing, toileting, bed-to-chair transfer, walking, standing, or climbing stairs. Is there any use of wheelchair, prostheses, or mobility aids?

Record leisure activities enjoyed and the exercise pattern (type, amount per day or week, method of warm-up session, method of monitoring the response of the body to exercise).

Sleep/Rest. Sleep patterns, daytime naps, any sleep aids used.

Nutrition/Elimination. Record the diet by a recall of all food and beverages taken over the past 24 hours (see Chapter 11 for suggested method of inquiry). Ask, "Is that menu typical of most days?" Describe eating habits and current appetite. Ask, "Who buys food and prepares food? Are your finances adequate for food? Who is present at mealtimes?" Indicate any food allergy or intolerance. Record daily intake of caffeine (coffee, tea, cola drinks).

Ask about usual pattern of bowel elimination and urinating, including problems with mobility or transfer in toileting, continence, use of laxatives.

Interpersonal Relationships/Resources. Social roles: Ask, "How would you describe your role in the family? How would you say you get along with family, friends, and co-workers?" Ask about support systems composed of family and significant others: "To whom could you go for support with a problem at work, your health, or a personal problem?" Include contact with spouse, siblings, parents, children, friends, organizations, workplace. "Is time spent alone pleasurable and relaxing, or is it isolating?"

Spiritual Resources. Many people believe in a relationship between spirituality and health, and they may wish to have spiritual matters addressed in the traditional health care setting. Use the **F**aith, **I**nfluence, **C**ommunity, and **A**ddress (FICA) questions to incorporate the person's spiritual values into the health history.[15] *Faith:* "Does religious faith or spirituality play an important part in your life? Do you consider yourself to be a religious or spiritual person?" *Influence:* "How does your religious faith or spirituality influence the way you think about your health or care for yourself?" *Community:* "Are you a part of any religious or spiritual community or congregation?" *Address:* "Would you like me to address any religious or spiritual issues or concerns with you?"

Coping and Stress Management. Types of stresses in life, especially in the past year; any change in lifestyle or any current stress; methods tried to relieve stress and whether these have been helpful.

Personal Habits. Tobacco, alcohol, street drugs: Ask, "Do you smoke cigarettes (pipe, use chewing tobacco)? At what age did you start? How many packs do you smoke per day? How many years have you smoked?" Record the number of packs smoked per day (PPD) and duration (e.g., 1 PPD × 5 years). Then ask, "Have you ever tried to quit?" and "How did it go?" to introduce plans about smoking cessation.

Alcohol. Health care professionals often fail to question about alcohol unless problems are obvious. However, alcohol interacts adversely with all medications; is a factor in many social problems such as assaults, rapes, high-risk sexual behavior, and child abuse; contributes to half of all fatal traffic accidents; and accounts for 5% of all deaths in the United States. The latter figure is actually an underestimate because alcohol-related conditions are underreported on death certificates.

Therefore be alert to early signs of hazardous alcohol use. Ask whether the person drinks alcohol. If yes, ask specific questions about the amount and frequency of alcohol use: Ask, "When was your last drink of alcohol? How much did you drink that time? In the past 30 days, about how many days would you say that you drank alcohol? Has anyone ever said that you had a drinking problem?"

You may wish to use a screening questionnaire to identify excessive or uncontrolled drinking such as the **C**ut down, **A**nnoyed, **G**uilty, and **E**ye-opener (**CAGE**) test[6]:

- Have you ever thought you should **C**ut down your drinking?
- Have you ever been **A**nnoyed by criticism of your drinking?
- Have you ever felt **G**uilty about your drinking?
- Do you drink in the morning? (i.e., an **E**ye opener?)

If the person answers "yes" to two or more CAGE questions, you should suspect alcohol abuse and continue with a more complete substance-abuse assessment (see Chapter 6, p. 89). If the person answers "no" to drinking alcohol, ask the reason for this decision (psychosocial, legal, health). Any history of alcohol treatment? Involved in recovery activities? History of a family member with problem drinking?

Illicit or Street Drugs. Ask specifically about prescription painkillers such as OxyContin or Vicodin, cocaine, crack cocaine, amphetamines, heroin, and marijuana. Indicate frequency of use and how use has affected work or family.

Environment/Hazards. Housing and neighborhood (living alone, knowledge of neighbors), safety of area, adequate heat and utilities, access to transportation, and involvement in community services. Note environmental health, including hazards in workplace, hazards at home, use of seatbelts, geographic or occupational exposures, and travel or residence in other countries, including time spent abroad during military service.

Intimate Partner Violence. Begin with open-ended questions: "How are things at home?" and "Do you feel safe?" These are valuable initial screening questions because some people may not recognize that they are in abusive situations or may be reluctant to admit it because of guilt, fear, shame, or denial. If the person responds to feeling unsafe, follow up with closed-ended questions: "Have you ever been emotionally or physically abused by your partner or someone important to you? Within the past year, have you been hit, slapped, kicked, pushed, or shoved or otherwise physically hurt by your partner or ex-partner?" If yes, ask: "By whom? How many times? Does your partner ever force you into having sex? Are you afraid of your partner or ex-partner?" See Chapter 7 for more information.

Occupational Health. Ask the person to describe his or her job. Ever worked with any health hazard such as asbestos, inhalants, chemicals, repetitive motion? Wear any protective equipment? Any work programs in place that monitor exposure? Aware of any health problems now that may be related to work exposure?

Note the timing of the reason for seeking care and whether it may be related to change in work or home activities, job titles, or exposure history. Take a careful smoking history, which may contribute to occupational hazards. Finally ask the person what he or she likes or dislikes about the job.

Perception of Health

Ask the person questions such as: "How do you define health? How do you view your situation now? What are your concerns? What do you think will happen in the future? What are your health goals? What do you expect from us as nurses, physicians (or other health care providers)?"

❖ DEVELOPMENTAL COMPETENCE

Children

The health history is adapted to include information specific for the age and developmental stage of the child (e.g., the mother's health during pregnancy, labor and delivery, the perinatal period, and the family unit) (Fig. 4-6). Note that the developmental history and nutritional data are listed as separate sections because of their importance for current health.

4-6

Biographic Data

Include the child's name, nickname, address and phone number, parents' names and work numbers, child's age and birth date, birthplace, sex, race, ethnic origin, and information about other children and family members at home.

Source of History

1. Person providing information and relation to child
2. Your impression of reliability of information
3. Any special circumstances (e.g., the use of an interpreter)

Reason for Seeking Care

Record the parent's spontaneous statement. Because of the frequency of well-child visits for routine health care, there will be more reasons such as "time for the child's checkup" or "she needs the next baby shot." Reasons for health problems may be initiated by the child, the parent, or a third party such as a classroom teacher or social worker.

Sometimes the reason stated may not be the real reason for the visit. A parent may have a "hidden agenda," such as the mother who brought her 4-year-old child in because "she looked pale." Further questioning revealed that the mother had heard recently from a former college friend whose 4-year-old child had just been diagnosed with leukemia.

Present Health or History of Present Illness

If the parent or child seeks routine health care, include a statement about the usual health of the child and any common health problems or major health concerns.

Describe any presenting symptom or sign, using the same format as for the adult. Some additional considerations include:

- Severity of pain: "How does your child behave when he or she is in pain?" (e.g., pulling at ears alerts parent to ear pain). Note the effect of pain on usual behavior (e.g., does it stop child from playing?).
- Associated factors such as relation to activity, eating, and body position.
- The parent's intuitive sense of a problem. As the constant caregiver, this intuitive sense is very accurate. Even if proved otherwise, this factor gives you an idea of the parent's area of concern.
- Parent's coping ability and reaction of other family members to child's symptoms or illness.

Past Health

Prenatal Status. Start with an open-ended question: "Tell me about this pregnancy." Then ask: "How was this pregnancy spaced? Was it planned? What was the mother's attitude toward the pregnancy? What was the father's attitude? Was there medical supervision for the mother? At what month was the supervision started? What was the mother's health during pregnancy? Were there any complications (bleeding, excessive nausea and vomiting, unusual weight gain, high blood pressure, swelling of hands and feet, falls, infections—rubella or sexually transmitted infections)? During which month were diet and medications prescribed and/or taken during pregnancy (dose and duration)?" Record the mother's use of alcohol, street drugs, or cigarettes and any x-ray studies taken during pregnancy.

Labor and Delivery. Parity of the mother, duration of the pregnancy, name of the hospital, course and duration of labor, use of anesthesia, type of delivery (vertex, breech, cesarean section), birth weight, Apgar scores, onset of breathing, any cyanosis, need for resuscitation, and use of special equipment or procedures.

Postnatal Status. Any problems in the nursery, length of hospital stay, neonatal jaundice, whether the baby was discharged with the mother, whether the baby was breastfed or bottle-fed, weight gain, any feeding problems, "blue spells," colic, diarrhea, patterns of crying and sleeping (Fig. 4-7), the mother's health postpartum, the mother's reaction to the baby, placement on back when sleeping.

Childhood Illnesses. Age and any complications of measles, mumps, rubella, chickenpox, whooping cough, strep throat, and frequent ear infections; any recent exposure to illness.

Serious Accidents or Injuries. Age of occurrence, extent of injury, how the child was treated, and complications of auto accidents, falls, head injuries, fractures, burns, and poisonings.

Serious or Chronic Illnesses. Age of onset, how the child was treated, and complications of meningitis or encephalitis; seizure disorders; asthma, pneumonia, and other chronic lung conditions; rheumatic fever; scarlet fever; diabetes; kidney problems; sickle cell anemia; high blood pressure; and allergies.

4-7

Operations or Hospitalizations. Reason for care, age at admission, name of surgeon or primary care providers, name of hospital, duration of stay, how child reacted to hospitalization, any complications. (If child reacted poorly, he or she may be afraid now and will need special preparation for the examination that is to follow.)

Immunizations. Age when administered, date administered, and any reactions following immunizations (Fig. 4-8). Because of outbreaks of measles across the United States, the American Academy of Pediatrics recommends two doses of the measles-mumps-rubella vaccine, one at 12 to 15 months and one at age 4 to 6 years.[3]

Pertussis (whooping cough) also is on the rise, with periodic epidemics every 3 to 5 years.[2b] The young infant is at high risk because of an immature immune system and because the schedule for the primary series of vaccinations does not start until 6 to 8 weeks of age. Therefore the *cocooning strategy* is recommended—vaccinating parents, especially the mother, siblings, grandparents, and others in close contact with the baby.[2b]

The CDC recommends routine immunizations to protect against 15 childhood and adolescent diseases and cancers.[2] The impact of routine immunizations in the United States is enormous: 42,000 lives saved annually for each cohort of babies born and 20 million disease episodes avoided each year.[2] Yet many children are underimmunized: those living in poverty, certain ethnic subgroups, even attentive parents who gain misinformation from the Internet and have unwarranted concerns. You should acknowledge these parents' concerns in a respectful way, yet teach what science says about immunizations.[2, 14]

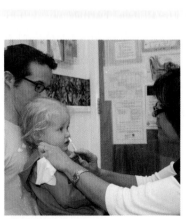

4-8

Allergies. Any drugs, foods, contact agents, and environmental agents to which the child is allergic and the reaction to the allergens. A true *food allergy* is an immune response caused by exposure to a food substance. Common pediatric food allergies include cow's milk, eggs, peanuts, soybean, wheat, tree nuts, and fish. A true food allergy can be life threatening but should be differentiated from a *food intolerance,* which causes distress and illness yet is a nonimmunologic response and not life threatening.[7] Also note allergic reactions particularly common in childhood, such as allergic rhinitis, insect hypersensitivity, eczema, and urticaria.

Medications. Any prescription and OTC medications (or vitamins) that the child takes, including the dosage, daily schedule, why the medication is given, and any problems.

Developmental History

Growth. Height and weight at birth and at 1, 2, 5, and 10 years; any periods of rapid gain or loss (Fig. 4-9); process of dentition (age of tooth eruption and pattern of loss).

Milestones. Age when child first held head erect, rolled over, sat alone, walked alone, cut his or her first tooth, said his or her first words with meaning, spoke in sentences, was toilet trained, tied shoes, dressed without help. Does the parent believe this development has been normal? How does this child's development compare with that of siblings or peers?

Current Development (Children 1 Month Through Preschool). Gross motor skills (rolls over, sits alone, walks alone, skips, climbs), fine motor skills (inspects hands, brings hands to mouth, has pincer grasp, stacks blocks, feeds self, uses crayon to draw, uses scissors), language skills (vocalizes, first words with meaning, sentences, persistence of baby talk, speech problems), and personal-social skills (smiles, tracks movement with eyes to midline, past midline, attends to sound by turning head, recognizes own name). If the child is undergoing toilet training, indicate the method used, age of bladder/bowel control, parents' attitude toward toilet training, and terms used for toileting.

School-Age Child. Gross motor skills (runs, jumps, climbs, rides bicycle, general coordination), fine motor skills (ties shoelace, uses scissors, writes name and numbers, draws pictures), and language skills (vocabulary, verbal ability, able to tell time, reading level).

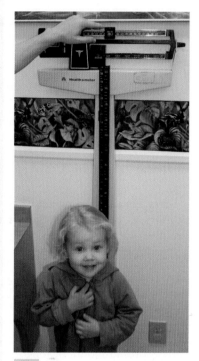

4-9

Nutritional History

The amount of nutritional information needed depends on the child's age; the younger the child, the more detailed and specific the data should be. For the infant, record whether breastfeeding or bottle-feeding. If the child is breastfed, record nursing frequency and duration, any supplements (vitamin, iron, fluoride, bottles), family support for nursing, and age and method of weaning. If the child is bottle-fed, record type of formula used, frequency and amount, any problems with feeding (spitting up, colic, diarrhea), and supplements used; discourage any bottle propping. Record introduction of solid foods (age when the child began eating solids, which foods, whether foods are home or commercially made, amount given, child's reaction to new food, parent's reaction to feeding).

For preschool and school-age children and adolescents, record the child's appetite, 24-hour diet recall (meals, snacks, amounts), vitamins taken, how much junk food is eaten, who eats with the child, food likes and dislikes, and parent's perception of child's nutrition.

A week-long diary of food intake may be more accurate than a spot 24-hour recall. Also consider cultural practices in assessing child's diet.

Family History

As with the adult, diagram a family tree for the child, including siblings, parents, and grandparents (see p. 53). Ask specifically for the family history of heart disease, high blood pressure, diabetes, blood disorders, cancer, sickle cell anemia, arthritis, allergies, obesity, cystic fibrosis, mental illness, seizure disorder, kidney disease, mental retardation, learning disabilities, birth defects, and sudden infant death. (When interviewing the mother, ask about the "child's father," not "your husband," in case of the separation of the child's biologic parents.)

Review of Systems

General. Significant gain or loss of weight, failure to gain weight appropriate for age, frequent colds, ear infections, illnesses, energy level, fatigue, overactivity, and behavioral change (irritability, increased crying, nervousness).

Skin. Birthmarks, skin disease, pigment or color change, mottling, change in mole, pruritus, rash, lesion, acne, easy bruising or petechiae, easy bleeding, and changes in hair or nails.

Head. Headache, head injury, dizziness.

Eyes. Strabismus, diplopia, pain, redness, discharge, cataracts, vision changes, reading problems. Is the child able to see the board at school? Does the child sit too close to the television?
Health Promotion. Use of eyeglasses, date of last vision screening.

Ears. Earaches, frequency of ear infections, myringotomy tubes in ears, discharge (characteristics), cerumen, ringing or crackling, and whether parent perceives any hearing problems.
Health Promotion. How does the child clean his or her ears?

Nose and Sinuses. Discharge and its characteristics, frequency of colds, nasal stuffiness, nosebleeds, and allergies.

Mouth and Throat. History of cleft lip or palate, frequency of sore throats, toothache, caries, sores in mouth or tongue, tonsils present, mouth breathing, difficulty chewing, difficulty swallowing, and hoarseness or voice change.
Health Promotion. Child's pattern of brushing teeth and last dental checkup.

Neck. Swollen or tender glands, limitation of movement, or stiffness.

Breast. For preadolescent and adolescent girl, when did she notice that her breasts were changing? What is the girl's self-perception of development? Does the female older adolescent perform breast self-examination? (See Chapter 17 for suggested phrasing of questions.)

Respiratory System. Croup or asthma, wheezing or noisy breathing, shortness of breath, chronic cough.

Cardiovascular System. Congenital heart problems, history of murmur, and cyanosis (what prompts this condition). Is there any limitation of activity, or can the child keep up with peers? Is there any dyspnea on exertion, palpitations, high blood pressure, or coldness in the extremities?

Gastrointestinal System. Abdominal pain, nausea and vomiting, history of ulcer, frequency of bowel movements, stool color and characteristics, diarrhea, constipation or stool holding, rectal bleeding, anal itching, history of pinworms, and use of laxatives.

Urinary System. Painful urination, polyuria/oliguria, narrowed stream, urine color (cloudy, dark), history of urinary tract infection, whether toilet trained, when toilet training was planned, any problems, bed-wetting (when the child started, frequency, associated with stress, how child feels about it).

Male Genital System. Penile or testicular pain, whether told if testes are descended, any sores or lesions, discharge, hernia or hydrocele, or swelling in scrotum during crying. Has the preadolescent or adolescent boy noticed any change in the penis and scrotum? Is the boy familiar with normal growth patterns, nocturnal emissions, and sex education? Screen for sexual abuse. (See Chapter 24 for suggested phrasing of questions.)

Female Genital System. Has the girl noted any genital itching, rash, vaginal discharge? For the preadolescent and adolescent girl, when did menstruation start? Was she prepared? Screen for sexual abuse. (See Chapter 26 for suggested phrasing of questions.)

Sexual Health. What is the child's attitude toward the opposite sex? Who provides sex education? How does the family deal with sex education, masturbation, dating patterns? Is the adolescent in a relationship involving intercourse? Does he or she have information on birth control and sexually transmitted infections? (See Chapters 24 and 26 for suggested phrasing of questions.)

Musculoskeletal System. In bones and joints: arthritis, joint pain, stiffness, swelling, limitation of movement, gait strength and coordination. In muscles: pain, cramps, and weakness. In the back: pain, posture, spinal curvature, and any treatment.

Neurologic System. Numbness and tingling. (Behavioral and cognitive issues are covered in the sections on development and interpersonal relationships.)

Hematologic Systems. Excessive bruising, lymph node swelling, and exposure to toxic agents or radiation.

Endocrine System. History of diabetes or thyroid disease; excessive hunger, thirst, or urinating; abnormal hair distribution; and precocious or delayed puberty.

Functional Assessment (Including Activities of Daily Living)

Interpersonal Relationships. Within the family constellation, record the child's position in family; whether the child is adopted; who lives with the child; who is the primary caregiver; who is the caregiver if both parents work outside the home; any support from relatives, neighbors, or friends; and the ethnic or cultural milieu.

Indicate family cohesion. Does the family enjoy activities as a unit? Has there been a recent family change or crisis (death, divorce, move)? Record information on child's self-image and level of independence. Does the child use a security blanket or toy? Is there any repetitive behavior (bed-rocking, head-banging), pica, thumb-sucking, or nail-biting? Note method of discipline used. Indicate type used at home. How effective is it? Who disciplines the child? Is there any occurrence of negativism, temper tantrums, withdrawal, or aggressive behavior?

Provide information on the child's friends: whether the child makes friends easily. How does the child get along with friends? Does he or she play with same-age or older or younger children?

Activity and Rest. Record the child's play activities. Indicate amount of active and quiet play, outdoor play, time watching television, and special hobbies or activities. Record sleep and rest. Indicate pattern and number of hours at night and during the day and the child's routine at bedtime. Is the child a sound sleeper, or is he or she wakeful? Does the child have nightmares, night terrors, or somnambulation? How does the parent respond? Does the child have naps during the day?

Record school attendance. Any experience with daycare or nursery school? In what grade is the child in school? Has the child ever skipped a grade or been held back? Does the child seem to like school? What is his or her school performance? Are the parent and child satisfied with the performance? Were days missed in school? Provide a reason for the absence. (These questions give an important index to the child's functioning outside the home.)

Economic Status. Ask about the mother's and father's occupations. Indicate the number of hours each parent is away from home. Do parents perceive their income to be adequate? What is the effect of illness on financial status?

Home Environment. Where does family live (house, apartment)? Is the size of the home adequate? Is there access to an outdoor play area? Does the child share a room, have his or her own bed, and have toys appropriate for his or her age?

Environmental Hazards. Inquire about home safety (precautions for poisons, medications, household products, presence of gates for stairways, and safe yard equipment). Inquire about the home structure (adequate heating, ventilation, bathroom facilities), neighborhood (residential or industrial, age of neighbors, safe play areas, playmates available, distance to school, amount of traffic, whether area remote or congested and overcrowded, if crime is a problem, presence of air or water pollution), and automobile (child safety seat, seatbelts).

Coping/Stress Management. Is the child able to adapt to new situations? Record recent stressful experiences (death, divorce, move, loss of special friend). How does the child cope with stress? Any recent change in behavior or mood? Has counseling ever been sought?

Habits. Has the child ever tried cigarette smoking? How much did he or she smoke? Has the child ever tried alcohol? How much alcohol did he or she drink weekly or daily? Has the child ever tried other drugs (marijuana, cocaine, amphetamines, barbiturates)?

Health Promotion. Who is the primary health care provider? When was the child's last checkup? Who is the dental care provider and when was the last dental checkup? Provide date and result of screening for vision, hearing, urinalysis, phenylketonuria, hematocrit, TB skin test, sickle cell trait, blood lead, and other tests specific for high-risk populations.

The Adolescent

This section presents a psychosocial review of symptoms intended to maximize communication with youth. The **HEEADSSS** method of interviewing focuses on assessment of the **H**ome environment, **E**ducation and employment, **E**ating, peer-related **A**ctivities, **D**rugs, **S**exuality, **S**uicide/depression, and **S**afety from injury and violence (Fig. 4-10). The tool minimizes adolescent stress because it moves from expected and less-threatening questions to those that are more personal. It presents the questions in three colors: green are considered essential to explore with every adolescent; blue are important for you to ask if time permits; red questions delve more deeply if the situation demands it.[10] Interview the youth alone while the parent waits outside and fills out past health questionnaires.

In addition ask, "How many hours of sleep do you get on most nights of the week? What time do you actually go to bed? What time do you wake up on school days? What time would you wake up if left alone? Which activities are you in at or after school? Do your activities change the time that you go to bed or get up in the morning?"[8] Note that teens need about 9 hours of sleep per night, yet most U.S. teens get far less than that. Older teens report < 6.5 to 7 hours per night; younger teens report 7.7 hours per night.[8]

Ask about driving; stress the importance of keeping hands on the wheel and paying attention to the road. Evidence shows the risk of crash increases significantly among novice drivers when they perform secondary tasks (e.g., dialing or reaching for a cell phone, texting, eating, reaching for another object, looking at a roadside object).[12a]

The HEEADSSS Psychosocial Interview for Adolescents

Home

Who lives with you? Where do you live? Do you have your own room?
What are relationships like at home?
To whom are you closest at home?
To whom can you talk at home?
Is there anyone new at home? Has someone left recently?
Have you moved recently?
Have you ever had to live away from home? (Why?)
Have you ever run away? (Why?)
Is there any physical violence at home?

Education and Employment

What are your favorite subjects at school? Your least favorite subjects?
How are your grades? Any recent changes? Any dramatic changes in the past?
Have you changed schools in the past few years?
What are your future education/employment plans/goals?
Are you working? Where? How much?
Tell me about your friends at school.
Is your school a safe place? (Why?)
Have you ever had to repeat a class? Have you ever had to repeat a grade?
Have you ever been suspended? Expelled? Have you ever considered dropping out?
How well do you get along with the people at school? Work?
Have your responsibilities at work increased?
Do you feel connected to your school? Do you feel as if you belong?
Are there adults at school you feel you could talk to about something important? (Who?)

Eating

What do you like and not like about your body?
Have there been any recent changes in your weight?
Have you dieted in the past year? How? How often?
Have you done anything else to try to manage your weight?
How much exercise do you get in an average day? Week?
What do you think would be a healthy diet? How does that compare with your current eating patterns?
Do you worry about your weight? How often?
Do you eat in front of the TV? Computer?
Does it ever seem as though your eating is out of control?
Have you ever made yourself throw up on purpose to control your weight?
Have you ever taken diet pills?
What would it be like if you gained (lost) 10 pounds?

Activities

What do you and your *friends* do for fun? (with whom, where, and when?)
What do you and your *family* do for fun? (with whom, where, and when?)
Do you participate in any sports or other activities?
Do you regularly attend a church group, club, or other organized activity?
Do you have any hobbies?
Do you read for fun? (What?)
How much TV do you watch in a week? How about video games?
What music do you like to listen to?

Drugs

Do any of your friends use tobacco? Alcohol? Other drugs?
Does anyone in your family use tobacco? Alcohol? Other drugs?
Do you use tobacco? Alcohol? Other drugs?
Is there any history of alcohol or drug problems in your family?
Do you ever drink or use drugs when you're alone?
(Assess frequency, intensity, patterns of use or abuse, and how youth obtains or pays for drugs, alcohol, or tobacco.)

Sexuality

Have you ever been in a romantic relationship?
Tell me about the people that you've dated. *OR* Tell me about your sex life.
Have any of your relationships ever been sexual relationships?
Are your sexual activities enjoyable?
What does the term "safer sex" mean to you?
Are you interested in boys? Girls? Both?
Have you ever been forced or pressured into doing something sexual that you didn't want to do?
Have you ever been touched sexually in a way that you didn't want?
Have you ever been raped, on a date or any other time?
How many sexual partners have you had altogether?
Have you ever been pregnant or worried that you may be pregnant? (females)
Have you ever gotten someone pregnant or worried that that might have happened? (males)
What are you using for birth control? Are you satisfied with your method?
Do you use condoms every time you have intercourse?
Does anything ever get in the way of always using a condom?
Have you ever had a sexually transmitted infection (STI) or worried that you had an STI?

Suicide and Depression

Do you feel sad or down more than usual? Do you find yourself crying more than usual?
Are you "bored" all the time?
Are you having trouble getting to sleep?
Have you thought a lot about hurting yourself or someone else?
Does it seem that you've lost interest in things that you used to really enjoy?
Do you find yourself spending less and less time with friends?
Would you rather just be by yourself most of the time?
Have you ever tried to kill yourself?
Have you ever had to hurt yourself (by cutting yourself, for example) to calm down or feel better?
Have you started using alcohol or drugs to help you relax, calm down, or feel better?

Safety (Savagery)

Have you ever been seriously injured? (How?) How about anyone else you know?
Do you always wear a seatbelt in the car?
Have you ever ridden with a driver who was drunk or high? When? How often?
Do you use safety equipment for sports and/or other physical activities (e.g., helmets for biking or skateboarding)?
Is there any violence in your home? Does the violence ever get physical?
Is there a lot of violence at your school? In your neighborhood? Among your friends?
Have you ever been physically or sexually abused? Have you ever been raped, on a date or at any other time? (If not asked previously)
Have you ever been in a car or motorcycle accident? (What happened?)
Have you ever been picked on or bullied? Is that still a problem?
Have you gotten into physical fights in school or your neighborhood? Are you still getting into fights?
Have you ever felt that you had to carry a knife, gun, or other weapon to protect yourself? Do you still feel that way?

Green = essential questions
Blue = as time permits
Red = optional or when situation requires

4-10

(Goldenring, 2004.)

BIBLIOGRAPHY

1. Advisory Committee on Immunization Practices (ACIP). (2013). Recommended immunization schedule for adults aged 19 years and older—United States, 2013. *MMWR, 62,* 9-18.

2. Baker, D., & Niederhauser, V. (2012). Immunizations: how do your patients score? *Nurse Pract, 37*(11), 46-52.

2a. Blackwell, C. W. (2014). Vaccination guidelines for gay and bisexual men. *Nurse Pract, 39*(2):35-39.

2b. Carrico, C. A., & O'Keefe, C. (2013). Protecting infants against pertussis: the cocooning strategy. *Nurse Pract, 38*(3), 40-44.

3. Centers for Disease Control and Prevention (CDC). (2013). *Immunization schedules for health care professionals.* Available at http://www.cdc.gov/vaccines/schedules/index.html.

4. Diekema, D. S. (2012). Improving childhood vaccination rates. *N Engl J Med 366*(5), 391-393.

5. Dreneth-van Maanen, C., Spee, J., van Hensbergen, L., et al. (2011). Structured history taking of medication use reveals iatrogenic harm due to discrepancies in medication histories in hospital and pharmacy records. *J Am Geriatr Soc, 59*(10), 1976-1977.

6. Ewing, J. A. (1984). Detecting alcoholism: the CAGE questionnaire. *JAMA, 252,* 1905-1907.

7. Garzon, D. L., Kempker, T., & Piel, P. (2011). Primary care management of food allergy and food intolerance. *Nurse Pract, 36*(12), 34-40.

8. George, N. M, & Davis, J. E. (2013). Assessing sleep in adolescents through a better understanding of sleep physiology. *Am J Nurs, 113*(6), 26-32.

9. Gerlock, A. A., Grimesey, J. L., Pisciotta, A. K., et al. (2011). Ask a few more questions (intimate partner violence). *Am J Nurs, 111*(11), 35-39.

10. Goldenring, J. M., & Rosen, D. S. (2004). Getting into adolescent heads: an essential update. *Contemp Pediatr, 21*(1), 64-75.

11. Gordon, M. (2009). *Manual of nursing diagnosis* (12th ed.). Burlington: Jones Bartlett.

12. Holcomb, S. S. (2009). Common herb drug interactions. *Nurse Pract, 34*(5), 21-29.

12a. Klauer, S. G., Gue, F., Simmons-Morton, B. G., et al. (2014). Distracted driving and risk of road crashes among novice and experienced drivers. *N Engl J Med 370*(1):54-58.

12b. Lehne, R. A. (2013). *Pharmacology for nursing care* (8th ed.). St. Louis: Saunders.

13. Matthews, R., & Moore, A. (2013). Babies are still dying of SIDS. *Am J Nurs, 113*(2), 59-64.

14. Merchant, N., & Waldrop, J. (2012). The safety advantages of pentavalent vaccines. *Nurse Pract, 37*(4), 48-53.

15. Post, S. G., Puchalski, C. M., Larson, D. B., et al. (2000). Physician and patient spirituality: professional boundaries, competency, and ethics. *Ann Intern Med, 132,* 578-583.

16. Qureshi, N., Armstrong, S., Dhiman, P., et al. (2012). Effect of adding systematic family history enquiry to cardiovascular disease risk assessment in primary care. *Ann Intern Med, 156*:253-262.

17. Schuster, M. A., Elliott, M. N., & Kanouse, D. E. (2012). Racial and ethnic health disparities among fifth-graders in three cities. *N Engl J Med, 367*(8), 735-744.

18. Simon, M. A., Ragas, D. M., Nonzee, N. J., et al. (2013). Perceptions of patient-provider communication in breast and cervical cancer-related care. *J Commun Health 38,* 700-715.

19. Zurakowski, T. (2009). The practicalities and pitfalls of polypharmacy. *Nurse Pract, 34*(4), 36-41.

CHAPTER 5

Mental Status Assessment

http://evolve.elsevier.com/Jarvis/

STRUCTURE AND FUNCTION

5-1

DEFINING MENTAL STATUS

Mental status is a person's emotional (feeling) and cognitive (knowing) function. Optimal functioning aims toward simultaneous life satisfaction in work, in caring relationships, and within the self (Fig. 5-1). Mental health is "a state of well-being in which every individual realizes his or her own potential, can cope with normal stresses of life, can work productively and fruitfully, and is able to make a contribution to her or his community."[26,38] Mental health is relative and ongoing. Everyone has "good" days and "bad" days. We all have days when we feel anxious or depressed or feel as if we cannot cope. Usually these feelings migrate and we return to healthy function socially and occupationally.

The stress surrounding a traumatic life event (death of a loved one, serious illness) tips the balance, causing transient dysfunction. This is an expected response to a trauma. For example, grieving after the death of a loved one is painful, but it is a normal and expected emotional response to major loss.[13] Most grieving people feel sadness, tearfulness, loss of appetite, and insomnia; these feelings last 2 to 6 months. The survivor needs social support but no medical treatment.

Mental status assessment during a traumatic life event can identify remaining strengths and help the individual mobilize resources and use coping skills.

A **mental disorder** is apparent when a person's response is much greater than the expected reaction to a traumatic life event. It is a clinically significant behavioral, emotional, or cognitive *syndrome* that is associated with significant distress (a painful symptom) or disability (impaired functioning) involving social, occupational, or key activities.[3a] For example, major depression has feelings that are unrelenting or include delusional or suicidal thinking, feelings of low self-esteem or worthlessness, or loss of ability to function.[13]

Mental disorders include **organic disorders** (caused by brain disease of *known* specific organic cause [e.g., delirium, dementia, alcohol and drug intoxication, and withdrawal]) and **psychiatric mental disorders** (in which an organic etiology has not yet been established [e.g., anxiety disorder or schizophrenia]). Mental status assessment documents a dysfunction and determines how that dysfunction affects self-care in everyday life.

Mental status cannot be scrutinized directly like the characteristics of skin or heart sounds. Its functioning is *inferred* through assessment of an individual's behaviors:

Consciousness: Being aware of one's own existence, feelings, and thoughts and of the environment. This is the most elementary of mental status functions.

Language: Using the voice to communicate one's thoughts and feelings. This is a basic tool of humans, and its loss has a heavy social impact on the individual.

Mood and affect: Both of these elements deal with the prevailing feelings. **Affect** is a temporary expression of feelings or state of mind, and **mood** is more durable, a prolonged display of feelings that color the whole emotional life.

Orientation: The awareness of the objective world in relation to the self. Able to name own person, place, and time.

Attention: The power of concentration, the ability to focus on one specific thing without being distracted by many environmental stimuli.

Memory: The ability to lay down and store experiences and perceptions for later recall. *Recent* memory evokes day-to-day events; *remote* memory brings up years' worth of experiences.

Abstract reasoning: Pondering a deeper meaning beyond the concrete and literal.

Thought process: The *way* a person thinks; the logical train of thought.

Thought content: *What* the person thinks—specific ideas, beliefs, the use of words.

Perceptions: An awareness of objects through the five senses.

⬧ DEVELOPMENTAL COMPETENCE

Infants and Children

Emotional and cognitive functioning mature progressively from simple reflex behavior into complex logical and abstract thought. It is difficult to separate and trace the development of just one aspect of mental status. All aspects are interdependent. For example, consciousness is rudimentary at birth because the cerebral cortex is not yet developed; the infant cannot distinguish the self from the mother's body. Consciousness gradually develops along with language so that, by 18 to 24 months, the child learns that he or she is separate from objects in the environment and has words to express this. We also can trace language development: from the differentiated crying at 4 weeks, the cooing at 6 weeks, through one-word sentences at 1 year, to multiword sentences at 2 years. The concept of language as a social tool of communication occurs around 4 to 5 years of age, coincident with the child's readiness to play cooperatively with other children.

Attention gradually increases in span through preschool years so that by school age most children are able to sit and concentrate on their work for a period of time. Some children are late in developing concentration. School readiness coincides with the development of the thought process; around age 7 years thinking becomes more logical and systematic, and the child is able to reason and understand. Abstract thinking, the ability to consider a hypothetical situation, usually develops between ages 12 and 15 years, although a few adolescents never achieve it.

The Centers for Disease Control and Prevention (CDC) estimates "that 13% to 20% of children living in the United States (up to 1 of 5 children) experience a mental disorder in a given year."[8] A childhood mental disorder is one that is diagnosed and begins in childhood (e.g., attention-deficit/hyperactivity disorder [ADHD]), behavioral or conduct problems, anxiety, depression, autism spectrum disorders). Adolescents ages 12 to 17 years also experience illicit drug use or alcohol use disorder and cigarette dependence. These disorders present as "serious changes in the ways children typically learn, behave, or handle their emotions."[8] These disorders can interact with other factors, resulting in suicide, the second leading cause of death among adolescents ages 12 to 17 years.[9]

The Aging Adult

The aging process leaves the parameters of mental status mostly intact. There is no decrease in general knowledge and little or no loss in vocabulary. Response time is slower than in youth; it takes a bit longer for the brain to process information and react to it. Thus performance on timed intelligence tests may be lower for the aging person—not because intelligence has declined, but because it takes longer to respond to the questions. The slower response time affects new learning; if a new presentation is rapidly paced, the older person does not have time to respond to it.[30]

Recent memory, which requires some processing (e.g., medication instructions, 24-hour diet recall, names of new acquaintances), is somewhat decreased with aging. Remote memory is not affected.

Age-related changes in sensory perception can affect mental status. For example, vision loss (as detailed in Chapter 14) may result in apathy, social isolation, and depression. Hearing changes are common in older adults (see the discussion of presbycusis in Chapter 15). Age-related hearing loss involves high-frequency sounds. Consonants are high-frequency sounds; therefore older people who have difficulty hearing them have problems with normal conversation. This problem produces frustration, suspicion, and social isolation and makes the person look confused.

The era of older adulthood contains more potential for loss (e.g., loss of loved ones, job status and prestige, income, and an energetic and resilient body) than do earlier eras. In addition, living with chronic diseases (heart failure, cancer, diabetes, osteoporosis) includes the fear of loss of life itself. The grief and despair surrounding these losses can affect mental status. The losses can result in disorientation, disability, or depression.

In a given year mental disorders affect an estimated 26.2% of U.S. adults ages 18 years and older.[20] A smaller group, approximately 6%, suffers a serious mental illness. In addition, almost half of adults (45%) with any mental disorder meet the criteria for two or more disorders.[20] The global impact of mental illness is enormous, with an estimated 7.4% of the measurable burden of disease in the world.[4] The problem is lack of access to good-quality mental health services, both in the United States for poor, homeless, uninsured, or underinsured people and in the rest of the world for low- and middle-income countries.

COMPONENTS OF THE MENTAL STATUS EXAMINATION

The full mental status examination is a systematic check of emotional and cognitive functioning. However, the steps described here rarely need to be taken in their entirety. Usually you can assess mental status through the context of the health history interview. During that time keep in mind the four main headings of mental status assessment:

**Appearance, Behavior, Cognition,
and Thought processes,
or A, B, C, T**

Integrating the mental status examination into the health history interview is sufficient for most people. You will collect ample data to be able to assess mental health strengths and coping skills and to screen for any dysfunction.

It is necessary to perform a full mental status examination when you discover any abnormality in affect or behavior and in the following situations:

- Patients whose initial brief screening suggests an anxiety disorder or depression.
- Family members concerned about a person's behavioral changes such as memory loss or inappropriate social interaction.
- Brain lesions (trauma, tumor, stroke). A mental status assessment documents any emotional or cognitive change associated with the lesion. Not recognizing these changes hinders care planning and creates problems with social readjustment.
- Aphasia (the impairment of language ability secondary to brain damage). A mental status examination assesses language dysfunction and any emotional problems associated with it such as depression or agitation.
- Symptoms of psychiatric mental illness, especially with acute onset.

In every mental status examination, note these factors from the health history that could affect your interpretation of the findings:

- Any known illnesses or health problems such as alcohol use disorders or chronic renal disease
- Current medications with side effects that may cause confusion or depression
- The usual educational and behavioral level—note that factor as the normal baseline and do not expect performance on the mental status examination to exceed it
- Responses to personal history questions indicating current stress, social interaction patterns, sleep habits, drug and alcohol use

In the following examination the sequence of steps forms a *hierarchy* in which the most basic functions (consciousness, language) are assessed first. The first steps must be assessed accurately to ensure validity for the steps to follow (i.e., if consciousness is clouded, the person cannot be expected to have full attention and to cooperate with new learning). Or if language is impaired, subsequent assessment of new learning or abstract reasoning (anything that requires language functioning) can give erroneous conclusions.

OBJECTIVE DATA

Objective Data

EQUIPMENT NEEDED
(Occasionally)
Pencil, paper, reading material

Normal Range of Findings	Abnormal Findings

Appearance

Posture. *Posture* is erect, and *position* is relaxed.

Sitting on edge of chair or curled in bed, tense muscles, frowning, darting and watchful eyes, and restless pacing occur with anxiety and hyperthyroidism. Sitting slumped in chair, slow walk, dragging feet occur with depression and some organic brain diseases.

Body Movements. *Body movements* are voluntary, deliberate, coordinated, and smooth and even.

Restless, fidgety movement or hyperkinetic appearance occurs with anxiety.
Apathy and psychomotor slowing occur with depression and dementia.
Abnormal posturing and bizarre gestures occur with schizophrenia.
Facial grimaces.

Dress. *Dress* is appropriate for setting, season, age, gender, and social group. Clothing fits and is worn appropriately.

Inappropriate dress can occur with organic brain syndrome.
Eccentric dress combination and bizarre makeup occur with schizophrenia or manic syndrome.

Normal Range of Findings	Abnormal Findings
Grooming and Hygiene. The person is clean and well groomed; hair is neat and clean; women have moderate or no makeup; men are shaved, or beard or mustache is well groomed. Nails are clean (although some jobs leave nails chronically dirty). NOTE: A disheveled appearance in a previously well-groomed person is significant. Use care in interpreting clothing that is disheveled, bizarre, or in poor repair; piercings; and tattoos because these sometimes reflect the person's economic status or a deliberate fashion trend (especially among adolescents).	Unilateral neglect (total inattention to one side of body) occurs following some strokes. Inappropriate dress, poor hygiene, and lack of concern with appearance occur with depression and severe Alzheimer disease. Meticulously dressed and groomed appearance and fastidious manner may occur with obsessive-compulsive disorders.

Behavior

Level of Consciousness. The person is awake, alert, and aware of stimuli from the environment and within the self and responds appropriately and reasonably soon to stimuli.	Loses track of conversation, falls asleep. Lethargic (drowsy), obtunded (confused) (see Table 5-1, Levels of Consciousness, p. 79).
Facial Expression. The look is appropriate to the situation and changes appropriately with the topic. There is comfortable eye contact unless precluded by cultural norm.	Flat, masklike expression occurs with parkinsonism and depression.
Speech. Judge the quality of speech by noting that the person makes laryngeal sounds effortlessly and shares conversation appropriately.	Dysphonia is abnormal volume, pitch (see Table 5-2, Speech Disorders, p. 80). Monopolizes interview. Silent, secretive, or uncommunicative.
The pace of the conversation is moderate, and stream of talking is fluent.	Slow, monotonous speech with parkinsonism, depression. Rapid-fire, pressured, and loud talking occurs with manic syndrome.
Articulation (ability to form words) is clear and understandable.	Dysarthria is distorted speech (see Table 5-2). Misuses words; omits letters, syllables, or words; transposes words; occurs with aphasia. Circumlocution, or repetitious abnormal patterns: neologism, echolalia (see Table 5-6, p. 84).
Word choice is effortless and appropriate to educational level. The person completes sentences, occasionally pausing to think.	Unduly long word-finding or failure in word search occurs with aphasia.
Mood and Affect. Judge this by body language and facial expression and by asking directly, "How do you feel today?" or "How do you usually feel?" The mood should be appropriate to the person's place and condition and change appropriately with topics. The person is willing to cooperate with you.	See Table 5-3, Mood and Affect Abnormalities, p. 81, and Table 5-5, Delirium, Dementia, and Depression, p. 83.

Cognitive Functions

Orientation. You can discern orientation through the course of the interview by asking about the person's address, phone number, and health history. Or ask for it directly, using tact, by saying, "Some people have trouble keeping up with the dates while in the hospital. Do you know today's date?" Assess:

Objective Data

Normal Range of Findings	Abnormal Findings

Time: Day of week, date, year, season
Place: Where person lives, present location, type of building, name of city and state
Person: Own name, age, who examiner is, type of worker

Many hospitalized people normally have trouble with the exact date but are fully oriented on the remaining items.

Disorientation occurs with delirium and dementia. Orientation is usually lost in this order: first to time, then to place, and rarely to person.

Attention Span. Check the person's ability to concentrate by noting whether he or she completes a thought without wandering. Note any distractibility or difficulty attending to you. Or give a series of directions to follow and note the correct sequence of behaviors, such as, "Please take this glass of water with your left hand, drink from it, shift it to your right hand, and set it on the table." Note that attention span commonly is impaired in people who are anxious, fatigued, or drug intoxicated.

Digression from initial thought. Irrelevant replies to questions. Easily distracted; "stimulus bound" (i.e., any new stimulus quickly draws attention). Confusion, negativism.

Recent Memory. Assess recent memory in the context of the interview by the 24-hour diet recall or by asking the time the person arrived at the agency. Ask questions you can corroborate. This screens for the occasional person who confabulates or makes up answers to fill in the gaps of memory loss.

Recent memory deficit occurs with delirium, dementia, amnestic syndrome, or Korsakoff syndrome in chronic alcoholism.

Remote Memory. In the context of the interview, ask the person verifiable past events (e.g., ask to describe past health, the first job, birthday and anniversary dates, and historical events that are relevant for that person).

Remote memory is lost when cortical storage area for that memory is damaged (e.g., Alzheimer dementia or any disease that damages the cerebral cortex).

New Learning—The Four Unrelated Words Test. This tests the person's ability to lay down new memories. It is a highly sensitive and valid memory test. It requires more effort than does the recall of personal or historic events. It also avoids the danger of unverifiable material.

To the person, say, "I am going to say four words. I want you to remember them. In a few minutes I will ask you to recall them." To be sure the person has understood, have the words repeated. Pick four words with semantic and phonetic diversity:

1. brown	1. fun
2. honesty	2. carrot
3. tulip	3. ankle
4. eyedropper	4. loyalty

After 5 minutes ask for the recall of the four words. To test the duration of memory, ask for a recall at 10 minutes and at 30 minutes. The normal response for people younger than 60 years is an accurate three- or four-word recall after a 5-, 10-, and 30-minute delay.[33a]

People with Alzheimer dementia score a zero- or one-word recall. Impaired new learning ability also occurs with anxiety (because of inattention and distractibility) and depression (because of lack of effort mobilized to remember).

Additional Testing for Persons with Aphasia

Word Comprehension. Point to articles in the room, parts of the body, or articles from pockets and ask the person to name them.

Reading. Ask the person to read available print. Be aware that reading is related to educational level. Use caution that you are not just testing literacy.

Aphasia is the loss of the ability to speak or write coherently or to understand speech or writing as a result of a stroke (see Table 5-2, p. 80).

Writing. Ask the person to make up and write a sentence. Note coherence, spelling, and parts of speech (the sentence should have a subject and a verb).

Reading and writing are important in planning health teaching and rehabilitation.

Objective Data

Normal Range of Findings	Abnormal Findings

Thought Processes and Perceptions

Thought Processes. Ask yourself, "Does this person make sense? Can I follow what the person is saying?" The *way* a person thinks should be logical, goal directed, coherent, and relevant. The person should complete a thought.

Illogical, unrealistic thought processes. Digression from initial thought. Ideas run together. Evidence of blocking (person stops in middle of thought) (see Table 5-6, Thought Process Abnormalities, p. 84).

Thought Content. *What* the person says should be consistent and logical.

Obsessions, compulsions (see Table 5-7, Thought Content Abnormalities).

Perceptions. The person should be consistently aware of reality. The perceptions should be congruent with yours. Ask the following questions:
- How do people treat you?
- Do other people talk about you?
- Do you feel like you are being watched, followed, or controlled?
- Is your imagination very active?
- Have you heard your name when alone?

Illusions, hallucinations (see Table 5-8, Perception Abnormalities, p. 85). Auditory and visual hallucinations occur with psychiatric and organic brain disease and psychedelic drugs. Tactile hallucinations occur with alcohol withdrawal.

Screen for Anxiety Disorders. Anxiety and depression are the two most common mental health problems seen in people seeking general medical care. Anxiety disorders are common, disabling, and often untreated. However, you can screen for core anxiety symptoms by asking the first two questions from the 7-item generalized anxiety disorder (GAD) scale listed in Fig. 5-2.[19b] Scores on this GAD subscale range from 0 to 6; a score of 0 suggests that no anxiety disorder is present.

The four most common anxiety disorders: GAD, panic disorder, social anxiety disorder, posttraumatic stress disorder (PTSD) (see Table 5-4, Anxiety Disorders, p. 82).

GAD-7

Over the last 2 weeks, how often have you been bothered by the following problems?	Not at all	Several days	More than half the days	Nearly every day
1. Feeling nervous, anxious, or on edge	0	1	2	3
2. Not being able to stop or control worrying	0	1	2	3
3. Worrying too much about different things	0	1	2	3
4. Trouble relaxing	0	1	2	3
5. Being so restless that it is hard to sit still	0	1	2	3
6. Becoming easily annoyed or irritable	0	1	2	3
7. Feeling afraid as if something awful might happen	0	1	2	3

Total score ____ = Add columns ____ + ____ + ____

If you checked off any problems, how difficult have these problems made it for you to do your work, take care of things at home, or get along with other people?

Not difficult at all	Somewhat difficult	Very difficult	Extremely difficult
☐	☐	☐	☐

5-2 Screen for anxiety symptoms.   (Kroenke, 2007.)

Objective Data

Normal Range of Findings

If these first two items yield positive results, Kroenke et al. suggest following with the other five items. The full scale identifies probable presentations of GAD and also is a severity measure in that increasing scores are associated with increasing impairment and disability.

Screen for Depression. Many formal screening tools are available. However, a shorter method is the Patient Health Questionnaire-2 (PHQ-2), which entails asking two simple questions about depressed mood and anhedonia (little interest or pleasure in doing things) that will detect a majority of depressed patients. Thus you can ask: "Over the past 2 weeks have you felt down, depressed, or hopeless?" and "Over the past 2 weeks, have you felt little interest or pleasure in doing things?"[6]

The PHQ-2 works as a screening tool for depression, and it measures the severity of depression. If the person answers "several days" or higher, proceed with the rest of the nine questions of the PHQ-9[19a] (Fig. 5-3). Add the totals for each of the three columns together to obtain the severity score. If question 10 is answered "somewhat difficult" or greater, it indicates functional impairment.

Abnormal Findings

A score of 10 on the GAD-7 identifies GAD; scores of 5, 10, and 15 represent mild, moderate, and severe levels of anxiety.

Finding positive answers to these questions then requires further diagnostic tools to assess specific depressive disorders (see Table 5-5).

PHQ-9 scores: 5 to 9 = minimal symptoms; if present ≥2 years, it = chronic depression. Scores of 10 to 14 = minor depression; 15 to 19 = major depression, moderately severe; ≥20 = major depression, severe. Note treatment recommendations for each score in the complete tool.[19a]

PATIENT HEALTH QUESTIONNAIRE-9 (PHQ-9)

Over the last 2 weeks, how often have you been bothered by any of the following problems? (Use "✓" to indicate your answer)	Not at all	Several days	More than half the days	Nearly every day
1. Little interest or pleasure in doing things	0	1	2	3
2. Feeling down, depressed, or hopeless	0	1	2	3
3. Trouble falling or staying asleep, or sleeping too much	0	1	2	3
4. Feeling tired or having little energy	0	1	2	3
5. Poor appetite or overeating	0	1	2	3
6. Feeling bad about yourself — or that you are a failure or have let yourself or your family down	0	1	2	3
7. Trouble concentrating on things, such as reading the newspaper or watching television	0	1	2	3
8. Moving or speaking so slowly that other people could have noticed? Or the opposite — being so fidgety or restless that you have been moving around a lot more than usual	0	1	2	3
9. Thoughts that you would be better off dead or of hurting yourself in some way	0	1	2	3

FOR OFFICE CODING _0_ + ___ + ___ + ___

=Total Score: ___

If you checked off any problems, how difficult have these problems made it for you to do your work, take care of things at home, or get along with other people?

Not difficult at all	Somewhat difficult	Very difficult	Extremely difficult
☐	☐	☐	☐

5-3

Objective Data

Normal Range of Findings	Abnormal Findings

Screen for Suicidal Thoughts. When a person expresses feelings of sadness, hopelessness, despair, or grief, it is important to assess for any possible risk of physical harm to himself or herself. Begin with more general questions. If you hear affirmative answers, continue with more specific questions:

- Have you ever felt that life is not worth living?
- Have you ever felt so blue that you thought of hurting yourself?
- Do you feel like hurting yourself now?
- Do you have a plan to hurt yourself?
- How would you do it?
- What would happen if you were dead?
- How would other people react if you were dead?
- Whom could you tell if you felt like killing yourself?

It is very difficult, especially for beginning examiners, to question people about possible suicidal wishes. Examiners fear an invasion of privacy and may have their own normal denial of death and suicide. However, the risk is *far greater* if you skip these questions when you have the slightest clue that they are appropriate. You may be the only health professional to pick up clues of suicide risk. You are responsible for encouraging the person to talk about suicidal thoughts.

Depression is painful and debilitating, and sometimes a depressed person really wishes to kill himself or herself. However, most suicidal people are ambivalent, and for them you can buy time so they can be helped to find an alternate route to the stressful situation. Asking about suicidal thoughts does not increase suicidal behavior. Promptly share any concerns you have about a person's suicide ideation with a mental health professional.

Suicide is preventable, but it is the 10th leading cause of death in the United States and the 3rd leading cause among those ages 15 to 24 years. Between 20% and 33% of suicide victims test positive for alcohol, antidepressants, or opiates. Although females are more likely to have suicidal thoughts, males are 4 times more likely to commit suicide (most often by firearms).[7,21]

A precise suicide plan to take place in the next 24 to 48 hours using a lethal method constitutes high risk. Important clues and warning signs of suicide:

Prior suicide attempts
Depression, hopelessness
Firearms in the home
Family history of suicide
Incarceration
Family violence, including physical or sexual abuse
Self-mutilation
Anorexia
Verbal suicide messages (defeat, failure, worthlessness, loss, giving up, desire to kill self)
Death themes in art, jokes, writing, behaviors
Saying goodbye (giving away prized possessions)

Judgment

A person exercises judgment when he or she can compare and evaluate the alternatives in a situation and reach an appropriate course of action. You are interested in the person's judgment about daily or long-term life goals, the likelihood of acting in response to delusions or hallucinations, and the capacity for violent or suicidal behavior.

To assess judgment in the context of the interview, note what the person says about job plans, social or family obligations, and plans for the future. Job and future plans should be realistic, considering the person's health situation. In addition, ask the person to describe the rationale for personal health care and how he or she decided whether or not to comply with prescribed health regimens. The person's actions and decisions should be realistic.

Impaired judgment (unrealistic or impulsive decisions, wish fulfillment) occurs with mental retardation, emotional dysfunction, schizophrenia, and organic brain disease.

Supplemental Mental Status Examination

The Mini-Mental State Examination (MMSE) is a simplified scored form of the cognitive functions of the mental status examination (memory, orientation to time and place, naming, reading, copying or visuospatial orientation, writing, and the ability to follow a three-stage command). It requires paper and pencil; the person must be able to write and have no vision impairment. The MMSE is copyrighted and available for purchase from Psychological Assessment Resources, Inc.

The MMSE is used with caution with people with low education, who may have problems copying intersecting pentagons, spelling "world" backward, or performing serial 7s.[12]

Normal Range of Findings

The MMSE is quick and easy, includes a standard set of only 11 questions, and requires only 5 to 10 minutes to administer. It is useful for both initial and serial measurement; therefore you can demonstrate worsening or improvement of cognition over time and with treatment. It concentrates only on cognitive functioning, not on mood or thought processes. It is a valid detector of organic disease; thus it is a good screening tool to detect dementia and delirium and to differentiate these from psychiatric mental illness.

The maximum score on the test is 30; people with normal mental status average 27. Scores between 24 and 30 indicate no cognitive impairment.

❖ DEVELOPMENTAL COMPETENCE

Infants and Children
The mental status assessment of infants and children covers behavioral, cognitive, and psychosocial development and examines how the child is coping with his or her environment. Essentially you follow the same A-B-C-T guidelines as for the adult, with special consideration for developmental milestones. Your best examination "technique" arises from thorough knowledge of developmental milestones. Abnormalities are often problems of *omission*; the child does not achieve a milestone you would expect.

The parent's health history, especially the sections on the developmental history and personal history, yields most of the mental status data.

In addition, the **Denver II screening** test gives you a chance to interact directly with the young child to assess mental status. The Denver II is designed to detect developmental delays in infants and preschoolers within four functions: gross motor, language, fine motor–adaptive, and personal-social skills. For mental status assessment, the Denver II helps identify young children who may be slow in development in behavioral, language, cognitive, and psychosocial areas. The test has 125 items arranged in chronologic order and displayed in groupings corresponding to recommended ages for health maintenance visits.

As you talk to the parent, listen for signs of irritability in the child (i.e., overreacting to a stimulus, leading to excitability or anger). This is expected in a child who is ill with a medical condition. Some irritability also is expected in some developmental stages: (i.e., age 2 years and in adolescence as the teen struggles for independence).

For a list of common screen tools used for the pediatric population, please note websites in the bibliography.

For the adolescent, follow the same A-B-C-T guidelines as described for the adult. Keep your beginning questions open ended (i.e., how are things at school? At home? How about friends—anyone close?). Then you can ask more specific questions: Do you feel any extra stress or anxiety at school? At home? With friends? How about your parents—Do they think you act worried or anxious?

Abnormal Findings

Scores that occur with dementia and delirium are classified as follows: 18-23 = mild cognitive impairment; 0-7 = severe cognitive impairment.

Denver II scoring avoids diagnostic labeling (e.g., mental retardation, language disorder). Instead the child's performance is scored either "normal," "abnormal," or "questionable."

See Table 5-10, Childhood Mental Disorders, p. OO.

In children and teens note irritability that is more constant or obstructs performance in school or in social and family relationships.[37] Note that irritability is a common sign in four common mental health disorders in childhood: anxiety, depression, ADHD, oppositional defiant disorder (ODD), and autism spectrum disorders.[37]

Anxiety disorders are common in the teen years and are associated with GAD, social phobia, ADHD, PTSD (see Table 5-4, p. 82). In addition, anxiety and depression are seen together, two sides of a double-edged sword.

Objective Data

Normal Range of Findings	**Abnormal Findings**

The Aging Adult

It is important to conduct even a brief examination of all older people admitted to the hospital. Confusion is common in aging people and is easily misdiagnosed. Up to 25% of older adults are hospitalized with acute delirium, and up to 56% develop acute delirium during their hospitalization.[18a] Delirium is common following cardiac surgery (46%) and is noticeable as an initial decline in cognitive ability, with prolonged impairment lasting up to 1 year.[28] In comparison, 14.7% of U.S. adults over 70 years of age have dementia. At increased risk are racial or ethnic groups other than Whites, women, singles, those at an older age, people with a lower income level, and those with a lower educational level.[18]

Check sensory status before assessing any aspect of mental status. Vision and hearing changes caused by aging may alter alertness and leave the person looking confused. When older people cannot hear your questions, they may test worse than they actually are. Older people with mental health disorders test significantly better when wearing hearing aids.

Follow the same A-B-C-T guidelines as described for the younger adult with these *additional* considerations:

Behavior

Level of Consciousness. In a hospital or extended-care setting, the Glasgow Coma Scale (see Chapter 23) is a quantitative tool that is useful in testing consciousness in aging people in whom confusion is common. It gives a numeric value to the person's response in eye opening, best verbal response, and best motor response. This system avoids ambiguity when numerous examiners care for the same person.

Cognitive Functions

Orientation. Many aging persons experience social isolation, loss of structure without a job, a change in residence, or some short-term memory loss. These factors affect orientation, and this person may not provide the precise date or complete name of the agency. You may consider aging persons oriented if they know *generally* where they are and the present period (i.e., consider them oriented to time if the year and month are stated correctly). Orientation to place is accepted with the correct identification of the type of setting (e.g., the hospital) and the name of the town.

New Learning

In people of normal cognitive function, an age-related decline occurs in performance in the Four Unrelated Words Test described on p. 71. People in their 70s average two of four words recalled over 5 minutes. They will improve their performance at 10 and 30 minutes after being reminded by verbal cues (e.g., "one word was a color; a common flower in Holland is _____").

Supplemental Mental Status Examination

The Mini-Cog. Because the MMSE described earlier is available only by copyright, the Mini-Cog is a newly developed, reliable, quick, and easily available instrument to screen for cognitive impairment in otherwise healthy older adults (Fig. 5-4).[4b] It can be used with various language, culture, and literacy levels and takes only 3 to 5 minutes to administer.

Delirium is an acute confusional change or loss of consciousness and perceptual disturbance, may accompany acute illness (e.g., pneumonia, alcohol/drug intoxication), and is usually resolved when the underlying cause is treated.

In contrast, **dementia** is a gradual, progressive process, causing decreased cognitive function even though the person is fully conscious and awake; it is not reversible. Alzheimer disease accounts for about two thirds of cases of dementia in older adults (see Table 5-5). Dementia is not part of normal aging.

People with Alzheimer dementia do not improve their performance on subsequent trials.

Normal Range of Findings

Abnormal Findings

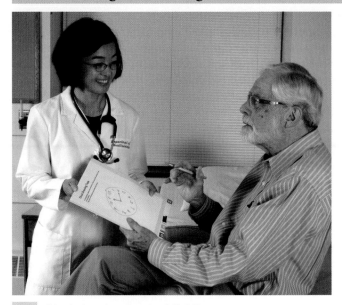

5-4   Clock drawing for the Mini-Cog.

The Mini-Cog consists of a 3-item recall test and a clock-drawing test. Begin by asking the older adult to listen carefully to, remember, and then repeat three words that you will say. Make sure that the person can hear you and that no distracting noises are present. Keep the words short and unrelated: "*Listen carefully, I am going to say three words. Say them back after I stop. Ready? Cup (pause), train (pause), blue. Now repeat those words to me. Good.*" Next give the adult a blank sheet of paper, saying, "*Now I want you to draw the face of a clock and write the numbers on the clock face. That's fine. Next I want you to draw the hands of the clock so it shows the time of 11:10.*" "*Remember the three words I told you earlier? Now I want you to repeat them.*"

The Mini-Cog tests the person's executive function, including the ability to plan, manage time, organize activities, and manage working memory.[10a] A person with no cognitive impairment or dementia can recall all three words and draw a complete, round, closed clock circle, with all face numbers present and in correct position and sequence and with the hour and minute hands indicating the time you requested.

Recalling 1 or 2 words indicates possible dementia; recalling none of the words indicates dementia. Drawing an abnormal clock (numbers misplaced, crowded, or out of sequence; short hour hand or long minute hand in wrong spot) indicates cognitive impairment.

DOCUMENTATION AND CRITICAL THINKING

Sample Charting

Appearance: Person's posture is erect, with no involuntary body movements. Dress and grooming are appropriate for season and setting.

Behavior: Person is alert, with appropriate facial expression and fluent, understandable speech. Affect and verbal responses are appropriate.

Cognitive functions: Oriented to time, person, place. Able to attend cooperatively with examiner. Recent and remote memory intact. Can recall four unrelated words at 5-, 10-, and 30-minute testing intervals. Future plans include returning home and to local university once individual therapy is established and medication is adjusted.

Thought processes: Perceptions and thought processes are logical and coherent. No suicide ideation.

Score on Mini-Mental State Examination is 28.

Clinical Case Study 1

L.P. is a 79-year-old married Caucasian woman, with a recent hospitalization for evaluation of increasing memory loss, confusion, and socially inappropriate behavior. Her family reports that Mrs. P.'s hygiene and grooming have decreased; she eats very little and has lost weight, does not sleep through the night, has angry emotional outbursts that are unlike her former demeanor, and does not recognize her younger grandchildren. Her husband reports that she has drifted away from the stove while cooking, allowing food to burn on the stovetop. He has found her wandering through the house in the middle of the night, unsure of where she was. She used to "talk on the phone for hours," but now he has to push her into conversations. During this hospitalization Mrs. P. has undergone a series of medical tests, including a negative lumbar puncture test, normal electroencephalogram (EEG), and a negative head computed tomography (CT) scan. Her physician now suggests a diagnosis of Alzheimer dementia.

Appearance: Sitting quietly, somewhat slumped, picking on loose threads on her dress. Hooded, zippered sweatshirt top worn over dress. Hair is gathered in loose ponytail with stray wisps. No makeup.

Behavior: Awake and gazing at hands and lap. Expression is flat and vacant. Will make eye contact when called by name, although gaze quickly shifts back to lap. Speech is a bit slow but articulate; some trouble with word choice.

Cognitive functions: Oriented to person and place. Can state the season but not the day of the week or the year. Is not able to repeat the correct sequence of complex directions involving lifting and shifting glass of water to the other hand. Scores a one-word recall on the Four Unrelated Words Test. Cannot tell examiner how she would plan a grocery shopping trip.

Thought processes: Experiences blocking in train of thought. Thought content is logical. Acts cranky and suspicious with family members. No suicide ideation.

Mini-Mental State Examination score is 17 and shows poor recall ability and marked difficulty with serial 7s.

ASSESSMENT

Chronic confusion
Impaired social interaction
Impaired memory
Wandering

Clinical Case Study 2

I.E. is a 64-year-old Caucasian man with chronic hypertension who was admitted to the hospital 3 days ago with acute coronary syndrome. He underwent coronary artery bypass surgery 2 days ago and has been in the ICU. His preoperative score on the Mini-Mental State Examination was 26.

Appearance Moves restlessly in hospital bed. Responds with quieting during family visits.

Behavior Restlessness increases during evening and night hours. Speech is incoherent and rambling.

Cognitive Function Oriented to own name but not to time, place. No memory of surgery or recent events. Wants to leave and "get back to the plant." Verbalizes that nurses are keeping him here against his will. "They are in it together." Unable to recall words on Four Unrelated Words Test. Believes "little bugs" are crawling up wall by his bed.

Thought Process Thought content is illogical. Experiences hallucinations. Appears angry and suspicious with nurses.

ASSESSMENT

Postoperative delirium
Acute confusion
Impaired memory

ABNORMAL FINDINGS

TABLE 5-1   Levels of Consciousness

These terms are commonly used in clinical practice. They spread over a continuum from full alertness to deep coma. The terms are qualitative and therefore are not always reliable. (A *quantitative* tool that serves the same purpose and eliminates ambiguity is the Glasgow Coma Scale in Chapter 23.) However, these terms are widely accepted and are useful as long as all co-workers agree on definitions and are consistent in their application. To increase clarity when using these terms, record also:

1. The level of stimulus used, ranging progressively from:
   a. Name called in normal tone of voice
   b. Name called in loud voice
   c. Light touch on person's arm
   d. Vigorous shake of shoulder
   e. Pain applied
2. The person's response
   a. Amount and quality of movement
   b. Presence and coherence of speech
   c. Opening of eyes and making eye contact
3. What the person does on cessation of your stimulus

(1) Alert

Awake or readily aroused; oriented, fully aware of external and internal stimuli and responds appropriately; conducts meaningful interpersonal interactions.

(2) Lethargic (or Somnolent)

Not fully alert; drifts off to sleep when not stimulated; can be aroused to name when called in normal voice but looks drowsy; responds appropriately to questions or commands but thinking seems slow and fuzzy; inattentive; loses train of thought; spontaneous movements are decreased.

(3) Obtunded

(Transitional state between lethargy and stupor; some sources omit this level.)
Sleeps most of time; difficult to arouse—needs loud shout or vigorous shake; acts confused when is aroused; converses in monosyllables; speech may be mumbled and incoherent; requires constant stimulation for even marginal cooperation.

(4) Stupor or Semi-Coma

Spontaneously unconscious; responds only to persistent and vigorous shake or pain; has appropriate motor response (i.e., withdraws hand to avoid pain); otherwise can only groan, mumble, or move restlessly; reflex activity persists.

(5) Coma

Completely unconscious; no response to pain or any external or internal stimuli (e.g., when suctioned, does not try to push the catheter away); light coma has some reflex activity but no purposeful movement; deep coma; has no motor response.

Delirium (Acute Confusional State)

Clouding of consciousness (dulled cognition, impaired alertness); inattentive; incoherent conversation; impaired recent memory and confabulatory for recent events; often agitated and having visual hallucinations; disoriented, with confusion worse at night when environmental stimuli are decreased.

Adapted from Strub, R. L., & Black, F. W. (2000). *Mental status examination in neurology.* (4th ed.). Philadelphia: Davis, with permission.

TABLE 5-2	Speech Disorders	
Condition	Disorder of	Description
Dysphonia	Voice	Difficulty or discomfort in talking, with abnormal pitch or volume, caused by laryngeal disease. Voice sounds hoarse or whispered, but articulation and language are intact.
Dysarthria	Articulation	Distorted speech sounds; speech may sound unintelligible; basic language (word choice, grammar, comprehension) intact.
Aphasia	Language comprehension and production secondary to brain damage	True language disturbance; defect in word choice and grammar or defect in comprehension; defect is in *higher* integrative language processing.

Types of Aphasia

An earlier dichotomy classified aphasias as *expressive* (difficulty producing language) or *receptive* (difficulty understanding language). Because all people with aphasia have some difficulty with expression, beginning examiners tend to classify them all as expressive. The following system is more descriptive.

Condition	Description
Global aphasia	The most common and severe form. Spontaneous speech is absent or reduced to a few stereotyped words or sounds. Comprehension is absent or reduced to only the person's own name and a few select words. Repetition, reading, and writing are severely impaired. Prognosis for language recovery is poor. Caused by a large lesion that damages most of combined anterior and posterior language areas.
Broca aphasia	Expressive aphasia. The person can understand language but cannot express himself or herself using language. This is characterized by nonfluent, dysarthric, and effortful speech. The speech is mostly nouns and verbs (high-content words) with few grammatic fillers, termed *agrammatic* or *telegraphic* speech. Repetition and reading aloud are severely impaired. Auditory and reading comprehensions are surprisingly intact. Lesion is in anterior language area called the *motor speech cortex* or *Broca area*.
Wernicke aphasia	Receptive aphasia. The linguistic opposite of Broca aphasia. The person can hear sounds and words but cannot relate them to previous experiences. Speech is fluent, effortless, and well articulated but has many paraphasias (word substitutions that are malformed or wrong) and neologisms (made-up words) and often lacks substantive words. Speech can be totally incomprehensible. Often there is a great urge to speak. Repetition, reading, and writing also are impaired. Lesion is in posterior language area called the *association auditory cortex* or *Wernicke area*.

(For a discussion of other types of aphasia [e.g., conduction, anomic, transcortical], please consult a neurology text.)

TABLE 5-3 Mood and Affect Abnormalities

Type of Mood or Affect	Definition	Clinical Example
Flat affect (blunted affect)	Lack of emotional response; no expression of feelings; voice monotonous and face immobile	Topic varies, expression does not
Depression	Sad, gloomy, dejected; symptoms may occur with rainy weather, after a holiday, or with an illness; if the situation is temporary, symptoms fade quickly	"I've got the blues."
Depersonalization (lack of ego boundaries)	Loss of identity, feels estranged, perplexed about own identity and meaning of existence	"I don't feel real." "I feel like I'm not really here."
Elation	Joy and optimism, overconfidence, increased motor activity; not necessarily pathologic	"I'm feeling very happy."
Euphoria	Excessive well-being; unusually cheerful or elated, which is inappropriate considering physical and mental condition; implies a pathologic mood	"I'm high." "I feel like I'm flying." "I feel on top of the world."
Anxiety	Worried, uneasy, apprehensive from the anticipation of a danger whose source is unknown	"I feel nervous and high-strung." "I worry all the time." "I can't seem to make up my mind."
Fear	Worried, uneasy, apprehensive; external danger is known and identified	Fear of flying in airplanes
Irritability	Annoyed, easily provoked, impatient	Person internalizes a feeling of tension, and a seemingly mild stimulus "sets him (or her) off"
Rage	Furious, loss of control	Person has expressed violent behavior toward self or others
Ambivalence	The existence of opposing emotions toward an idea, object, person	A person feels love and hate toward another at the same time
Lability	Rapid shift of emotions	Person expresses euphoric, tearful, angry feelings in rapid succession
Inappropriate affect	Affect clearly discordant with content of person's speech	Laughs while discussing admission for liver biopsy

TABLE 5-4 Anxiety Disorders

Panic Attack

A defined period of intense fear, anxiety, and dread accompanied by signs of dyspnea, choking, chest pain, increased heart rate, palpitations, nausea, and sweating. Also has fear of going crazy or dying or impending doom. Sudden onset, lasts about 10 minutes, then subsides.

Agoraphobia

An irrational fear of being out in the open or in a place from which escape is difficult (airport or airplane, car or bus, elevator, bridge). Fear of anxiety is so intense that these places are avoided and person is reluctant to leave safe place (home).

Specific Phobia

A pattern of debilitating fear when faced with a particular object or situation (e.g., dogs, spiders, thunder or storms, enclosed spaces, heights, blood). Person knows it is irrational yet studiously avoids the feared object, thus becoming restricted in social or occupational activities.

Social Anxiety Disorder (Social Phobia)

A persistent and irrational fear of speaking or performing in public in which the person anticipates being judged or criticized, feeling or looking foolish, feeling embarrassment, being unable to answer questions, or being unable to remember the lines or notes. Person studiously avoids such situations or endures them with intense anxiety.

Generalized Anxiety Disorder (GAD)

A pattern of excessive worrying and morbid fear about anticipated "disasters" in the job, personal relationships, health, or finances. Characterized by restlessness, muscle tension, diarrhea, palpitations, tachypnea, hypervigilance, fatigue, or sleep disturbance. Person devotes much time to preparing for anticipated catastrophe, has difficulty making decisions, and practices avoidance.

Obsessive-Compulsive Disorder (OCD)

A pattern of recurrent obsessions (intrusive, uncontrollable thoughts) and compulsions (repetitive ritualistic actions) done to decrease anxiety and prevent a catastrophe (e.g., contamination [fear of germs], violence, perfectionism, and superstitions). Intrusive thoughts and actions are time consuming, interfere with daily activities, and make the person feel humiliated or ashamed for giving in to them.

Posttraumatic Stress Disorder (PTSD)

This follows a traumatic event outside the range of usual human experience involving actual or threatened death (e.g., military combat, natural disaster [flood, tornado, earthquake], plane or train accident, violence [mugging, rape, bombing]). The person relives the trauma many times, intrusively and unwillingly. The same feelings of helplessness, fear, or horror recur. Avoidance of any trigger associated with the trauma occurs, and the person has hypervigilance, sleep problems, and difficulty concentrating, leading to feelings of being permanently damaged.

Adapted from Halter, M. J. (2014). *Varcarolis' foundations of psychiatric mental health nursing.* (7th ed.). St. Louis: Elsevier; and *Stedman's medical dictionary.* (28th ed.). (2005). Philadelphia: Lippincott Williams & Wilkins.

TABLE 5-5 Delirium, Dementia, and Depression

Delirium is an acute confusional state, potentially preventable in hospitalized persons. (See Table 5-1.) Characterized by disorientation, disordered thinking and perceptions (illusions and hallucinations), defective memory, agitation, inattention.

Dementia is a chronic progressive loss of cognitive and intellectual functions, although perception and consciousness are intact. Characterized by disorientation, impaired judgment, memory loss. (See Table 23-2, 10 Warning Signs of Alzheimer Disease).

Depression is a long-term depressed mood (≥previous 2 weeks), with lack of pleasure; disturbed sleep and appetite; feelings of hopelessness, guilt, worthlessness, sadness, loneliness and despair; suicide ideation. See the following comparisons.

	Delirium	Dementia	Depression
Onset	Sudden, over hours to days	Slowly, over months	May have been gradual, with exacerbation during crisis or stress
Cause or contributing factors	Hypoglycemia, fever, dehydration, hypotension; infection, other conditions that disrupt body homeostasis; adverse drug reaction; head injury; change in environment (e.g., hospitalization); pain; emotional stress; substance abuse	Alzheimer disease, vascular disease, human immunodeficiency virus infection, neurological disease, chronic alcoholism, head trauma	Lifelong history, losses, loneliness, crises, declining health, medical conditions
Cognition	Impaired memory, judgment, calculations, attention span; can fluctuate through the day	Impaired memory, judgment, calculations, attention span, abstract thinking; agnosia	Difficulty concentrating, forgetfulness, inattention
Level of consciousness	Altered	Not altered	Not altered
Activity level	Can be increased or reduced; restlessness, behaviors may worsen in evening (sundowning); sleep/wake cycle may be reversed	Not altered; behaviors may worsen in evening (sundowning)	Usually decreased; lethargy, fatigue, lack of motivation; may sleep poorly and awaken in early morning
Emotional state	Rapid swings; can be fearful, anxious, suspicious, aggressive, have hallucinations and/or delusions	Flat; agitation	Extreme sadness, apathy, irritability, anxiety, paranoid ideation
Speech and language	Rapid, inappropriate, incoherent, rambling	Incoherent, slow (sometimes due to effort to find the right word), inappropriate, rambling, repetitious	Slow, flat, low
Prognosis	Reversible with proper and timely treatment	Not reversible; progressive	Reversible with proper and timely treatment

From Halter, M. J. (2014). *Varcarolis' foundations of psychiatric mental health nursing.* (7th ed.). St. Louis: Elsevier.

ABNORMAL FINDINGS
FOR ADVANCED PRACTICE

TABLE 5-6   Thought Process Abnormalities

Type of Process	Definition	Clinical Example
Blocking	Sudden interruption in train of thought, unable to complete sentence, seems related to strong emotion.	"Forgot what I was going to say."
Confabulation	Fabricates events to fill in memory gaps.	Gives detailed description of his long walk around the hospital although you know Mr. J. remained in his room all afternoon.
Neologism	Coining a new word; invented word has no real meaning except for the person; may condense several words.	"I'll have to turn on my thinkilator."
Circumlocution	Round-about expression, substituting a phrase when cannot think of name of object.	Says "the thing you open the door with" instead of "key."
Circumstantiality	Talks with excessive and unnecessary detail, delays reaching point; sentences have a meaningful connection but are irrelevant (this occurs normally in some people).	"When was my surgery? Well I was 28, I was living with my aunt, she's the one with psoriasis, she had it bad that year because of the heat, the heat was worse then than it was the summer of '92. ...."
Loosening associations	Shifting from one topic to an unrelated topic; person seems unaware that topics are unconnected.	"My boss is angry with me, and it wasn't even my fault. (pause) I saw that movie too, Lassie. I felt really bad about it. But she kept trying to land the airplane and she never knew what was going on."
Flight of ideas	Abrupt change, rapid skipping from topic to topic, practically continuous flow of accelerated speech; topics usually have recognizable associations or are plays on words.	"Take this pill? The pill is blue. I feel blue. (sings) She wore blue velvet."
Word salad	Incoherent mixture of words, phrases, and sentences; illogical, disconnected, includes neologisms.	"Beauty, red-based five, pigeon, the street corner, sort of."
Perseveration	Persistent repeating of verbal or motor response, even with varied stimuli.	"I'm going to lock the door, lock the door. I walk every day, and I lock the door. I usually take the dog, and I lock the door."
Echolalia	Imitation, repeats others' words or phrases, often with a mumbling, mocking, or mechanical tone	Nurse: "I want you to take your pill." Patient (mocking): "Take your pill. Take your pill."
Clanging	Word choice based on sound, not meaning, includes nonsense rhymes and puns.	"My feet are cold. Cold, bold, told. The bell tolled for me."

TABLE 5-7 Thought Content Abnormalities

Type of Content	Definition	Clinical Example
Phobia	Strong, persistent, irrational fear of an object or situation; feels driven to avoid it	Cats, dogs, heights, enclosed spaces
Hypochondriasis	Morbid worrying about his or her own health; feels sick with no actual basis for that assumption	Preoccupied with the fear of having cancer; any symptom or physical sign means cancer
Obsession	Unwanted, persistent thoughts or impulses; logic will not purge them from consciousness; experienced as intrusive and senseless	Violence (parent having repeated impulse to kill a loved child); contamination (becoming infected by shaking hands)
Compulsion	Unwanted repetitive, purposeful act; driven to do it; behavior thought to neutralize or prevent discomfort or some dreaded event	Handwashing, counting, checking and rechecking, touching
Delusions	Firm, fixed, false beliefs; irrational; person clings to delusion despite objective evidence to contrary	Grandiose—Person believes that he or she is God; famous, historical, or sports figure; or other well-known person Persecution—"They're out to get me."

TABLE 5-8 Perception Abnormalities

Type of Perception	Definition	Clinical Example
Hallucination	Sensory perceptions for which there are no external stimuli; may strike any sense: visual, auditory, tactile, olfactory, gustatory	Visual: seeing an image (ghost) of a person who is not there; auditory: hearing voices or music
Illusion	*Mis*perception of an actual existing stimulus, by any sense	Folds of bedsheets appear to be animated

TABLE 5-9 Characteristics of Eating Problems

Anorexia Nervosa	Bulimia Nervosa	Binge Eating

• Intense fear of weight gain
• Distorted body image
• Restricted calories with significantly low body mass index
• Subtypes:
  • Restricting (no consistent bulimic features)
  • Binge eating/purging type (primarily restriction, some bulimic behaviors)
	• Recurrent episodes of uncontrollable binging
	• Inappropriate compensatory behaviors: vomiting, laxatives, diuretics, or exercise
	• Self-image largely influenced by body image
		• Recurrent episodes of uncontrollable binging without compensatory behaviors
		• Binging episodes induce guilt, depression, embarrassment, or disgust

From Halter, M. J. (2014). *Varcarolis' foundations of psychiatric mental health nursing.* (7th ed.). St. Louis: Elsevier.

TABLE 5-10   Childhood Mental Disorders

Attention-Deficit/Hyperactivity Disorder (ADHD)

A common behavioral disorder with inappropriate inattention (short attention span, unable to complete tasks or follow directions, easily distracted), impulsiveness, and hyperactivity (restlessness and fidgeting, excess talking). Present in two settings, home and school. Nearly 8% children ages 5-11 years and 12% of adolescents ages 12-17 years have ADHD.[9]

Autism Spectrum Disorder

A complex neurologic and biologic development disorder characterized by problems in social interactions and verbal and nonverbal communication. Dysfunctions range from mild to severe and include problems making and maintaining friends, strict adherence to rituals or routines, resistance to change, repetitive speech, poor eye contact, motor mannerisms. Autism has a genetic component, appears in early childhood (by 2 or 3 years), is 4 times more common in boys than girls, and is not affected by race, family income, or educational level.

Oppositional Defiant Disorder (ODD)

A disruptive set of behaviors characterized by negative, aggressive, angry, and irritable mood. Children with ODD lose their temper, argue with adults, refuse to obey adults' requests or rules, deliberately annoy others, and blame their actions on others. They may be spiteful, vindictive, or malicious. Because they violate social norms, presence in school is difficult. It is also hard to make friends or to fit well in the family.

Eating Disorder

A group of serious and complex psychologic disorders affecting primarily adolescents. (1) Anorexia nervosa presents as a severely low body weight for height (low body mass index) and an intense fear of gaining weight. The person may eat very little food or binge and then purge food by vomiting. (2) Bulimia nervosa is the hallmark of a young person who binge eats, then compensates with self-induced vomiting, misuse of laxatives or diuretics, fasting, or excessive exercise. Both disorders leave the person severely underweight and at risk for electrolyte disturbances and other medical comorbidities (see Table 5-9). (3) People with binge eating disorder use excessive food for comfort or to relieve stress and then feel extreme remorse. This leads to obesity.

Data from CDC. (2013). *Children's mental health—new report.* Available at http://www.cdc.gov/features/childrensmentalhealth; Halter, M. J. (2014). *Varcarolis' foundations of psychiatric mental health nursing.* (7th ed.). St. Louis: Elsevier; and *Stedman's medical dictionary.* (28th ed.). (2006). Philadelphia: Lippincott Williams & Wilkins.

Summary Checklist: Mental Status Assessment

1. **Appearance**
   Posture
   Body movements
   Dress
   Grooming and hygiene
2. **Behavior**
   Level of consciousness
   Facial expression
   Speech (quality, pace, articulation, word choice)
   Mood and affect

3. **Cognitive functions**
   Orientation
   Attention span
   Recent and remote memory
   New learning—the Four Unrelated Words Test
   Judgment
4. **Thought processes**
   Thought processes
   Thought content
   Perceptions

   Screen for suicidal thoughts (when indicated)
5. **Perform the Mini-Mental State Examination or the Mini-Cog**

BIBLIOGRAPHY

1. Acee, A. M., & Fahs, M. C. (2012). Can treating depression improve diabetic management? *Nurse Pract 37*(1), 46-52.

2. Acee, A. M. (2012). Type 2 diabetes and vascular dementia. *Medsurg Nurs 21*(6), 349-53.

3. ADHD/ODD. *Assesses symptom presence and severity in home, classroom, and social settings in children ages 6 to 12.* Available at http://dcf.psychiatry.ufl.edu/files/2011/05/VanderbiltEvaluation-Parent-and-Teacher.pdf.

3a. American Psychiatric Association. (2013). *Diagnostic and statistical manual of mental disorders* (5th ed.). Washington, DC: The Association.

4. Becker, A. E., & Kleinman, A. (2013). Mental health and the global agenda. *N Engl J Med, 369*(1), 66-73.

4a. Birren, J. E., & Schaie, K. W. (Eds.). (2010). *Handbook of the psychology of aging* (7th ed.). San Diego: Academic Press.

4b. Borson, S., Scanlan, J. M., Watanabe, J., et al. (2006). Improving identification of cognitive impairment in primary care. *Int J Geriatr Psychiatr, 21*(4), 349-355.

5. Boydston, L., Hsiao, R. C., & Varley, C. K. (2012). Anxiety disorders in adolescents. *Contemp Pediatr, July*, 36-42.

6. Cahoon, C. G. (2012). Depression in older adults. *Am J Nurs, 112*(11), 22-30.

7. Centers for Disease Control and Prevention (CDC). (2012). *Suicide: facts at a glance.* Available at http://www.cdc.gov/violenceprevention/pdf/suicide-datasheet-a.pdf.

8. Centers for Disease Control and Prevention (CDC). (2013). *Children's mental health—new report.* Available at http://www.cdc.gov/features/childrensmentalhealth.

9. Centers for Disease Control and Prevention (CDC). (May 2013). *Mental health surveillance among children—United States, 2005-2011.* Available at http://www.cdc.gov/mmwr/preview/mmwrhtml/sub202a1.htm?s_cid=sub202a1_w.

10. Center for Epidemiological Studies. Depression Scale Modified for Children (CES-DC). Available at http://www.brightfutures.org/mentalhealth/pdf/professionals/bridges/ces_dc.pdf.

10a. Doerflinger, D. M. C. (2007). The Mini-Cog. *Am J Nurs, 107*(12), 62-72.

11. Feldman, H. M., & Reiff, M. I. (2014). Attention deficit-hyperactivity disorder in children and adolescents. *N Engl J Med, 370*(9):838-845.

12. Fong, T. G., Jones, R. N., Rudolph, J. L., et al. (2011). Development and validation of a brief cognitive assessment tool: the sweet 16. *Arch Int Med, 171*(5), 432-437.

13. Friedman, R. A. (2012). Grief, depression, and the DSM-5. *N Engl J Med, 366*(20), 1855-1857.

14. Garzon, D. L., & Figgemeier, M. E. (2011). Dying to be thin: identifying and managing eating disorders. *Nurse Pract, 36*(10), 45-51.

15. Halter, M. J. (2014). *Varcarolis' foundations of psychiatric mental health nursing.* (7th ed.). St. Louis: Elsevier.

16. Hamrin, V., Antenucci, M., & Magorno, M. (2012). Evaluation and management of pediatric and adolescent depression. *Nurse Pract, 37*(3), 22-30.

17. Hedges, C., & Ruggiero, J. S. (2012). Treatment options for insomnia. *Nurse Pract, 37*(1), 14-19.

18. Hurd, M. D., Martorell, P., Delavande, A., et al. (2013). Monetary costs of dementia in the United States. *N Engl J Med, 368*(14), 1326-1334.

18a. Inouye, S. K. (2006). Delirium in older persons. *N Engl J Med, 354*(11), 1157-1165.

19. Johnson, B. S., Boudiab, L. D., Freundl, M., et al. (2013). Enhancing veteran-centered care. *Am J Nurs, 113*(7):24-39.

19a. Kroenke, K., & Spitzer, R. L. (2002). The PHQ9: a new depression diagnostic and severity index. *Psychiatr Ann, 32*(9), 1-7.

19b. Kroenke, K., Spitzer, R. L., Williams, J. B., et al. (2007). Anxiety disorders in primary care: prevalence, impairment, comorbidity, and detection. *Ann Intern Med, 146*(5), 317-325.

19c. McCravy, S., Johnson, A., Wetsel, M. A., et al. (2010). Speak the language of autism. *Nurse Pract, 35*(4), 26-33.

20. National Institutes of Health (NIH). *The numbers count: mental disorders in America.* Available at http://www.nimh.nih.gov/health/publications/the-numbers-count-mental-disorders-in-america/index.shtml.

21. Nock, M. K., Green, J. G., Hwang, I., et al. (2013). Prevalence, correlates, and treatment of lifetime suicidal behavior among adolescents. *JAMA Psychiatry, 70*(3), 300-310.

22. O'Brien, P. G., & Fleming, L. (2012). Recognizing anxiety disorders. *Nurse Pract, 37*(10), 35-42.

23. Reade, M. C., Phil, D., & Finfer, S. (2014). Sedation and delirium in the intensive care unit. *N Engl J Med, 370*(5):444-454.

24. Sabella, D. (2012a). PTSD among our returning veterans. *Am J Nurs, 112*(11), 48-52.

25. Sabella, D. (2012b). When caring for the body isn't enough. *Am J Nurs, 112*(2), 50-51.

26. Sabella, D. (2013). Where's the 'health' in mental health? *Am J Nurs, 113*(4), 62-65.

27. Sabella, D. (2014). Mental illness and violence. *Am J Nurs, 114*(1), 49.

28. Saczynski, J. S., Marcantonio, E. R., Quach, L., et al. (2012). Cognitive trajectories after postoperative delirium. *N Engl J Med, 367*(1), 30-39.

29. SCARED. Screens adolescents >8 years for anxiety disorders. Available at http://www.psychiatry.pitt.edu/sites/default/files/Documents/assessments/SCARED%20Child.pdf.

30. Schaie, K. W., & Willis, S. L. (2011). *Handbook of the psychology of aging* (7th ed.). London: Academic Press, Elsevier.

31. Schmid, A. M., Truog, A. W., & Damian, F. J. (2011). Care of the suicidal pediatric patient in the ED. *Am J Nurs, 111*(9), 34-43.

32. SNAP-IV Rating Scale-Revised (SNAP-IV-R). *Assesses children and adolescents 6 to 18 years for symptoms of ADHD, ODD, and aggression.* Available at http://adhd.net.

33. Stedman's. (2005). *Stedman's medical dictionary.* (28th ed.). Philadelphia: Lippincott Williams & Wilkins.

33a. Strub, R. L., & Black, F. W. (2000). *Mental status examination in neurology* (4th ed.). Philadelphia: Davis.

34. Struble, L. M., & Sullivan, B. J. (2011). Cognitive health in older adults. *Nurse Pract, 36*(4), 24-34.

35. Valente, S. M. (2010). Evaluating and managing adult PTSD in primary care. *Nurse Pract, 35*(11), 41-47.

36. Valente, S., & Kennedy, B. L. (2012). Recognizing and treating adult ADHD. *Nurse Pract, 37*(3), 41-46.

37. Vause, H. E., & Chapman, M. (2013). Irritability in the pediatric population. *Nurse Pract, 38*(1), 10-16.

38. World Health Organization (WHO). (December 2013). *Mental health: a state of well-being.* Available at http://www.who.int/features/mental_health/en/index.html.

CHAPTER 6

Substance Use Assessment

http://evolve.elsevier.com/Jarvis/

6-1   (© Shevs, Shutterstock.com.)

ALCOHOL USE AND ABUSE

Over half (52.1%) of Americans ages 12 and older report being current alcohol drinkers.[40] For adults ages 18 to 25 years, almost 40% reported binge drinking ≥5 drinks/occasion, and almost 13% reported heavy alcohol use (binge drinking on ≥5 days in past 30 days) (Fig. 6-1). Thus alcohol is the most used and abused psychoactive drug. People like to drink! Given the rates of alcohol use, it is not surprising that many patients in the hospital and in primary care offices find themselves with alcohol-related disorders.

Morbidity and mortality data reflect the adverse consequences of excessive alcohol use. Alcohol-related traffic deaths have been cut in half since the 1980s, but still 37% of traffic deaths are alcohol related in youth ages 16 to 20 years.[24] The prevalence of alcohol-related emergency department (ED) visits has nearly doubled within the last 15 years,[7] and one quarter of ED drug-abuse visits involve alcohol taken together with other drugs. Over 150 medications are additive or interactive with alcohol, especially drugs that depress the central nervous system (CNS) (e.g., heroin, opiate pain relievers, benzodiazepines, antihistamines, antidepressants).[41]

In the global population drinking an average volume of alcohol (Table 6-1) has a causal impact on many diseases: tuberculosis; oral-pharyngeal and esophageal cancer; cancers of colon, rectum, liver, female breast; diabetes mellitus; depression; hypertension; heart disease and stroke; cirrhosis; pneumonia; alcohol use disorders; and fetal alcohol syndrome.[28] These relationships are dose dependent; the more a person drinks, the higher the risk.

There is no safe drinking threshold for cancer risk.[26] Up to one alcohol drink/day increases risk of breast cancer by 4%, and heavy drinking (≥3 drinks/day) increases risk by 40% to 50%.[32] The presumptive mechanism is that alcohol increases estrogen levels, which affect breast tissue directly or through estrogen receptors.[4,8] Alcohol abuse and viral hepatitis are the most common causes of liver cirrhosis, which is the 12th leading cause of death in the United States.[34]

Alcohol has multiple effects on the heart. Even moderate drinking leads to hypertension by stimulating the sympathetic nervous system, which constricts blood vessels and increases contractility. With hypertension the increased afterload may cause cardiomyopathy.[43] Heavy drinking and binge drinking are associated with increased risk of atrial fibrillation, but even moderate drinking increases the atrial fibrillation risk in people over 55 years with cardiovascular disease or diabetes.[21]

Because of alcohol-related morbidity, many patients you encounter in primary care settings and in the hospital will have a significant drinking history. People visiting primary care providers have a significantly higher rate of past or present alcohol abuse than those in the general population. Alcohol abuse and alcohol withdrawal are involved in trauma, violence, suicides, motor vehicle accidents, and other conditions leading to intensive care unit (ICU) admissions. Once in ICU, alcohol withdrawal syndrome occurs in 16% of postsurgical patients and 31% of trauma patients.[31,39]

TABLE 6-1   What Is a Standard Drink?

A standard drink in the United States is any drink that contains about 14 grams of pure alcohol (about 0.6 fl oz or 1.2 tbsp). Below are U.S. standard drink equivalents. These are approximate because different brands and types of beverages vary in their actual alcohol content.

12 oz of beer or cooler	**8-9 oz of malt liquor** 8.5 oz shown in a 12-oz glass that, if full, would hold about 1.5 standard drinks of malt liquor	**5 oz of table wine**	**3-4 oz of fortified wine** (such as sherry or port) 3.5 oz shown	**1.5 oz of spirits** (a single jigger of 80-proof gin, vodka, whiskey, etc.) Shown straight and in a highball glass with ice to show the level before adding a mixer*	**3 oz martini = 2 standard drinks**
~5% alcohol	~7% alcohol	~12% alcohol	~17% alcohol	~40% alcohol	~40% alcohol
12 oz	8.5 oz	5 oz	3.5 oz	1.5 oz	3 oz

Many people do not know what counts as a standard drink; therefore they do not realize how many standard drinks are in the containers in which these drinks are often sold. Some examples:

For **beer,** the approximate number of standard drinks in:
12 oz = 1
16 oz = 1.3
22 oz = 2
40 oz = 3.3

For **malt liquor,** the approximate number of standard drinks in:
12 oz = 1.5
16 oz = 2
22 oz = 2.5
40 oz = 4.5

For **table wine,** the approximate number of standard drinks in:
A standard 750-mL (25-oz) bottle = 5

For **80-proof spirits,** or "hard liquor," the approximate number of standard drinks in:
A mixed drink = 1 to 3 or more*
A pint (16 oz) = 11
A fifth (25 oz) = 17
1.75 L (59 oz) = 39

Adapted from National Institute on Alcohol Abuse and Alcoholism (NIAAA). (Reprinted 2007). *Helping patients who drink too much: a clinician's guide.* Available at http://pubs.niaaa.nih.gov/publications/Practitioner/CliniciansGuide2005/clinicians_guide.htm.
***Note:** It can be difficult to estimate the number of standard drinks in a single mixed drink made with hard liquor. Depending on factors such as the type of spirits and the recipe, a mixed drink can contain from 1 to 3 or more standard drinks.

DEFINING ILLICIT DRUG USE

There are 9 categories of illicit drug use: marijuana; cocaine; heroin; hallucinogens; inhalants; and the nonmedical use of prescription pain relievers, tranquilizers, stimulants, and sedatives. The prevalence of Americans ages 12 or older reporting the use of any of the 9 categories is 9.2%.[40] Marijuana use is the most common, used by almost 80% of illicit drug users, although many of these also used other drugs. Among youth ages 12 to 17 years, 9.5% were current illicit drug users, which represents 1 out of 10 adolescents. This warrants our attention and intervention. Any amount of illicit drug use has serious legal consequences and consequences for health, trauma, brain maturation, relationships, school, and career.

The abuse of prescription drugs is the fastest-growing drug problem in the United States. After marijuana use, the nonmedical use of psychotherapeutic drugs (pain relievers, tranquilizers, stimulants, sedatives) is the second most common form of illicit drug use. These users are 3.4% of people ages 12 or older.[40] Of those who used pain relievers nonmedically, 54% got the drug free from a friend or relative, 11% bought it from a friend or relative, and almost 20% got it from a doctor's prescription.[40] Contributing factors include inappropriate prescribing, aggressive marketing by drug companies for off-label use, belated government response, and an increase in prescriptions for pain relief in response to the past practices of undertreatment of pain.[22] The three most frequently abused prescription opioid pain relievers were products using oxycodone, hydrocodone, and methadone. The misuse of prescription drugs has a huge impact not only on health and safety but also on burdens to the ED system.

TABLE 6-2 Categories and Definitions for Patterns of Alcohol Use

Category	Organization	Definition
Moderate drinking	NIAAA	Men, ≤2 drinks/day; women, ≤1 drink/day; >65 years, ≤1 drink/day
At-risk drinking	NIAAA	Men, >14 drinks/wk or >4 drinks/occasion; women, >7 drinks/wk or >3 drinks/occasion
Hazardous drinking	WHO	At risk for adverse consequences from alcohol
Harmful drinking	WHO	Alcohol is causing physical or psychological harm
Alcohol use disorder	APA	≥2 of the following events in a year: tolerance (increased amounts to achieve effect; diminished effect from same amount); withdrawal; a great deal of time spent obtaining alcohol, using it, or recovering from its effect; craving to use alcohol; important activities given up or reduced because of alcohol; drinking more or longer than intended; persistent desire or unsuccessful efforts to cut down or control alcohol use; use continued despite knowledge of having a psychological problem caused or exacerbated by alcohol

APA, American Psychiatric Association; *DUI,* driving under the influence; *NIAAA,* National Institute on Alcohol Abuse and Alcoholism; *WHO,* World Health Organization.

DIAGNOSING SUBSTANCE ABUSE

The rate of Americans classified with substance abuse or dependence is 8.5 % of the population ages 12 years and older; 6.8% were dependent on or abused alcohol but not illicit drugs, and 2.8% had illicit drug dependence or abuse.[40] The continuum of alcohol drinking ranges from special occasion use through moderate drinking to harmful drinking (Table 6-2). Alcohol dependence, or alcoholism, is a chronic progressive disease that is not curable but is highly treatable. Accurate diagnosis is needed to provide advice, brief intervention, appropriate treatment, and follow-up. The gold standard of diagnosis is well defined by the American Psychiatric Association (APA) in its *Diagnostic and Statistical Manual of Mental Disorders,* 5th edition. Table 6-3 gives the criteria for Alcohol Use Disorder. Unfortunately alcohol

TABLE 6-3 Alcohol Use Disorder

Diagnostic Criteria

A. A problematic pattern of alcohol use leading to clinically significant impairment or distress, as manifested by at least two of the following occurring within a 12-month period:
   1. Alcohol is often taken in larger amounts or over a longer period than was intended.
   2. There is a persistent desire or unsuccessful efforts to cut down or control alcohol use.
   3. A great deal of time is spent in activities necessary to obtain alcohol, use it, or recover from its effects.
   4. Craving or a strong desire or urge to use alcohol.
   5. Recurrent alcohol use results in a failure to fulfill major role obligations at work, school, or home.
   6. Continued alcohol use despite having persistent or recurrent social or interpersonal problems caused or exacerbated by the effects of alcohol.
   7. Important social, occupational, or recreational activities are given up or reduced because of alcohol use.
   8. Recurrent alcohol use in situations in which it is physically hazardous.
   9. Alcohol use is continued despite knowledge of having a persistent or recurrent physical or psychological problem that is likely to have been caused or exacerbated by alcohol.
   10. Tolerance, as defined by either of the following:
       a. A need for markedly increased amounts of alcohol to achieve intoxication or desired effect
       b. A markedly diminished effect with continued use of the same amount of alcohol
   11. Withdrawal, as manifested by either of the following:
       a. The characteristic withdrawal syndrome for alcohol
       b. Alcohol (or a closely related substance such as a benzodiazepine) taken to relieve or avoid withdrawal symptoms

Specify if:

In early remission: After full criteria for alcohol use disorder were previously met, none of the criteria for alcohol use disorder have been met for at least 3 months but for less than 12 months (with the exception that criterion A4, "Craving, or a strong desire or urge to use alcohol," may be met).

In sustained remission: After full criteria for alcohol use disorder were previously met, none of the criteria for alcohol use disorder have been met at any time during a period of 12 months or longer (with the exception that criterion A4, "Craving, or a strong desire or urge to use alcohol," may be met).

Specify if:

In a controlled environment: This additional specifier is used if the individual is in an environment where access to alcohol is restricted.

Specify current severity:

Mild: Presence of 2-3 symptoms.

Moderate: Presence of 4-5 symptoms.

Severe: Presence of 6 or more symptoms.

From American Psychiatric Association (2013). *Diagnostic and statistical manual of mental disorders.* (5th ed.). Washington, DC: The Association.

problems are underdiagnosed in both primary care settings and hospitals. Excessive alcohol use often is unrecognized until patients develop serious complications.

❖ DEVELOPMENTAL COMPETENCE

Adolescents

Here are the estimates for youth who are current alcohol users: 2.2% of youth ages 12 or 13 years, 11% of those ages 14 or 15, 25% of those ages 16 or 17, almost 46% of those ages 18 to 20, and almost 70% of those ages 21 to 25.[40] It is well known that alcohol retards brain development and maturity levels in adolescents. It is estimated that 4.7% of 16- or 17-year-olds and nearly 13% of 18- to 20-year-olds drive under the influence of alcohol. Youth who abuse alcohol also engage in high-risk sexual behavior, have academic problems in school, injuries from trauma, and alcohol problems that carry over to adulthood.[37]

The Pregnant Woman

The dangers of alcohol use to the growing fetus during pregnancy are well known. Alcohol slips easily through the placenta; a defined dose that is easily metabolized by an adult woman is toxic to a fetus who weighs only grams or a few pounds. Alcohol toxicity results in physical, learning, and behavioral problems in a fetus that are defined in the Fetal Alcohol Spectrum Disorder (see Table 13-2, p. 274). Public awareness and health teaching have reduced the number of U.S. pregnant women who drink alcohol. Yet close to 18% of pregnant women drink during the first trimester,[30] perhaps not knowing that they are pregnant. Alcohol use decreases during the 2nd and 3rd trimesters to 4.2% and 3.7%.[30] The bottom line is that no amount of alcohol is safe during pregnancy.

The Aging Adult

Among adults ages 65 years or older, the prevalence of current alcohol use (41.2%), binge drinking (8.2%), and heavy alcohol use (2%) is lower than among other adult groups.[40]

However, older adults have numerous characteristics that can increase the risk for alcohol use. Liver metabolism and kidney function are decreased, which increases the bioavailability of alcohol in the blood for longer time periods. Aging people lose muscle mass; less tissue to which the alcohol can be distributed means an increased alcohol concentration in the blood. Older adults may be on multiple medications, which can interact adversely with alcohol (e.g., benzodiazepines, antidepressants, antihypertensives, aspirin). Drinking alcohol increases risk for falls, depression, and gastrointestinal problems. Older adults may avoid detection of their alcohol problems; they may avoid alcohol-related consequences such as driving under the influence (DUI) because they no longer drive, or they may avoid job problems because they no longer work.

In addition, the prevalence of dementia in older adults with alcohol use disorders is 5 times higher than in older adults who are not alcoholic.[6] One positive note is that older adults may adhere to rehabilitation better than younger adults; over 20% of treated older-adult alcoholics remained abstinent after 4 years, with women maintaining abstinence better than men.[6]

SUBJECTIVE DATA

If the patient currently is intoxicated or going through substance withdrawal, collecting any history data is difficult and unreliable. However, when sober, most people are willing and able to give reliable data, provided the setting is private, confidential, and nonconfrontational.

Examiner Asks	Rationale
1. Ask about alcohol use: "Do you sometimes drink beer, wine, or other alcoholic beverages?" If the answer is "Yes," ask the screening question about heavy drinking days: "How many times in the past year have you had 5 or more drinks a day *(for men)* or 4 or more drinks a day?" *(for women)*	One or more heavy drinking days means that this person is an "at-risk" drinker.
To complete a picture of the person's drinking pattern, ask: "On average, how many days a week do you have an alcoholic drink?" and "On a typical drinking day, how many drinks do you have?" Recommend that the person stay at **moderate** drinking patterns: for men, ≤2 drinks/day; for women, ≤1 drink/day; for older than 65 years, ≤1 drink/day.[24] Recommend even lower limits or abstinence for patients who take medications that interact with alcohol, have a health condition exacerbated by alcohol, or are pregnant (advise abstinence here).	For men, ≥14 drinks/week or ≥4 drinks/occasion = **at-risk** drinking. For women, ≥7 drinks/week or ≥3 drinks/occasion = **at-risk** drinking.[24]

Examiner Asks	Rationale

2. Use brief screening instruments to help identify problem drinking and people who need a more thorough assessment. Ask the patient to respond to the AUDIT questionnaire (Table 6-4). A quantitative form has the advantage of letting you document a number for a response so it is not open to individual interpretation. The AUDIT helps to detect both less severe alcohol problems (hazardous and harmful drinking) and alcohol abuse and dependence disorders. It is helpful with ED and trauma patients because it is sensitive to current as opposed to past alcohol problems. It is useful in primary care settings with adolescents and older adults. It is relatively free of gender and cultural bias.

Hazardous drinking—Pattern is high risk for future damage to physical or mental health. Harmful drinking—Alcohol use already results in problems.

TABLE 6-4 The Alcohol Use Disorders Identification Test—AUDIT*

Questions	0	1	2	3	4
1. How often do you have a drink containing alcohol?	Never	Monthly or less	2-4 times a month	2-3 times a week	4 or more times a week
2. How many drinks containing alcohol do you have on a typical day when you are drinking?	1 or 2	3 or 4	5 or 6	7 to 9	10 or more
3. How often do you have 5 or more drinks on one occasion?	Never	Less than monthly	Monthly	Weekly	Daily or almost daily
4. How often during the last year have you found that you were not able to stop drinking once you had started?	Never	Less than monthly	Monthly	Weekly	Daily or almost daily
5. How often during the last year have you failed to do what was normally expected of you because of drinking?	Never	Less than monthly	Monthly	Weekly	Daily or almost daily
6. How often during the last year have you needed a first drink in the morning to get yourself going after a heavy drinking session?	Never	Less than monthly	Monthly	Weekly	Daily or almost daily
7. How often during the last year have you had a feeling of guilt or remorse after drinking?	Never	Less than monthly	Monthly	Weekly	Daily or almost daily
8. How often during the last year have you been unable to remember what happened the night before because of your drinking?	Never	Less than monthly	Monthly	Weekly	Daily or almost daily
9. Have you or someone else been injured because of your drinking?	No		Yes, but not in the last year		Yes, during the last year
10. Has a relative, friend, doctor, or other health care worker been concerned about your drinking or suggested that you cut down?	No		Yes, but not in the last year		Yes, during the last year
					Total

*NOTE: This questionnaire (the AUDIT) is reprinted with permission from the World Health Organization. To reflect standard drink sizes in the United States, the number of drinks in question 3 was changed from 6 to 5. A free AUDIT manual with guidelines for use in primary care settings is available online at www.who.org.

Subjective Data

Examiner Asks	Rationale

Note that the AUDIT covers three domains: alcohol consumption (questions 1 to 3); drinking behavior or dependence (questions 4 to 6); and adverse consequences from alcohol (questions 7 to 10). Record the score at the end of each line and total; the maximum total is 40.

A cut point of ≥8 points for men or ≥4 points for women, adolescents, and those older than 60 years indicates hazardous alcohol consumption.

The AUDIT-C is a shorter form that is helpful for acute and critical care units. The AUDIT-C is a valid screening test for heavy drinking and/or active alcohol abuse.[5] It uses the three alcohol consumption questions (numbers 1 to 3), including question number 3, which is itself a brief screening test for heavy drinking. This helps examiners discriminate heavy, at-risk drinking from low-risk drinking in a very short time (less than 2 minutes). The possible score is 0 to 12; a low-risk response is ≤2 points.

A cut point of ≥3 is a measure of heavy or at-risk drinking. In addition, a "Yes" to drinking 6 or more drinks on one occasion *ever* in the past year warrants further assessment.

The CAGE questionnaire (**C**ut down, **A**nnoyed, **G**uilty, **E**ye-opener) described in Chapter 4, (p. 58) works well in busy primary care settings because it takes less than 1 minute to complete and the 4 straightforward yes/no questions are easy for clinicians to remember. The CAGE tests for lifetime alcohol abuse and/or dependence but does not distinguish past problem drinking from active present drinking.[5] It may not detect low but risky levels of drinking and is less effective with women and minority groups.[35]

Answering "Yes" to ≥2 CAGE questions signals possible alcohol abuse and a need for further assessment.

3. Assess for alcohol use disorders using the standard clinical diagnostic criteria. Determine whether there is a maladaptive pattern of alcohol use causing clinically significant impairment or distress.[25] Ask, "In the past 12 months has your drinking repeatedly caused or contributed to:
   - **Risk** for bodily harm (drinking and driving, operating machinery, swimming)?
   - **Relationship** trouble (family or friends)?
   - **Role failure** (interference with home, work, or school obligations)?
   - **Run-ins** with the law (arrests or other legal problems)?"

If "Yes" to one or more points, it means that the person has been abusing alcohol. Warrants advice and brief intervention for assistance.

Ask, "In the past 12 months have you:
   - Not been able to stick to drinking limits (repeatedly gone over them)?
   - **Not been able to cut down or stop** (repeated failed attempts)?
   - **Shown tolerance** (needed to drink a lot more to get the same effect)?
   - **Shown signs of withdrawal** (tremors, sweating, nausea, or insomnia when trying to quit or cut down)?
   - **Kept drinking despite problems** (recurrent physical or psychological problems)?
   - **Spent a lot of time drinking** (or anticipating or recovering from drinking)?
   - **Spent less time on other matters** (activities that had been important or pleasurable)?"

If "Yes" to 2 or more →, person may have alcohol use disorder. Warrants counseling and brief intervention for treatment or mutual help meetings (AA, NA).

If "No" →, patient still at risk for developing alcohol-related problems. Warrants advice and brief intervention for assistance and close follow-up.

Ask about use of illicit substances: "Do you sometimes take illicit or street drugs such as marijuana, cocaine, hallucinogens, narcotics?" If "Yes," "When was the last time you used drugs? How much did you take that time?"

Screening Women for Alcohol Problems

The TWEAK questions[29] are a combination of items of two other questionnaires that help identify at-risk drinking in women, especially pregnant women. Instead of the guilt question from the CAGE questionnaire, the TWEAK includes a question that measures tolerance:
   - **Tolerance:** How many drinks can you hold? Or how many drinks does it take to make you feel high?

Taking ≥3 drinks to feel high = Tolerance.

Examiner Asks	Rationale

- **Worry:** Have close friends or relatives worried or complained about your drinking in the past year?
- **Eye-opener:** Do you sometimes take a drink in the morning when you first get up?
- **Amnesia:** Has a friend or family member ever told you about things you said or did that you could not remember?
- **Kut down:** Do you sometimes feel the need to cut down on your drinking?

Score 2 points each for Tolerance and Worry, 1 point each for the rest. A low-risk response is ≤1 point.

≥2 points = a drinking problem.

Screening Aging Adults

Use the SMAST-G questionnaire for older adults who report social or regular drinking of any amount of alcohol. Older adults have specific emotional responses and physical reactions to alcohol, and the 10 questions with yes/no responses address these factors. A low-risk response is zero or 1 point (Table 6-5).

Scoring ≥2 points indicates an alcohol problem and a need for more in-depth assessment.

4. Advise and Assist (brief intervention). Although it is beyond the scope of this text to present treatment plans, the consequences of substance abuse are so debilitating and destructive to patients and their families that a short statement of assistance and concern is given here. If your assessment has determined the patient to have at-risk drinking or illicit substance use, state your conclusion and recommendation clearly.[24]

"You're drinking more than is medically safe." Relate to the person's concerns and medical findings, if present. "I strongly recommend that you cut down (or quit), and I'm willing to help."

Or, if you determine the person to have an alcohol use disorder, state your conclusion and recommendation clearly:

"I believe that you have an alcohol use disorder. I strongly recommend that you quit drinking, and I'm willing to help." Relate to the person's concerns and medical findings if present.

Subjective Data

TABLE 6-5 Short Michigan Alcoholism Screening Test—Geriatric Version (SMAST-G)

	Yes (1)	No (0)
1. When talking with others, do you ever underestimate how much you drink?		
2. After a few drinks, have you sometimes not eaten or been able to skip a meal because you didn't feel hungry?		
3. Does having a few drinks help decrease your shakiness or tremors?		
4. Does alcohol sometimes make it hard for you to remember parts of the day or night?		
5. Do you usually take a drink to relax or calm your nerves?		
6. Do you drink to take your mind off your problems?		
7. Have you ever increased your drinking after experiencing a loss in your life?		
8. Has a doctor or nurse ever said they were worried or concerned about your drinking?		
9. Have you ever made rules to manage your drinking?		
10. When you feel lonely, does having a drink help?		
TOTAL SMAST-G-SCORE (0-10)		‾‾‾‾‾

SCORING: 2 OR MORE "**YES**" RESPONSES IS INDICATIVE OF AN ALCOHOL PROBLEM.

©The Regents of the University of Michigan, 1991. Source: University of Michigan Alcohol Research Center. Reprinted with permission.

OBJECTIVE DATA

Normal Range of Findings	Abnormal Findings

Clinical laboratory findings (called *biomarkers)* give objective evidence of problem drinking. These are less sensitive than self-report questionnaires, but they are useful data to corroborate the subjective data and are unbiased. The serum protein *gamma glutamyl transferase (GGT)* is the most commonly used biomarker of alcohol drinking. Occasional alcohol drinking does not raise this measure, but chronic heavy drinking does. Be aware that nonalcoholic liver disease also can increase GGT levels in the absence of alcohol.

The GGT is helpful in detecting relapses for alcohol-dependent people who are in recovery.

The carbohydrate-deficient transferrin (CDT) is used together with the GGT, which may increase detection of alcohol abuse. Healthy women have higher CDT levels than men; therefore combining it with GGT may improve accuracy.[38]

Serum aspartate aminotransferase (AST) is an enzyme found in high concentrations in the heart and liver.

From the complete blood count, the mean corpuscular volume (MCV) is an index of red blood cell (RBC) size. MCV is not sensitive enough to use as the only biomarker for problem drinking.

Breath alcohol analysis detects any amount of alcohol in the end of exhaled air following a deep inhalation until all ingested alcohol is metabolized. This measure can be correlated with blood alcohol concentration (BAC) and is the basis for legal interpretation of drinking. Normal values indicating no alcohol are 0.00.

When caring for people experiencing alcohol withdrawal, the Clinical Institute Withdrawal Assessment (CIWA) is the most sensitive scale for objective measurement (Table 6-6). It is quantified to measure the progress of withdrawal. Intervention with appropriate pharmacotherapy avoids advanced withdrawal stages such as delirium tremens. Most withdrawing persons do not progress to advanced stages; thus using the CIWA scale also avoids overmedicating.

Take the vital signs: blood pressure (BP), pulse, respirations, oxygen saturation. Assess and rate each of the 10 criteria of the CIWA scale. Each criterion has a range from 0 to 7, except for "Orientation," which is rated 0 to 4. Add the scores for the total CIWA-Ar score. A score of 0 to 7 means that you can assess every 4 hours for 72 hours. If all the scores are <8 for 72 hours, you can safely discontinue use of the CIWA assessment.

Clinical appearance and behavioral signs of commonly abused substances are presented in Table 6-7. Note that clinical signs are described for both the intoxicated person and the person in withdrawal.

Abnormal Findings

Chronic alcohol drinking of ≥4 drinks/day for 4 to 8 weeks significantly raises GGT. It takes 4 to 5 weeks of abstinence for GGT levels to return to normal range.[19]

A sudden elevated GGT after a period of normal GGT levels may indicate relapse and should prompt discussion with the person.

CDT is elevated in people who drink 50 to 80 g alcohol/day for 1 week.[19] CDT normalizes during abstinence with a half-life of 15 days.

Chronic drinking for months increases AST.

Heavy alcohol drinking for 4 to 8 weeks increases MCV.

A BAC ≥0.08% = legal intoxication in most states (3 standard drinks), with loss of balance and motor coordination.

Withdrawal symptoms: craving for alcohol, irritability, anorexia, abdominal pain, fatigue. Signs are chills, muscle cramps, palpitations, tachycardia, hypertension, fever, disorientation, slurred speech, staggered gait, poor dexterity.

Scores of 0 to 9 = absent or minimal withdrawal; 10 to 19 = mild-to-moderate withdrawal; ≥20 = severe withdrawal.

If initial score is ≥8, take vital signs every hour for 8 hours. A score of 8 may trigger PRN medication. A score of ≥15 triggers scheduled medication.

ABNORMAL FINDINGS

TABLE 6-6 Clinical Institute Withdrawal Assessment of Alcohol Scale, Revised (CIWA-Ar)

Patient: _____ Date: _____ Time: _____:_____

Pulse (1 minute): _____ Blood pressure: _____/_____ Resp _____ O$_2$ Sat _____

Nausea and vomiting. Ask, "Do you feel sick to your stomach? Have you vomited?" Observation:
0 – No nausea and no vomiting
1 – Mild nausea with no vomiting
2 –
3 –
4 – Intermittent nausea with dry heaves
5 –
6 –
7 – Constant nausea, frequent dry heaves, and vomiting

Tremor. Ask patient to extend arms and spread fingers apart. Observation:
0 – No tremor
1 – Tremor not visible but can be felt, fingertip to fingertip
2 –
3 –
4 – Moderate tremor with arms extended
5 –
6 –
7 – Severe tremor, even with arms not extended

Paroxysmal sweats. Observation:
0 – No sweat visible
1 – Barely perceptible sweating; palms moist
2 –
3 –
4 – Beads of sweat obvious on forehead
5 –
6 –
7 – Drenching sweats

Anxiety. Ask, "Do you feel nervous?" Observation:
0 – No anxiety (at ease)
1 – Mildly anxious
2 –
3 –
4 – Moderately anxious or guarded; thus anxiety is inferred
5 –
6 –
7 – Equivalent to acute panic states as occur in severe delirium or acute schizophrenic reactions

Agitation. Observation:
0 – Normal activity
1 – Somewhat more than normal activity
2 –
3 –
4 – Moderately fidgety and restless
5 –
6 –
7 – Paces back and forth during most of the interview or constantly thrashes about

Tactile Disturbances. Ask, "Do you have any itching, pins-and-needles sensations, burning, or numbness, or do you feel like bugs are crawling on or under your skin?" Observation:
0 – None
1 – Very mild itching, pins-and-needles sensation, burning, or numbness
2 – Mild itching, pins-and-needles sensation, burning, or numbness
3 – Moderate itching, pins-and-needles sensation, burning, or numbness
4 – Moderately severe hallucinations
5 – Severe hallucinations
6 – Extremely severe hallucinations
7 – Continuous hallucinations

Auditory disturbances. Ask, "Are you more aware of sounds around you? Are they harsh? Do they frighten you? Are you hearing anything that is disturbing to you? Are you hearing things you know are not there?" Observation:
0 – Not present
1 – Very mild harshness or ability to frighten
2 – Mild harshness or ability to frighten
3 – Moderate harshness or ability to frighten
4 – Moderately severe hallucinations
5 – Severe hallucinations
6 – Extremely severe hallucinations
7 – Continuous hallucinations

Continued

TABLE 6-6   Clinical Institute Withdrawal Assessment of Alcohol Scale, Revised (CIWA-Ar)—cont'd

Visual disturbances. Ask, "Does the light appear to be too bright? Is its color different? Does it hurt your eyes? Are you seeing anything that is disturbing to you? Are you seeing things you know are not there? Observation:
0 – Not present
1 – Very mild sensitivity
2 – Mild sensitivity
3 – Moderate sensitivity
4 – Moderately severe hallucinations
5 – Severe hallucinations
6 – Extremely severe hallucinations
7 – Continuous hallucinations

Headache, fullness in head. Ask, "Does your head feel different? Does it feel like there is a band around your head?" Do not rate for dizziness or light-headedness; otherwise rate severity.
0 – Not present
1 – Very mild

2 – Mild
3 – Moderate
4 – Moderately severe
5 – Severe
6 – Very severe
7 – Extremely severe

Orientation and clouding of sensorium. Ask, "What day is this? Where are you? Who am I?" Observation:
0 – Oriented and can do serial additions
1 – Cannot do serial additions or is uncertain about date
2 – Date disorientation by no more than 2 calendar days
3 – Date disorientation by more than 2 calendar days
4 – Disorientated for place and/or person
Total score: _____ (Maximum = 67)
Rater's initials: _____

From Bayard, M., McIntyre, J., Hill, K.R., et al. (2004). Alcohol withdrawal syndrome. *Am Fam Physician, 69*(6), 1443-1550.

TABLE 6-7   Clinical Signs of Substance Use Disorders

"Substances" refer to agents taken nonmedically to alter mood or behavior.

Intoxication: Ingestion of substance produces maladaptive behavioral changes because of effects on the central nervous system
Abuse: Daily use needed to function, inability to stop, impaired social and occupational functioning, recurrent use when it is physically hazardous, substance-related legal problems

Dependence: Physiologic dependence on substance
Tolerance: Requires increased amount of substance to produce same effect
Withdrawal: Cessation of substance produces syndrome of physiologic symptoms

Substance	Intoxication	Withdrawal
Alcohol	**Appearance.** Unsteady gait, incoordination, nystagmus, flushed face **Behavior.** Sedation; relief of anxiety; dulled concentration; impaired judgment; expansive, uninhibited behavior; talkativeness; slurred speech; impaired memory; irritability; depression; emotional lability	**Uncomplicated.** (Shortly after cessation of drinking, peaks at 2nd day, improves by 4th to 5th day.) Coarse tremor of hands, tongue, eyelids; anorexia; nausea and vomiting; malaise; autonomic hyperactivity (tachycardia, sweating, elevated blood pressure); headache; insomnia; anxiety; depression or irritability; transient hallucinations or illusions **Withdrawal delirium, "delirium tremens."** (Much less common than uncomplicated, occurs within 1 week of cessation.) Coarse, irregular tremor; marked autonomic hyperactivity (tachycardia, sweating); vivid hallucinations; delusions; agitated behavior; fever

TABLE 6-7   Clinical Signs of Substance Use Disorders—cont'd

Substance	Intoxication	Withdrawal
Sedatives, hypnotics (benzodiazepines)	Similar to alcohol **Appearance.** Unsteady gait, incoordination **Behavior.** Talkativeness, slurred speech, inattention, impaired memory, irritability, emotional lability, sexual aggressiveness, impaired judgment, impaired social or occupational functioning	Anxiety or irritability; nausea or vomiting; malaise; autonomic hyperactivity (tachycardia, sweating); orthostatic hypotension; coarse tremor of hands, tongue, and eyelids; marked insomnia; grand mal seizures
Nicotine	**Appearance.** Alert, increased systolic blood pressure, increased heart rate, vasoconstriction **Behavior.** Nausea, vomiting, indigestion (first use); loss of appetite; head rush; dizziness; jittery feeling; mild stimulant	Vasodilation, headaches, anger, irritability, frustration, anxiety, nervousness, awakening at night, difficulty concentrating, depression, hunger, impatience or restlessness, desire to smoke
Cannabis (marijuana)	**Appearance.** Reddened eyes; tachycardia; dry mouth; increased appetite, especially for "junk" food; loss of coordination and balance **Behavior.** Euphoria, pleasant state of relaxation and tranquility, slowed time perception, increased perceptions, impaired judgment, social withdrawal, anxiety, suspiciousness or paranoid ideation	No withdrawal with occasional use. Chronic heavy use may → mild withdrawal: irritability, sleep disturbances, weight loss, loss of appetite, sweating
Cocaine (including crack)	**Appearance.** Pupillary dilation, tachycardia or bradycardia, elevated or lowered blood pressure, sweating, chills, nausea, vomiting, weight loss **Behavior.** Euphoria, talkativeness, hypervigilance, pacing, psychomotor agitation, impaired social or occupational functioning, fighting, grandiosity, visual or tactile hallucinations	Dysphoric mood (anxiety, depression, irritability), fatigue, insomnia or hypersomnia, psychomotor agitation
Amphetamines	Similar to cocaine **Appearance.** Pupillary dilation, tachycardia or bradycardia, elevated or lowered blood pressure, sweating or chills, nausea and vomiting, weight loss **Behavior.** Elation, talkativeness, hypervigilance, psychomotor agitation, fighting, grandiosity, impaired judgment, impaired social and occupational functioning	Dysphoric mood (anxiety, depression, irritability), fatigue, insomnia or hypersomnia, psychomotor agitation
Opiates (morphine, heroin, meperidine)	**Appearance.** Pinpoint pupils; decreased blood pressure, pulse, respirations, and temperature **Behavior.** Lethargy; somnolence; slurred speech; initial euphoria followed by apathy, dysphoria, and psychomotor retardation; inattention; impaired memory; impaired judgment; impaired social or occupational functioning	Dilated pupils, lacrimation, runny nose, tachycardia, fever, elevated blood pressure, piloerection, sweating, diarrhea, yawning, insomnia, restlessness, irritability, depression, nausea, vomiting, malaise, tremor, muscle and joint pains; symptoms remarkably similar to clinical picture of influenza

PROMOTING A HEALTHY LIFESTYLE

Prescription Drug Abuse: An Epidemic Among Teens and Young Adults

Prescription drug abuse occurs when an individual takes a medication that was prescribed for someone else *or* takes a prescription in a manner or dosage other than what was prescribed. This type of drug abuse is a growing problem, especially among teens and young adults. A 2013 national survey shows that 1 in 4 teens has misused or abused a prescription drug at least once in his or her lifetime, which is a 33% increase over the past 5 years (http://www.drugfree.org/). Of particular note is the abuse of drugs normally prescribed for the treatment of attention-deficit/hyperactivity disorder (ADHD) (e.g., Adderall, Ritalin). According to the survey's findings, 1 in 8 teens (i.e., approximately 2.7 million teens) report having taken Ritalin or Adderall when it was not prescribed. Some have even declared prescription drug abuse to be an epidemic (Spoth et al., 2013).

This finding is not isolated. *Monitoring the Future* is an ongoing study of behaviors, attitudes, and values of American secondary school and college students and young adults, funded by the National Institute on Drug Abuse (NIDA). In their 2012 survey, prescription and over-the-counter drugs were also noted among the top substances being abused by 12th graders, with Adderall leading the list.

This group of drugs is known to health care providers by either the *chemical* names, *dextroamphetamine* and *methylphenidate*, or by their *brand* names, *Dexedrine, Adderall, Ritalin*, or *Concerta*. However, they also have *street* names, including but certainly not limited to: *Skippy, Vitamin R, Cramming Drug, R-Ball, The Smart Drug, Bennies, Black Beauties, Roses, Speed*, or *Uppers*.

The therapeutic action of these stimulant medications is a slow and steady increase in dopamine, a neurotransmitter associated with attention. The prescription doses are typically started at low levels and increased gradually until a therapeutic effect is achieved for the individual that mimics levels in the brain unaffected by ADHD and allows individuals with ADHD to focus. When these medications are taken in doses and/or routes other than those prescribed, such as crushing the pill and snorting or injecting it, dopamine levels increase in a rapid, highly amplified manner, disrupting normal neurotransmission and often creating a state of euphoria. When prescription ADHD medications are taken orally either in higher doses or by individuals without ADHD, students report that they can stay awake and maintain abnormally high levels of concentration for long nights of studying. However, continued abuse or an overdose of stimulants can cause anxiety, panic, tremors, irregular heartbeat, dangerously high body temperatures, and even heart attack. Further, teens and young adults who stop taking stimulants may suffer from fatigue and depression, which may set the stage for further medication use, abuse, and addiction.

One of the additional findings in the survey conducted by the Partnership at Drugfree.org was the apparent oversight or missed opportunity for conversation about prescription drug abuse. In their study teens reported that during the last conversation they had with their parents regarding substance abuse, only 16% said they discussed the misuse or abuse of prescription drugs, whereas 81% reported that they had discussed the risks of marijuana use with their parents, 80% had discussed alcohol, and 30% had discussed crack/cocaine.

The primary mission of NIDA is to bring the power of science to bear on drug abuse and addiction. NIDA offers various resources, including its InfoFacts series (e.g., *InfoFacts: Stimulant ADHD Medications: Methylphenidate and Amphetamines)*, which provides current science and use and abuse. It is available at: http://www.nida.nih.gov/infofacts/ADHD.html. NIDA also has a site *for teens* about prescription medication abuse and the science behind addiction. Of note is that this site also includes information aimed at parents: http://teens.drugabuse.gov/facts/facts_rx1.php.

Start or encourage conversations about this serious and growing problem early and often. Even brief universal interventions during middle school have potential to reduce prescription drug abuse in teens and young adults (Spoth, 2013).

References

Spoth, R., Trudeau, L., Shin, C., et al. (2013). *American Journal of Public Health, 103*(4), 665-672.
The Partnership at Drugfree.org.
Full report. http://www.drugfree.org/wp-content/uploads/2013/04/PATS-2012-FULL-REPORT2.pdf.
Key findings. http://www.drugfree.org/wp-content/uploads/2013/04/PATS-2012-KEY-FINDINGS.pdf.
Monitoring the Future.
http://www.monitoringthefuture.org//pubs/monographs/mtf-overview2012.pdf.

BIBLIOGRAPHY

1. American College of Obstetricians and Gynecologists. (2012). Nonmedical use of prescription drugs. *Obstet Gynecol, 120*(4), 977-982.
2. Babor, T. F., Higgins-Biddle, J. C., Saunders, J. B., et al. (2001). *AUDIT: the alcohol use disorders identification test: guidelines for use in primary care* (2nd ed.). Geneva, Switzerland: World Health Organization.
3. Benzer, T. I., Nejad, S. H., & Flood, J. G. (2013). Case 40-2013: a 36-year-old man with agitation and paranoia. *N Engl J Med, 369*(26), 2536-2545.
4. Brooks, P. J., & Zakhari, S. (2013). Moderate alcohol consumption and breast cancer in women. *Alcohol Clin Exp Res, 37*(1), 23-30.
5. Bush, K., Kivlahan, D. R., McDonell, M. B., et al. (1998). The AUDIT alcohol consumption questions. *Arch Intern Med, 158*, 1789-1795.

6. Caputo, F., Vignoli, T., Leggio, L., et al. (2012). Alcohol use disorders in the elderly. *Exp Gerontol, 47*(6), 411-416.

7. Cherpitel, C. J., & Ye, Y. (2012). Trends in alcohol- and drug-related emergency department and primary care visits. *J Stud Alcohol Drug, 73*(3), 454-458.

8. Demark-Wahnefried, W., & Goodwin, P. J. (2013). How does the latest research on alcohol and breast cancer inform clinical practice? *J Clin Oncol, 31*(16), 1917-1919.

9. Elliott, D. Y., Geyer, C., Lionetti, T., et al. (2012). Managing alcohol withdrawal in hospitalized patients. *Nursing2013, 42*(4), 22-30.

10. Ewing, J. A. (1984). Detecting alcoholism: the CAGE questionnaire. *JAMA, 252*(14), 1905-1907.

11. Finnell, D. S., & Nowzari, S. (2013). Providing information about the neurobiology of alcohol use disorders to close the 'referral to treatment gap.' *Nurs Clin N Am 48*(3), 373-383.

12. Friedmann, P. D. (2013). Alcohol use in adults. *N Engl J Med 368*(4), 365-373.

13. Geneste, J., Pereira, B., Arnaud, B., et al. (2012). CAGE, RAPS4, RAPS4-QF and AUDIT screening tests for men and women admitted for acute alcohol intoxication to an emergency department. *Alcohol Alcohol, 47*(3), 273-281.

14. Hingson, R. W., Zha, W., Iannotti, R. J., et al. (2013). Physician advice to adolescents about drinking and other health behaviors. *Pediatrics, 131*(2), 249-257.

15. Jones, S. N., & Waite, R. L. (2013). Underage drinking: an evolutionary concept analysis. *Nurs Clin N Am 48*(3), 401-413.

16. Jones, L. A. (2011). Systematic review of alcohol screening tools for use in the emergency department. *Emerg Med J 28*:182-191.

17. Reference deleted in proofs.

18. Keegan, J., Parva, M., Finnegan, M., et al. (2010). Addiction in pregnancy. *J Addict Dis, 29*(2), 175-191.

19. Kessenich, C. R., & Cronin, K. (2012). GGT and alcohol consumption. *Nurse Pract, 37*(8), 9-11.

20. Kim, J. W., Lee, B. C., Lee, D. Y., et al. (2013). The 5-Item Alcohol Use Disorders Identification Test (AUDIT-5). *Alcohol Alcohol, 48*(1), 68-73.

21. Liang, Y., Mente, A., Yusuf, S., et al. (2012). Alcohol consumption and the risk of incident atrial fibrillation among people with cardiovascular disease. *Can Med Assoc J 184*(16), E857-E866.

22. Maxwell, J. C. (2011). The prescription drug epidemic in the United States. *Drug Alcohol Rev, 30*(3), 264-270.

23. May, P. A., & Phillip Gossage, J. (2011). Maternal risk factors for fetal alcohol spectrum disorders. *Alcohol Res Health, 34*(1), 15-26.

24. National Institutes of Health. (October 2010). *Fact sheet: alcohol-related traffic deaths.* Available at http://report.nih.gov/nihfactsheets/Pdfs/AlcoholRelatedTrafficDeaths(NIAAA).pdf .

25. National Institute on Alcohol Abuse and Alcoholism. (2005). (Reprinted 2007). *Helping patients who drink too much: a clinician's guide.* Available at http://pubs.niaaa.nih.gov/publications/Practitioner/CliniciansGuide2005/Clinicians_guide.htm.

26. Nelson, D. E., Jarman, D. W., Rehm, J., et al. (2013). Alcohol-attributable cancer deaths and years of potential life lost in the United States. *Am J Public Health, 103*(4), 641-648.

27. O'Malley, P. M., & Johnston, L. D. (2013). Driving after drug or alcohol use by US high school seniors, 2001–2011. *Am J Public Health, 103*(11), 2027-2034.

28. Rehm, J., Baliunas, D., Borges, G. L., et al. (2010). The relation between different dimensions of alcohol consumption and burden of disease. *Addiction, 105*(5), 817-843.

29. Russell, M., Materier, S. S., & Sokol, R. J. (1994). Screening for pregnancy risk-drinking. *Alcohol Clin Exp Res, 18*(5), 1156-1161.

30. SAMHSA. (September 2013). *18 percent of pregnant women drink alcohol during early pregnancy.* Available at http://www.samhsa.gov/data/spotlight/spot123-pregnancy-alcohol-2013.pdf.

31. Sarff, M., & Gold, J. A. (2010). Alcohol withdrawal syndromes in the intensive care unit. *Crit Care Med, 38*(9), S494-S501.

32. Seitz, H. K., Pelucchi, C., Bagnardi, V., et al. (2012). Epidemiology and pathophysiology of alcohol and breast cancer. *Alcohol Alcohol, 47*(3), 204-212.

33. Shapiro, B., Coffa, D., & McCance-Katz, E. F. (2013). A primary care approach to substance misuse. *Am Fam Phys, 88*(2), 113-121.

34. Starr, S. P., & Raines, D. (2011). Cirrhosis: diagnosis, management, and prevention. *Am Fam Phys, 84*(12), 1353-1359.

35. Steinbauer, J. R., Cantor, S. B., Holzer, C. E., et al. (1998). Ethnic and sex bias in primary care screening tests for alcohol use disorders. *Ann Int Med, 129*(5), 353-362.

36. Strobbe, S. (2013). Addressing substance use in primary care. *Nurse Pract, 38*(10), 45-53.

37. Tadros, A., Davidov, D. M., Coleman, J., et al. (2013). Pediatric visits to United States emergency departments for alcohol-related disorders. *J Emerg Med 44*(5), 1034-1038.

37a. Talbert, J. (2014). Club drugs: coming to a patient near you. *Nurse Pract 39*(3):20-25.

38. Tavakoll, H. R., Hull, M., & Okashski, L. M. (2011). Review of current clinical biomarkers for the detection of alcohol dependence. *Innov Clinical Neurosci, 8*(3), 26-33.

39. Ungur, L. A., Neuner, B., John, S., et al. (2013). Prevention and therapy of alcohol withdrawal on intensive care units. *Alcoholism: Clin Exper Res 37*(4), 675-686.

40. U.S. Department of Health and Human Services. (2012). *Results from the 2012 National Survey on Drug Use and Health.* Available at http://www.samhsa.gov/data/NSDUH/2012SummNatFindDetTables/NationalFindings/NSDUHresults2012.pdf.

41. U.S. Department of Health and Human Services. (2011). *National estimates of drug-related emergency department visits.* Accessed January 2014 from http://www.samhsa.gov/data/2k13/DAWN2k11ED/DAWN2k11ED.pdf.

42. U.S. Preventive Services Task Force. (2013). Screening and behavioral counseling interventions in primary care to reduce alcohol misuse. Available at http://www.uspreventiveservicestaskforce.org/uspstf/uspsdrin.htm.

43. Walker, R. K., Cousins, V. M., Umoh, N. A., et al. (2013). The good, the bad, and the ugly with alcohol use and abuse on the heart. *Alcoholism: Clin Exper Res, 37*(8), 1253-1260.

CHAPTER 7

Domestic and Family Violence Assessments

Intimate partner violence, dating violence, child abuse, and **elder abuse** are important health problems that health care professionals must recognize and assess. The Joint Commission has set standards that all health care settings have policies and procedures to assess, document, and make referrals for family violence, including child abuse, intimate partner abuse, and elder abuse.

TYPES OF VIOLENCE

Intimate Partner Violence

The Centers for Disease Control and Prevention (CDC)* definition for intimate partner violence (IPV) identifies four types of IPV:

- **Physical violence** (intentional use of physical force)
- **Sexual violence** (use of physical force to compel one to engage in a sex act against one's will; attempted or completed sex act to a person unable to consent because of illness, disability, or the influence of alcohol/drugs; and abusive sexual contact)
- **Threats of physical or sexual violence**
- **Psychological/emotional abuse and/or coercive tactics** when there has been prior physical and/or sexual violence between people who are spouses or nonmarital partners (dating, boyfriend/girlfriend) or former spouses or nonmarital partners that includes name calling, public embarrassment or humiliation, stalking, and harassment

Child Abuse and Neglect

Child abuse and neglect are defined at both the federal and state levels. The Child Abuse and Prevention Treatment Act (2010) dictates the minimum definitions that must be incorporated into state-defined standards. Some general definitions of child abuse and neglect include[11]:

- **Neglect** is the failure to provide for a child's basic needs (physical, educational, medical, and emotional). Prenatal drug exposure, child abandonment, and the manufacturing of methamphetamines in the presence of a child are considered neglect in some states.

- **Physical abuse** is nonaccidental physical injury caused by punching, beating, kicking, biting, burning, shaking, or otherwise harming a child. Even if the parent or caregiver did not intend to harm the child, such acts are considered abuse when done purposefully.
- **Sexual abuse** includes fondling a child's genitals, incest, penetration, rape, sodomy, indecent exposure, and commercial exploitation through prostitution or the production of pornographic materials.
- **Emotional abuse** is any pattern of behavior that harms a child's emotional development or sense of self-worth. It includes frequent belittling, rejection, threats, and withholding of love and support.

Adolescent Relationship Violence

Adolescent dating violence has been referred to in the literature as relationship violence, teen or "tween" dating violence, dating abuse, or relationship abuse. The CDC definition for adolescent dating violence* is:

> **Physical, sexual, or psychological/emotional violence within a dating relationship, and includes stalking**

The abuse may occur in person or electronically and may occur between a current or former dating partner.

It is important to note that, with advances of technology, new types of relationship violence are emerging such as 'sexting' or cyber abuse, which can be perpetrated 24/7 from a distance.

Elder Abuse and Neglect

The CDC definition for elder abuse[†] defines four types of elder abuse:

- **Physical abuse** is when an elder is intentionally injured, assaulted, threatened with a weapon, or inappropriately restrained.
- **Sexual abuse or abusive sexual contact** includes any sexual contact against the elder's will, including sexual

---

*http://www.cdc.gov/violenceprevention/intimatepartnerviolence/definitions.html.

---

*http://www.cdc.gov/violenceprevention/intimatepartnerviolence/teen_dating_violence.html.
[†]http://www.cdc.gov/violenceprevention/elderabuse/definitions.html.

contact with a person unable to understand the act or communicate consent.

- **Psychological or emotional abuse** is when an elder experiences trauma after exposure to threats or coercive tactics. It includes humiliation, embarrassment, controlling behavior, social isolation, and damaging/destroying property.
- **Financial abuse or exploitation** is the unauthorized or improper use of the elder's resources for monetary or personal benefit, profit, or gain such as forgery, theft, or improper use of guardianship or power of attorney.

Almost every state has some form of mandatory reporting of abused older adults and other vulnerable patients (the developmentally disabled and the mentally ill). You need to be familiar with the reporting requirements in the state in which you practice. Those who work in communities that border two states need to be informed about mandatory reporting statutes in both states. In some communities the reporting mechanism is established county by county, whereas other states have a statewide hotline. As mandatory reporters of abuse, you need only have suspicion that elder abuse and/or neglect may have occurred to generate a call to the authorities. Many nurses, physicians, and social workers are erroneously under the assumption that they must have proof of abuse before calling the hotline.

HEALTH EFFECTS OF VIOLENCE

Although estimates vary, approximately 1 million women in the United States report being physically and/or sexually assaulted by an intimate partner annually. Lifetime estimates of intimate violence against women are 31%, and the figure for men is 26%.[36] Women are significantly more likely to be physically or sexually assaulted by a current or former intimate partner than by an acquaintance, family member, friend, or stranger. The CDC's National Intimate Partner Violence and Sexual Violence Summary reported similar rates of abuse among men and women: 29% of men experienced rape, physical violence, and/or stalking in comparison to 36% of women when comparing lifetime prevalence rates[7]; but it is well known that women experience more severe adverse consequences as a result of IPV.[36]

Adolescents experience similar rates of relationship violence. According to the 2011 CDC's Youth Risk Behavior Survey, 1 of 10 high school students nationwide report experiencing purposeful physical violence by a boyfriend or girlfriend, and 8% report being victims of sexual violence in the past year. Prevalence rates of adolescent relationship violence range from 25% to 60% when assessing for lifetime abuse.[9]

In 2011 approximately 677,000 children in the United States were determined by Child Protective Services to have been maltreated. Of these children, approximately 79% were neglected, 18% were physically abused, 9% were sexually abused, and 10% were victims of other types of maltreatment (e.g., parental substance abuse, abandoned newborn). Some children were victims of multiple forms of maltreatment,

accounting for the total greater than 100%.[48] Although a number of children are injured by nonrelated caregivers, approximately 80% of injuries and fatalities caused by maltreatment are perpetrated by a parent or parents. Of the 1570 estimated fatalities, most were children younger than 4 years of age.[48]

Aside from minor differences, the reporting laws across the United States are essentially the same. As in cases of elder abuse, you need only a reasonable suspicion that a child has been maltreated to make a report to the appropriate authorities. Waiting until a conclusive diagnosis of abuse is made can put children at risk of further abuse and injury.

Violent experiences have significant immediate and long-term effects on the health of women and children. The most obvious immediate health care problem is injury. Cutaneous injuries can be caused by blunt, squeezing, and/or sharp mechanisms of injury.[5,46-48] Blunt-force injury is the most common form of IPV, with being struck by a hand (closed fist or slap) the most common mechanism of blunt-force trauma.[46-48] When blunt injuries cause the skin to tear, the wound is best described as a *laceration*.[5,46-48] When a sharp instrument (knife, razor, scalpel, glass) slices through the tissue, the wound is best described as a *cut* or *incision*.[5,46-48] *Strangulation* (often referred to by patient as "being choked") can be caused by the manual compression of the neck by any body part (usually hands) or by tightening a cordlike object around the neck (ligature compression).[5,46-48] Many of the mechanisms of injury just mentioned leave particular patterns to the skin that can be recognized.[5,46-48,51]

Abused women also have been found to have significantly more chronic health problems, including significantly more neurologic, gastrointestinal, and gynecologic symptoms and chronic pain.[39,55] Abused women have also been shown to visit health care professionals more often than women not battered and to incur more health care costs. In terms of mental health, abused women also have significantly more depression, suicidality, posttraumatic stress disorder (PTSD) symptoms, and problems with substance abuse.[39,55] Forced sex, which occurs in 40% to 45% of IPV cases, contributes to a host of reproductive health problems, including chronic pelvic pain, unintended pregnancy, sexually transmitted infections (STIs) including HIV, and urinary tract infections.[10,39] Abuse during pregnancy is also a significant health problem, with serious consequences for both the pregnant mother (e.g., depression, substance abuse) and infant (low birth weight, increased risk of child abuse).[7,10,12,19,36,43]

Although more than half of battered women report being injured during an assault, only 25% to 30% of abused women report that they have actually sought health care for one of the injuries.[43] Even so, the majority of abused women (80%) say they have been in the health care setting for some reason, either for regular checkups or for one of the long-term health problems described previously. Because many abused women are not yet ready to seek help from a shelter or the criminal justice system, the health care system can be an extremely important early point of contact. By uncovering abuse in its early stages, it is hoped that the pattern of violence can be stopped and long-term health problems avoided or minimized.

Abused adolescents are at risk for adverse health outcomes similar to those of adult women. Short-term consequences of relationship violence include depression, suicidal ideation, anxiety, alcohol abuse, cigarette and drug use, unintended pregnancies, and other sexual risky behaviors.[13,27] Long-term consequences include decreased self-esteem, poor academic performance, disordered eating behaviors, substance dependence, and poor mental health outcomes. Adolescent relationship violence can be fatal. Intimate partners of adolescents are responsible for nearly half (44%) of homicides of females ages 15 to 18 years.[33]

The health effects of elder abuse are not nearly as well studied. Complications from intentional injury can range from minor pain and discomfort to life-threatening injuries.[4,5,17,24,41,56] Bleeding from intentional trauma can cause significant changes in circulatory homeostasis, leading to marked fluctuations in blood pressure and pulse, shock, and then death. Localized infections can progress to generalized sepsis and then death in aging patients who are immunocompromised. The actual assault or the stress leading up to or following an assault can contribute to cardiac complications. All of the STIs and sexually related complications that are sequelae of abuse for younger women are present in older sexually assaulted women. In addition, postmenopausal women have more friable vaginal mucosal tissue secondary to deestrogenation.[41]

Abuse of older adults often is coupled with neglect. Neglect can manifest itself with symptoms of dehydration, malnutrition, and skin breakdown. It can be intentional or unintentional. Many family members or caregivers working with an aging person consciously and with malice withhold food, water, medication, and appropriate necessities while often stealing the financial assets of the older, dependent person. By definition this type of neglect is often criminal in nature.

Other family members or caregivers working with an older person may struggle with their own severe physical and cognitive health challenges. Their intentions are good; however, the older patient may experience profound unintentional neglect. Although unintentional neglect is usually not viewed as a crime, it is still reportable to adult protective service agencies. Self-neglect raises often unanswerable questions about one's right to live autonomously versus the obligation of society to care for a person who is not able to care for herself or himself. Suspected self-neglect is also a mandatory reportable activity to adult protective services.

There are many possible long-term physical and psychological effects of child maltreatment. The immediate consequences can include a spectrum of physical injuries such as bruises, fractures, and lacerations and can involve more severe injury such as abusive head trauma. More severe forms of maltreatment can lead to death or long-term disability such as mental retardation, blindness, and physical disability.

Child maltreatment can have deleterious effects on a child's quality of life and may lead to overall poor health, which can last into adulthood. Child maltreatment, including chronic maltreatment and exposures to multiple types of maltreatment, has shown to be a predictor of negative health outcomes for children that can persist into adulthood (e.g., mental health issues, incidence of suicide attempts, substance abuse, and the risk of perpetrating abuse as an adult).[23] Childhood physical abuse is reported to be the most consistent predictor of youth violence.[30]

The following are examples of risk factors that may contribute to child maltreatment[17]:

- Disabilities or chronic illnesses in children that may increase caregiver burden
- Social isolation of families
- Parents' lack of understanding of children's needs and of child development
- Poverty and other socioeconomic disadvantages such as unemployment and low educational achievement
- Family disorganization, dissolution, and violence, including IPV
- Substance abuse in family
- Young, single, nonbiological parents
- Poor parent-child relationships and negative interactions
- Parental thoughts and emotions supporting maltreatment behaviors
- Parental stress and distress, including depression or other mental health conditions
- Community violence

ASSESSMENT OF VIOLENCE

Intimate Partner Violence

Routine, universal assessments for IPV mean asking every woman at every health care encounter whether she has been abused by a husband, boyfriend, or other intimate partner or ex-partner. The majority of both abused and nonabused women support routine abuse assessments and believe it would assist women in getting help for the problem.[3] Despite this, nurses continue to have myths and stereotypes about when and whom they should screen such as the following: IPV is not a health problem; the patient will not be truthful about being abused; the patient will never leave the abusive relationship; and patients will be upset if the nurse asks questions about abuse.[42]

The U.S. Preventive Services Task Force (USPSTF) now states that there is sufficient research supporting the positive benefits of routine screening for IPV and recommends that screening be done. However, the USPSTF said that there has been so little research in screening for elder abuse that they could not yet make a recommendation about whether it is beneficial.[36]

How To Assess

The Abuse Assessment Screen (AAS) has been used in many different health care settings, has been translated into at least

Child Abuse and Neglect

Child abuse is part of the continuum of family violence, which includes IPV and elder abuse.[17] Assessing for child-abuse risk can be incorporated into the continuum of care in the child. You can use various developmental screening tools that identify risk factors for abuse and provide a platform for guidance to parents about expected development and upcoming developmental changes (i.e., the normal periods of excessive crying in the newborn period). This time is also important to emphasize the strengths of the family to reinforce positive interactions and behaviors.

When an injury is present or reported, an important part of the evaluation is to determine the child's age and developmental level. Could the child have suffered this injury based on his or her developmental level? Because you may not be able to directly observe the child's motor and cognitive milestones during the history taking, it is important to ask the caregivers directly. Is your child crawling, pulling to stand, or walking? Which other developmental issues are currently being faced at home (e.g., tantrums, potty training)?

If the child is verbal, a history should be obtained away from the caregivers through open-ended questions or spontaneous statements. It is important to remember that children may have suffered significant trauma yet respond only minimally to open-ended questions. Keeping the questions short and using age-appropriate language and familiar words can help enrich the history taking. Children older than 11 years can generally be expected to provide a history at the level of most adults.

The medical history is also an important part of your evaluation. Has the child had previous hospitalizations or injuries, or does he or she suffer from any chronic medical conditions? Does the child take any medication that may cause easy bruising? Does the child have a history of repeated visits to the hospital? Was there a delay in seeking care for anything other than a minor injury? Is there a history of substance abuse in the family or any financial or social stressors in the home? What are the typical methods of discipline used in the home?

HISTORY

It is important also to assess and document prior abuse, including prior IPV, childhood physical and sexual abuse, and prior rapes of all kinds (stranger, date, intimate partner). Cumulative trauma has been associated with more severe mental and physical health problems.[55] Also important to determine is the history of traumatic injuries because these may have an impact on the current health condition. For example, a woman may have experienced prior episodes of head trauma and strangulation, both of which may be related to chronic but subtle neurologic symptoms and problems. Another extremely important area of history and examination in cases of IPV or elder abuse is a mental status examination, both for potential head trauma and neurologic symptoms and also for mental health problems. All survivors

of violence should be given a mental status examination, with particular attention to the most frequent mental health problems associated with violence: depression, suicidality, PTSD, substance abuse, and anxiety. Chapter 5 gives direction for conducting this part of the history.

PHYSICAL EXAMINATION

Important components of the physical examination of the known survivor of IPV and/or elder abuse include a complete head-to-toe visual examination, especially if the patient is receiving health services secondary to reported abuse. When the examination reveals physical findings, knowledge of basic medical forensic terminology is essential in all documentation. Table 7-1 lists the most common forensic terms with definitions. Note that the most commonly misused terms are *ecchymosis* and *laceration*. Ecchymoses are not directly related to blunt-force trauma that results in bruising, and not all open wounds (only those related to splitting of tissue from blunt-force impact and/or tearing of tissue) should be called *lacerations*.

Keep in mind the following guidelines when documenting the physical examination[5,44-46]:

- *Bruise* can be used interchangeably with *contusion*.
- *Laceration* is related to *avulsion*.
- *Ecchymosis* is related to *(senile) purpura*.
- *Petechia* is related to *purpura*.
- *Rug burn* is more accurately described as a *friction abrasion*.
- *Incision* can be used interchangeably with *cut*.
- *Cut* can be used interchangeably with *sharp injury*.
- *Stab wounds* are penetrating, deep, sharp injuries.
- *Hematoma* is a collection of blood that is often but not always caused by blunt-force trauma.

Many practitioners try to date bruises based on the color; however, there is no scientific evidence to support the accurate dating of injuries based on color of the contusion.[37] Therefore trying to date injuries accurately solely by examination is forensically futile. However, some guidelines can help to determine if the approximate age of the bruise is consistent with the history being provided by the patient and/or caregiver.

A new bruise is usually red and often develops a purple or purple-blue appearance 12 to 36 hours after blunt-force trauma. The color of bruises (and ecchymoses) generally progresses from purple-blue to bluish-green to greenish-brown to brownish-yellow before fading away. This process is the same on all people; however, depending on the color of a person's skin, the process may be more or less visible and more or less able to be photographed. In general, newer bruises are mostly reddish-purple, whereas bruises that are beginning to age will be more greenish-brown or brownish-yellow.[37]

Multiple factors can contribute to older adults bruising more readily or more severely than younger people. Medications and abnormal blood values related to medication side effects and underlying hematologic disorders can affect ease

TABLE 7-1	**Forensic Terminology**

Abrasion A wound caused by rubbing the skin or mucous membrane.

Avulsion The tearing away of a structure or part.

Bruise Superficial discoloration caused by hemorrhage into the tissues from ruptured blood vessels beneath the skin surface, without the skin itself being broken; also called a *contusion*.

Contusion A bruise; injury to tissues without breakage of skin; blood from broken blood vessels accumulates, producing pain, swelling, tenderness.

Cut See "Incision."

Ecchymosis A hemorrhagic spot or blotch, larger than petechia, in the skin or mucous membrane, forming a nonelevated, rounded or regular blue or purplish patch.

Hematoma A localized collection of extravasated blood, usually clotted in an organ, space, or tissue.

Hemorrhage The escape of blood from a ruptured vessel, which can be external, internal, and/or into the skin or other organ.

Incision A cut or wound made by a sharp instrument; the act of cutting.

Laceration The act of tearing or splitting; a wound produced by the tearing and/or splitting of body tissue, usually from blunt impact over a bony surface.

Lesion A broad term referring to any pathologic or traumatic discontinuity of tissue or loss of function of a part.

Patterned injury An injury caused by an object that leaves a distinct pattern on the skin and/or organ (e.g., being whipped with an extension cord) or an injury caused by a unique mechanism of injury (e.g., immersion burns to the hands [glove burns] or feet [sock burns]).

Pattern of injuries Usually bruises and fractures in various stages of healing.

Petechiae Minute, pinpoint, nonraised, perfectly round purplish-red spots caused by intradermal or submucous hemorrhage, which later turn blue or yellow.

Puncture The act of piercing or penetrating with a pointed object or instrument.

Stab wound A penetrating, sharp, cutting injury that is deeper than it is wide.

Traumatic alopecia Loss of hair from pulling and yanking or by other traumatic means.

Wound A general term referring to a bodily injury caused by physical means.

Adapted from Merriam-Webster's *Medical Desk Dictionary Revised Edition.* (2005). Springfield, MA: Merriam-Webster; and Sheridan, D. J., & Nash, K. R. (2007). Acute injury patterns of intimate partner violence. *Trauma Violence Abuse, 8*(3), 281-289.

of bruising or the formation of ecchymosis. Common medications that increase risk for bruising or bleeding complications include but are not limited to aspirin, ibuprofen, any of the nonsteroidal antiinflammatory drugs, warfarin, heparin, valproic acid, prednisone, and clopidogrel. Vitamin nutritional supplements also may contribute to hematologic complications, especially if the person is already taking a blood-thinning or platelet-altering medication. Bilberry, garlic, ginger, and ginkgo are among the more common supplements linked to increased risk of bruising and/or bleeding complications.

Any health evaluation for known or suspected elder abuse and neglect should include these baseline laboratory tests: a complete blood count (CBC) with platelet level, basic blood chemistries (including blood urea nitrogen [BUN], creatinine, protein, and albumin), serum liver function tests, a coagulation panel, and a urinalysis. In a young child a radiologic survey to look for occult injuries may be warranted. This includes a skeletal survey (series of x-ray images of all bones) or a bone scan (nuclear medicine).

Physical Examination of Children

A visual inspection of the child from head to toe is important in any physical examination. Significant injuries can be hidden under clothing, diapers, socks, and long hair. The American Academy of Pediatrics[2] defines significant trauma as any injury beyond temporary redness of the skin. Bruising in children is one of the most common physical findings in child abuse. Unfortunately it can be easily overlooked and may be a missed opportunity for intervention and prevention of further injury. Accidental bruising in healthy, active children is common; yet the presence of bruises in babies has significance in evaluating a child for abuse. Children who are not yet walking with support—"cruising"—typically should not have bruises. Bruising in infants who are not yet cruising, usually infants younger than 9 months, should alert you to possible abusive mechanisms to the injury or an underlying medical illness. One study[40] found that bruising was a missed warning sign in up to 44% of fatal and near-fatal cases of physical child abuse.

Bruising is a common finding in children who are walking. Although any area of the body can be injured intentionally, certain locations are more concerning for inflicted injury. Bruising in "atypical" places, such as the buttocks, hands, feet, and abdomen, is exceedingly rare and should arouse concern. In children younger than 4 years, bruising on the torso, ears, and neck and any bruising on a precruising infant are significantly correlated with abuse in the absence of a compelling history.[40] Any bruise that takes the shape of an object is highly concerning for abuse. Bruising found in nonmobile children should raise your concern for further injury (i.e., fractures and intracranial injury) and should be the basis for a comprehensive evaluation for an underlying medical condition.

Health care providers are often asked to estimate the age of bruises, particularly as it relates to an inflicted injury. As with adults, avoid this because published evidence does not support the ability to date a bruise by color alone, either by visual assessment or photography.[37]

In addition to bruising, lacerations, abrasions, bite marks, and burns are commonly seen in abused children. These findings, taken into context with the child's developmental level, the history and mechanism of injury, location of injury, and social history, can help guide if an injury is a concern for abuse.

Many dermatologic conditions can mimic traumatic skin injuries of abuse; consider these when evaluating skin findings in children. Mongolian spots (dermal melanosis) are common in children of Asian, African, or Mediterranean descent. The lesions typically have a blue-gray appearance and are often found on the lower back and buttocks, although the distribution can be much more extensive. Mongolian spots often fade over time, do not cause pain (as with a bruise), and are present since birth. Some purpural diseases, which cause hemorrhage into underlying skin, can mimic bruising. Henoch Schönlein purpura, a vasculitis of the small blood vessels, can present with a maculopapular rash that often starts on the lower part of the body and can mimic inflicted bruises. Other prodromal symptoms such as malaise, abdominal pain, and arthralgias can be present as well. Drug eruptions can manifest as a variety of skin reactions, which can mimic bruises, burns, and blisters.[8]

DOCUMENTATION

Documentation of IPV, adolescent relationship violence, and elder abuse must include detailed, nonbiased progress notes, the use of injury maps, and photographic documentation in the health record. Note the examples of photographic documentation (Figs. 7-3 through 7-9).

Written documentation of histories of IPV and elder abuse need to be verbatim but within reason. It is clinically unrealistic to chart verbatim every statement made by an abused patient. However, it is critical to document exceptionally poignant statements made by the victim that identify the reported perpetrator and severe threats of harm made by the reported perpetrator. Other aspects of the abuse history, including reports of past abusive incidents, can be paraphrased with the use of partial direct quotations.

When quoting or paraphrasing the history, you should not sanitize the words reportedly heard by the victim. Verbatim documentation of the reported perpetrator's threats interlaced with curses and expletives can be extremely useful in future court proceedings. Also be careful to use the exact

7-4   Patterned punchlike abrasion to the mid-forehead from an assailant wearing a ring with a stone; sutured laceration to the left eyebrow; sutured partial-avulsion injury to the nose, punchlike contusion to the left eye involving the sclera, and manual strangulation–related abrasion to the neck. (Courtesy Daniel J. Sheridan.)

terms that an abused patient may use to describe sexual organs or sexually assaultive behaviors.

Digital photographic documentation in the medical record can be invaluable. Prior written consent to take photographs should be obtained from all cognitively intact, competent adults. Most health facilities have standardized consent-to-photograph forms. If a patient is unconscious or cognitively impaired, taking photographs without consent is generally viewed as ethically sound because it is a noninvasive, painless intervention that has high potential to help a suspected abuse victim.

7-3   Patterned fingernail-like scratch abrasions to the left lateral neck from a manual strangulation mechanism of injury. (Courtesy Daniel J. Sheridan.)

7-5   Newer patterned looped, cordlike contusions to the right upper posterior shoulder and left lower posterior shoulder; patterned looped, cordlike scar to the right mid-lateral back; scabbed, cordlike abrasions to the mid-back; patterned kick/stomplike heel contusion to the left mid-back; and patterned foot/kick/stomplike heel and sole bruise imprint to the upper left posterior shoulder. (Courtesy Daniel J. Sheridan.)

7-6 Multiple patterned punchlike contusions to the right upper arm. (Courtesy Daniel J. Sheridan.)

7-7 Multiple patterned "hidden" punchlike contusions to the upper abdomen and lower anterior chest. (Courtesy Daniel J. Sheridan.)

When documenting the history and physical findings of child abuse and neglect, use the words the child has given to describe how his or her injury occurred. Remember that the possibility arises that the abuser may be accompanying the child. If the child is nonverbal, use statements from caregivers. It is important to know your employer/institutional protocol for obtaining a history in cases of suspected child maltreatment. Some protocols may delay a full interview until it can be done by a forensically trained interviewer.

ASSESSING FOR RISK OF HOMICIDE

Women in this country are more often killed by a husband, boyfriend, or ex-husband than by anyone else, and battering during pregnancy is a major risk for domestic homicide.[1a] Failing to routinely assess for IPV in medical settings is a missed opportunity for health care professionals to identify

7-8 Patterned defensive posture–like bruises to the right forearm. (Courtesy Daniel J. Sheridan.)

7-9 Series of two photographs to illustrate how photographs can be used to demonstrate mechanisms of injuries. **A,** Victim has obvious facial trauma to her left eyelid, left lateral nose, and mouth. The left lateral nose contusion was caused by the nosepiece of her glasses being forcefully pushed into her skin from a punch injury to the left eye. The patient's glasses absorbed much of the punch force and were broken (not pictured). A second punch produced the mouth trauma. **B,** The force of the mouth punch caused the upper teeth to leave patterned contusions, abrasions, and minor lacerations to the oral mucosa of the upper lip. (Courtesy Daniel J. Sheridan.)

IPV and intervene to decrease the danger. The Danger Assessment (DA) (http://www.dangerassessment.org/) is a 19-item yes/no instrument that has been used extensively by nurses in health care settings and advocates in other settings with battered women[12] (Fig. 7-10). The instrument starts with a calendar so women can see for themselves more accurately how frequent and severe the violence has become over the past year. This is also an excellent assessment of frequency and severity for the health care provider. Although there are no predetermined cutoff scores on the DA, the more "yes" answers there are, the more serious the danger of the woman's situation.

The DA has been incorporated into an anonymous free application for smart phones and other electronic devices for college-aged women called One Love MyPlan. Completing the app can help a woman determine if a relationship is unsafe and helps create an action plan based on the woman's unique characteristics and values. The tool can be found at http://www.joinonelove.org/resources-help.

CULTURE AND GENETICS

Domestic violence is a phenomenon that occurs universally in all populations.[54] However, lifetime prevalence of IPV (including rape, physical violence, and stalking) is significantly higher among ethnic and racial minorities than among non-Hispanic White women (34.6%), with the exception of Asians and Pacific Islanders (19.6%).[7] The highest rates of IPV are among multiracial women (54%), followed by American Indians or Alaska natives (46%), Blacks (44%), and Hispanics (37%).[7] Deaths from IPV are significantly higher among refugee and immigrant women.[1,26,28] In spite of these overwhelming statistics, little research exists about the effectiveness of screening and prevention efforts among racial and ethnic minority women and the effectiveness of therapeutic interventions to help survivors with resultant mental health problems.[41a]

Although there are wide differences among distinct cultural groups and within any given culture, some common

---

DANGER ASSESSMENT Jacquelyn C. Campbell, Ph.D., R.N. Copyright 1985, 1988, 2001

Several risk factors have been associated with homicides (murders) of both batterers and battered women in research conducted after the murders have taken place. We cannot predict what will happen in your case, but we would like you to be aware of the danger of homicide in situations of severe battering and for you to see how many of the risk factors apply to your situation.

Using the calendar, please mark the approximate dates during the past year when you were beaten by your husband or partner. Write on that date how bad the incident was according to the following scale:

1. Slapping, pushing; no injuries and/or lasting pain
2. Punching, kicking; bruises, cuts, and/or continuing pain
3. "Beating up"; severe contusions, burns, broken bones
4. Threat to use weapon; head injury, internal injury, permanent injury
5. Use of weapon; wounds from weapon

(If **any** of the descriptions for the higher number apply, use the higher number.)

Mark **Yes** or **No** for each of the following. ("He" refers to your husband, partner, ex-husband, ex-partner, or whoever is currently physically hurting you.)

_____ 1. Has the physical violence increased in severity or frequency over the past year?
_____ 2. Has he ever used a weapon against you or threatened you with a weapon?
_____ 3. Does he ever try to choke you?
_____ 4. Does he own a gun?
_____ 5. Has he ever forced you to have sex when you did not wish to do so?
_____ 6. Does he use drugs? By drugs, I mean "uppers" or amphetamines, speed, angel dust, cocaine, "crack," street drugs or mixtures.
_____ 7. Does he threaten to kill you and/or do you believe he is capable of killing you?
_____ 8. Is he drunk every day or almost every day? (In terms of quantity of alcohol.)
_____ 9. Does he control most or all of your daily activities? (For instance, does he tell you who you can be friends with, when you can see your family, how much money you can use, or when you can take the car?)
 (If he tries, but you do not let him, check here: _____)
_____ 10. Have you ever been beaten by him while you were pregnant? (If you have never been pregnant by him, check here: _____)
_____ 11. Is he violently and constantly jealous of you? (For instance, does he say, "If I can't have you, no one can"?)
_____ 12. Have you ever threatened or tried to commit suicide?
_____ 13. Has he ever threatened or tried to commit suicide?
_____ 14. Does he threaten to harm your children?
_____ 15. Do you have a child that is not his?
_____ 16. Is he unemployed?
_____ 17. Have you left him during the past year? (If you have *never* lived with him, check here: _____)
_____ 18. Do you currently have another (different) intimate partner?
_____ 19. Does he follow or spy on you, leave threatening notes, destroy your property, or call you when you don't want him to?

_____ Total "Yes" Answers

Thank you. Please talk to your nurse, advocate, or counselor about what the Danger Assessment means in terms of your situation.

7-10 Danger Assessment.   (Courtesy Jacquelyn C. Campbell.)

themes create barriers to treatment for all. These barriers are societal stressors (poverty, discrimination, legal systems), regulations, lack of access to care and culturally responsive care, cultural values, and gender roles.

Societal stressors contribute to daily struggles and conflict in relationships. For example, poverty is a risk factor for domestic violence.[36] All ethnic and racial minority groups have poverty rates exceeding the national average for non-Hispanic Whites of 11.6%. In addition, help-seeking often is deferred because of fears of racism and discrimination. Because of past experiences of prejudice and discrimination by health care providers and lack of knowledge of the culture, many immigrants and members of racial and ethnic minorities are reluctant to seek help in the health care setting.[20,25,53] African-American and Native American women may be reluctant to call the police on their partners because they fear being perceived as disloyal by their families by participating in a racist criminal system that incarcerates minority men far more frequently than Caucasians.[20,53]

Legal status in the United States creates a barrier to care for many immigrant families. If a woman does not have legal status or citizenship within the United States, she may fear that she will be deported and lose her children.[6] Many immigrant women are unaware of their legal rights (e.g., the U.S. Violence Against Women Act [VAWA]) in situations of domestic violence.[22]

A **lack of access to care and culturally competent care** is a continual problem. In spite of the widespread growth of domestic violence services in the 1980s and 1990s and the widely distributed availability of translation services,[14] immigrants, Native Americans and African Americans are less likely than native-born Euro-Americans to use social service resources.[25] In mental health settings, social service settings, and primary care, often a conflict of values exists that leads to inappropriate care.[15,25]

Cultural values and gender roles are barriers. Among many ethnic and racial minority groups, domestic violence is viewed as something shameful and private that a person does not share outside the family.[15,20,25] Traditional gender roles reinforce dependency and may increase the risk for domestic violence.[15] Women are often financially dependent on their husbands, and this dependency is reinforced by religious and cultural values, which identify men as the providers within the family.[18] Women are expected to endure domestic violence to sacrifice for the sake of their children and out of fear of losing them.[29]

To address these barriers to care, recommendations for culturally sensitive approaches to screening and treatment are available.[25,31,53] These recommendations include access to bilingual bicultural providers, access to translators, education about legal rights, incorporation and acknowledgment of the importance of religion and training of religious leaders, and involvement of the family and outreach to the community to raise awareness of the prevalence of domestic violence. However, the most important aspects of treatment are to understand the meaning and experiences of IPV for each person and to account for her or his cultural beliefs and values.

BIBLIOGRAPHY

1. Abu-Ras, W. (2007). Cultural beliefs and service utilization by battered Arab immigrant women. *Violence Against Women, 13,* 1002-1028.

2. American Academy of Pediatrics. (2002). When inflicted skin injuries constitute child abuse. *Pediatrics, 110,* 644-645.

3. Anglin, D. (2009). Diagnosis through disclosure and pattern recognition. In Mitchell, C., & Anglin, D. (Eds.). *Intimate partner violence: a health-based perspective.* New York: Oxford University Press.

4. Arvanis, S. C., Adelman, R. D., Breckman, R., et al. (1993). Diagnostic and treatment guidelines on elder abuse and neglect. *Arch Fam Med, 2*(4), 371-388.

5. Besant-Matthews, P. E. (2006). Blunt and sharp injuries. In Lynch, V., & Duval, J. B. (Eds.) *Forensic nursing.* St. Louis: Mosby.

6. Bhuyan, R., & Senturia, K. (2005). Understanding domestic violence resource utilization and survivor solutions among immigrant and refugee women. *J Interpers Violence, 20*(8), 895-901.

7. Black, M. C., Basile, K. C., Breiding, M. J., et al. (2011). National Intimate Partner and Sexual Violence Survey: 2010 Summary Report. Available at http://www.cdc.gov/violenceprevention/nisvs/.

8. Brogdon, B. G., Shwayder, T., & Elifritz, J. (2013). *Child abuse and its mimics in skin and bone.* Boca Raton: Taylor & Francis Group.

9. Centers for Disease Control and Prevention (CDC) (2010). *Youth risk behavior surveillance system.* Available at http://www.cdc.gov/healthyyouth/partners/funded/yrbs.htm.

10. Reference deleted in proofs.

11. Child Welfare Information Gateway. (2008). *What is child abuse and neglect?* Available at https://www.childwelfare.gov/pubs/factsheets/whatiscan.cfm.

12. Clements, P. T., Holt, K. E., Hasson, C. M., et al. (2011). Enhancing assessment of interpersonal violence (IPV) pregnancy-related homicide risk within nursing curricula. *J Forensic Nurs, 7,* 195-202.

13. Cutter-Wilson, E., & Richmond, T. (2011). Understanding teen dating violence: practical screening and intervention strategies for pediatric and adolescent healthcare providers. *Curr Opin Pediatr, 23*(4), 379-383.

14. Douglas, E. M., & Hines, D. A. (2011). The reported availability of U.S. domestic violence services to victims who vary by immigration status, primary language, and disability. *Partner Abuse, 2*(4), 427-451.

15. Edelson, M. G., Hokoda, A., & Ramos-Lira, L. (2007). Differences in effects of domestic violence between Latina and non-Latina women. *J Fam Viol, 1*(22), 1-10.

16. Reference deleted in proofs.

17. Flaherty, E. G., Stirling, J., & The Committee on Child Abuse and Neglect (2010). The pediatrician's role in child maltreatment prevention. *Pediatrics, 126,* 833-841.

18. Gharaibeh, M., & Oweis, A. (2009). Why do Jordanian women stay in an abusive relationship. *J Nurs Scholarsh, 41*(4), 376-384.

19. Goodman, P. E. (2009). Intimate partner violence and pregnancy. In Mitchell, C., & Anglin, D. (Eds.). *Intimate partner violence: a health-based perspective.* New York: Oxford University Press.

20. Hamdy, S. L. (2004). *Sexual victimization in Indian country: barriers and resources for native women seeking help.* Harrisburg, PA: VAWnet. Available at http://www.vawnet.org.

21. Reference deleted in proofs.

22. Ingram, M., McClelland, D. J., Martin, J., et al. (2010). Experiences of immigrant women who self-petition under the Violence Against Women Act. *Violence Against Women, 16*(8), 858-880.

23. Jonson-Reid, M., Kohl, P. L., & Drake, B. (2012). Child and adult outcomes of child maltreatment. *Pediatrics, 129*(5), 8398-8345.

24. Koin, D. (2009). Intimate partner violence among the elderly and people with disabilities. In Mitchell, C., & Anglin, D. (Eds.). *Intimate partner violence: a health-based perspective.* New York: Oxford University Press.

25. Kulwicki, A., Aswad, B., Carmona, T., et al. (2010). Barriers in the utilization of domestic violence services among Arab immigrant women. *J Fam Violence, 25,* 727-735.

26. Lee, E. (2007). Domestic violence and risk factors among Korean immigrant women in the US. *J Fam Violence, 29,* 141-149.

27. Leshner, A. I. (2007). *NIDA probes the elusive link between child abuse and later drug use.* NIDA Notes (serial online). Available at www.nida.nih.gov/NIDA_Notes/NNVol13N2/DirrepVol13N2.html.

28. Liao, M. S. (2006). Domestic violence among Asian Indian immigrant women: risk factors, acculturation, and intervention. *Women Ther 29,* 23-39.

29. Reference deleted in proofs.

30. Maas, C., Herrenkohl, T. I., & Sousa, C. (2008). Review of research on child maltreatment and violence in youth. *Trauma, Violence Abuse, 9*(1), 56-67.

31. Marrs Fuchsel, C. L., & Hysjulien, B. (2013). Exploring a domestic violence intervention curriculum for immigrant Mexican women in a group setting. *Soc Work Groups, 36*(4), 304-320.

32. Martin, C. E., Houston, A. M., Mmari, K. N., et al. (2011). Urban teens and young adults describe drama, disrespect, dating violence, and help-seeking preferences. *Matern Child Health J, 16*(5), 957-966.

33. Martin, E. K., Taft, C. T., & Resick, P. A. (2007). A review of marital rape. *Aggress Viol Behav, 12,* 329-347. doi: 10.10116/j.avb2006.10.003.

34. Reference deleted in proofs.

35. Reference deleted in proofs.

36. Moyer, V. A. (2013). Screening for intimate partner violence and abuse of elderly and vulnerable adults: U.S. Preventative Task Force recommendation statement. *Ann Intern Med, 158*(16), 478-486.

37. Nash, K. R., & Sheridan, D. J. (2009). Can one accurately date a bruise: state of the science, *J Forensic Nurs 5,* 31-37.

38. Reference deleted in proofs.

39. Nicolaidis, C., & Liebschutz, J. (2009). Chronic physical symptoms in survivors of intimate partner violence. In Mitchell, C., & Anglin, D. (Eds.). *Intimate partner violence: a health-based perspective.* New York: Oxford University Press.

40. Pierce, M. C., Kaczor, K., Aldridge, S., et al. (2010). Bruising characteristics discriminating physical child abuse from accidental trauma. *Pediatrics, 125*(1), 67-74.

41. Poulos, C., & Sheridan, D. J. (2008). Genital injuries in postmenopausal women after sexual assault. *J Elder Abuse Neglect, 20*(4), 323-335.

41a. Rana, S. (2012). Addressing domestic violence in immigrant communities: critical issues for culturally competent services. Harrisburg, PA: VAWNet, a project of the National Resource Center on Domestic Violence. Available at http://www.vawnet.org.

42. Robinson, R. (2010). Myths and stereotypes: how registered nurses screen for intimate partner violence. *J Emerg Nurs, 36*(6), 572-576.

43. Saltzman, L. E., & Houry, D. (2009). Prevalence of nonfatal and fatal intimate partner violence in the United States. In Mitchell, C., & Anglin, D. (Eds.), *Intimate partner violence: a health-based perspective.* New York: Oxford University Press.

44. Reference deleted in proofs.

45. Shavers. C. A. (2013). Intimate partner violence: a guide for primary care providers. *Nurse Pract,38*(12):39-46.

46. Sheridan, D. J. (2007). Treating survivors of intimate partner abuse: forensic identification and documentation. In Olshaker, J. S., Jackson, M. C., & Smock, W. S. (Eds.). (2007). *Forensic emergency medicine* (2nd ed.). Philadelphia: Lippincott Williams & Wilkins.

47. Sheridan, D. J., & Nash, K. R. (2007). Acute injury patterns of intimate partner violence. *Trauma Violence Abuse, 8*(3), 281-289.

48. Sheridan, D. J., Nash, K. R., Poulos, C. A., et al. (2009). Soft tissue and cutaneous injury patterns. In Mitchell, C., & Anglin, D. (Eds.). *Intimate partner violence: a health-based perspective.* New York: Oxford University Press.

49. Snyder, R. L. (2013). A raised hand. *The New Yorker, 89,* 34-41. July 22.

50. Somes, J., & Donatelli, N. S. (2012). Sex and the older adult. *J Emerg Nurs, 38*(2), 166-167.

51. Taliaferro, E., Hawley, D., McClane, G., et al. (2009). Strangulation in intimate partner violence. In Mitchell, C., & Anglin, D. (Eds.). *Intimate partner violence: a health-based perspective.* New York: Oxford University Press.

52. Reference deleted in proofs.

53. Vann, A. A. (2003*). Developing culturally relevant responses to domestic abuse. Asha Family Services.* Harrisburg, PA: National Resource Center on Domestic Violence.

54. Warrier, S. (2009). Culture and cultural competency in addressing intimate partner violence. In Mitchell, C., & Anglin, D. (Eds.). *Intimate partner violence: a health-based perspective.* New York: Oxford University Press.

55. Warsaw, C., Brashler, P., & Gil, J. (2009). Mental health consequence of intimate partner violence. In Mitchell, C., & Anglin, D. (Eds.). *Intimate partner violence: a health-based perspective.* New York: Oxford University Press.

56. Yaffe, M. J., Wolfson, C., Lithwick, M., et al. (2008). Development and validation of a tool to improve physician identification of elder abuse: the Elder Abuse Suspicion Index (EASI). *J Elder Abuse Neglect, 20*(3), 276-300.

CHAPTER 8

Assessment Techniques and Safety in the Clinical Setting

CULTIVATING YOUR SENSES

The physical examination requires you to develop technical skills and a knowledge base. The technical skills are the tools to gather data. You use your senses—sight, smell, touch, and hearing—to gather data during the physical examination. The skills requisite for the physical examination are **inspection, palpation, percussion,** and **auscultation.** They are performed one at a time and in this order.

Inspection

Inspection is concentrated watching. It is close, careful scrutiny, first of the individual as a whole and then of each body system. Inspection begins the moment you first meet the person and develop a "general survey." (Specific data to consider for the general survey are presented in Chapter 9.) As you proceed through the examination, start the assessment of each body system with inspection.

Inspection always comes first. Initially you may feel embarrassed "staring" at the person without also "doing something." A focused inspection takes time and yields a surprising amount of data. Train yourself not to rush through inspection by holding your hands behind your back.

Learn to use each person as his or her own control and compare the right and left sides of the body. The two sides are nearly symmetric. Inspection requires good lighting, adequate exposure, and occasional use of certain instruments (otoscope, ophthalmoscope, penlight, nasal and vaginal specula) to enlarge your view.

Palpation

Palpation follows and often confirms points that you noted during inspection. Palpation applies your sense of touch to assess these factors: texture; temperature; moisture; organ location and size; and any swelling, vibration or pulsation, rigidity or spasticity, crepitation, presence of lumps or masses, and presence of tenderness or pain. Different parts of the hands are best suited for assessing different factors:

- Fingertips—Best for fine tactile discrimination, as of skin texture, swelling, pulsation, and determining presence of lumps
- A grasping action of the fingers and thumb—To detect the position, shape, and consistency of an organ or mass
- The dorsa (backs) of hands and fingers—Best for determining temperature because the skin here is thinner than on the palms

- Base of fingers (metacarpophalangeal joints) or ulnar surface of the hand—Best for vibration

Your palpation technique should be slow and systematic, calm and gentle. Warm your hands by kneading them together or holding them under warm water. Identify any tender areas and palpate them last.

Start with light palpation to detect surface characteristics and accustom the person to being touched. Then perform deeper palpation, perhaps by helping the person use relaxation techniques such as imagery or deep breathing. With deep palpation (as for abdominal contents), intermittent pressure is better than one long, continuous palpation. Avoid any situation in which deep palpation could cause internal injury or pain.

Bimanual palpation requires the use of both of your hands to envelop or capture certain body parts or organs such as the kidneys, uterus, or adnexa for more precise delimitation (see Chapters 21 and 26).

Percussion

Percussion is tapping the person's skin with short, sharp strokes to assess underlying structures. The strokes yield a palpable vibration and a characteristic sound that depicts the location, size, and density of the underlying organ. Why learn percussion when an x-ray image is so much more accurate? It's because your percussing hands are always available, are easily portable, and give instant feedback. Percussion has the following uses:

- Mapping out the *location* and *size* of an organ by exploring where the percussion note changes between the borders of an organ and its neighbors
- Signaling the *density* (air, fluid, or solid) of a structure by a characteristic note
- Detecting an abnormal mass if it is fairly superficial; the percussion vibrations penetrate about 5 cm deep— a deeper mass would give no change in percussion
- Eliciting a deep tendon reflex using the percussion hammer

The Stationary Hand

Hyperextend the middle finger (the *pleximeter)* and place its distal joint and tip *firmly* against the person's skin. Avoid the person's ribs and scapulae. Percussing over a bone yields no data because it always sounds "dull." Lift the rest of the stationary hand up off the person's skin (Fig. 8-1). Otherwise the resting hand will dampen off the produced vibrations, just as a drummer uses the hand to halt a drum roll.

8-1

characteristic waves and are heard as "notes" (Table 8-1), which are differentiated by the following components: (1) **amplitude** (or intensity), a loud or soft sound; (2) **pitch** (or frequency), the number of vibrations per second; (3) **quality** (timbre), a subjective difference caused by the distinctive overtones of a sound; and (4) **duration**, the length of time the note lingers.

A basic principle is that a structure with relatively more air (e.g., the lungs) produces a louder, deeper, and longer sound because it vibrates freely; whereas a denser, more solid structure (e.g., the liver) gives a softer, higher, shorter sound because it does not vibrate as easily. Although Table 8-1 describes five "normal" percussion notes, variations occur in clinical practice. The "note" you hear depends on the nature of the underlying structure, the thickness of the body wall, and your correct technique.

Auscultation

Auscultation is listening to sounds produced by the body, such as the heart and blood vessels and the lungs and abdomen. Likely you already have heard certain body sounds with your ear alone (e.g., the harsh gurgling of very congested breathing). However, most body sounds are very soft and must be channeled through a **stethoscope** for you to evaluate them. The stethoscope does not magnify sound but does block out extraneous room sounds. Of all the equipment you use, the stethoscope quickly becomes a very personal instrument. Take time to learn its features and to fit one individually to yourself.

The Striking Hand

Use the middle finger of your dominant hand as the *striking finger* (the *plexor*) (Fig. 8-2). Hold your forearm close to the skin surface, with your upper arm and shoulder steady. Scan your muscles to make sure that they are steady but not rigid. The action is all in the wrist, and it *must* be relaxed. Spread your fingers, swish your wrist, and bounce your middle finger off the stationary one. Aim for just behind the nail bed or at the distal interphalangeal joint; the goal is to hit the portion of the finger that is pushing the hardest into the skin surface. Flex the striking finger so its tip, not the finger pad, makes contact. It hits directly at right angles to the stationary finger.

Percuss 2 times in this location using even, staccato blows. Lift the striking finger off quickly; a resting finger dampens vibrations. Then move to a new body location and repeat, keeping your technique even. The force of the blow determines the loudness of the note. You do not need a very loud sound; use just enough force to achieve a clear note. The thickness of the person's body wall will be a factor. You need a stronger percussion stroke for people with obese or very muscular body walls.

Production of Sound

All sound results from vibration of some structure. Percussing over a body structure causes vibrations that produce

8-2

TABLE 8-1	Characteristics of Percussion Notes				
	Amplitude	Pitch	Quality	Duration	Sample Location
Resonant	Medium-loud	Low	Clear, hollow	Moderate	Over normal lung tissue
Hyperresonant	Louder	Lower	Booming	Longer	Normal over child's lung Abnormal in the adult, over lungs with increased amount of air as in emphysema
Tympany	Loud	High	Musical and drumlike (like the kettledrum)	Sustained longest	Over air-filled viscus (e.g., the stomach, the intestine)
Dull	Soft	High	Muffled thud	Short	Relatively dense organ as liver or spleen
Flat	Very soft	High	A dead stop of sound, absolute dullness	Very short	When no air is present, over thigh muscles or bone or over tumor

The fit and quality of the stethoscope are important. You cannot assess what you cannot hear through a poor instrument. The slope of the earpiece should point forward toward your nose. This matches the natural slope of your ear canal and efficiently blocks out environmental sound. If necessary, twist the earpieces to parallel the slope of your ear canals. The earpieces should fit snugly, but if they hurt, they are inserted too far. Adjust the tension, and experiment with different rubber or plastic earplugs to achieve the most comfort. The tubing should be of thick material, with an internal diameter of 4 mm ($\frac{1}{8}$ in), and about 36 to 46 cm (14 to 18 in) long. Longer tubing may distort the sound.

Choose a stethoscope with two endpieces—a diaphragm and a bell (Fig. 8-3). You will use the **diaphragm** most often because its flat edge is best for high-pitched sounds—breath, bowel, and normal heart sounds. Hold the diaphragm firmly against the person's skin, firm enough to leave a slight ring afterward. The **bell** endpiece has a deep, hollow, cuplike shape. It is best for soft, low-pitched sounds such as extra heart sounds or murmurs. Hold it lightly against the person's skin, just enough that it forms a perfect seal. Holding it any harder causes the person's skin to act as a diaphragm, obliterating the low-pitched sounds.

Some newer stethoscopes have one endpiece with a "tunable diaphragm." This enables you to listen to both low- and high-frequency sounds without rotating the endpiece. For low-frequency sounds (traditional bell mode), hold the endpiece very lightly on the skin; for high-frequency sounds (traditional diaphragm mode), press the endpiece firmly on the skin.

Before you can evaluate body sounds, you must eliminate any confusing artifacts:

- Any extra room noise can produce a "roaring" in your stethoscope; therefore the room must be quiet.
- Keep the examination room warm. If the person starts

shivering, the involuntary muscle contractions could drown out other sounds.

- Clean the stethoscope endpiece with an alcohol wipe. Then warm it by rubbing it in your palm. This avoids the "chandelier sign" elicited when placing a cold endpiece on a warm chest!
- The friction on the endpiece from a man's hairy chest causes a crackling sound that mimics an abnormal breath sound called *crackles*. To minimize this problem, wet the hair before auscultating the area.

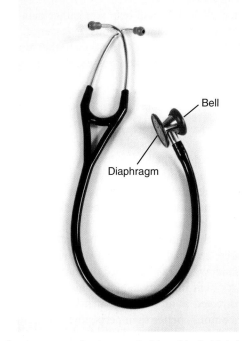

8-3 Stethoscope diaphragm *(left)* and bell *(right)*.

8-4

8-5

- **Never listen through a gown** (Fig. 8-4). Even though you see this on television, listening through clothing creates artifactual sound and muffles any diagnostically valuable sound from the heart or lungs. Therefore reach under a gown to listen, and take care that no clothing rubs on the stethoscope.
- Finally avoid your own "artifact," such as breathing on the tubing or the "thump" from bumping the tubing together.

Auscultation is a skill that beginning examiners are eager to learn but one that is difficult to master. First you must learn the wide range of normal sounds. Once you can recognize normal sounds, you can distinguish the abnormal and "extra" sounds. Be aware that in some body locations you may hear more than one sound; this can be confusing. You need to listen selectively to only one thing at a time. As you listen, ask yourself: What am I *actually hearing?* and What *should* I be hearing at this spot?

These technical skills will help you gather data to add to your knowledge base and previous experience. A sturdy knowledge base enables you to look *for* rather than merely look *at*. The chapters that follow present the content you will be looking *for*.

SETTING

The examination room should be warm and comfortable, quiet, private, and well lit. When possible, stop any distracting noises such as humming machinery, radio or television, or talking that could make it difficult to hear body sounds. Your time with the individual should be secure from interruptions from other health care personnel.

Lighting with natural daylight is best, although it is often not available; artificial light from two sources suffices and prevents shadows. A wall-mounted or gooseneck stand lamp is needed for high-intensity lighting. This provides *tangential* lighting (directed at an angle), which highlights pulsations and body contours better than perpendicular lighting.

Position the examination table so both sides of the person are easily accessible (Fig. 8-5). The table should be at a height

at which you can stand without stooping and should be equipped to raise the person's head up to 45 degrees. A roll-up stool is used for the sections of the examination for which you must be sitting. A bedside stand or table is needed to lay out all your equipment.

EQUIPMENT

During the examination you do not want to be searching for equipment or to have to leave the room to find an item. Have all your equipment at easy reach and laid out in an organized fashion (Fig. 8-6). The following items are usually needed for a screening physical examination:

- Platform scale with height attachment
- Sphygmomanometer
- Stethoscope with bell and diaphragm endpieces
- Thermometer
- Pulse oximeter (in hospital setting)
- Paper and pencil or pen
- Flashlight or penlight
- Otoscope/ophthalmoscope

8-6

8-7   Otoscope.

* Tuning fork
* Nasal speculum (if a short, broad speculum is not included with the otoscope)
* Tongue depressor
* Pocket vision screener
* Skin-marking pen
* Flexible tape measure and ruler marked in centimeters
* Reflex hammer
* Sharp object (split tongue blade)
* Cotton balls
* Bivalve vaginal speculum
* Clean gloves
* Alcohol wipes
* Hand sanitizer
* Materials for cytologic study
* Lubricant
* Fecal occult blood test materials

Most of the equipment is described as it comes into use throughout the text. However, consider these introductory comments on the otoscope and ophthalmoscope.

The **otoscope** funnels light into the ear canal and onto the tympanic membrane. The base serves both as the power source by holding a battery and as the handle. To attach the head, press it down onto the male adaptor end of the base and turn clockwise until you feel a stop. To turn the light on, press the red button rheostat down and clockwise. (Always turn it off after use to increase the life of the bulb and battery.) Five specula, each a different size, are available to attach to the head (Fig. 8-7). (The short, broad speculum is for viewing the nares.) Choose the largest one that will fit comfortably into the person's ear canal. See Chapter 15 for technique on use of the otoscope.

The **ophthalmoscope** illuminates the internal eye structures. Its system of lenses and mirrors enables you to look through the pupil at the fundus (background) of the eye, much like looking through a keyhole at a room beyond. The ophthalmoscope head attaches to the base male adaptor just as the otoscope head does (Fig. 8-8). The head has five different parts:

1. Viewing aperture, with five different apertures
2. Aperture selector dial on the front
3. Mirror window on the front
4. Lens selector dial
5. Lens indicator

Select the aperture to be used, most often the small spot for undilated pupils or the large full spot for dilated pupils.

Rotating the lens selector dial brings the object into focus. The lens indicator shows a number, or *diopter,* that indicates the value of the lens in position. The black numbers indicate a positive lens, from 0 to +40. The red numbers indicate a negative lens, from 0 to −20. The ophthalmoscope can compensate for myopia (nearsightedness) or hyperopia (farsightedness) but does not correct for astigmatism. See Chapter 14 for details on how to hold the instrument and what to inspect.

The following equipment occasionally will be used, depending on the individual's needs: goniometer to measure

8-8   Ophthalmoscope.

joint range of motion, Doppler sonometer to augment pulse or blood pressure measurement, pain rating scale (in numbers or faces), monofilament to test sensation in the foot, and bladder scanner to assess urine retention.

For a child you also will need appropriate pediatric-size endpieces for stethoscope and otoscope specula, materials for developmental assessment, age-appropriate toys, and a pacifier for an infant.

A Clean Field

Do not let your stethoscope become a *staph*-oscope! Stethoscopes and other equipment that are frequently used on many patients are common vehicles for transmission of infection. Clean your stethoscope endpiece with an alcohol wipe before and after every patient contact. The best routine is to combine stethoscope rubbing with every episode of hand hygiene.

Designate a "clean" versus a "used" area for handling your equipment. In a hospital setting you may use the bedside stand for your clean surface and the over-bed table for the used equipment surface. Or in a clinic setting use two separate areas of the pull-up table. Distinguish the clean area by one or two disposable paper towels. On the towels place all the new or newly alcohol-swabbed equipment that you will use for this patient (e.g., your stethoscope endpieces, the reflex hammer, ruler). As you proceed through the examination, pick up each piece of equipment from the clean area; and, after use on the patient, relegate it to the used area or (as in the case of tongue blades, gloves) throw it directly in the trash.

A SAFER ENVIRONMENT

In addition to monitoring the cleanliness of your equipment, take all steps to avoid any possible transmission of infection between patients or between patient and examiner (Table 8-2). A health care–associated (nosocomial) infection is a hazard because hospitals have sites that are reservoirs for virulent microorganisms. Some of these microorganisms are resistant to antibiotics such as methicillin-resistant *Staphylococcus aureus* (MRSA), vancomycin-resistant *Enterococcus* (VRE), or multidrug-resistant tuberculosis or are microorganisms for which there is currently no known cure such as human immunodeficiency virus (HIV).

The single most important step to decrease risk of microorganism transmission is to wash your hands promptly and thoroughly: (1) **before and after** every physical patient encounter; (2) after contact with blood, body fluids, secretions, and excretions; (3) after contact with any equipment contaminated with body fluids; and (4) after removing gloves (see Table 8-2). Using alcohol-based hand rubs takes less time than soap-and-water handwashing; it also kills more organisms more quickly and is less damaging to the skin because of emollients added to the product. Alcohol is highly effective against both gram-positive and gram-negative bacteria; *Mycobacterium tuberculosis*; and most viruses, including hepatitis B and C viruses, HIV, and enteroviruses.[1] Rub all hand surfaces with 3 to 5 mL of alcohol for 20 to 30 seconds. Use the mechanical action of soap-and-water handwashing when

hands are visibly soiled and when patients are infected with spore-forming organisms (e.g., *Clostridium difficile* and noroviruses).[8] Rub all hand surfaces for 40 to 60 seconds (Fig. 8-9).

Wear gloves when the potential exists for contact with any body fluids (e.g., blood, mucous membranes, body fluids, drainage, open skin lesions). However, wearing gloves is *not* a protective substitute for washing hands because gloves may have undetectable holes or become torn during use, or hands

---

TABLE 8-2 Standard Precautions for Use with All Patients

STANDARD PRECAUTIONS are based on the principle that all blood, body fluids, secretions, excretions (except sweat), nonintact skin, and mucous membranes may contain transmissible infectious agents. Precautions apply to all patients, regardless of suspected or confirmed infection status, and in any setting in which health care is delivered. Components are:

- **Hand hygiene.** (1) Avoid unnecessary touching of surfaces in close proximity to the patient. (2) When hands are visibly dirty, contaminated with proteinaceous material, or visibly soiled with blood or body fluids, wash them with soap and water. (3) If not visibly soiled, decontaminate hands with an alcohol-based hand rub. Perform hand hygiene: (a) before having direct contact with patients; (b) after contact with blood, body fluids or excretions, mucous membranes, nonintact skin, or wound dressings; (c) after contact with a patient's intact skin (e.g., taking a pulse or blood pressure or lifting a patient); (d) after contact with medical equipment in the immediate vicinity of the patient; (e) after removing gloves.
- **Use of gloves, gown, mask, eye protection, or face shield.** (1) Wear gloves when you anticipate that contact with blood or other potentially infectious materials, mucous membranes, nonintact skin, or potentially contaminated intact skin (e.g., patient incontinent of stool or urine) could occur. (2) Wear a gown to protect skin and clothing when you anticipate contact with blood, body fluids, secretions, or excretions. (3) Use mouth, nose, and eye protection to protect the mucous membranes during procedures that are likely to generate splashes or sprays of blood, body fluids, secretions, and excretions.
- **Respiratory hygiene/cough etiquette** is targeted at patients and accompanying persons with undiagnosed transmissible respiratory infections. Elements include: (1) education of staff, patients, and visitors; (2) posted signs in language(s) appropriate to the population; (3) source control measures (e.g., covering the mouth/nose with a tissue when coughing and promptly disposing of used tissues, using surgical masks on the coughing person); (4) hand hygiene after contact with respiratory secretions; and (5) spatial separation of >3 feet from people with respiratory infections in common waiting areas.

Adapted from Centers for Disease Control and Prevention. (2007). *Standard precautions—excerpt from the guidelines for isolation precautions: preventing transmissions of infectious agents in healthcare settings.* (2007). Available at www.cdc.gov/ncidod/dhqp/gl_isolation_standard.html.

8-9   (Zakus, 2001.)

may become contaminated as gloves are removed. Wear a gown, mask, and protective eyewear when the potential exists for any blood or body fluid spattering (e.g., suctioning, arterial puncture).

THE CLINICAL SETTING

General Approach

Consider your emotional state and that of the person being examined. The patient may be anxious about being examined by a stranger and the unknown outcome of the examination. Try to reduce any anxiety so the data will more closely describe the person's natural state. Anxiety can be reduced by an examiner who is confident and self-assured, considerate, and unhurried.

Usually a beginning examiner feels anything *but* self-assured! Most worry about their technical skill, missing something significant, or forgetting a step. Many are embarrassed themselves about encountering a partially dressed individual. All these fears are natural and common. The best way to minimize them is with much tutored practice on a healthy willing subject, usually a fellow student. You have to feel comfortable with your motor skills before you can absorb what you are actually seeing or hearing in a "real" patient. This comes with practice under the guidance of an experienced tutor and in an atmosphere in which it is acceptable to make mistakes and ask questions. Your subject should "act like a patient" so you can deal with the "real" situation while still in a safe setting. After you feel comfortable with the laboratory setting, accompany your tutor as he or she examines an actual patient so you can observe an experienced examiner.

Hands On

With this preparation it is possible to interact with your own patient in a confident manner. Begin by measuring the person's height, weight, blood pressure, temperature, pulse, and respirations (see Chapter 9). If needed, measure visual acuity at this time using the Snellen eye chart. All of these are familiar, relatively nonthreatening actions; they will gradually accustom the person to the examination. Sometimes an

icebreaker about an irrelevant topic will help the person feel he or she is seen as an individual. You might say, "Interesting cap. Does that mean you are a baseball fan?" or "I see you are from Michigan. How was the winter there?" These irrelevant openers signal that you have shared experiences and also that you are willing to have a conversation—a good warm-up for the examination data and shared decision making that come next.[8c]

Then ask the person to change into an examining gown, leaving his or her underpants on. This will feel more comfortable, and the underpants can easily be removed just before the genital examination. Unless your assistance is needed, leave the room as the person undresses. (Teens can remain in street clothes.)

As you reenter the room, clean your hands in the person's presence. This indicates that you are protective of this person and are starting fresh for him or her. Explain each step in the examination and how the person can cooperate. Encourage the person to ask questions. Keep your own movements slow, methodical, and deliberate.

Begin by touching the person's hands, checking skin color, nail beds, and metacarpophalangeal joints (Fig. 8-10; see Chapters 12 and 22). Again this is a less threatening way to ease a person into being touched. Most people are used to having relative strangers touch their hands.

As you proceed through the examination, avoid distractions and concentrate on one step at a time. The sequence of the steps may differ, depending on the age of the person and your own preference. However, you should establish a system that works for you and stick to it to avoid omissions. Organize the steps so the person does not change positions too often. Although proper exposure is necessary, use additional drapes to maintain the person's privacy and prevent chilling.

8-10

Do not hesitate to write out the examination sequence and refer to it as you proceed. The patient will accept this as quite natural if you explain that you are making brief notations to ensure accuracy. Many agencies use a printed form. You will find that you will glance at the form less and less as you gain experience. Even with a form, you sometimes may forget a step in the examination. When you realize this, perform the maneuver in the next logical place in the sequence. (See Chapter 27 for the sequence of steps in the complete physical examination.)

As you proceed through the examination, occasionally offer some brief teaching about the person's body. For example, you might say, "Everyone has two sounds for each heartbeat, something like this—lub-dup. Your own beats sound healthy and normal." Do not do this with every single step or you will be hard pressed to make a comment when you do come across an abnormality. But some sharing of information builds rapport and increases the person's confidence in you as an examiner. It also gives the person a little more control in a situation in which it is easy to feel completely helpless.

At some point you will want to linger in one location to concentrate on some complicated findings. To avoid anxiety, tell the person, "I always listen to heart sounds on a number of places on the chest. Just because I am listening a long time doesn't necessarily mean that anything is wrong with you." And it follows that sometimes you *will* discover a finding that may be abnormal and you want another examiner to double-check. You need to give the person some information, yet you should not alarm him or her unnecessarily. Say something like, "I don't have a complete assessment of your heart sounds. I want Ms. Wright to listen to you, too."

At the end of the examination, summarize your findings and share the necessary information with the person. Thank him or her for the time spent. In a hospital setting, apprise the person of what is scheduled next. Before you leave a hospitalized person, lower the bed to avoid risk for falls; make the person comfortable and safe; and return the bedside table, television, or any equipment to the way it was originally, with the call button available.

❖ DEVELOPMENTAL COMPETENCE

Children are different from adults. Their difference in size is obvious. Their bodies grow in a predictable pattern that is assessed during the physical examination. However, their behavior is also different. Behavior grows and develops through predictable stages, just as the body does.

With all children the goal is to increase their comfort in the setting. This approach reveals their natural state as much as possible and will give them a more positive memory of health care providers. Remember that a "routine" examination is anything but routine to the child. You can increase his or her comfort by attending to the following developmental principles and approaches. The *order* of the developmental stages is more meaningful than the exact chronologic age. Each child is an individual and will not fit exactly into one

category. For example, if your efforts to "play games" with the preschooler are rebuffed, modify your approach to the security measures used with the toddler.

The Infant

Erikson defines the major task of infancy as establishing trust. An infant is completely dependent on the parent for his or her basic needs. If these needs are met promptly and consistently, the infant feels secure and learns to trust others.

Position

- The parent always should be present to understand normal growth and development and for the child's feeling of security.
- Place the neonate or young infant flat on a padded examination table (Fig. 8-11). The infant also may be held against the parent's chest for some steps.
- Once the baby can sit without support (around 6 months), as much of the examination as possible should be performed while the infant is in the parent's lap.
- By 9 to 12 months the infant is acutely aware of the surroundings. Anything outside the infant's range of vision is "lost"; thus the parent must be in full view.

Preparation

- Timing should be 1 to 2 hours after feeding, when the baby is not too drowsy or too hungry.
- Maintain a warm environment. A neonate may require an overhead radiant heater.
- An infant will not object to being nude. Have the parent remove outer clothing, but leave a diaper on a boy.
- An infant does not mind being touched, but make sure that your hands and stethoscope endpiece are warm.
- Use a soft, crooning voice during the examination; the

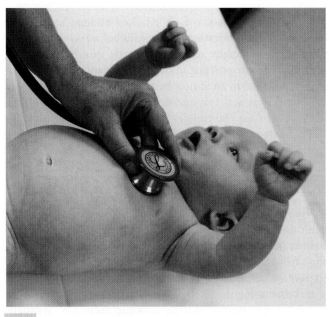

8-11

baby responds more to the feeling in the tone of the voice than to what is actually said.

- An infant likes eye contact; lock eyes from time to time.
- Smile; a baby prefers a smiling face to a frowning one. (Often beginning examiners are so absorbed in their technique that they look serious or stern.) Take time to play.
- Keep movements smooth and deliberate, not jerky.
- Use a pacifier for crying or during invasive steps.
- Offer brightly colored toys for a distraction when the infant is fussy.
- Let an older baby touch the stethoscope or tongue blade.

Sequence

- Seize the opportunity with a sleeping baby to listen to heart, lung, and abdominal sounds first.
- Perform least distressing steps first. (See the sequence in Chapter 27.) Save the invasive steps of examination of the eye, ear, nose, and throat until last.
- If you elicit the Moro or "startle" reflex, do it at the end of the examination because it may cause the baby to cry.

The Toddler

This is Erikson's stage of developing autonomy. However, the need to explore the world and be independent is in conflict with the basic dependency on the parent. This often results in frustration and negativism. The toddler may be difficult to examine; do not take this personally. Because he or she is acutely aware of the new environment, the toddler may be frightened and cling to the parent. The toddler also has fear of invasive procedures and dislikes being restrained (Fig. 8-12).

Position

- The toddler should be sitting up on the parent's lap for all of the examination. When he or she must be supine (as in the abdominal examination), move chairs to sit knee-to-knee with parent. Have the toddler lie in the parent's lap with his or her legs in your lap.
- Enlist the aid of a cooperative parent to help position the toddler during invasive procedures such as using the otoscope or taking a rectal temperature.

Preparation

- Children 1 or 2 years of age can understand symbols; thus a security object such as a special blanket or teddy bear is helpful.
- Begin by greeting the child and the accompanying parent by name, but with a child 1 to 6 years old focus more on the parent. By essentially "ignoring" the child at first, you allow him or her to adjust gradually and size you up from a safe distance. Then turn your attention gradually to the child, at first to a toy or object the child is holding or perhaps to compliment a dress, the hair, or what a big girl or boy the child is. If the child is ready, you will note these signals: eye contact with you, smiling, talking with you, or accepting a toy or a piece of equipment.

8-12

- A 2-year-old child does not like to take off his or her clothes; have the parent undress the child one part at a time.
- Children 1 or 2 years of age like to say "No." Do not offer a choice when there really is none. Avoid saying, "May I listen to your heart now?" When the 1- or 2-year-old child says "No" and you go ahead and do it anyway, you lose trust. Instead use clear, firm instructions in a tone that expects cooperation, "Now it is time for you to lie down so I can check your tummy."
- Also, 1- or 2-year-old children like to make choices. When possible, enhance autonomy by offering the *limited option:* "Shall I listen to your heart next or your tummy?"
- Demonstrate the procedures on the parent.
- Praise the child when he or she is cooperative.

Sequence

- Collect some objective data during the history, which is a less stressful time. While you are focusing on the parent, note the child's gross motor and fine motor skills and gait.
- Begin with "games" such as the Denver II test or cranial nerve testing.
- Start with nonthreatening areas. Save distressing procedures such as examination of the head, ear, nose, or throat for last.

The Preschool Child

The child at this stage displays developing initiative. The preschooler takes on tasks independently and plans the task and sees it through. A child of this age is often cooperative, helpful, and easy to involve. However, he or she may have fantasies and see illness as punishment for being "bad." The concept of body image is limited. The child fears any body injury or mutilation; therefore he or she will recoil from invasive procedures (e.g., tongue blade, rectal temperature, injection, and venipuncture).

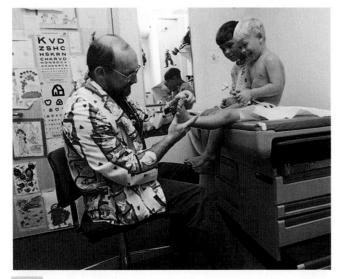

8-13

Position

- With a 3-year-old child the parent should be present and may hold the child on his or her lap.
- A 4- or 5-year-old child usually feels comfortable on the Big Girl or Big Boy (examining) table with the parent present (Fig. 8-13).

Preparation

- A preschooler can talk. Verbal communication becomes helpful now, but remember that the child's understanding is still limited. Use short, simple explanations.
- The preschooler is usually willing to undress. Leave underpants on until the genital examination.
- Talk to the child and explain the steps in the examination exactly.
- Do not allow a choice when there is none.
- As with the toddler, enhance the autonomy of the preschooler by offering choice when possible.
- Allow the child to play with equipment to reduce fears (see Fig. 8-13).
- A preschooler likes to help; have the child hold the stethoscope for you.
- Use games. Have the child "blow out" the light on the penlight as you listen to the breath sounds. Or pretend to listen to the heart sounds of the child's teddy bear first. One technique that is absorbing to a preschooler is to trace his or her shape on the examining table paper. You can comment on how big the child is, then fill in the outline with a heart or stomach and listen to the paper doll first. After the examination the child can take the paper doll home as a souvenir.
- Use a slow, patient, deliberate approach. Do not rush.
- During the examination give the preschooler needed feedback and reassurance: "Your tummy feels just fine."
- Compliment the child on his or her cooperation.

Sequence

- Examine the thorax, abdomen, extremities, and genitalia first. Although the preschooler is usually cooperative, continue to assess head, eye, ear, nose, and throat last.

The School-Age Child

During the school-age period the major task of the child is developing industry. The child is developing basic competency in school and social networks and desires the approval of parents and teachers. When successful, the child has a feeling of accomplishment. During the examination the child is cooperative and interested in learning about the body. Language is more sophisticated now, but do not overestimate and treat the school-age child as a small adult. The child's level of understanding does not match that of his or her speech.

Position

- The school-age child should be sitting or lying on the examination table (Fig. 8-14).
- A 5-year-old child has a sense of modesty. To maintain privacy, let the older child (an 11- or 12-year-old child) decide whether parents or siblings should be present.

Preparation

- Break the ice with small talk about family, school, friends, music, or sports.
- The child should undress himself or herself, leave underpants on, and use a gown and drape.
- Demonstrate equipment; a school-age child is curious to know how equipment works (Fig. 8-15).
- Comment on the body and how it works. An 8- or 9-year-old child has some understanding of the body and is

8-14

interested to learn more. It is rewarding to see the child's eyes light up when he or she hears the heart sounds.

Sequence

- As with the adult, progress from head to toes.

The Adolescent

The major task of adolescence is developing a self-identity. This takes shape from various sets of values and different social roles (son or daughter, sibling, and student). In the end each person needs to feel satisfied and comfortable with who he or she is. In the process the adolescent is increasingly self-conscious and introspective. Peer group values and acceptance are important.

Position

- The adolescent should be sitting on the examination table. Try to keep street clothes on and work around them as much as possible (Fig. 8-16).
- Examine the adolescent alone, without parent or sibling present.

Preparation

- The body is changing rapidly. During the examination the adolescent needs feedback that his or her own body is healthy and developing normally.
- The adolescent has keen awareness of body image, often comparing himself or herself to peers. Apprise the adolescent of the wide variation among teenagers on the rate of growth and development (see Sexual Maturity Rating [SMR], Chapters 17, 24, and 26).

8-16

- Communicate with some care. Do not treat the teenager like a child, but do not overestimate and treat him or her like an adult either.
- Because the person is idealistic at this age, the adolescent is ripe for health teaching. Positive attitudes developed now may last through adult life. Focus your teaching on ways the adolescent can promote wellness.

Sequence

- As with the adult, a head-to-toe approach is appropriate. Examine genitalia last and do it quickly.

The Aging Adult

During later years the tasks are developing the meaning of life and one's own existence and adjusting to changes in physical strength and health (Fig. 8-17).

Position

- The older adult should be sitting on the examination table; a frail older adult may need to be supine.
- Arrange the sequence to allow as few position changes as possible.
- Allow rest periods when needed.

Preparation

- Adjust examination pace to meet the possible slowed pace of the aging person. It is better to break the complete examination into a few visits than to rush through the examination and turn off the person.
- Use physical touch (unless there is a cultural contraindication). This is especially important with the aging person

8-15

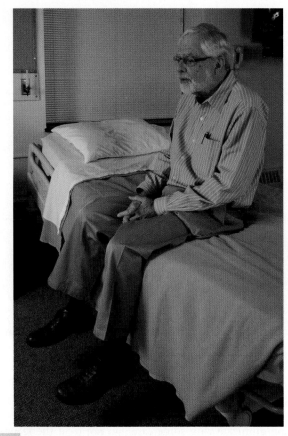

8-17

because other senses such as vision and hearing may be diminished.

- Do not mistake diminished vision or hearing for confusion. Confusion of sudden onset may signify a disease state. It is noted by short-term memory loss, diminished thought process, diminished attention span, and labile emotions (see Mental Status Assessment in Chapter 5).
- Be aware that aging years contain more life stress. Loss is inevitable, including changes in physical appearance of the face and body, declining energy level, loss of job through retirement, loss of financial security, loss of longtime home, and death of friends or spouse. How the person adapts to these losses significantly affects health assessment.

Sequence

- Use the head-to-toe approach as in the younger adult.

The Ill Person

For the person in some distress, alter the position during the examination. For example, a person with shortness of breath or ear pain may want to sit up, whereas a person with faintness or overwhelming fatigue may want to be supine. Initially it may be necessary just to examine the body areas appropriate to the problem, collecting a **mini-database.** You may return to finish a complete assessment after the initial distress is resolved.

BIBLIOGRAPHY

1. Boyce, J. M., & Pittet, D. (2002). Guideline for hand hygiene in health-care settings. *MMWR Recommendation and Reports,* 51(RR16), 1-44. Available at www.cdc.gov/mmwr/preview/mmwrhtml/rr5116a1.htm.
2. Centers for Disease Control and Prevention (CDC). (2007). *Standard precautions—excerpt from the guidelines for isolation precautions: preventing transmission of infectious agents in healthcare settings.* Available at http://cdc.gov/ncidod/dhqp/pdf/isolation2007.pdf.
3. Centers for Disease Control and Prevention (CDC). (2013). Antibiotic resistance threats in the United States. Atlanta: CDC.
4. Centers for Disease Control and Prevention (CDC). (2013). *Diseases and organisms in healthcare settings.* Available at http://www.cdc.gov/HAI/organisms/organisms.html.
5. Duderstadt, K. (2013). *Pediatric physical examination: an illustrated handbook.* St. Louis: Mosby.
6. Dufy, M. (2011). Patient privacy and company policy in online life. *Am J Nurs, 111*(9), 65-69.
7. Kane, R. L., Ouslander, J. G., Abrass, I. B., et al. (2013). *Essentials of clinical geriatrics* (7th ed.). New York: McGraw Hill.
8. KuKanich, K. S., Kaur, R., Freeman, L. C., et al. (2013). Evaluation of a hand hygiene campaign in outpatient health care clinics. *Am J Nurs, 113*(3), 36-43.
8a. Lim, F. A., Brown, D. V., Justin Kim, S. M. (2014). Addressing health care disparities in the lesbian, gay, bisexual, and transgender population. *Am J Nurs, 114*(6), 24-35.
8b. Riley, D. (2014). The art of a pediatric exam. *Nurse Pract, 39*(6), 50-54.
8c. Wolpaw, D. R., & Shapiro, D. (2014). The virtues of irrelevance. *N Engl J Med, 370*(13), 1282-1285.
9. World Health Organization. (2009). *WHO guidelines on hand hygiene in health care.* Geneva, Switzerland. Available at http://whqlibdoc.who.int/publications/2009/9789241597906_eng.pdf.
10. Zychowicz, M. E. (2012). Pre-participation physical evaluations for athletes. *Nurse Pract, 37*(11), 41-45.

CHAPTER 9

General Survey, Measurement, Vital Signs

ⓔ http://evolve.elsevier.com/Jarvis/

OBJECTIVE DATA

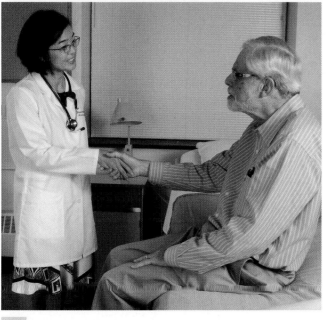

9-1

The general survey is a study of the whole person, covering the general health state and any obvious physical characteristics. It is an introduction for the physical examination that will follow; it gives an overall impression, a "gestalt," of the person (see Sample Charting on p. 154). The general survey includes objective parameters, but these apply to the whole person, not just to one body system.

Begin a general survey at the moment you first encounter the person. What leaves an immediate impression? Does the person stand promptly as his or her name is called and walk easily to meet you? Or does the person look sick, rising slowly or with effort, with shoulders slumped and eyes without luster or downcast? Is the hospitalized patient conversing with visitors, involved in reading or television, or lying perfectly still? Even as you introduce yourself and shake hands, you collect data (Fig. 9-1). Does the person fully extend the arm, shake your hand firmly, make eye contact, or smile? Are the palms dry or wet and clammy? As you proceed through the health history, the measurements, and the vital signs, consider and make note of these four areas: **physical appearance, body structure, mobility,** and **behavior.**

Normal Range of Findings	Abnormal Findings
The General Survey	
Physical Appearance	
Age—The person appears his or her stated age.	Appears older than stated age, as with chronic illness or chronic alcoholism.
Sex—Sexual development is appropriate for sex and age. If the individual is transgender, note the stage of transformation.	Delayed or precocious puberty.
Level of consciousness—The person is alert and oriented to person, place, time, and situation. Attends to and responds appropriately to your questions.	Confused, drowsy, lethargic (see Table 5-1, Levels of Consciousness, p. 79).
Skin color—Color tone is even, pigmentation varying with genetic background; skin is intact with no obvious lesions. Make note of tattoos and piercings and stage of healing.	Pallor, cyanosis, jaundice, erythema, any lesions (see Chapter 12, p. 208).

Normal Range of Findings	Abnormal Findings
Facial features—Facial features are symmetric with movement.	Immobile, masklike, asymmetric, drooping (see Table 13-5, Abnormal Facies with Chronic Illness, p. 278).
Overall appearance—No signs of acute distress are present.	Cardiac or respiratory signs— Diaphoresis, clutching the chest, shortness of breath, wheezing. Pain, indicated by facial grimace, holding body part.

Body Structure

Normal Range of Findings	Abnormal Findings
Stature—The height appears within normal range for age, genetic heritage (see Measurement, p. 130).	Excessively short or tall (see Table 9-5, Abnormalities in Body Height and Proportion, p. 156).
Nutrition—The weight appears within normal range for height and body build; body fat distribution is even.	Cachectic, emaciated. Simple obesity, with even fat distribution. Centripetal (truncal) obesity—Fat concentrated in face, neck, trunk, with thin extremities, as in Cushing syndrome (see Table 9-5).
Symmetry—Body parts look equal bilaterally and are in relative proportion to each other.	Unilateral atrophy or hypertrophy. Asymmetric location of a body part.
Posture—The person stands comfortably erect as appropriate for age. Note the normal "plumb line" through anterior ear, shoulder, hip, patella, ankle. Exceptions are the standing toddler, who has a normally protuberant abdomen ("toddler lordosis"), and the aging person, who may be stooped with kyphosis.	Rigid spine and neck; moves as one unit (e.g., arthritis). Stiff and tense, ready to spring from chair, fidgety movements. Shoulders slumped; looks deflated (e.g., depression).
Position—The person sits comfortably with arms relaxed at sides and head turned to examiner.	Tripod—Leaning forward with arms braced on chair arms; occurs with chronic pulmonary disease. Sits straight up and resists lying down (e.g., heart failure). Curled up in fetal position (e.g., acute abdominal pain).
Body build, contour—Proportions are: 1. Arm span (fingertip to fingertip) equals height. 2. Body length from crown to pubis roughly equal to length from pubis to sole.	Elongated arm span (e.g., Marfan syndrome, hypogonadism) (see Table 9-5).
Obvious physical deformities—Note any congenital or acquired defects.	Missing extremities or digits; webbed digits; shortened limb.

Mobility

Normal Range of Findings	Abnormal Findings
Gait—Feet approximately shoulder width apart; foot placement is accurate; walk is smooth and even, and person can maintain balance without assistance. Associated movements such as symmetric arm swing are present.	Exceptionally wide base. Staggering, stumbling. Shuffling, dragging, nonfunctional leg. Limping with injury. Propulsion—Difficulty stopping (see Table 23-7, Abnormal Gaits, p. 683).

Normal Range of Findings	Abnormal Findings
Range of motion—Note full mobility for each joint and that movement is deliberate, accurate, smooth, and coordinated. (See Chapter 22 for information on more detailed testing of joint range of motion.) No involuntary movement.	Limited joint range of motion. Paralysis—Absent movement. Jerky, uncoordinated movement. Tics, tremors, seizures (see Table 23-5, Abnormalities in Muscle Movement, p. 679).

Behavior

Normal Range of Findings	Abnormal Findings
Facial expression—The person maintains eye contact (if culturally appropriate); expressions are appropriate to the situation (e.g., thoughtful, serious, or smiling). (Note expressions both while the face is at rest and while the person is talking.)	Flat, depressed, angry, sad, anxious. However, note that anxiety is common in ill people. Also, some people smile when they are anxious.
Mood and affect—The person is comfortable and cooperative with the examiner and interacts pleasantly.	Hostile, distrustful, suspicious, crying.
Speech—Articulation (the ability to form words) is clear and understandable.	Dysarthria and dysphagia (see Table 5-2, Speech Disorders, p. 80). Speech defect, monotone, garbled speech.
Speech pattern—The stream of talking is fluent, with an even pace. The person conveys ideas clearly. Word choice is appropriate for culture and education. Communicates in prevailing language easily by himself or herself or with an interpreter.	Extremes of few words or constant talking.
Dress—Clothing is appropriate to the climate, looks clean and fits the body, and is appropriate to the person's culture and age-group (e.g., normally Amish women wear clothing from the 19th century; Indian women may wear saris). Culturally determined dress should not be labeled as inappropriate by Western standards or adult expectations.	Clothing too large and held up by belt suggests weight loss, as does the addition of new holes in belt. Clothing too tight may indicate obesity or ascites. Consistent wear of certain clothing may provide clues: long sleeves may conceal needle marks of drug abuse or thin arms of anorexia; Velcro fasteners instead of buttons may indicate chronic motor dysfunction.
Personal hygiene—The person appears clean and groomed appropriately for his or her age, occupation, and socioeconomic group. (Note that a wide variation of dress and hygiene is "normal." Many cultures do not include use of deodorant or women shaving legs.). Hair is groomed, brushed. Makeup is appropriate for age and culture.	Body odor, scent of alcohol. Unkempt appearance in an individual who previously had good hygiene may indicate depression, malaise, or illness.

Measurement

Weight

Normal Range of Findings	Abnormal Findings
Use a standardized *balance* or electronic standing scale (Fig. 9-2). Instruct the person to remove his or her shoes and heavy outer clothing before standing on the scale. When a sequence of repeated weights is necessary, aim for approximately the same time of day and the same type of clothing worn each time. Record the weight in kilograms and in pounds.	An unexplained weight loss may be a sign of a short-term illness (e.g., fever, infection, disease of the mouth or throat) or a chronic illness (e.g., endocrine disease, malignancy, depression, anorexia nervosa, bulimia). Unexplained weight gain may indicate fluid retention (e.g., heart failure).

Normal Range of Findings	Abnormal Findings

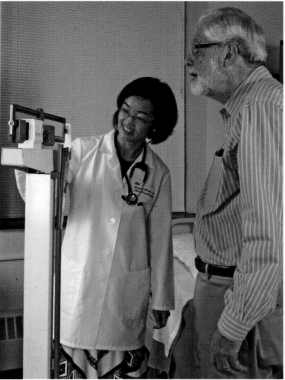

9-2

Height

Use a wall-mounted device or the measuring pole on the balance scale. Align the extended headpiece with the top of the head. The person should be shoeless, standing straight with gentle traction under the jaw, and looking straight ahead. Feet, shoulders, and buttocks should be in contact with the hard surface.

Body Mass Index

Body mass index (BMI) is a practical marker of optimal healthy weight for height and an indicator of obesity or malnutrition. Evidence supports the use of BMI in obesity risk assessment because it provides a more accurate measure of total body fat compared with the measure of body weight alone.[26]

The cause of weight gain is usually excess caloric intake; occasionally it is endocrine disorders, drug therapy (e.g., corticosteroids), or depression. BMI classifications for adults[26]:
  Underweight < 18.5 kg/m^2
  Normal weight 18.5 to 24.9 kg/m^2
  Overweight 25 to 29.9 kg/m^2
  Obesity (class 1) 30 to 34.9 kg/m^2
  Obesity (class 2) 35 to 39.9 kg/m^2
  Extreme obesity (class 3) ≥ 40

A healthy BMI is a level of 19 or greater to less than 25. Show the person how his or her own weight matches up to the national guidelines for optimal BMI (see Table 9-1). Compare the person's current weight with that from the previous health visit. A recent weight loss may be explained by successful dieting. A weight gain usually reflects overabundant caloric intake, unhealthy eating habits, and sedentary lifestyle. Note that BMI overestimates body fat in people who are very muscular and underestimates body fat in older adults who have lost muscle mass.

More than ⅔ of adults and ⅓ of children in the United States are overweight or obese. Overweight and obesity affect more Hispanics and non-Hispanic Blacks than non-Hispanic Whites, whereas Asian Americans have a much lower prevalence than other ethnic groups.[27]

Objective Data

TABLE 9-1 Body Mass Index Table

	NORMAL						OVERWEIGHT					OBESE									
BMI	19	20	21	22	23	24	25	26	27	28	29	30	31	32	33	34	35	36	37	38	39
HEIGHT (inches)	BODY WEIGHT (pounds)																				
58	91	96	100	105	110	115	119	124	129	134	138	143	148	153	158	162	167	172	177	181	186
59	94	99	104	109	114	119	124	128	133	138	143	148	153	158	163	168	173	178	183	188	193
60	97	102	107	112	118	123	128	133	138	143	148	153	158	163	168	174	179	184	189	194	199
61	100	106	111	116	122	127	132	137	143	148	153	158	164	169	174	180	185	190	195	201	206
62	104	109	115	120	126	131	136	142	147	153	158	164	169	175	180	186	191	196	202	207	213
63	107	113	118	124	130	135	141	146	152	158	163	169	175	180	186	191	197	203	208	214	220
64	110	116	122	128	134	140	145	151	157	163	169	174	180	186	192	197	204	209	215	221	227
65	114	120	126	132	138	144	150	156	162	168	174	180	186	192	198	204	210	216	222	228	234
66	118	124	130	136	142	148	155	161	167	173	179	186	192	198	204	210	216	223	229	235	241
67	121	127	134	140	146	153	159	166	172	178	185	191	198	204	211	217	223	230	236	242	249
68	125	131	138	144	151	158	164	171	177	184	190	197	203	210	216	223	230	236	243	249	256
69	128	135	142	149	155	162	169	176	182	189	196	203	209	216	223	230	236	243	250	257	263
70	132	139	146	153	160	167	174	181	188	195	202	209	216	222	229	236	243	250	257	264	271
71	136	143	150	157	165	172	179	186	193	200	208	215	222	229	236	243	250	257	265	272	279
72	140	147	154	162	169	177	184	191	199	206	213	221	228	235	242	250	258	265	272	279	287
73	144	151	159	166	174	182	189	197	204	212	219	227	235	242	250	257	265	272	280	288	295
74	148	155	163	171	179	186	194	202	210	218	225	233	241	249	256	264	272	280	287	295	303
75	152	160	168	176	184	192	200	208	216	224	232	240	248	256	264	272	279	287	295	303	311
76	156	164	172	180	189	197	205	213	221	230	238	246	254	263	271	279	287	295	304	312	320

	EXTREME OBESITY														
BMI	40	41	42	43	44	45	46	47	48	49	50	51	52	53	54
HEIGHT (inches)	BODY WEIGHT (pounds)														
58	191	196	201	205	210	215	220	224	229	234	239	244	248	253	258
59	198	203	208	212	217	222	227	232	237	242	247	252	257	262	267
60	204	209	215	220	225	230	235	240	245	250	255	261	266	271	276
61	211	217	222	227	232	238	243	248	254	259	264	269	275	280	285
02	210	224	229	235	240	240	251	250	202	207	273	270	204	209	295
63	225	231	237	242	248	254	259	265	270	278	282	287	293	299	304
64	232	238	244	250	256	262	267	273	279	285	291	296	302	308	314
65	240	246	252	258	264	270	276	282	288	294	300	306	312	318	324
66	247	253	260	266	272	278	284	291	297	303	309	315	322	328	334
67	255	261	268	274	280	287	293	299	306	312	319	325	331	338	344
68	262	269	276	282	289	295	302	308	315	322	328	335	341	348	354
69	270	277	284	291	297	304	311	318	324	331	338	345	351	358	365
70	278	285	292	299	306	313	320	327	334	341	348	355	362	369	376
71	286	293	301	308	315	322	329	338	343	351	358	365	372	379	386
72	294	302	309	316	324	331	338	346	353	361	368	375	383	390	397
73	302	310	318	325	333	340	348	355	363	371	378	386	393	401	408
74	311	319	326	334	342	350	358	365	373	381	389	396	404	412	420
75	319	327	335	343	351	359	367	375	383	391	399	407	415	423	431
76	328	336	344	353	361	369	377	385	394	402	410	418	426	435	443

Adapted from *Clinical guidelines on the identification, evaluation, and treatment of overweight and obesity in adults: the evidence report.* Available at www.nhlbi.nih.gov/guidelines/obesity/bmi_tbl.pdf.

You also may calculate BMI by using the BMI calculator at the NIH website.[26] Or you can calculate with the following formulae:

$$BMI = \frac{\text{Weight (in pounds)}}{\text{Height (in inches)}^2} \times 703 \quad Or \quad BMI = \frac{\text{Weight (in kilograms)}}{\text{Height (in meters)}^2}$$

Normal Range of Findings	Abnormal Findings

Normal Range of Findings

Waist Circumference

Excess abdominal fat is an important independent risk factor for disease, over and above that of BMI.[26] If most of the weight is carried around the waist instead of around the hips, the person is at higher risk for heart disease and type 2 diabetes.

With the person standing, locate the hip bone—the very top is the iliac crest. Place a measuring tape around the waist, parallel to the floor, at the level of the iliac crest. The tape should be snug but not pinch in the skin. Note the measurement at the end of a normal expiration (Fig. 9-3).

Iliac crest

Measuring tape position for abdominal circumference

9-3   © Pat Thomas, 2010.

Vital Signs

Temperature

Cellular metabolism requires a stable core, or "deep body," temperature of a mean of 37.2°C (99°F). The body maintains a steady temperature through a thermostat, or feedback mechanism, regulated in the hypothalamus of the brain. The thermostat balances heat production (from metabolism, exercise, food digestion, external factors) with heat loss (through radiation, evaporation of sweat, convection, conduction).

The various routes of temperature measurement reflect the core temperature of the body. The normal oral temperature in a resting person is 37°C (98.6°F), with a range of 35.8° to 37.3°C (96.4° to 99.1°F). The rectal temperature measures 0.4° to 0.5°C (0.7° to 1°F) higher.

Abnormal Findings

A waist circumference (WC) ≥35 inches in women and ≥40 inches in men increases the risk for type 2 diabetes, dyslipidemia, hypertension, and cardiovascular disease (CVD) in people with a BMI between 25 and 35.

The thermostatic function of the hypothalamus may become scrambled during illness or central nervous system (CNS) disorders.

Normal Range of Findings	Abnormal Findings

The normal temperature is influenced by:
- A diurnal cycle of 1° to 1.5° F, with the trough occurring in the early morning hours and the peak occurring in late afternoon to early evening.
- The menstruation cycle in women. Progesterone secretion, occurring with ovulation at midcycle, causes a 0.5° to 1° F rise in temperature that continues until menses.
- Exercise. Moderate-to-hard exercise increases body temperature.
- Age. Wider normal variations occur in the infant and young child because of less effective heat control mechanisms. In older adults temperature is usually lower than in other age-groups, with a mean of 36.2°C (97.2°F) via the oral route. Rectal temperatures remain 0.5°C higher than oral temperatures in older adults.[22]

The **oral temperature** is the most convenient and accurate site. The sublingual pocket has a rich blood supply from the carotid arteries that quickly responds to changes in inner core temperature.

Hyperthermia, or fever, is caused by pyrogens secreted by toxic bacteria during infections or from tissue breakdown such as that following myocardial infarction, trauma, surgery, or malignancy. Neurologic disorders (e.g., a stroke, cerebral edema, brain trauma, tumor, or surgery) also can reset the thermostat of the brain at a higher level, resulting in heat production and conservation.

Hypothermia is usually caused by accidental, prolonged exposure to cold. It also may be purposefully induced to lower the body's oxygen requirements during heart or peripheral vascular surgery or neurosurgery, amputation, postcardiac arrest, or gastrointestinal (GI) hemorrhage.

The Procedure: Oral Temperature

Shake a glass thermometer down to 35.5°C (96°F) and place it at the base of the tongue in either of the posterior sublingual pockets—*not* in front of the tongue. Instruct the person to keep his or her lips closed. Leave in place 3 to 4 minutes if the person is afebrile and up to 8 minutes if febrile. (Take other vital signs during this time.) Wait 15 minutes if the person has just taken hot or iced liquids and 2 minutes if he or she has just smoked.

The **electronic thermometer** has the advantages of swift and accurate measurement (usually in 20 to 30 seconds). The instrument must be fully charged and correctly calibrated. Most children enjoy watching their temperature numbers advance on the box. Electronic thermometers can be used for both oral and rectal temperatures. Blue-tipped probes are for the oral route, whereas red-tipped probes are rectal.

The Procedure: Rectal Temperature

Rectal temperatures are the most accurate route, and the result is as close to core temperature as possible without using more invasive measures reserved for the operating room and critical care environments. Although the rectal temperature provides the closest approximation to core temperature, it is more invasive than other measures; therefore you must weigh the risks and benefits. In children the temporal artery route misses fever in as many as 30% of children 6 to 36 months old[14]; therefore it may be advantageous to use rectal temperature in children with a suspected fever or infection.

The rectal temperature is the preferred route when the other routes are not practical (e.g., for the comatose or confused person; people in shock; or those who cannot close the mouth because of breathing or oxygen tubes, wired mandible, or other facial dysfunction). Wear gloves and insert a lubricated rectal probe cover on an electronic thermometer only 2 to 3 cm (1 in) into the adult rectum, directed toward the umbilicus. (For a glass thermometer, leave in place for 2½ minutes.) Do not let go of the temperature probe while it is inserted into the rectum. Disadvantages to the rectal route are patient discomfort and the invasive nature of the procedure.

Objective Data

Normal Range of Findings	Abnormal Findings

The Procedure: Tympanic Membrane Temperature

The **tympanic membrane thermometer (TMT)** senses infrared emissions of the tympanic membrane (eardrum). The tympanic membrane shares the same vascular supply that perfuses the hypothalamus (the internal carotid artery); thus it is an accurate measurement of core temperature.

The TMT is a noninvasive, nontraumatic device that is extremely quick and efficient. The probe tip has the shape of an otoscope, the instrument used to inspect the ear. Gently place the covered probe tip in the person's ear canal and aim the infrared beam at the tympanic membrane (see Fig. 9-17 on p. 148). Do not occlude the canal. Activate the device and read the temperature in 2 to 3 seconds.

There is minimal chance of cross-contamination with the tympanic thermometer because the ear canal is lined with skin and not mucous membrane. Current evidence is conflicting; some studies do not support use of tympanic thermometry in critically ill patients.[11a] TMT has fallen out of favor in many acute care settings but is still used by some clinics.

The Procedure: Temporal Artery Thermometer

The newest noninvasive temperature measurement method uses infrared emissions from the temporal artery. The temporal artery thermometer (TAT) is used by sliding the probe across the forehead and behind the ear. The thermometer works by taking multiple readings and providing an average. The reading takes approximately 6 seconds. This approach is well tolerated and is more accurate than TMTs; however, there are conflicting reports about its accuracy.[3,14,33]

Report the temperature in degrees Celsius unless your agency uses the Fahrenheit scale. Familiarize yourself with both scales. Note that it is far easier to learn to *think* in the centigrade scale than to take the time for paper-and-pencil conversions. Begin by memorizing these convenient equivalents:

$$104° = 40° C; \quad 98.6° F = 37° C; \quad 95° F = 35° C$$

Along with your results, make sure to note the route used to obtain the temperature reading.

Pulse

With every beat the heart pumps an amount of blood—the **stroke volume**—into the aorta. This is about 70 mL in the adult. The force flares the arterial walls and generates a pressure wave, which is felt in the periphery as the **pulse.** Palpating the peripheral pulse gives the rate and rhythm of the heartbeat and local data on the condition of the artery.

Using the pads of your first three fingers, palpate the radial pulse at the flexor aspect of the wrist laterally along the radius bone (Fig. 9-4). If the rhythm is regular, count the number of beats in 30 seconds and multiply by 2. Although the 15-second interval is frequently practiced, any one-beat error in counting results in a recorded error of 4 beats/min. The 30-second interval is most accurate and efficient when heart rates are normal or rapid and when rhythms are regular. However, if the rhythm is irregular, count for a full minute. As you begin the counting interval, start your count with "zero" for the first pulse felt. The second pulse felt is "one," and so on. Assess the pulse, including (1) rate, (2) rhythm, and (3) force.

Normal Range of Findings	Abnormal Findings

9-4

Rate

In the adult at physical and mental rest, recent clinical evidence shows the normal resting heart range of 95% of healthy persons at 50 to 95 beats/min.[24] Traditional resting heart rate limits established in the 1950s are 60 to100 beats/min. This range is still used; however, no research evidence supports it.

The rate normally varies with age, being more rapid in infancy and childhood and more moderate during adult and older years. The rate also varies with gender; after puberty females have a slightly faster rate than males.

In the adult a resting heart rate less than 50 beats/min is **bradycardia.** Heart rates in the 50s/min occur normally in the well-trained athlete whose heart muscle develops along with the skeletal muscles. The stronger, more efficient heart muscle pushes out a larger stroke volume with each beat, thus requiring fewer beats per minute to maintain a stable cardiac output.

A more rapid heart rate, variably defined as over 95 beats/min or over 100 beats/min, is **tachycardia.** Rapid rates occur normally with anxiety or with increased exercise to match the body's demand for increased metabolism.

Many medications also affect heart rate, with nearly all heart disease patients taking at least one medication that slows the heart rate.

For descriptions of abnormal rates and rhythms, see Table 20-1, Variations in Pulse Contour on p. 530).

Tachycardia occurs with fever and also with sepsis, pneumonia, myocardial infarction, and pancreatitis. This evidence predicts complications and worse survival rates in the latter conditions.[24]

Rhythm

The pulse normally has a regular, even tempo. One irregularity that is commonly found in children and young adults is **sinus arrhythmia.** In sinus arrhythmia the heart rate varies with the respiratory cycle, speeding up at the peak of inspiration and slowing to normal with expiration. Inspiration momentarily causes a decreased stroke volume from the left side of the heart; to compensate the heart rate increases. (See Chapter 19 for a full discussion on sinus arrhythmia.) If any other irregularities are felt, auscultate heart sounds for a more complete assessment (see Chapter 19).

Objective Data

Normal Range of Findings	**Abnormal Findings**

Force

The force of the pulse shows the strength of the heart's stroke volume. A "full, bounding" pulse denotes an increased stroke volume (e.g., as with anxiety, exercise, and some abnormal conditions). The pulse force is recorded using a three-point scale:

  3+—Full, bounding
  2+—Normal
  1+—Weak, thready
  0—Absent

Some agencies use a four-point scale; make sure that your system is consistent with that used by the rest of your staff. Either scale is somewhat subjective. Experience will increase your clinical judgment. Most healthy adults have a force of 2+.

A "weak, thready" pulse reflects a decreased stroke volume (e.g., as occurs with hemorrhagic shock).

Respirations

Normally a person's breathing is relaxed, regular, automatic, and silent. Because most people are unaware of their breathing, do not mention that you will be counting the respirations, because sudden awareness may alter the normal pattern. Maintain your position of counting the radial pulse and unobtrusively count the respirations. Count for 30 seconds, but count for a full minute if you suspect an abnormality. Avoid the 15-second interval. The result can vary by a factor of +4 or −4, which is significant with such a small number. If you are having difficulty seeing the chest rise, which can be especially difficult in obese individuals and children, you can place a hand on the upper chest or abdomen to help you "feel" the respiratory rate. Report the number of breaths per minute.

Report additional objective data (e.g., labored, shallow, or deep breathing; retractions in infants and children; and accessory muscle use in adults).

Note that respiratory rates presented in Table 9-2 normally are more rapid in infants and children. Also, a fairly constant ratio of pulse rate to respiratory rate exists, which is about 4:1. Normally both pulse and respiratory rates rise as a response to exercise or anxiety. More detailed assessment on respiratory status is presented in Chapter 18.

TABLE 9-2	Normal Respiratory Rates
AGE	**BREATHS PER MINUTE**
Neonate	30-40
1 yr	20-40
2 yr	25-32
8-10 yr	20-26
12-14 yr	18-22
16 yr	12-20
Adult	10-20

Blood Pressure

Blood pressure (BP) is the force of the blood pushing against the side of its container, the vessel wall. The strength of the push changes with the event in the cardiac cycle. The **systolic** pressure is the maximum pressure felt on the artery during left ventricular contraction, or systole. The **diastolic** pressure is the elastic

| **Normal Range of Findings** | **Abnormal Findings** |

recoil, or resting, pressure that the blood exerts constantly between each contraction. The **pulse pressure** is the difference between the systolic and diastolic pressures and reflects the stroke volume (Fig. 9-5).

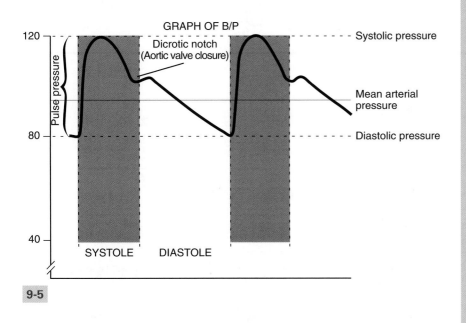

9-5

The **mean arterial pressure (MAP)** is the pressure forcing blood into the tissues averaged over the cardiac cycle. This is not an arithmetic average of systolic and diastolic pressures because diastole lasts longer. Rather it is a value closer to diastolic pressure plus one third the pulse pressure.

The average BP in the young adult varies with many factors such as:

- **Age.** Normally a gradual rise occurs through childhood and into the adult years.
- **Sex.** Before puberty no difference exists between males and females. After puberty females usually show a lower BP reading than do male counterparts. After menopause BP in females is higher than in male counterparts.
- **Race.** In the United States an African-American adult's BP is often higher than that of a White person of the same age. The incidence of hypertension is twice as high in African Americans as in Whites. The reasons for this difference are not understood fully, but we do know that genetic profile and environmental factors are involved.
- **Diurnal rhythm.** A daily cycle of a peak and a trough occurs: the BP climbs to a high in late afternoon or early evening and then declines to an early-morning low.
- **Weight.** BP is higher in obese people than in people of normal weight of the same age (including adolescents).
- **Exercise.** Increasing activity yields a proportionate increase in BP. Within 5 minutes of terminating the exercise, the BP normally returns to baseline.
- **Emotions.** The BP momentarily rises with fear, anger, and pain as a result of stimulation of the sympathetic nervous system.
- **Stress.** The BP is elevated in people feeling continual tension because of lifestyle, occupational stress, or life problems.

Objective Data

Normal Range of Findings			Abnormal Findings
FACTOR	FACTORS CONTROLLING BLOOD PRESSURE CONDITION		RESULT
Cardiac output	↑	with heavy exercise to meet body demand for increased metabolism	↑ BP
	↓	with pump failure (weak pumping action after myocardial infarction, or in shock)	↓ BP
Vascular resistance	↑	resistance (vasoconstriction)	↑ BP
	↓	resistance (vasodilation)	↓ BP
Volume	↓	volume (hemorrhage)	↓ BP
	↑	volume (increased sodium and water retention, intravenous fluid overload)	↑ BP
Viscosity	↑	viscosity (increased hematocrit in polycythemia)	↑ BP
Elasticity of arterial walls	↑	rigidity, hardening as in arteriosclerosis (heart pumping against greater resistance)	↑ BP

9-6   © Pat Thomas, 2006.

The level of BP is determined by five factors (Fig. 9-6):

1. **Cardiac output.** If the heart pumps more blood into the container (i.e., the blood vessels), the pressure on the container walls increases.
2. **Peripheral vascular resistance.** Peripheral vascular resistance is the opposition to blood flow through the arteries. When the container becomes smaller (e.g., with constricted vessels), the pressure needed to push the contents becomes greater. Conversely, if the container becomes larger (e.g., vasodilation), less pressure is needed.
3. **Volume of circulating blood.** Volume of circulating blood refers to how tightly the blood is packed into the arteries. Increasing the contents in the container increases the pressure.
4. **Viscosity.** The "thickness" of blood is determined by its formed elements, the blood cells. When the contents are thicker, the pressure increases.
5. **Elasticity of vessel walls.** When the container walls are stiff and rigid, the pressure needed to push the contents increases.

BP is measured with a stethoscope and an aneroid *sphygmomanometer*. The aneroid gauge is subject to drift; it must be recalibrated at least once each year, and it must rest at zero.

The cuff consists of an inflatable rubber bladder inside a cloth cover. The width of the rubber bladder should equal 40% of the circumference of the person's arm. The length of the bladder should equal 80% of this circumference.

Many medications used in the treatment of critically ill people affect peripheral vascular resistance.

Blood volume is increased via blood transfusions or volume expanders and decreased through hemorrhage.

If the gauge doesn't rest at zero, the readings obtained will either be high or low, depending on the direction of the drift.

Normal Range of Findings	Abnormal Findings

Thigh cuff or large arm cuff

Standard adult arm cuff

9-7

Available cuffs include 6 sizes that fit newborn infants to the extra-large adult and tapered cuffs for the cone-shaped obese arm and thigh cuffs. Match the appropriate-size cuff to the person's arm size and shape and not to his or her age (Fig. 9-7).

The cuff size is important; using a cuff that is too narrow yields a falsely high BP because it takes extra pressure to compress the artery.

The Procedure: Arm Pressure

A comfortable, relaxed person yields a valid BP. Many people are anxious at the beginning of an examination; allow at least a 5-minute rest before measuring the BP. Then take two or more BP measurements separated by 2 minutes.

For each person, verify BP in both arms once, either on admission or for the first complete physical examination. It is not necessary to continue to check both arms for screening or monitoring. Occasionally a 5- to 10-mm Hg difference may occur in BP in the two arms (if values are different, use the higher value), which is caused by artifact or subtle differences in technique.

A reproducible difference in the two arms of more than 10 to 15 mm Hg may indicate arterial obstruction on the side with the lower reading. This warrants referral.

The person may be sitting or lying, with the **bare arm** supported at heart level. When sitting, the patient's feet should be flat on the floor because BP has a false-high measurement when legs are crossed versus uncrossed.[10]

Palpate the brachial artery, which is located just above the antecubital fossa, medial to the biceps tendon. With the cuff deflated, center it about 2.5 cm (1 in) above the brachial artery and wrap it evenly.

Now palpate the brachial or radial artery (Fig. 9-8). Inflate the cuff until the artery pulsation is obliterated and then 20 to 30 mm Hg beyond. This helps you to avoid missing an **auscultatory gap,** which is a period when Korotkoff sounds disappear during auscultation (Table 9-3).

An auscultatory gap occurs in about 5% of people, most often in hypertension caused by a noncompliant arterial system.

9-8

Objective Data

Normal Range of Findings   **Abnormal Findings**

TABLE 9-3   Korotkoff Sounds

PHASE	QUALITY	DESCRIPTION	RATIONALE
Cuff correctly inflated	No sound		Cuff inflation compresses brachial artery. Cuff pressure exceeds heart systolic pressure, occluding brachial artery blood flow.
I	Tapping	Soft, clear tapping, increasing in intensity	**Systolic** pressure. As cuff pressure lowers to reach intraluminal systolic pressure, artery opens, and blood first spurts into brachial artery. Blood is at very high velocity because of small opening of artery and large pressure difference across opening. This creates turbulent flow, which is audible.
Auscultatory gap	No sound	Silence for 30 to 40 mm Hg during deflation; an abnormal finding	Sounds temporarily disappear during end of phase I and reappear in phase II. Common with hypertension. If undetected, results in falsely low systolic or falsely high diastolic reading.
II	Swooshing	Softer murmur follows tapping	Turbulent blood flow through still partially occluded artery.
III	Knocking	Crisp, high-pitched sounds	Longer duration of blood flow through artery. Artery closes just briefly during late diastole.
IV	Abrupt muffling	Sound mutes to a low-pitched, cushioned murmur; blowing quality	Artery no longer closes in any part of cardiac cycle. Change in quality, not intensity.
V	Silence		Decreased velocity of blood flow. Streamlined blood flow is silent. The last audible sound (marking the disappearance of sounds) is **diastolic** pressure. The fifth Korotkoff sound is now used to define diastolic pressure in all age-groups.[7]

Brachial artery occluded by cuff,
no blood flow

Artery intermittently compressed,
blood spurts into artery

Cuff deflated,
artery flows freely

| | I | IV | V |
| Auscultatory sound | Silence | Clear tapping | Abrupt muffling | Silence |

Normal Range of Findings	Abnormal Findings

Normal Range of Findings

Deflate the cuff quickly and completely; then wait 15 to 30 seconds before reinflating so the blood trapped in the veins can dissipate. Place the bell or diaphragm of the stethoscope over the site of the brachial artery, making a light but airtight seal (Fig. 9-9). The diaphragm endpiece is usually adequate, but the bell is designed to pick up low-pitched sounds such as the sounds of a BP reading. Most novice practitioners find it easier to use the diaphragm than the bell. You can use either side to obtain an accurate reading.[17]

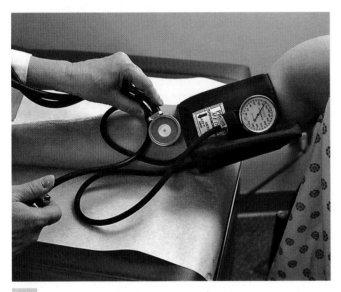

9-9

Rapidly inflate the cuff to the maximal inflation level that you determined. Then deflate the cuff slowly and evenly, about 2 mm Hg per heartbeat. Note the points at which you hear the first appearance of sound, the muffling of sound, and the final disappearance of sound. These are phases I, IV, and V of **Korotkoff sounds,** which are the components of a BP reading first described by a Russian surgeon in 1905 (see Table 9-3).

For all age-groups the fifth Korotkoff phase is now used to define diastolic pressure.[7] However, when a variance greater than 10 to 12 mm Hg exists between phases IV and V, record *both* phases along with the systolic reading (e.g., 142/98/80). Clear communication is important because the results significantly affect diagnosis and planning of care. See Table 9-4 for a list of common errors in BP measurement.

Abnormal Findings

Hypotension, abnormally low BP; **hypertension,** abnormally high BP (see parameters in Table 9-6, Abnormalities in Blood Pressure on p. 158).

Objective Data

Normal Range of Findings	Abnormal Findings

Objective Data

TABLE 9-4 Common Errors in Blood Pressure Measurement

COMMON ERROR	RESULT	RATIONALE
Taking blood pressure reading when person is anxious or angry or has just been active	Falsely high	Sympathetic nervous system stimulation
Faulty arm position:		
Above level of heart	Falsely low	Eliminates effect of hydrostatic pressure
Below level of heart	Falsely high	Additional force of gravity added to brachial artery pressure
Person supports own arm	Falsely high diastolic	Sustained isometric muscular contraction
Faulty leg position (e.g., person's legs are crossed)	Falsely high systolic and diastolic	Translocation of blood volume from dependent legs to thoracic area
Inaccurate cuff size (most common error):		
Cuff too narrow for extremity	Falsely high	Needs excessive pressure to occlude brachial artery
Cuff wrap is too loose or uneven, or bladder balloons out of wrap	Falsely high	Needs excessive pressure to occlude brachial artery
Failure to palpate radial artery while inflating:		
Inflating cuff not high enough	Falsely low systolic	Misses initial systolic tapping or may tune in during *auscultatory gap* (tapping sounds disappear for 10 to 40 mm Hg and then return; common with hypertension)
Inflating cuff too high	Pain	
Pushing stethoscope too hard on brachial artery	Falsely low diastolic	Excessive pressure distorts artery, and sounds continue
Deflating cuff:		
Too quickly	Falsely low systolic or falsely high diastolic	Insufficient time to hear tapping
Too slowly	Falsely high diastolic	Venous congestion in forearm makes sounds less audible
Halting during descent and reinflating cuff to recheck systolic	Falsely high diastolic	Venous congestion in forearm
Failure to wait 1-2 min before repeating entire reading	Falsely high diastolic	Venous congestion in forearm
Any observer error:		
Examiner's "subconscious bias"; a preconceived idea of what BP reading *should* be because of person's age, race, gender, weight, history, or condition	Error anywhere	Never assume that because a person appears healthy, his or her BP will be within normal limits
Examiner's haste	Error anywhere	
Faulty technique		
Examiner's digit preference; "hears" more results that end in zero than would occur by chance alone (e.g., 130/80)		
Diminished hearing acuity		
Defective or inaccurately calibrated equipment		

Orthostatic (or Postural) Vital Signs

Take serial measurements of pulse and BP when (1) you suspect volume depletion; (2) when the person is known to have hypertension or is taking antihypertensive medications; or (3) when the person reports fainting or syncope. Have the person rest supine for 2 or 3 minutes, take baseline readings of pulse and

Normal Range of Findings

BP, and repeat the measurements with the person sitting and then standing. For the person who is too weak or dizzy to stand, assess supine and then sitting with legs dangling. When the position is changed from supine to standing, normally a slight decrease (less than 10 mm Hg) in systolic pressure may occur.

Record the BP using even numbers. Also record the person's position, the arm used, and the cuff size if different from the standard adult cuff. Record the pulse rate and rhythm, noting whether the pulse is regular.

Thigh Pressure

When BP measured at the arm is excessively high, particularly in adolescents and young adults, compare it with the thigh pressure to check for **coarctation** of the aorta (a congenital form of narrowing). Normally the *thigh pressure is higher* than that in the arm. If possible, help the person to a prone position. (If the person must remain in the supine position, bend the knee slightly.) Wrap a large cuff, 18 to 20 cm, around the lower third of the thigh, centered over the popliteal artery on the back of the knee. Auscultate the popliteal artery for the reading (Fig. 9-10). Normally the systolic value is 10 to 40 mm Hg higher in the thigh than in the arm, and the diastolic pressure is the same.

9-10

✤ DEVELOPMENTAL COMPETENCE

Infants and Children
General Survey

Physical appearance, body structure, mobility—Note the same basic elements as for the adult, with consideration to age and development. Remember that children just learning to walk have a wide gait and normal toddler posture shows a protruding abdomen (lordosis).

Behavior—Note the response to stimuli and level of alertness appropriate for age. Infants usually look toward your voice and may mimic facial expressions.

Abnormal Findings

Orthostatic hypotension, a drop in systolic pressure of ≥20 mm Hg or increase in pulse of ≥20 beats/min occurs with a quick change to a standing position. These changes are caused by abrupt peripheral vasodilation without a compensatory increase in cardiac output. Orthostatic changes occur with prolonged bed rest, older age, hypovolemia, and some medications.

With **coarctation of the aorta,** arm pressures are high. Thigh pressure is *lower* because the blood supply to the thigh is below the constriction.

Objective Data

Normal Range of Findings	Abnormal Findings

Parental bonding—Note the child's interactions with parents, (i.e., that parent and child show a mutual response and are warm and affectionate, appropriate to the child's condition). The parent provides appropriate physical care of child and promotes new learning.

Some signs of child abuse are that the child avoids eye contact; the child exhibits no separation anxiety when you would expect it for age; the parent is disgusted by child's odor, sounds, drooling, or stools.

Deprivation of physical or emotional care (see Chapter 7).

Measurement

Weight. Weigh an infant on a platform-type balance scale (Fig. 9-11). To check calibration, set the weight at zero and observe the beam balance. Guard the baby so he or she does not fall. Weigh to the nearest 10 g (½ oz) for infants and 100 g (¼ lb) for toddlers.

9-11

By age 2 or 3 years use the upright scale. Leave underpants on the child. Some young children are fearful of the rickety standing platform and may prefer sitting on the infant scale. Use the upright scale with preschoolers and school-age children, maintaining modesty with light clothing (Fig. 9-12).

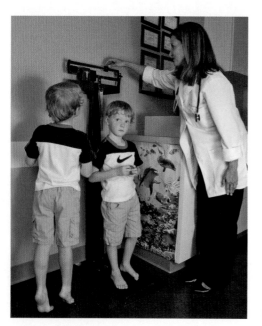

9-12

Objective Data

Normal Range of Findings	Abnormal Findings

Length. Until age 2 years measure the infant's body length supine by using a horizontal measuring board (Fig. 9-13). One person holds the top of the head against the head plate. Because the infant normally has flexed legs, extend them momentarily by gently stretching the spine and legs with the feet touching the perpendicular footplate. You may need to repeat the measure to ensure accuracy.

9-13

Measure the child's height by standing against a ruler mounted on the scale or wall (Fig. 9-14). Encourage the child to stand straight and tall and to look straight ahead without tilting the head. The shoulders, buttocks, and heels ideally should touch the ruler. Hold a level on the child's head at a right angle and note the measure to the nearest 1 mm (⅛ in).

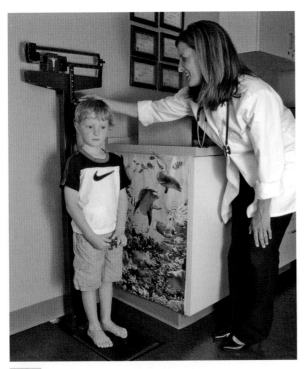

9-14

Normal Range of Findings

Physical growth is perhaps the best index of a child's general health. The child's height and weight are recorded at every health care visit to determine normal growth patterns. The results are plotted on growth charts based on data from the Centers for Disease Control and Prevention (CDC).[5] You can view these charts at www.cdc.gov. In addition to the weight, height, and head circumference charts, BMI-for-age charts are available for boys and girls ages 2 to 20 years.

Healthy childhood growth is continuous but uneven, with rapid growth spurts occurring during infancy and adolescence. Growth chart results are more reliable when comparing numerous growth measures over a long time. These charts also compare the individual child's measurements against the general population. Normal limits range from the 5th to the 95th percentile on the standardized charts.

Use your judgment and consider the genetic background of the small-for-age child. Explore the growth patterns of the parents and siblings. The differences in size and growth among the major racial/ethnic groups in the United States appear to be small and inconsistent.[5] You can use the revised 2000 CDC growth charts on all infants and children in the United States, regardless of race or ethnicity. The CDC notes that the most important evidence for growth potential appears to be economic, nutritional, and environmental.[5]

Head Circumference. Measure the infant's head circumference at birth and at each well-child visit up to age 2 years and then annually up to 6 years (Fig. 9-15). A retractable plastic tape measure is more accurate than a paper tape measure. Circle the tape around the head aligned with the eyebrows at the prominent frontal and occipital bones; the widest span is correct. Plot the measurement on standardized growth charts. Compare the infant's head size with that expected for age. A series of measurements is more valuable than a single figure to show the *pattern* of head growth.

Abnormal Findings

Further explore any growth measure that:
- Falls below the 5th or above the 95th percentile with no genetic explanation
- Shows a wide percentile difference between height and weight (e.g., a 10th percentile height with a 95th percentile weight)
- Shows that growth has suddenly stopped when it had been steady
- Fails to show normal growth spurts during infancy and adolescence

9-15

Normal Range of Findings	**Abnormal Findings**

The newborn's head measures about 32 to 38 cm (average around 34 cm) and is about 2 cm larger than the chest circumference. The chest grows at a faster rate than the cranium; at some time between 6 months and 2 years both measurements are about the same; after age 2 years the chest circumference is greater than the head circumference.

Measurement of the chest circumference is valuable in a comparison with the head circumference but not necessarily by itself. Encircle the tape around the chest at the nipple line. It should be snug but not so tight that it leaves a mark (Fig. 9-16).

Enlarged head circumference occurs with increased intracranial pressure (see Chapter 13).

9-16

Vital Signs

Measure vital signs with the same purpose and frequency as you would in an adult. With an *infant,* reverse the order of vital sign measurement to respiration, pulse, and temperature. Taking a rectal temperature may cause the infant to cry, which will increase the respiratory and pulse rate, thus masking the normal resting values. A *preschooler's* normal fear of body mutilation is increased with any invasive procedure. Whenever possible avoid the rectal route and take a tympanic or temporal artery temperature. Remember that you may have to use the rectal route for an accurate core measure. It is important to weigh risks and benefits when deciding on the appropriate temperature route for a child. Promote the cooperation of the *school-age child* by explaining the procedure completely and encouraging the child to handle the equipment. Your approach to measuring vital signs with the *adolescent* is much the same as with the adult.

Temperature

Tympanic. TMT and TAT measurements are useful with toddlers who squirm at the restraint needed for the rectal route and with preschoolers who are not yet able to cooperate for an oral temperature yet fear the disrobing and invasion of a rectal temperature. These measurements are so rapid that they are over before the child realizes it (Fig. 9-17).

Objective Data

Normal Range of Findings	Abnormal Findings

9-17

Axillary. The axillary route is safer and more accessible than the rectal route; however, its accuracy and reliability have been questioned. When cold receptors are stimulated, brown fat tissue in the area releases heat through chemical energy, which artificially raises skin temperature. When the axillary route is used, place the tip well into the axilla and hold the child's arm close to the body.

Oral. Use the oral route when the child is old enough to keep his or her mouth closed. This is usually at age 5 or 6 years, although some 4-year-old children can cooperate. When available, use an electronic thermometer because it is unbreakable and it registers quickly.

Rectal. Use this route with infants or other age-groups when other routes are not feasible, such as with the child who is unable to cooperate or is agitated, unconscious, or critically ill. An infant may be supine or side-lying, with the examiner's hand flexing the knees up onto the abdomen. (When supine, cover the boy's penis with a diaper.) An infant also may lie prone across the adult's lap. Separate the buttocks with one hand, and insert the lubricated electronic rectal probe *no farther than* 2.5 cm (1 in). Any deeper insertion risks rectal perforation because the colon curves posteriorly at 3 cm (1¼ in). (With a glass thermometer a temperature registers by 3 minutes.)

Normally rectal temperatures measure higher in infants and young children than in adults, with an average of 37.8°C (100°F) at 18 months. In addition, the temperature normally may be elevated in the late afternoon, after vigorous playing, or after eating.

Pulse

Palpate or auscultate an apical rate with infants and toddlers. (See Chapter 19 for location of apex and technique.) In children older than 2 years, use the radial site. Count the pulse for a full minute to take into account normal irregularities such as sinus arrhythmia. The heart rate normally fluctuates more with infants and children than with adults in response to exercise, emotion, and illness.

Up to ages 6 to 8 years, children have higher fevers with illness than adults do. Even with minor infections, fevers may elevate to 39.5° to 40.5°C (103° to 105°F).

Normal Range of Findings	Abnormal Findings

Respirations

Watch the infant's abdomen for movement because an infant's respirations are normally more diaphragmatic than thoracic (Fig. 9-18). The sleeping respiratory rate is the most accurate. Count a full minute because the pattern varies significantly from rapid breaths to short periods of apnea. Note the normal rate in Table 9-2 on p. 136.

> Tachypnea, or rapid respiratory rate, is >60/min for newborns to 2 months, and >50/min for 2 to 12 months. This occurs with fever and may indicate infection. Tachypnea and labored respirations may indicate pneumonia.

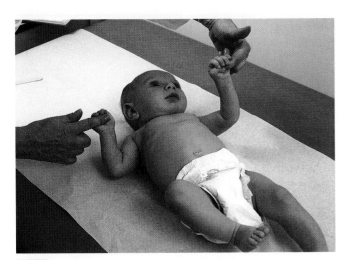

9-18

Blood Pressure

In children ages 3 years and older and in younger children at risk, measure a routine BP at least annually. For accurate measurement in children, make some adjustment in the choice of equipment and technique. The most common error is to use the incorrect size cuff. The cuff width must cover two thirds of the upper arm, and the cuff bladder must encircle it completely.

Use a pediatric-size endpiece on the stethoscope to locate the sounds. If possible, allow a crying infant to become quiet for 5 to 10 minutes before measuring the BP; crying may elevate the systolic pressure by 30 to 50 mm Hg. Use the disappearance of sound (phase V Korotkoff) for the diastolic reading in both children and adults. Note the guidelines for BP standards based on sex, age, and height.[25] These standards give a more precise classification of BP according to body size and avoid misclassifying children who are very tall or very short.

> Developing evidence shows that primary hypertension is detectable in children and occurs commonly.[31] BP between the 90th and 95th percentiles is prehypertension. In adolescents BP ≥ 120/80 mm Hg is prehypertension, even if this is <90th percentile. BP > 95th percentile may be hypertension. It should be measured again on two more occasions. But if BP is >99th percentile, make a prompt referral for evaluation and therapy. Similar to adults, hypertension in children and adolescents is associated with obesity, hyperlipidemia, and diabetes.[11,31]

Children younger than 3 years have such small arm vessels that it is difficult to hear Korotkoff sounds with a stethoscope. Instead use an electronic BP device that uses *oscillometry*, such as Dinamap, and gives a digital readout for systolic, diastolic, and MAP and pulse. Or use a *Doppler* ultrasound device to amplify the sounds. This instrument is easy to use and can be used by one examiner. (Note the technique for using the Doppler device on p. 153.)

Objective Data

Normal Range of Findings	Abnormal Findings

The Aging Adult

General Survey

Physical appearance—By the eighth and ninth decades, body contour is sharper with more angular facial features, and body proportions are redistributed. (See measuring weight and height, p. 130.)

Posture—A general flexion occurs by the eighth or ninth decade.

Kyphosis is the humpback appearance common in the very old and with osteoporosis.

Gait—Older adults often use a wider base to compensate for diminished balance, arms may be held out to help balance, and steps may be shorter or uneven.

Measurement

Weight. The aging person appears sharper in contour with more prominent bony landmarks than the younger adult. Body weight decreases during the 80s and 90s. This factor is more evident in males, perhaps because of greater muscle shrinkage. The distribution of fat also changes during the 80s and 90s. Even with good nutrition, subcutaneous fat is lost from the face and periphery (especially the forearms), whereas additional fat is deposited on the abdomen and hips (Fig. 9-19).

9-19 (Rossman, 1986.)

This change in fat distribution and loss in muscle mass can affect the BMI interpretation in older adults. For any given BMI, an older adult has more fat tissue than lean tissue when compared with a younger adult. As an aging person becomes shorter, the BMI reflecting the shorter height may overestimate the body fat content. However, these factors do not affect the validity of BMI classification to monitor the person's weight status.[26]

Height. By their 80s and 90s many people are shorter than they were in their 70s because of thinning of the vertebral disks, shortening of the individual vertebrae, postural changes of kyphosis, and slight flexion in the knees and hips. Because long bones do not shorten with age, the overall body proportion looks different—a shorter trunk with relatively long extremities (see Fig. 9-19).

Normal Range of Findings	**Abnormal Findings**

Vital Signs

Temperature. Changes in the body's temperature regulatory mechanism leave the aging person less likely to have fever but at a greater risk for hypothermia. Thus the temperature is a less reliable index of the older person's true health state. Sweat gland activity is also diminished.

Pulse. The normal range of heart rate is 50 to 95 beats/min, but the rhythm may be slightly irregular. The radial artery may feel stiff, rigid, and tortuous in an older person, although this condition does not necessarily imply vascular disease in the heart or brain. The increasingly rigid arterial wall needs a faster upstroke of blood, so the pulse is actually easier to palpate.

Respirations. Aging causes a decrease in vital capacity and a decreased inspiratory reserve volume. You may note a shallower inspiratory phase and an increased respiratory rate.

Blood Pressure. The aorta and major arteries tend to harden with age. As the heart pumps against a stiffer aorta, the systolic pressure increases, leading to a widened pulse pressure. With many older people, both the systolic and diastolic pressures increase, making it difficult to distinguish expected aging values from abnormal hypertension.

Additional Techniques

Measurement of Oxygen Saturation

The **pulse oximeter** is a noninvasive method to assess arterial oxygen saturation (SpO_2). A sensor attached to the person's finger or earlobe has a diode that emits light and a detector that measures the relative amount of light absorbed by oxyhemoglobin (HbO_2) and unoxygenated (reduced) hemoglobin (Hb). The pulse oximeter compares the ratio of light emitted with light absorbed and converts this ratio into the percentage of oxygen saturation. Because it only measures light absorption of pulsatile flow, the result is SpO_2. A healthy person with no lung disease normally has an SpO_2 of 97% to 99%, but a value of >95% is clinically acceptable in the presence of a normal hemoglobin.[2]

Select the appropriate pulse oximeter probe. The finger probe is spring loaded and feels like a clothespin attached to the finger, but it does not hurt (Fig. 9-20). An infant has a probe taped to the large toe. Some clinics use single-use probes that stick to the finger or ear instead of the multipatient-use spring-loaded model. If you are using a finger, make sure that the hand is warm to prevent false low readings caused by vasoconstriction. At lower oxygen saturations, the earlobe probe is more accurate.

9-20

©Pat Thomas, 2014.

The probe will show both the oxygen saturation and the pulse. Make sure that the pulse reading you see on the pulse oximeter matches the palpated pulse. If it does not correlate with the palpated pulse, question the accuracy of the result.

Objective Data

Normal Range of Findings	Abnormal Findings

Electronic Vital Signs Monitor

An automated vital signs monitor is in frequent use in hospital and clinic settings, especially when frequent BP measurement is needed. The artery pulsations create vibrations that are detected by an electronic sensor. The BP mode is non-invasive and fast and has automatic measurement intervals and a bright numeric display. As with manual BP equipment, accuracy depends on correct cuff selection and placement.

The electronic BP monitor cannot sense vibrations of low BP; do not use it with a patient who has a systolic BP of <90 mm Hg or conditions of an irregular heart rate, shivering, tremors, or seizures. If the numeric display does not fit with the patient's clinical picture, always validate the measurement with a manual sphygmomanometer and your own stethoscope. Evidence suggests that automatic BP devices are not reliable for high-risk patients, including those with hypotension or hypertension, recent trauma, or a dysrhythmia.[32] Some electronic BP devices also have probes for thermometry and pulse oximetry (Fig. 9-21).

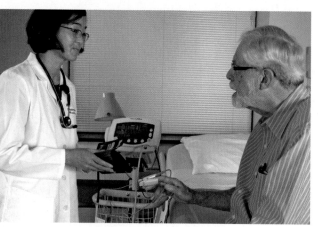

9-21

The Doppler Technique

In many situations pulse and BP measurement are enhanced by using an electronic device, the *Doppler ultrasonic flowmeter*. The Doppler technique works by a principle discovered in the 19th century by an Austrian physicist, Johannes Doppler. Sound varies in pitch in relation to the distance between the sound source and the listener; the pitch is higher when the distance is small, and the pitch lowers as the distance increases. Think of a railroad train speeding toward you; its train whistle sounds higher the closer it gets, and the pitch of the whistle lowers as the train fades away.

In this case the sound source is the blood pumping through the artery in a rhythmic manner. A handheld transducer picks up changes in sound frequency as the blood flows and ebbs, and it amplifies them. The listener hears a whooshing pulsatile beat.

The Doppler technique is used to locate the peripheral pulse sites (see Chapter 20 for further discussion). For BP measurement the Doppler technique will augment Korotkoff sounds (Fig. 9-22). Through this technique you can evaluate sounds that are hard to hear with a stethoscope such as those in critically ill individuals with a low BP, infants with small arms, and obese persons in whom the sounds are muffled by layers of fat. In addition, proper cuff placement is difficult on the obese person's cone-shaped upper arm. In this situation you can place the cuff on the more even forearm and hold the Doppler probe over the radial artery. For either location, use the following procedure:

Normal Range of Findings	Abnormal Findings

9-22

- Apply coupling gel to the transducer probe.
- Turn Doppler flowmeter on.
- Touch the probe to the skin, holding it perpendicular to the artery.
- A pulsatile whooshing sound indicates location of the artery. You may need to rotate the probe, but maintain contact with the skin. Do not push the probe too hard or you will occlude the pulse.
- Inflate the cuff until the sounds disappear; then proceed another 20 to 30 mm Hg beyond that point.
- Slowly deflate the cuff, noting the point at which the first whooshing sounds appear. This is the systolic pressure.
- It is difficult to hear the muffling of sounds or a reliable disappearance of sounds indicating the diastolic pressure (phases IV and V of Korotkoff sounds). However, the systolic pressure alone gives valuable data on the level of tissue perfusion and blood flow through patent vessels.

CULTURE AND GENETICS

General Appearance

Genetic differences are found in the body proportions of individuals. In general, White males are 1.27 cm (0.5 in) taller than Black males, whereas White women and Black women are, on the average, the same height. Sitting-to-standing height ratios reveal that Blacks of both sexes have longer legs and shorter trunks than Whites.[5] Because proportionately most of the weight is in the trunk, White men appear more obese than Black men. Asians are markedly shorter, weigh less, and have smaller body frames.

However, genes are not destiny. In the 20th century people grew taller in developed countries than they did in developing countries, largely because of environmental influences. This is most apparent among children of immigrants[4]:

Japanese-born men living in Japan are shorter than those living in Hawaii and shorter still than those living in California, and Hawaiian-born children of Japanese immigrants were significantly taller than their parents. Similarly, Guatemala Mayan refugee children born in the United States were significantly taller than their peers born in Guatemala or in Mexico en route to the United States. In total, Mayan children growing up in the United States are on average 5.5 cm taller than their cohort remaining in Guatemala. In general, subsequent generations of children of immigrants tend to increase in stature until they attain the height of the host population.

On average, Asians and American Indians have proportionately longer trunks and shorter limbs than Whites. Blacks tend to be wide shouldered and narrow hipped, whereas Asians tend to be wide hipped and narrow shouldered. Shoulder width is largely produced by the clavicle. Because the clavicle is a long bone, taller people have wide shoulders, whereas shorter people have narrower shoulders.

Obesity

Data from the most recent National Health and Nutrition Examination Survey (NHANES) show that 36% of U.S. adults are obese.[27] Obesity rates by racial groups include 34.3% non-Hispanic White adults; 49.5% non-Hispanic Blacks; and 39.1% Mexican Americans. When studied by sex, among adult men no differences in weight are found between racial/ethnic groups. However, Mexican-American and non-Hispanic Black women are significantly more likely to be obese than non-Hispanic White women. Trends in children over the past 30 years show that Black children have had larger increases in BMI, weight, and height than White children, with increases for Mexican-American children in between. What causes the increase in obesity? It is probably an interaction of biologic and social factors, but notably a U.S. environment with few opportunities for physical activity and an overabundance of inexpensive high-calorie food. This is now termed an **obesogenic environment**.

Objective Data

DOCUMENTATION AND CRITICAL THINKING

Sample Charting

K.A. is a 56-year-old Hispanic male construction worker who appears healthy and stated age. Alert, oriented, cooperative, with no signs of distress. Ht 170 cm (5'7"). Wt 83 kg (182 lbs). BMI 28.5 (overweight). Temp 98.6° F (37° C). Pulse 84 bpm. Resp 14/min. BP 146/84 mm Hg right arm, sitting.

Clinical Case Study 1*

G.S. is a 76-year-old Black female retired secretary, previously in good health, who is brought to the ED by her 83-year-old husband. G.S. and her husband report nausea, vomiting, diarrhea, and abdominal cramping since last night. Symptoms began after eating "bad food" at a buffet-style restaurant. G.S.'s husband reports that his symptoms have improved. G.S. continues to have diarrhea and dry heaving.*

*Please note that space does not allow a detailed plan for each clinical case study in this text. Please use these case studies as critical-thinking exercises and consult the appropriate text for current treatment plan.

SUBJECTIVE

G.S. reports extreme fatigue, weakness, and dizziness with position changes: "Feels like I'm going to black out." Severe nausea and vomiting; thirsty but cannot keep anything down; even sips of water result in "dry heaves." Cramping, intermittent abdominal pain. Watery brown diarrhea, profuse during the night, somewhat diminished now.

OBJECTIVE

Vital signs: Temp 100.1° F (37.8° C). BP (supine) 102/64 mm Hg. Pulse (supine) 70 bpm, regular rhythm. Resp 18/min. Helped to seated, leg-dangling position. Vitals: BP 74/52 mm Hg. Pulse 138 bpm, regular rhythm. Resp 20/min. Skin pale and moist (diaphoretic). Reports light-headed and dizzy in seated position. Returned to supine.

Respiratory: Breath sounds clear in all fields; no adventitious sounds.

Cardiovascular: Regular rate (70 bpm) and rhythm when supine, S_1 and S_2 are not accentuated or diminished, no extra sounds. All pulses present, 2+ and equal bilaterally. Carotids 2+ with no carotid bruit.

Abdomen: Bowel sounds hyperactive, skin pale and moist, abdomen soft and mildly tender to palpation. No enlargement of liver or spleen.

Neuro: Level of consciousness alert and oriented; pupils equal, round, react to light and accommodation. Sensory status normal. Mild weakness in arms and legs. Gait and standing leg strength not tested because of weakness. Deep tendon reflexes 2+ and equal bilaterally. Babinski reflex → down-going toes.

ASSESSMENT

Orthostatic hypotension, orthostatic pulse increase, and syncopal symptoms R/T hypovolemia
Diarrhea, possibly R/T ingestion of contaminated food
Risk for hyperthermia R/T dehydration and aging
Deficient fluid volume

Clinical Case Study 2

G.H. is a 31-year-old African-American male with no significant past medical history. Family history includes a mother with diabetes; father with hypertension diagnosed at age 40 years; and paternal grandfather with myocardial infarction at age 50, stroke at age 62, and heart failure diagnosed at age 51. G.H. presents to the ED with blurred vision and headache for the past 24 hours. He appears anxious but denies pain other than his headache.

SUBJECTIVE

Blurred vision for the past 24 hours that gets worse with activity. Frontal lobe headache that "comes and goes" for the past 24 hours. Denies nausea, vomiting. Reports occasional dizziness.

OBJECTIVE

Vital signs: Temp 98.6°F (37°C). BP 210/112 mm Hg right arm, sitting; 220/120 mm Hg left arm, sitting. Pulse 110 bpm. RR 20/min.

Respiratory: Breath sounds clear throughout; no adventitious sounds.

Cardiovascular: Regular rate and rhythm. S_1 and S_2 not accentuated or diminished, no extra sounds. Pulses bounding 3+ bilateral. 2+ pitting edema bilateral lower extremities.

Abdomen: Rounded abdomen. Bowel sounds active. Abdomen soft, nontender.

Neuro: Level of consciousness alert and oriented. Pupils equal; sluggish reaction to light. Optic disc swollen. Deep tendon reflexes 2+ and equal bilaterally. Babinski reflex → down-going toes.

ASSESSMENT

Hypertensive urgency

Risk for stroke R/T severe hypertension

Risk for myocardial ischemia R/T severe hypertension

Acute pain R/T increased cerebral vascular pressure

Decreased cardiac output R/T altered stroke volume due to hypertensive urgency

Knowledge deficit R/T hypertension

Clinical Case Study 3

J.T. is a 4-month-old Asian-American girl brought to the pediatric clinic by her mother. Until 2 days PTA, she has been in good health. She has had diarrhea, vomiting, and decreased intake for 2 days PTA. J.T.'s mother, father, and 3-year-old brother all had the same symptoms but are now improved.

SUBJECTIVE

J.T. has less diarrhea and no vomiting today, but she doesn't want to breastfeed and still appears to be "more sleepy than usual and just not herself." Her mother reports, "Now that I think about it, J.T. has only had 1 or 2 wet diapers since yesterday."

OBJECTIVE

Vital signs: Temp 99.5°F (37.5°C, rectally). BP 68/46 mm Hg (while lying being held). Pulse (apical) while sleeping 164 bpm. Resp 56/min. Weight 11 lbs, 4 oz (5.2 kg).

General appearance: Listless, pale; appears to be sleeping in mother's arms and awakens to physical stimuli but doesn't cry.

HEENT: Anterior fontanel sunken; dry oral mucosa; no tear production.

Cardiovascular: Tachycardia; no abnormal heart sounds; femoral pulses + 1 = bilat.

Respiratory: Tachypnea. Pulse oximetry 94% on room air. Breath sounds clear in all fields and = bilat; no adventitious sounds.

Abdomen: Hyperactive bowel sounds; no palpable masses.

Extremities: Cool, decreased pulse, cap refill 4 sec.

ASSESSMENT

Dehydration

Diarrhea R/T infectious process

Risk for electrolyte imbalance R/T diarrhea, fluid imbalance, and vomiting

Risk for ineffective thermoregulation R/T illness

ABNORMAL FINDINGS

TABLE 9-5 Abnormalities in Body Height and Proportion

Hypopituitary Dwarfism

Deficiency in growth hormone in childhood results in retardation of growth below the 3rd percentile, delayed puberty, hypothyroidism, and adrenal insufficiency. The 9-year-old girl at left appears much younger than her chronologic age, with infantile facial features and chubbiness. The age-matched girl at right shows increased height, more mature facial features, and loss of infantile fat.

Gigantism

Excessive secretion of growth hormone by the anterior pituitary results in overgrowth of the entire body. When this occurs during childhood before closure of bone epiphyses in puberty, it causes increased height (here 2.09 m, or 6 ft 9 in) and weight and delayed sexual development.

◀ Acromegaly (Hyperpituitarism)

Excessive secretion of growth hormone in adulthood after normal completion of body growth causes overgrowth of bone in face, head, hands, and feet but no change in height. Internal organs also enlarge (e.g., cardiomegaly); and metabolic disorders (e.g., diabetes mellitus) may be present.

See illustration credits for source information.

TABLE 9-5   Abnormalities in Body Height and Proportion—cont'd

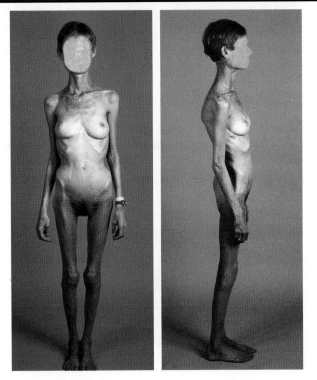

Achondroplastic Dwarfism

A genetic disorder in converting cartilage to bone results in normal trunk size, short arms and legs, and short stature. It is characterized by a relatively large head with frontal bossing; midplace hypoplasia; and often thoracic kyphosis, prominent lumbar lordosis, and abdominal protrusion. The mean adult height in men is about 131.5 cm (4 ft 4 in) and in women about 125 cm (4 ft 1 in).

Anorexia Nervosa

This serious mental health disorder is characterized by severe and life-threatening weight loss in an otherwise healthy person. Behavior is characterized by fanatic concern about weight, aversion to food, distorted body image (perceives self as fat despite skeletal appearance), starvation diets, frenetic exercise patterns, and striving for perfection. Results in amenorrhea in females.

◄ Endogenous Obesity—Cushing Syndrome

Either administration of adrenocorticotropin (ACTH) or excessive production of ACTH by the pituitary stimulates the adrenal cortex to secrete excess cortisol. This causes Cushing syndrome, characterized by weight gain and edema with central trunk and cervical obesity (buffalo hump) and round, plethoric face (moon face). Excessive catabolism causes muscle wasting; weakness; thin arms and legs; reduced height; and thin, fragile skin with purple abdominal striae, bruising, and acne. Note that the obesity here is markedly different from *exogenous obesity* caused by excessive caloric intake, in which body fat is evenly distributed and muscle strength is intact.

Continued

TABLE 9-5   Abnormalities in Body Height and Proportion—cont'd

◀ Marfan Syndrome

This inherited connective tissue disorder is characterized by tall, thin stature (≥95th percentile), arachnodactyly (long, thin fingers), hyperextensible joints, arm span greater than height, pubis-to-sole measurement exceeding crown-to-pubis measurement, sternal deformity (note pectus excavatum), high-arched narrow palate, narrow face, and pes planus (flat feet). Early morbidity and mortality occur as a result of cardiovascular complications such as mitral regurgitation and aortic dissection.

TABLE 9-6   Abnormalities in Blood Pressure

Hypotension

In normotensive adults: <95/60 mm Hg
In hypertensive adults: <The person's average reading, but >95/60 mm Hg
In children: <Expected value for age

Occurs With	*Rationale*
Acute myocardial infarction	Decreased cardiac output
Shock	Decreased cardiac output
Hemorrhage	Decrease in total blood volume
Vasodilation	Decrease in peripheral vascular resistance
Addison disease (hypofunction of adrenal glands)	Decrease in circulating aldosterone

Associated Symptoms and Signs

In conditions of decreased cardiac output, a low BP is accompanied by an increased pulse, dizziness, diaphoresis, confusion, and blurred vision. The skin feels cool and clammy because the superficial blood vessels constrict to shunt blood to the vital organs. An individual having an acute MI may also complain of crushing substernal chest pain, high epigastric pain, and shoulder or jaw pain.

Hypertension

Essential or Primary Hypertension

This occurs from no known cause but is responsible for about 95% of cases of hypertension in adults.

TABLE 9-6 Abnormalities in Blood Pressure—cont'd

Classification and Follow-Up of Blood Pressure for Adults Ages 18 and Older*

BP Classification	SBP (mm Hg)†	DBP (mm Hg)†	Lifestyle Modification	INITIAL DRUG THERAPY	
				Without Compelling Indication	With Compelling Indication
Normal	<120	and <80	Encourage		
Prehypertension	120-139	or 80-89	Yes	No antihypertensive drug indicated	Drug(s) for the compelling indications
Stage 1 hypertension	140-159	or 90-99	Yes	Thiazide-type diuretics for non-Blacks; may consider ACEI, ARB, CCB, or combination. Thiazide-type diuretic or CCB for Blacks.	Drug(s) for the compelling indications; other antihypertensive drugs (diuretics, ACEI, ARB, BB, CCB) as needed
Stage 2 hypertension	≥160	or ≥100	Yes	Two-drug combination for most‡; usually thiazide-type diuretic and ACEI, ARB, or CCB	Drug(s) for the compelling indications; other antihypertensive drugs (diuretics, ACEI, ARB, CCB) as needed§

Cardiovascular Risk Stratification in Patients With Hypertension

Major Risk Factors
Smoking
Dyslipidemia
Diabetes mellitus
Age > 60 yr
Gender (men and postmenopausal women)
Family history of cardiovascular disease: women
    < 65 yr or men < 55 yr

Target Organ Damage/Clinical Cardiovascular Disease
Heart diseases
Left ventricular atrophy
Angina or prior myocardial infarction
Prior coronary revascularization
Heart failure
Stroke or transient ischemic attack
Nephropathy
Peripheral arterial disease
Retinopathy

Lifestyle Modifications for Hypertension Prevention and Management

- Lose weight if overweight
- Limit alcohol intake to no more than 1 oz (30 mL) of ethanol (e.g., 24 oz [720 mL] of beer, 10 oz [300 mL] of wine, or 2 oz [60 mL] of 100-proof whiskey) per day or 0.5 oz (15 mL) of ethanol per day for women and lighter-weight people.
- Increase aerobic physical activity (30-45 min most days of the week).
- Reduce sodium intake to no more than 100 mmol/day (2.4 g of sodium or 6 g of sodium chloride).
- Maintain adequate intake of dietary potassium (approximately 90 mmol/day).
- Maintain adequate intake of dietary calcium and magnesium for general health.
- Stop smoking and reduce intake of dietary saturated fat and cholesterol for overall cardiovascular health.

Data on classification of hypertension in adults adapted from Chobanian et al. (2003). The JNC 7 report. *JAMA 289*, 2560-2572; and James, P.A. et al. (2013). 2014 Evidence-based guidelines for the management of high blood pressure in adults report from the panel members appointed to the Eighth Joint National Committee (The JNC 8 Report). *JAMA*, Published online December 18, 2013. doi: 10.1001/jama.2013.284427.
ACEI, Angiotensin-converting enzyme inhibitor; *ARB*, angiotensin receptor blocker; *BB*, beta-blocker; *BP*, blood pressure; *CCB*, calcium channel blocker; *DBP*, diastolic blood pressure; *MI*, myocardial infarction; *SBP*, systolic blood pressure.
*Please review full JNC 8 Guidelines for treatment in adults ≥ 60 years of age.
†Treatment determined by highest BP category.
‡Initial combined therapy should be used cautiously in those at risk for orthostatic hypotension.
§If BP goal is not attained with a diuretic and two additional medications (ARB, ACEI, and/or CCB), add an additional medication class (e.g., beta blocker, aldosterone antagonist) and/or refer to a hypertension specialist.

BIBLIOGRAPHY

1. Allen, D. B., & Cuttler, L. (2013). Short stature in childhood—challenges and choices. *N Engl J Med, 368*(13), 1220-1228.
2. American Association of Critical Care Nurses. (2011). *AACN procedure manual for critical care.* (6th ed.). St. Louis: Saunders.
3. Barringer, L. B., Evans, C. W., Ingram, L. L., et al. (2011). Agreement between temporal artery, oral, and axillary temperature measurements in the perioperative period. *J PeriAnesth Nurs, 26*(3), 143-150.
4. Beard, A. S., & Blaser, M. J. (2002). The ecology of height: the effect of microbial transmission on human height. *Perspect Biol Med, 45*(4), 475-498.
5. Centers for Disease Control and Prevention (CDC). (2002). *2000 CDC growth charts for the United States: methods and development.* Available at: www.cdc.gov.
6. Chester, J. G., & Rudolph, J. L. (2011). Vital signs in older patients: age-related changes. *J Am Med Dir Assoc, 12*(5), 337-343.
7. Chobanian, A. V., Bakris, G. L., Black, H. R., et al. National Heart, Lung, and Blood Institute (2003). The seventh report of the Joint National Committee on Prevention, Detection, Evaluation and Treatment of High Blood Pressure: the JNC 7 report. *JAMA, 289*(19), 2560-2572.
8. Davis, R. A. (2012). The big chill: accidental hypothermia. *Am J Nurs, 112*(1), 38-46.
9. Falkenstern, S. K., & Bauer, L. A. (2009). Helping kids grow. *Nurse Pract, 34*(3), 31-41.
10. Flegal, K. M., Carroll, M. D., Kit, B. K., et al. (2012). Prevalence of obesity and trends in the distribution of body mass index among US adults, 1999-2010. *JAMA, 307*(5), 491-497.
11. Flynn, J. T. (2010). Pediatric hypertension update. *Curr Opin Nephrol Hypertens, 19*, 292-297.
11a. Fountain, C., Goins, L., Hartman, M., et al. (2008). Evaluating the accuracy of four temperature instruments on an adult inpatient oncology unit. *Clin J Oncol Nurs 12*(6), 983-987.
12. Fryar, C. D., Gu, Q., & Ogden, C.L. (2012). *Anthropometric reference data for children and adults: United States 2007-2010.* National Center for Health Statistics, 11, 1-40.
13. Garzon, D. L., & Figgemeier, M. E. (2011). Dying to be thin: identifying and managing eating disorders. *Nurse Pract, 36*(10), 45-51.
14. Holzhauer, J. K., Reith, V., Sawin, K. J., et al. (2009). Evaluation of temporal artery thermometry in children 3-36 months old. *J Spec Pediatr Nurs, 14*(4), 239-244.
15. Hwu, Y. J., Coates, V. E., & Lin, F. Y. (2000). A study of the effectiveness of different measuring times and counting methods of human radial pulse rates. *J Clin Nurs, 9*(1), 146-152.
15a. Ingelfinger, J. R. (2014). The child or adolescent with elevated blood pressure. *N Engl J Med, 370*(24), 2316-2325.
16. Jones, B. G. (2013). Developing a vital sign alert system. *Am J Nurs, 113*(8), 36-44.
17. Kantola, I., Vesalainen, R., Kangassalo, K., et al. (2005). Bell or diaphragm in measurement of blood pressure? *J Hypertens, 23*, 499-503.
18. Keele-Smith, R., & Price-Daniel, C. (2001). Effects of crossing legs on blood pressure measurement. *Clin Nurs Res, 10*(2), 202-213.
19. Kiekkas, P., & Brokalaki, H. (2008). Physical antipyresis in critically ill adults. *Am J Nurs, 108*(7), 40-50.
20. Ledbetter, C. (2011). Fever of unknown origin: an evidence-based approach. *Nurse Pract, 36*(8), 46-52.
21. Lewis, C. E., McTigue, K. M., Burke, L. E., et al. (2009). Mortality, health outcomes, and body mass index in the overweight range. *Circulation, 119*(25), 3263.
22. Lu, S., Leasure, A., & Dai, Y. (2009). A systematic review of body temperature variations in older people. *J Clin Nurs 19*, 4-16.
23. Mattis, J. G., & Yates, A. M. (2011). Heat stroke: helping patients keep their cool. *Nurse Pract, 36*(5), 48-52.
24. McGee, S. (2012). *Evidence-based physical diagnosis.* (3rd ed.). Philadelphia: Saunders.
25. National High Blood Pressure Education Program (NHBPEP). (2004). The fourth report on the diagnosis, evaluation, and treatment of high blood pressure in children and adolescents. *Pediatrics, 114*(2), 555-576.
26. National Institutes of Health (NIH). (2000). *The practical guide to identification, evaluation, and treatment of overweight and obesity in adults.* Available at www.nhlbi.nih.gov/guidelines/obesity/ob_home_htm.
27. National Institutes of Health Weight-Control Information Network. (2012). *Overweight and obesity statistics.* Available at www.win.niddk.nih.gov.
28. Ogden, C. L., Carroll, M. D., Kit, B. K., et al. (2012). Prevalence of obesity and trends in body mass index among US children and adolescents, 1999-2010. *JAMA, 307*(5), 483-490.
29. Parkes, R. (2011). Rate of respiration: the forgotten vital sign. *Emerg Nurse, 19*(2), 12-7.
30. Pesola, G. R., Pesola, H. R., Nelson, M. J., et al. (2001). The normal difference in bilateral indirect blood pressure recordings in normotensive individuals. *Am J Emerg Med, 19*(1), 43-45.
31. Riley, M., & Bluhm, B. (2012). High blood pressure in children and adolescents. *Am Fam Phys, 85*(7), 693-700.
31a. Scordo, K. A., & Pickett, K. A. (2014). Hypertension in 2014: making sense of the guidelines. *Nurse Pract, 39*(6), 19-23.
32. Skirton, H., Chamberlain, W., Lawson, C., et al. (2011). A systematic review of variability and reliability of manual and automated blood pressure readings. *J Clin Nurs, 20*, 602-614.
33. Stelfox, H. T., Straus, S. E., Ghali, W. A., et al. (2010). Temporal artery versus bladder thermometry during adult medical-surgical intensive care monitoring: an observational study. *BMC Anesthesiol, 10*(1), 13.
34. Valdez-Lowe, C., Ghareeb, S. A., & Artinian, N. T. (2009). Pulse oximetry in adults. *Am J Nurs, 109*(6), 52-59.

CHAPTER 10

Pain Assessment: The Fifth Vital Sign

STRUCTURE AND FUNCTION

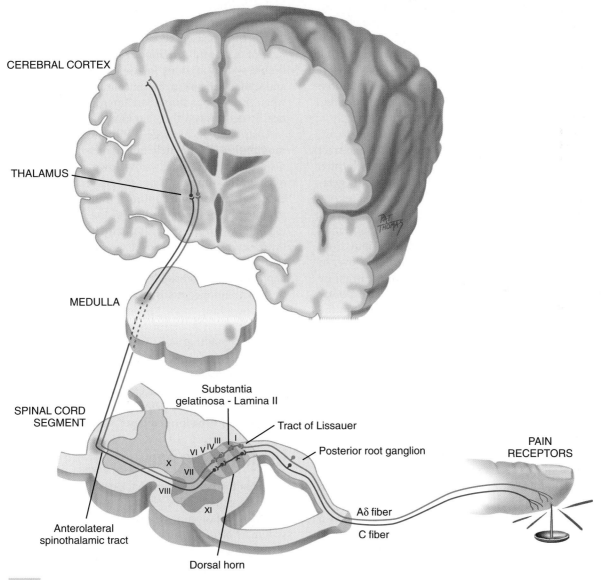

CEREBRAL CORTEX

THALAMUS

MEDULLA

SPINAL CORD SEGMENT

Substantia gelatinosa - Lamina II

Tract of Lissauer

Posterior root ganglion

PAIN RECEPTORS

Aδ fiber

C fiber

Anterolateral spinothalamic tract

Dorsal horn

10-1

Pathologic pain develops by two main processes: **nociceptive** (Fig. 10-1) and/or **neuropathic** processing. It is important to understand how these two types of pain develop because patients present with distinguishing sensations and respond differently to analgesics. An accurate pain assessment allows clinicians to more accurately select effective pharmacologic and nonpharmacologic strategies to interrupt the pain processing along multiple points within the pain messaging system and ultimately provide improved pain relief.

NEUROANATOMIC PATHWAY

Pain is a highly complex and subjective experience that originates from the central nervous system (CNS) and/or peripheral nervous system (PNS). Specialized nerve endings called **nociceptors** are designed to detect painful sensations from the periphery and transmit them to the CNS. Nociceptors are located primarily within the skin; joints; connective tissue; muscle; and thoracic, abdominal, and pelvic viscera. These nociceptors can be stimulated directly by mechanical or thermal trauma or secondarily by chemical mediators that are released from the site of tissue damage.

Nociceptors carry the pain signal to the CNS by two primary sensory (or afferent) fibers: **Aδ and C fibers** (see Fig. 10-1). Aδ fibers are myelinated and larger in diameter; thus they transmit the pain signal rapidly to the CNS. The sensation is very localized, short term, and sharp in nature because of the Aδ fiber stimulation. In contrast, C fibers are unmyelinated and smaller, and they transmit the signal more slowly. The "secondary" sensations are diffuse and aching, and they last longer after the initial injury.

Peripheral sensory Aδ and C fibers enter the spinal cord by posterior nerve roots within the dorsal horn by the tract of Lissauer. The fibers synapse with **interneurons** located within a specified area of the cord called the **substantia gelatinosa.** A cross section shows that the gray matter of the spinal cord is divided into a series of consecutively numbered laminae (layers of nerve cells) (see Fig. 10-1). The substantia gelatinosa is lamina II, which receives sensory input from various areas of the body. The pain signals then cross over to the other side of the spinal cord and ascend to the brain by the **anterolateral spinothalamic tract.** When pain is poorly controlled over an extended period of time, cells within the dorsal horn become altered in size and function, and this damage ultimately turns future pain signals into more exaggerated or hypersensitive processing.[36]

NOCICEPTIVE PAIN

Nociceptive pain develops when *functioning and intact* nerve fibers in the periphery and the CNS are stimulated. It is triggered by events outside the nervous system from actual or potential tissue damage. Nociception can be divided into four phases: (1) transduction, (2) transmission, (3) perception, and (4) modulation (Fig. 10-2).

Initially the first phase of **transduction** occurs when a noxious stimulus in the form of traumatic or chemical injury, burn, incision, or tumor takes place in the periphery. The periphery includes the skin and the somatic and visceral structures. These injured tissues then release a variety of chemicals, including substance P, histamine, prostaglandins, serotonin, and bradykinin. These chemicals are neurotransmitters that transmit a pain message, or action potential, along sensory afferent nerve fibers to the spinal cord. These nerve fibers terminate in the dorsal horn of the spinal cord. Because the initial afferent fibers stop in the dorsal horn, a second set of neurotransmitters carries the pain impulse across the synaptic cleft to the dorsal horn neurons. These neurotransmitters include substance P, glutamate, and adenosine triphosphate (ATP).

In the second phase, known as **transmission,** the pain impulse moves from the level of the spinal cord to the brain. Within the spinal cord, at the site of the synaptic cleft, are opioid receptors that can block this pain signaling with our own endogenous opioids or with exogenous opioids if they are administered. However, if not stopped, the pain impulse moves to the brain via various ascending fibers within the spinothalamic tract to the thalamus. Once the pain impulse moves through the thalamus, the message is dispersed to higher cortical areas via mechanisms that are not clearly understood at this time.

The third phase, **perception,** signifies the conscious awareness of a painful sensation. Cortical structures such as the limbic system account for the emotional response to pain, and somatosensory areas can characterize the sensation. Only when the noxious stimuli are interpreted in these higher cortical structures can this sensation be identified as "pain."

Last, the pain message is inhibited through the phase of **modulation.** Fortunately our bodies have a built-in mechanism that will eventually slow down and stop the processing of a painful stimulus. If not for pain modulation, the experience of pain would continue from childhood injuries to adulthood. To inhibit and block the pain impulse, descending pathways from the brainstem to the spinal cord release a third set of neurotransmitters that produce an analgesic effect. These neurotransmitters include serotonin, norepinephrine, neurotensin, γ-aminobutyric acid (GABA), and our own endogenous opioids—β-endorphins, enkephalins, and dynorphins.

This type of nociceptive processing is protective.[7] It is a warning signal that injury is about to or has taken place. We quickly learn to move our hand away from a burning flame. Other examples of nociceptive pain include a skinned knee, kidney stones, menstrual cramps, muscle strain, venipuncture, or arthritic joint pain. Nociceptive pain is typically predictable and time limited based on the extent of the injury.

NEUROPATHIC PAIN

Neuropathic pain is pain that does not adhere to the typical and rather predictable phases in nociceptive pain. It is "pain caused by a lesion or disease of the somatosensory nervous system."[19] Neuropathic pain implies an abnormal processing of the pain message from an injury to the nerve fibers. This type of pain is the most difficult to assess and treat. Pain is often perceived long after the site of injury heals, and it evolves into a chronic condition.

Nociceptive pain can change into a neuropathic pain pattern over time when pain has been poorly controlled. This is because of the constant irritation and inflammation caused by a pain stimulus, which alters nerve cells, making them more sensitive to any future stimulus. The constant irritation

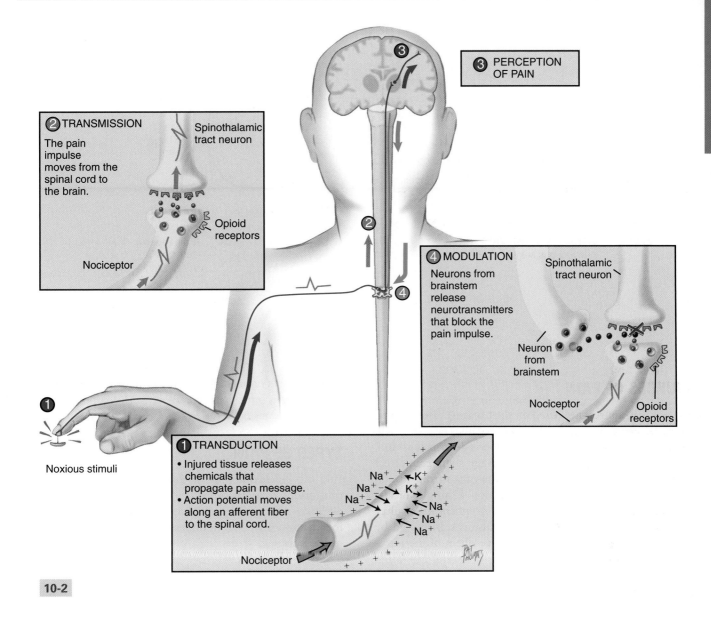

10-2

from uncontrolled pain also decreases the number of opioid receptors in the spinal cord.[4] Neurons in the spinal cord dorsal horn may experience excitotoxic and apoptotic cell death. There is significant depletion of GABAergic interneurons; because GABA is an inhibitory neurotransmitter, this may cause hyperalgesia and allodynia.[9]

Conditions that may cause neuropathic pain include diabetes mellitus, herpes zoster (shingles), HIV/AIDS, sciatica, trigeminal neuralgia, phantom limb pain, and chemotherapy. Further examples include CNS lesions such as stroke, multiple sclerosis, and tumor. Pain sustained on a neurochemical level cannot be identified by x-ray image, computerized axial tomography (CAT) scan, or traditional magnetic resonance imaging (MRI). Recent advances in noninvasive neuroimaging techniques allow us to study the structural, functional, and neurochemical changes on the brain caused by nociception.[23] Pain researchers are using functional MRI (fMRI) to visualize changes in brain activity while patients experience pain. When these images are shown to patients in real time, they can be used to help pain sufferers control their pain and improve their pain experience. Patients viewing fMRI of their brains are taught strategies such as meditation, guided imagery, and cognitive behavioral therapy to alter the response of their brains to pain; they can see the impact of these therapies on their brains.[25,38]

The abnormal processing of the neuropathic pain impulse can be continued by the PNS or CNS. An injury to peripheral neurons can result in spontaneous and repetitive firing of nerve fibers, almost seizurelike in activity (Fig. 10-3). Neuropathic pain may be sustained centrally in a phenomenon known as neuronal "wind-up." Within the dorsal horn of the spinal cord, neurons are converted into a hyperexcitable state, causing a minor stimulus to spiral into a much larger painful effect.[4]

Structure and Function

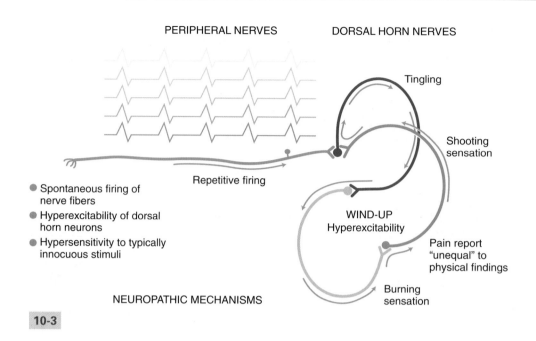

PERIPHERAL NERVES   DORSAL HORN NERVES

Tingling

Shooting
sensation

Repetitive firing

● Spontaneous firing of
   nerve fibers
● Hyperexcitability of dorsal
   horn neurons
● Hypersensitivity to typically
   innocuous stimuli

WIND-UP
Hyperexcitability

Pain report
"unequal" to
physical findings

NEUROPATHIC MECHANISMS

Burning
sensation

10-3

SOURCES OF PAIN

Physical pain sources are based on their origin. **Visceral** pain originates from the larger internal organs (i.e., stomach, intestine, gallbladder, pancreas). It often is described as dull, deep, squeezing, or cramping. The pain can stem from direct injury to the organ or stretching of the organ from tumor, ischemia, distention, or severe contraction. Examples of visceral pain include ureteral colic, acute appendicitis, ulcer pain, and cholecystitis. The pain impulse is transmitted by ascending nerve fibers along with nerve fibers of the autonomic nervous system (ANS). That is why visceral pain often presents along with autonomic responses such as vomiting, nausea, pallor, and diaphoresis.

Somatic pain originates from musculoskeletal tissues or the body surface. **Deep somatic pain** comes from sources such as the blood vessels, joints, tendons, muscles, and bone. Pain may result from pressure, trauma, or ischemia. **Cutaneous pain** is derived from skin surface and subcutaneous tissues. Deep somatic pain often is described as aching or throbbing, whereas cutaneous pain is superficial, sharp, or burning. Whether somatic pain is sharp or dull, it is usually well localized and easy to pinpoint. Somatic pain, like visceral pain, can be accompanied by nausea, sweating, tachycardia, and hypertension caused by the ANS response.

Pain that is felt at a particular site but originates from another location is known as **referred pain.** Both sites are innervated by the same spinal nerve, and it is difficult for the brain to differentiate the point of origin. Referred pain may originate from visceral or somatic structures. Various structures maintain their same embryonic innervation. For example, an inflamed appendix in the right lower quadrant of the abdomen may have referred pain in the periumbilical area, or the pain from acute coronary syndrome may be felt in the left arm or neck. Please know the areas of referred pain for diagnostic purposes (see Table 21-3, Common Sites of Referred Abdominal Pain).

TYPES OF PAIN

Pain can be classified by its duration into acute or chronic categories (*chronic* is called *persistent* because it carries a less negative, malingering connotation). The duration provides information on possible underlying mechanisms and treatment decisions.

Acute pain is short term and self limiting, often follows a predictable trajectory, and dissipates after an injury heals. Examples of acute pain include surgery, trauma, and kidney stones. Acute pain has a self-protective purpose; it warns the individual of actual or threatened tissue damage. *Incident pain* is an acute type that happens predictably when certain movements take place. Examples include pain in the lower back on standing or whenever turning a hospitalized patient from side to side.

In contrast, **chronic (persistent) pain** is diagnosed when the pain continues for 6 months or longer. It can last 5, 15, or 20 years and beyond. Chronic pain can be divided into *malignant* (cancer-related) and *nonmalignant*. Malignant pain often parallels the pathology created by the tumor cells. The pain is induced by tissue necrosis or stretching of an organ by the growing tumor. It fluctuates within the course of the disease. Chronic nonmalignant pain is often associated with musculoskeletal conditions such as arthritis, low back pain, or fibromyalgia.

Chronic pain does not stop when the injury heals. It persists after the predicted trajectory. It outlasts its protective purpose, and the level of pain intensity does not correspond with the physical findings. Unfortunately many chronic pain sufferers are not believed by clinicians and are labeled as malingerers, attention seekers, or drug seekers. Chronic pain originates from abnormal processing of pain fibers from peripheral or central sites.

Finally *breakthrough pain* is a transient spike in pain level, moderate to severe in intensity, in an otherwise controlled pain syndrome. It can result from end-of-dose medication failure. This occurs when a patient taking a long-acting opioid has a recurrence of pain before the next scheduled dose. Treatment of end-of-dose failure includes shortening the interval between doses or increasing the dose of medication. Breakthrough pain can also be the result of incident or episodic pain. This is a predictable breakthrough pain that may be triggered by a physical stimulus such as a return to activity after a surgery or from a psychosocial event.

The experience of pain is a complex biopsychosocial phenomenon. Because pain is transmitted on a cellular level, our current technology cannot reliably detect this process. Therefore the most important and reliable indicator for pain is the patient's self-report. When treating patients with acute or chronic pain, it is important to frequently reassess pain scores to evaluate the effectiveness of the therapy used.

DEVELOPMENTAL COMPETENCE

Infants have the same capacity for pain as adults. In fetal development ascending sensory fibers, neurotransmitters, and connections to the thalamus are developed by 20 weeks' gestation.[24] However, the immaturity of the cortex and lack of conscious awareness may prevent the fetus from experiencing emotional "pain" until 30 weeks' gestation. Conscious or not, pain-producing invasive fetal procedures elicit a stress response, and pain during gestation should be avoided until more is known about fetal pain.

Inhibitory neurotransmitters are insufficient until birth at full term. Therefore the preterm infant is rendered more sensitive to painful stimuli. Preverbal infants are at high risk for undertreatment of pain in part because of persistent myths and beliefs that infants do not remember pain. In fact, current evidence suggests that repetitive and poorly controlled pain in skin-breaking procedures in infants (e.g., daily heel sticks, venipunctures) can result in pain hypersensitivity later in life. This suggests use of analgesics during routine painful procedures.[22]

The Aging Adult

No evidence exists to suggest that older individuals perceive pain to a lesser degree or that sensitivity is diminished. Although pain is a common experience among individuals 65 years of age and older, it is *not* a normal process of aging. Pain indicates pathology or injury. It should never be considered something to tolerate or accept in one's later years.

Unfortunately many clinicians and older adults wrongfully assume that pain should be expected in aging, which leads to underreporting of pain and less aggressive treatment.

Older adults may have additional fears about becoming dependent, undergoing invasive procedures, taking pain medications, and having a financial burden. The most common pain-producing conditions for aging adults include pathologies such as osteoarthritis, osteoporosis, peripheral vascular disease, cancer, peripheral neuropathies, angina, and chronic constipation.

People with dementia do feel pain. The somatosensory cortex is generally unaffected by dementia of the Alzheimer type. Sensory discrimination is preserved in cognitively intact and impaired adults.[1] Because the limbic system is affected by Alzheimer disease, current research focuses on how the person interprets and reports these pain messages.[17] In patients with dementia we can assess body language instead of verbal communication (e.g., a clenched fist may indicate pain; agitation may mean hunger or cold). Other causes include fatigue, urinary tract or other infections, constipation, or medication side effects. See further discussion on pain assessment with dementia on p. 174.

Gender Differences

Gender differences are influenced by societal expectations, hormones, and genetic makeup. Traditionally men have been raised to be more stoic about pain, and more affective or emotional displays of pain are accepted for women. Hormonal changes have strong influences on pain sensitivity for women. Regarding migraine, the prevalence is equal in prepubertal girls and boys, but after puberty it increases to 18% for women and 6% for men.[13] Women may have more postoperative and procedural pain than men and are more likely to have chronic fibromyalgia.[13]

CULTURE AND GENETICS

Genetic differences between both sexes may account for the differences in pain perception. However, how many pain genes exist? There is no one clear genetic pain link such as there is between breast cancer and BRCA1. In animal models many hundreds of pain genes have been discovered. Humans are more complicated in that there are genetic links to pain variability, susceptibility to painful diseases such as arthritis, the development of nociceptors, and the neurotransmitter signaling systems such as glutamate of GABA.[29] Pharmacogenetics is the effort to tailor pharmacologic agents to improve pain treatment based on genetic sequencing, but today this is not close to guiding individualized pain therapy.[29]

When clinicians speak a language or belong to a culture different from their patient in pain, the risk increases for misunderstanding, underreporting, and undertreating. Please review the methods for working with an interpreter in Chapter 3 and the discussion on cultural variations in Chapter 2. Also adopt the habit of asking each patient how he or she typically behaves when in pain.

Most of the research conducted on racial differences and pain has focused on the disparity in management of pain for various racial groups (i.e., comparing pain treatment for individuals of color [e.g., African Americans, Asians, Latinos] with the standard treatment for all individuals with similar injuries or diseases). Pain-related disparities continue to exist for present minority groups "in acute, chronic, cancer, and palliative pain care across the lifespan and treatment settings," with members of minorities receiving less quality pain care than non-Hispanic Whites receive.[3] Poorly treated pain has devastating results for the patient, with huge costs to society in losses of wages and productivity.

The experience of pain is more layered than just physical suffering. Pain and the expression of pain are influenced by social, cultural, emotional, and spiritual concerns. A culturally competent practitioner includes an aspect of cultural assessment with pain assessment to paint a fuller picture of the individual experience of pain.[6,30,35]

SUBJECTIVE DATA

Pain is defined as an "unpleasant sensory and emotional experience associated with actual or potential tissue damage or described in terms of such damage. Pain is always subjective."[2]

The subjective report is the most reliable indicator of pain. Because pain occurs on a neurochemical level, the diagnosis of pain cannot be made exclusively on physical examination findings, although these findings can lend support. Self-report is the "gold standard" of pain assessment.

Examiner Asks	Rationale
Initial Pain Assessment	
1. **Do you have pain?** Discomfort or soreness? Ouch? Tell me in your own words.	Some people report pain only when it is severe. Try a variety of words.
2. **Where is your pain?** Tell me about *all* of the places that have pain.	Pain may be localized or occur in *multiple* sites.
3. **When did your pain start?** What were you doing then? Is it constant or does it come and go?	Identifies onset and duration. Chronic pain persists after injury heals; it is pain that occurs for 6 months or longer.
4. **What does your pain feel like?** • Burning, stabbing, aching • Throbbing, firelike, squeezing • Cramping, sharp, itching, tingling • Shooting, crushing, sharp, dull	Identifies quality of pain and helps differentiate between nociceptive and neuropathic pain mechanisms. Neuropathic pain is described as burning, shooting, and tingling. Nociceptive pain originating from visceral sites is described as aching if localized and cramping if poorly localized; from somatic sites, it is described as throbbing/aching.
5. **How much pain do you have now?**	Identifies intensity (refer to various intensity scales).
6. **What makes your pain better or worse?** (Include behavioral, pharmacologic, and nonpharmacologic interventions.) What medications control your pain? Are doses accurate? How often do you take pain medication?	Identifies alleviating and aggravating factors. Evaluates effectiveness of current treatment.
7. **How does pain limit your function or activities?** What does pain prevent you from doing?	Identifies degree of impairment and quality of life.

Examiner Asks	Rationale
8. **How do you usually react when you are in pain?** Any other symptoms along with the pain (nausea, vomiting, dizziness, heart racing)? How would others know that you are in pain?	Nonverbal behaviors are extremely variable, especially for chronic pain syndromes. Aids in detection and assessment.
9. **What does this pain mean to you?** Why do you think you are having pain?	Can identify myths, misconceptions, beliefs such as "I'm getting old"; "It's a punishment from God."

Alternatively you can collect a complete pain health history using the PQRST mnemonic described in Table 10-1.

TABLE 10-1 PQRST Method of Pain Assessment

P = Provocation/Palliation

What were you doing when the pain started? What caused it? What makes it better? Worse? What seems to trigger it? Stress? Position? Certain activities?

What relieves it? Medications, massage, heat/cold, changing position, being active, resting?

What aggravates it? Movement, bending, lying down, walking, standing?

Q = Quality/Quantity

What does it feel like? Use words to describe the pain such as sharp, dull, stabbing, burning, crushing, throbbing, nauseating, shooting, twisting, or stretching.

R = Region/Radiation

Where is the pain located? Does it radiate? Where? Does it feel as if it travels/moves around? Did it start elsewhere and is now localized to one spot?

S = Severity Scale

How severe is the pain on a scale of 0 to 10, with zero being no pain and 10 being the worst pain ever? Does it interfere with activities? How bad is it at its worst? Does it force you to sit down, lie down, slow down? How long does an episode last?

T = Timing

When/at what time did the pain start? How long did it last? How often does it occur: hourly? daily? weekly? monthly? Is it sudden or gradual? What were you doing when you first experienced it? When do you usually experience it: daytime? night? early morning? Are you ever awakened by it? Does it lead to anything else? Is it accompanied by other signs and symptoms? Does it ever occur before, during, or after meals? Does it occur seasonally?

From Crozer Keystone Center for Nursing Excellence: Best practices: PQRST method facilitates accurate pain assessment. Available at www.crozerkeystone.org/healthcare-professionals/nursing.

PAIN ASSESSMENT TOOLS

Pain is multidimensional in scope, encompassing physical, affective, and functional domains. Various tools have been developed to capture unidimensional aspects (i.e., intensity) or multidimensional components. Select the pain assessment tool based on its purpose, time involved in administration, and the patient's ability to comprehend and complete the tool.

First teach patients how to use each tool, with practice sessions to strengthen the validity and reliability of the response. Enlarge the print when appropriate for individuals with impaired vision. The printed language should be translated to the patient's native language. All words should be direct and free of medical jargon, at a 6th-grade reading level.

Ask the patient to rate and evaluate all of the pain sites. Some forms allow for only one number; therefore be sure to add to your documentation. Finally use the pain tool consistently before and after treatment to see if the treatment has been effective. Reassessment of pain following intervention, whether pharmacologic or nonpharmacologic, is essential to document pain trajectories alongside various treatments to achieve optimum pain control.

Standardized **overall pain assessment tools** are more useful for chronic pain conditions or particularly problematic acute pain problems. A few examples include the Initial Pain Assessment, the Brief Pain Inventory, and the McGill Pain Questionnaire.

The **Initial Pain Assessment**[26] asks the patient to answer 8 questions concerning location, duration, quality, intensity, and aggravating/relieving factors. Further, the clinician adds

questions about the manner of expressing pain and the effects of pain that impair one's quality of life (Fig. 10-4).

The **Brief Pain Inventory**[11] asks the patient to rate the pain within the past 24 hours using graduated scales (0 to 10) with respect to its impact on areas such as mood, walking ability, and sleep (Fig. 10-5). **The short-form McGill Pain**

Initial Pain Assessment Tool

Patient's Name_____ Age _____ Date_____
Diagnosis _____ Physician_____ Room _____
Nurse _____

1. LOCATION: Patient or nurse mark drawing.

2. INTENSITY: Patient rates the pain. Scale used _____
   Present:_____
   Worst pain gets:_____
   Best pain gets:_____
   Acceptable level of pain:_____

3. QUALITY: (Use patient's own words, e.g., prick, ache, burn, throb, pull, sharp.)_____

4. ONSET, DURATION, VARIATION, RHYTHMS:_____

5. MANNER OF EXPRESSING PAIN:_____

6. WHAT RELIEVES THE PAIN?_____

7. WHAT CAUSES OR INCREASES THE PAIN?_____

8. EFFECTS OF PAIN: (Note decreased function, decreased quality of life.)
   Accompanying symptoms (e.g., nausea) _____
   Sleep _____
   Appetite_____
   Physical activity_____
   Relationship with others (e.g., irritability)_____
   Emotions (e.g., anger, suicidal, crying)_____
   Concentration_____
   Other _____

9. OTHER COMMENTS:_____

10. PLAN:_____

10-4

Brief Pain Inventory

Date:____/____/____   Time:_____

Name:_____

        Last   First   Middle initial

1. Throughout our lives, most of us have had pain from time to time (such as minor headaches, sprains, and toothaches). Have you had pain other than these everyday kinds of pain today?
   1. Yes   2. No

2. On the diagram, shade in the areas where you feel pain. Put an X on the area that hurts the most.

Right   Left   Left   Right

3. Please rate your pain by circling the one number that best describes your pain at its **worst** in the past 24 hours.

   0   1   2   3   4   5   6   7   8   9   10
   No   Pain as bad as
   pain   you can imagine

4. Please rate your pain by circling the one number that best describes your pain at its **least** in the past 24 hours.

   0   1   2   3   4   5   6   7   8   9   10
   No   Pain as bad as
   pain   you can imagine

5. Please rate your pain by circling the one number that best describes your pain on the **average**.

   0   1   2   3   4   5   6   7   8   9   10
   No   Pain as bad as
   pain   you can imagine

6. Please rate your pain by circling the one number that tells how much pain you have **right now**.

   0   1   2   3   4   5   6   7   8   9   10
   No   Pain as bad as
   pain   you can imagine

7. What treatments or medications are you receiving for your pain?

   _____

   _____

8. In the past 24 hours, how much **relief** have pain treatments or medications provided? Please circle the one percentage that most shows how much relief you have received.

   0% 10 20 30 40 50 60 70 80 90 100%
   No   Complete
   relief   relief

9. Circle the one number that describes how, during the past 24 hours, pain has **interfered** with your:
   A: General activity

   0   1   2   3   4   5   6   7   8   9   10
   Does not   Completely
   interfere   interferes

   B: Mood

   0   1   2   3   4   5   6   7   8   9   10
   Does not   Completely
   interfere   interferes

   C: Walking ability

   0   1   2   3   4   5   6   7   8   9   10
   Does not   Completely
   interfere   interferes

   D: Normal work (includes both work outside the home and housework)

   0   1   2   3   4   5   6   7   8   9   10
   Does not   Completely
   interfere   interferes

   E: Relations with other people

   0   1   2   3   4   5   6   7   8   9   10
   Does not   Completely
   interfere   interferes

   F: Sleep

   0   1   2   3   4   5   6   7   8   9   10
   Does not   Completely
   interfere   interferes

   G: Enjoyment of life

   0   1   2   3   4   5   6   7   8   9   10
   Does not   Completely
   interfere   interferes

Subjective Data

10-5

Questionnaire[27] (not illustrated) asks the patient to rank a list of descriptors in terms of their intensity and to give an overall intensity rating to his or her pain.

Pain-rating scales are unidimensional and intended to reflect pain intensity. They come in various forms. They can indicate baseline intensity, track changes, and give some degree of evaluation to a treatment modality. **Numeric rating scales** ask the patient to choose a number that rates the level of pain for each painful site, with 0 being no pain and the highest anchor 10 indicating the worst pain ever experienced (Fig. 10-6). This makes recording of results easy and consistent with those of numerous clinicians. The **Verbal Descriptor Scale** uses words to describe the patient's feelings and the meaning of the pain for the person. The **Visual Analogue**

0-10 Numeric Pain Intensity Scale*

| 0 | 1 | 2 | 3 | 4 | 5 | 6 | 7 | 8 | 9 | 10 |
| No pain | | | | | Moderate pain | | | | | Unbearable pain |

Simple Descriptive Pain Intensity Scale*

| No pain | Mild pain | Moderate pain | Severe pain | Very severe pain | Worst possible pain |

Visual Analogue Scale (VAS)†

| No pain | | Pain as bad as it could possibly be |

* If used as a graphic rating scale, a 10-cm baseline is recommended.

† A 10-cm baseline is recommended for VAS scales.

10-6 (Acute Pain Management Guideline Panel, 1992.)

Scale lets the patient make a mark along a 10-cm horizontal line from "no pain" to "worst pain imaginable."

In general older adults find the numeric rating scale abstract and have difficulty responding, especially with a fluctuating chronic pain experience. An alternative is the simple **descriptor scale** that lists words that describe different levels of pain intensity such as *no pain, mild pain, moderate pain,* and *severe pain.* Older adults often respond to scales in which

words are selected. Again it is essential to teach the person how to use the scale to enhance accuracy.

Tools for Infants and Children

Because infants are preverbal and incapable of self-report, pain assessment depends on behavioral and physiologic cues. Refer to the Objective Data section. It is important to underscore the point that infants *do* feel pain.

Children 2 years of age can report pain and point to its location. They cannot rate pain intensity at this developmental level. It is helpful to ask the parent or caregiver what words the child uses to report pain (e.g., boo–boo, owie). Be aware that some children try to be "grown up and brave" and often deny having pain in the presence of a stranger or if they are fearful of receiving a "shot."

Rating scales can be introduced at 4 to 5 years of age. The Faces Pain Scale–Revised (FPS-R) has six drawings of faces that show pain intensity, from "no pain" on the left (score of 0) to "very much pain" on the right (score of 10) (Fig. 10-7). Numbers are not shown to children, but the number scoring makes this tool compatible with the widely used 0-to-10 metric for numeric pain scales.[16] This revised drawing has more realistic facial expressions, with a furrowed brow and horizontal mouth stretch to rate pain. It avoids smiles or tears so children will not confuse pain intensity with happiness or sadness.

Similarly the Oucher Scale[5] has six photographs of young boys' faces with different expressions of pain, ranked on a 0-to-5 scale of increasing intensity. The child is asked to point at the face that best matches his or her hurt/pain. You may use Oucher Scale variations for girls and diverse ethnic groups.

Faces Pain Scale — Revised (FPS-R)

In the following instructions, say "hurt" or "pain," whichever seems right for a particular child.

"These faces show how much something can hurt. This face [point to left-most face] **shows no pain. The faces show more and more pain** [point to each from left to right] **up to this one** [point to right-most face] **— it shows very much pain. Point to the face that shows how much you hurt** [right now]."

Score the chosen face 0, 2, 4, 6, 8, or 10, counting left to right, so '0' = 'no pain' and '10' = 'very much pain.' Do not use words like 'happy' and 'sad.' This scale is intended to measure how children feel inside, not how their face looks.

Permission for use. Copyright in the FPS-R is held by the International Association for the Study of Pain (IASP) © 2001. This material may be photocopied for non-commercial clinical and research use. To request permission from IASP to reproduce the FPS-R in a publication, or for any commercial use, please e-mail **iaspdesk@iasp-pain.org**. For all other information regarding the FPS-R contact **Tiina.Jaaniste@sesiahs.health.nsw.gov.au** (Pain Medicine Unit, Sydney Children's Hospital, Randwick, NSW 2031, Australia).

Sources. Hicks, C. L., von Baeyer, C. L., Spafford, P. van Korlaar, I., Goodenough, B. The Faces Pain Scale—Revised: toward a common metric in pediatric pain measurement. *Pain, 93,* 173-183. Bieri, D., Reeve, R., Champion, G. D. et al. The Faces Pain Scale for the self-assessment of the severity of pain experienced by children: development, initial validation and preliminary investigation for ratio scale properties. *Pain, 41,* 139-150.

10-7

OBJECTIVE DATA

PREPARATION

The physical examination process can help you understand the nature of the pain. Consider whether this is an acute or a chronic condition. Recall that physical findings may not always support the patient's pain reports, particularly for chronic pain syndromes. Based on the patient's pain report, make every effort to reduce or eliminate the pain with appropriate analgesic and nonpharmacologic intervention. According to the American Pain Society[2]:

> In cases in which the cause of acute pain is uncertain, establishing a diagnosis is a priority, but symptomatic treatment of pain should be given while the investigation is proceeding. With occasional exceptions (e.g., the initial examination of the patient with an acute condition of the abdomen), it is rarely justified to defer analgesia until a diagnosis is made. In fact, a comfortable patient is better able to cooperate with diagnostic procedures. (p. 3)

EQUIPMENT NEEDED

Tape measure to measure circumference of swollen joints or extremities
Tongue blade
Penlight

NORMAL RANGE OF FINDINGS

Joints

Note the size and contour of the joint. Measure the circumference of the involved joint for comparison with baseline. Check active or passive range of motion (see discussion of complete technique beginning on p. 590 in Chapter 22). Joint motion normally causes no tenderness, pain, or crepitation.

Observe posture; normally it is erect and relaxed.

Muscles and Skin

Inspect the skin and tissues for color, swelling, and any masses or deformity.

To assess for changes in sensation, ask the person to close his or her eyes. Test the person's ability to perceive sensation by breaking a tongue blade in two lengthwise. Lightly press the sharp and blunted ends on the skin in a random fashion and ask to identify it as sharp or dull (see Fig. 23-23). This test will help you identify location and extent of altered sensation.

Abdomen

Observe for contour and symmetry. Palpate for muscle guarding and organ size (see discussion of complete technique beginning on p. 555 in Chapter 21). Note any areas of referred pain (see Table 21-3).

ABNORMAL FINDINGS

Swelling, inflammation, injury, deformity, diminished range of motion, increased pain on palpation (crepitation is an audible and palpable crunching that accompanies movement)
Slumped posture or abdominal guarding with pain.

Bruising, lesions, open wounds, tissue damage, atrophy, bulging, change in hair distribution
Absent pain sensation (analgesia); increased pain sensation (hyperalgesia); or if a severe pain sensation is evoked with a stimulus that does not normally induce pain (e.g., the blunt end of the tongue blade, cotton ball, clothing) (allodynia)

Swelling, bulging, herniation, inflammation, organ enlargement

Objective Data

TABLE 10-2   Physiologic Changes from Poorly Controlled Pain

Pain is not a benign symptom. Poorly controlled acute and chronic pain have a negative impact on physiologic systems.

PHYSIOLOGIC SYSTEM	ACUTE PAIN RESPONSES
Cardiac	Tachycardia Elevated blood pressure Increased myocardial oxygen demand Increased cardiac output
Pulmonary	Hypoventilation Hypoxia Decreased cough Atelectasis
Gastrointestinal	Nausea Vomiting Ileus
Renal	Oliguria Urinary retention
Musculoskeletal	Spasm Joint stiffness
Endocrine	Increased adrenergic activity
Central nervous system	Fear Anxiety Fatigue
Immune	Impaired cellular immunity Impaired wound healing
Poorly controlled chronic pain	Depression Isolation Limited mobility and function Confusion Family distress Diminished quality of life

Table 10-2 lists physiologic changes resulting from poorly controlled pain. Be aware that tachycardia and tachypnea also occur with anxiety and fear and are not specific to pain.[10]

NONVERBAL BEHAVIORS OF PAIN

When the individual cannot verbally communicate the pain, you can (to a limited extent) identify it using behavioral cues. Recall that individuals react to painful stimuli with a wide variety of behaviors. Behaviors are influenced by a wide variety of factors, including the nature of the pain (acute versus chronic), age, and cultural and gender expectations.

Acute Pain Behaviors

Because acute pain involves autonomic responses and has a protective purpose, individuals experiencing moderate-to-intense levels of pain *may* exhibit the following behaviors: guarding, grimacing, vocalizations such as moaning, agitation, restlessness, stillness, diaphoresis, or change in vital signs. This list of behaviors is not exhaustive because they should not be used exclusively to deny or confirm the presence of pain. For example, in a postoperative patient pulse and blood pressure can be altered by fluid volume, medications, and blood loss.

Persistent (Chronic) Pain Behaviors

People with persistent pain live with the experience for months and years. One cannot function physiologically and go on with life in a repetitive state of behaviors such as grimacing, diaphoresis, and guarding. The person adapts over time, and clinicians cannot look for or anticipate the same acute pain behaviors to exist to confirm a pain diagnosis.

Chronic pain behaviors have even more variability than acute pain behaviors. People with chronic pain typically try to give little indication that they are in pain and therefore are at higher risk for underdetection (Fig. 10-8). Behaviors that have been associated with chronic pain include bracing, rubbing, diminished activity, sighing, and change in appetite. Whenever possible, it is best to ask the person how he or she acts or behaves when in pain. Chronic pain behaviors such as spending time with other people, movement, exercise, prayer, sleeping, or inactivity underscore the more subtle, less anticipated ways in which people behave when they are experiencing chronic pain (e.g., they use sleeping to self-distract). Unfortunately clinical staff may inadvertently interpret this behavior as "comfort" and fail to follow up with an appropriate pharmacologic intervention.

10-8   (From Rick Brady, Riva, MD.)

CRIES Neonatal Postoperative Pain Measurement Score

	0	1	2
Crying	No	High-pitched	Inconsolable
Requires O₂ for sat >95%	No	<30% from baseline	>30% from baseline
Increased vital signs	HR and BP = or < preop	HR or BP ↑ <20% of preop	HR or BP ↑ >20% of preop
Expression	None	Grimace	Grimace/grunt
Sleepless	No, continuously asleep	Wakes at frequent intervals	Constantly awake

10-9   (Krechel, 1995.)

❖ DEVELOPMENTAL COMPETENCE

Infants

Most pain research on infants has focused on acute procedural pain. We have a limited understanding of how to assess chronic pain in the infant. At this time no one assessment tool adequately identifies pain in the infant. Using a multidimensional approach for the whole infant is encouraged. Changes in facial activity and body movements may help. Much effort and time is spent on decoding facial expressions (e.g., taut tongue, bulging brow, closing of eye fissures), which may be difficult for the general practitioner to carry out in a busy clinical setting.

The CRIES score is one tool for postoperative pain in preterm and term neonates.[21] It measures physiologic and behavioral indicators on a three-point scale (Fig. 10-9).

A second tool often used is the FLACC scale.[28] This is a nonverbal assessment tool for infants and young children under 3 years. The FLACC scale is designed to be simple for practitioners to administer while providing a reliable and objective assessment of pain in young children. The tool assesses five behaviors of pain: facial expression, leg movement, activity level, cry, and consolability (Fig 10-10). You can summarize the scores as: 0 = relaxed and comfortable; 1-3 = mild discomfort; 4-6 = moderate pain; 7-10 = severe discomfort/pain.[33]

Because the sympathetic nervous system is engaged particularly in acute episodes of pain, physiologic changes take place that may indicate the presence of pain. These include sweating, increases in blood pressure and heart rate, vomiting, nausea, and changes in oxygen saturation. However, as in the adult, these physiologic changes cannot be used

Objective Data

	DATE/TIME					
Face 0 - No particular expression or smile 1 - Occasional grimace or frown, withdrawn, disinterested 2 - Frequent to constant quivering chin, clenched jaw						
Legs 0 - Normal position or relaxed 1 - Uneasy, restless, tense 2 - Kicking, or legs drawn up						
Activity 0 - Lying quietly, normal position, moves easily 1 - Squirming, shifting back and forth, tense 2 - Arched, rigid, or jerking						
Cry 0 - No cry (awake or asleep) 1 - Moans or whimpers; occasional complaint 2 - Crying steadily, screams or sobs, frequent complaints						
Consolability 0 - Content, relaxed 1 - Reassured by occasional touching, hugging or being talked to, distractible 2 - Difficult to console or comfort						
TOTAL SCORE						

10-10   FLACC Behavioral Pain Scale.   (Voepel-Lewis, 2010.)

exclusively to confirm or deny pain because of other factors such as stress, medications, and fluid changes.

Note that these measures target acute pain. No biological markers have been identified for long-term chronic pain in infants or children. Therefore evaluate the whole individual. Look for changes in temperament, expression, and activity. If a procedure or disease process is known to induce pain in adults (e.g., circumcision, surgery, sickle cell disease, cancer), it *will* induce pain in the infant or child.

The Aging Adult

Although pain should not be considered a "normal" part of aging, it is prevalent. When an older adult reports a history of conditions such as osteoarthritis, peripheral vascular disease, cancer, osteoporosis, angina, or chronic constipation, be alert and anticipate a pain problem. Older adults often deny having pain for fear of dependency, further testing or invasive procedures, cost, and fear of taking pain killers or becoming a drug addict. During the interview you must establish an empathic and caring rapport to gain trust.

When you look for behavioral cues, look at changes in functional status. Observe for changes in dressing, walking, toileting, or involvement in activities. A slowness and rigidity may develop, and fatigue may occur. Look for a sudden onset of acute confusion, which may indicate poorly controlled pain. However, you will need to rule out other competing explanations such as infection or adverse reaction from medications.

People with dementia become less able to identify and describe pain over time, although pain is still present and destructive. They communicate pain through their behavior. Agitation, pacing, and repetitive yelling may indicate pain and not a worsening of the dementia. People who are comfortable do not yell, cry, moan, hit, or kick. When these behaviors occur, consider pain as a primary explanation.

When asked whether they are having pain, people with dementia may say "no" when in fact they are very uncomfortable. Words have lost their meaning. Use the PAINAD scale (Fig. 10-11), which evaluates five common behaviors: breathing, vocalization, facial expression, body language, and consolability.[39] Specific behaviors in these categories are quantified from 0 to 2, with a total score ranging from 0 to 10. This is consistent with the commonly used 0-to-10 metric on other pain tool scores. For the PAINAD a score of 4 or more indicates a need for pain management.

Pain Assessment In Advanced Dementia (PAINAD) Scale

	0	1	2	Score
Breathing Independent of Vocalization	Normal	Occasional labored breathing, short period of hyperventilation	Noisy labored breathing, long period of hyperventilation, Cheyne-Stokes respirations	
Negative Vocalization	None	Occasional moan or groan, low level of speech with a negative or disapproving quality	Repeated troubled calling out, loud moaning or groaning, crying	
Facial Expression	Smiling or inexpressive	Sad, frightened, frown	Facial grimacing	
Body Language	Relaxed	Tense, distressed pacing, fidgeting	Rigid, fists clenched, knees pulled up, pulling or pushing away, striking out	
Consolability	No need to console	Distracted or reassured by voice or touch	Unable to console, distract, or reassure	
			TOTAL	

10-11 A score of 4 or greater should be reported to the RN for pain intervention. (Warden, 2003.)

DOCUMENTATION AND CRITICAL THINKING

Sample Charting

SUBJECTIVE

Starting within the past 2 weeks, states having severe epigastric pain within a half-hour of eating greasy, fatty foods. Pain is stabbing and squeezing in nature with radiation to right shoulder blade. Rates pain as a 10 on a 0-to-10 scale. Nausea accompanies pain. Takes antacids with minimal relief. Pain diminishes after bringing knees to chest and "not moving" for a 1-hour period.

OBJECTIVE

Patient diaphoretic, grimacing, and having difficulty concentrating. Breathless during history. Arms guarding upper abdominal area. Abdomen distended. Severe tenderness noted on light LUQ and epigastric palpation. Bowel sounds hyperactive in all 4 quadrants.

ASSESSMENT

Acute episodic pain

Clinical Case Study 1

J.T. is an 18-year-old African-American male living with sickle cell anemia. Admitted to the ED by his parents following 4 hours of increasing pain at home.

SUBJECTIVE

Within the past 48 hours J.T. reports increasing pain in upper- and lower-extremity joints and swelling of right knee. States having "stomach flu" 1 week before with periods of vomiting and diarrhea. Pain is aching and constant in nature. Rates pain as +10 on a 0-to-10 scale. Reports difficulty walking and climbing stairs. Taking acetaminophen, two tablets every 4 hours, and using ice packs with no relief. States, "I have had these before. I always need Dilaudid."

OBJECTIVE

Temp 98.6° F (37° C) oral. BP 118/68 mm Hg. Pulse 112 bpm. Resp 24/min.
Facial grimacing and moaning.
Requiring assistance to sit on exam table. Unable to bear weight on right leg. Affect flat; clenches jaw during position changes. Tenderness localized in elbow, wrist, finger, and knee joints. Diminished ROM in wrists and knees (right knee 36 cm, left knee 30 cm circumference). Right knee warm and boggy to touch.
Lungs: Clear to auscultation and percussion.
Heart: S_1 and S_2 not diminished or accentuated; no murmur.
Abdomen: Bowel sounds present, guarding with tenderness to palpation, RUQ pain with enlarged spleen at anterior axillary line.
Lab: Hb 9 g/dL. Hct 30%. Indices show sickling with RBCs of varying shapes.
Metabolic panel: Serum bilirubin 2 mg/dL, rest in normal limits.

ASSESSMENT

Acute pain
Risk for venous or arterial thromboembolism
Anemia R/T sickle cell crisis
Fear R/T outcome of acute pain episode

Clinical Case Study 2

H.S. is a 78-year-old Irish-American female with a 10-year history of osteoarthritis. Comes to routine checkup today with, "feeling pain in right knee now, and pain pills not working."

SUBJECTIVE

H.S. reports increased pain and stiffness in her neck, lower back, and right knee for the past month. Denies radiation of pain. Denies tingling or numbness in upper or lower extremities.

Having difficulty getting in and out of bathtub and dressing herself. Describes pain as aching, with good and bad days. Becomes frustrated when asked to rate her pain intensity. Replies, "I don't know what number to give; it hurts a lot, on and off." Takes acetaminophen, extra strength, two tablets, when the pain "really gets the best of me," with some degree of relief. Does not take part in "field trips" offered by assisted-living facility because she "hurts too much." Does not use cane or walker. No physical therapy.

OBJECTIVE

Localized tenderness noted on palpation to C3 and C4; unable to flex neck to chest. Crepitus noted in both shoulder joints. No swelling noted. Muscle strength 1+ and equal for upper extremities. Lumbar area tender to moderate palpation. Rubs lower back frequently; limited flexion at the waist. Right knee swollen with circumference 2 cm > left knee but no redness or warmth. Left knee not enlarged, and normal ROM. Gait slow and unsteady. Facial expression stoic.

ASSESSMENT

Chronic pain that is now increased in intensity
Decreased ROM in neck, shoulders, back, R knee
Decreased quality of life R/T lack of mobility and pain

Clinical Case Study 3

T.H. is a 7-year-old boy who has just experienced a laparoscopic appendectomy. On entering the room you see that he is awake but with his eyes closed and lying flat on the bed without movement.

SUBJECTIVE

When asked if he is in pain, T.H. states "a little"; however, he rates pain as a +8 using a Faces Pain Scale.

OBJECTIVE

Requires assistance to move in the bed. Speaks only when spoken to.
Vital signs: Temp 98.6°F (37°C) (oral). BP: 122/72 mm Hg (supine). Pulse 126 bpm (while quiet but awake). Resp 22/min.
General appearance: Diaphoretic, flushed, grimaces with slight touch.
Cardiovascular: Tachycardic at rest; no abnormal heart sounds.
Respiratory: Tachypneic at rest; pulse ox 98% on room air; breath sounds clear in all fields, no adventitious sounds.
ABD: Hypoactive bowel sounds, tenderness localized to abdomen, dressing dry and intact at surgical site.

ASSESSMENT

Acute pain R/T surgery

Clinical Case Study 4

J.Y. is a 53-year-old Caucasian male who fell approximately 10 feet from a ladder. Landed in a "funny" sitting position and is now experiencing severe back pain. Imaging studies in ED show herniated lumbar disk.

SUBJECTIVE

J.Y. reports pain rated at 10/10. Pain is sharp, constant, and shoots down left leg. Reports bilateral leg weakness.

OBJECTIVE

J.Y. required assistance to sit on exam table. Clenches jaw with position changes. Supports lower back with hands. Significant tenderness of lumbar spine. Unable to perform hip flexion/extension or spinal ROM because of pain.

ASSESSMENT

Herniated lumbar disk
Acute pain
Impaired physical mobility R/T pain and weakness

ABNORMAL FINDINGS

TABLE 10-3   Summary of Pain Types

Types of Pain	Etiology	Pain Descriptors	Associated Disorders	Treatment Options
Nociceptive (somatic or visceral)	Activity of nociceptors in cutaneous and deep musculoskeletal tissue in response to tissue-damaging stimuli Inflammation	**Somatic:** Dull Aching Well-localized Nocturnal **Visceral:** Deep, squeezing pressure Local tenderness and referred Poorly localized	**Somatic:** Postoperative pain Bone metastases Arthritis Sports injury Mechanical back pain **Visceral:** Liver metastases Pancreatic cancer	Treat the underlying cause Nonsteroidal anti-inflammatory drug (NSAID) Opioid Muscle relaxant Corticosteroid Bisphosphonate
Neuropathic	Primary lesion (neuroma) or dysfunction in nervous system causing ectopic charges within the nervous system	Constant dull ache Burning Stabbing Vicelike Electric shocklike Numbness Tingling Allodynia Hyperalgesia Hyperpathia	Distal polyneuropathy (diabetes, HIV) Central poststroke pain Herpes zoster Trigeminal neuralgia Neuropathic back pain Complex regional pain syndrome	Tricyclic antidepressant (TCA) Anticonvulsant Antidepressant Antineuroleptic Local anesthetic Bisphosphonate Corticosteroid Opioid Interventional techniques
Cancer pain	Infiltration of lesion Nerve injury from periphery or central nervous system	Dependent on underlying pathology	Bone metastases neuropathy	Symptom control—any of the above

Data from Miller-Saultz, D. (2008). Identifying chronic pain: awareness important. *Nurse Pract*, 33(9), 7.

TABLE 10-4   Peripheral Neuropathy

Peripheral neuropathy (PN) is symmetric damage to peripheral nerves (feet or hands) resulting in pain without stimulation of the nerves. This is a common neuropathic pain characterized by numbness and tingling, with interspersed shooting or lancinating pain that is not attributed to a specific nociceptive source.[14] Diabetic neuropathy is a common complication of diabetes and may relate to demyelination of the larger peripheral nerves, with an increase in smaller myelinated nerves. Other etiologies may include ischemic damage to nerves or hyperglycemia, causing changes in nerve microenvironment.[9] Patients experience burning pain in feet bilaterally, which is often worse at night.

Chemotherapy-induced PN (CIPN) occurs after chemotherapy treatment for cancer. The risk increases with the number of agents used in the course of treatment, higher cumulative doses of neurotoxic agents, preexisting neuropathy from diabetes or other causes, and older age.[12,14] A symptom is numbness or burning, shooting pain in a glove-and-stocking distribution. NOTE: With any cancer survivor, you must address new onset of pain promptly to rule out pathologic recurrence of the cancer because this is what survivors most fear.[12]

TABLE 10-5   Reflexive Sympathetic Dystrophy

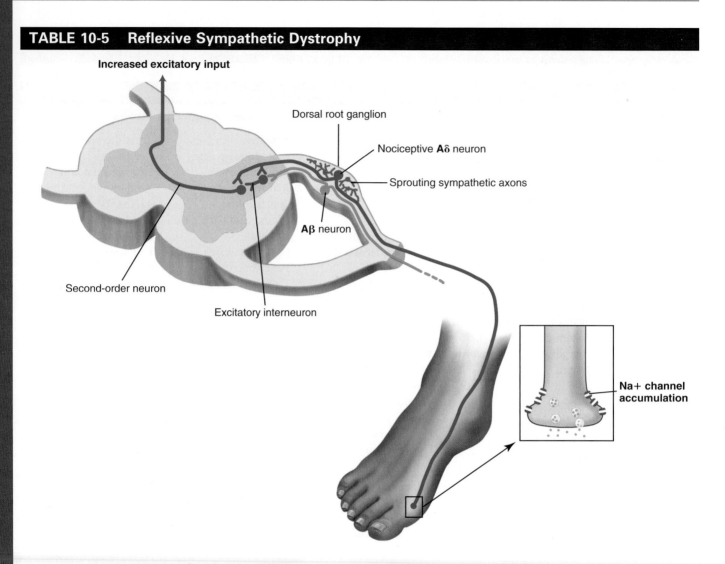

Increased excitatory input

Dorsal root ganglion

Nociceptive **Aδ** neuron

Sprouting sympathetic axons

Aβ neuron

Second-order neuron

Excitatory interneuron

Na+ channel accumulation

Complex Regional Pain Syndrome (CRPS) or Reflexive Sympathetic Dystrophy (RSD)

RSD/CRPS is a chronic progressive nerve condition, characterized by burning pain, swelling, stiffness, and discoloration of the affected extremity. It affects both men and women, usually around 40 to 60 years old, and occurs weeks to months after a nerve injury (e.g., carpal tunnel syndrome, broken leg, cerebral lesions). Pathophysiology involves a complex interaction of sensory, motor, and autonomic nerves and the immune system. The nerve injury may modify the usual pain pathway, causing a neuropathic "wind-up" or "short-circuit" mechanism.

A key feature is that a typically innocuous stimulus (e.g., a light brush of a cotton ball or clothing) can create a severe, intense painful response. Other subjective data include burning pain often disproportionate to the degree of injury and joint pain during movement. Objective data include swelling, disappearance of skin wrinkles, cool skin temperature, discoloration, brittle nails, and finally atrophic changes (pale, dry, shiny skin and muscle atrophy). Treatment includes high doses of drugs (e.g., prednisone, amitriptyline, pregabalin, clonidine) to decrease symptoms and physical therapy to regain limb function.

Image © Pat Thomas, 2010.

BIBLIOGRAPHY

1. American Geriatrics Society. (2009). Pharmacological management of persistent pain in older persons. *J Am Geriatr Soc*, 57(8), 1331-1346.

2. American Pain Society (APS). (2009). *Principles of analgesic use in the treatment of acute and cancer pain*. (6th ed.). Glenview, IL: American Pain Society.

3. Anderson, K. O., Green, C. R., & Payne, R. (2009). Racial and ethnic disparities in pain: causes and consequences of unequal care. *J Pain*, 10(12), 1187-1204.

4. Apkarian, A. V., Hashmi, J. A., & Baliki, M. N. (2011). Pain and the brain: specificity and plasticity of the brain in clinical chronic pain. *Pain*, 152(3 Suppl), S49-S64.

5. Beyer, J. E. (1983). *The Oucher: a user's manual and technical report*. Evanston, IL: Judson.

6. Bhui, K., & Dinos, S. (2008). Health beliefs and culture: essential considerations for outcome management. *Dis Manage Health Outcomes*, 16(6), 411-419.

7. Cervero, F. (2009). Pain: friend or foe? A neurobiologic perspective—the 2008 Bonica Award lecture. *Reg Anesth Pain Med*, 34(6), 569-574.

8. City of Hope Pain & Palliative Care Resource Center. *Pain assessment tools*. Available at http://prc.coh.org/pain assessment.

9. Copstead, L., & Banasik, J. (2013). *Pathophysiology*. (5th ed.). St. Louis: Elsevier.

10. D'Arcy, Y. (2012). Treating acute pain in the hospitalized patient. *Nurse Pract*, 37(8):23-30.

11. Daut, R. L., & Cleeland, C. S. (1982). The prevalence and severity of pain in cancer. *Cancer*, 50, 1913-1918.

12. Davies, P. S. (2013). Chronic pain management in the cancer survivor. *Nurse Pract*, 38(6):28-38.

13. Fillingim, R. B., King, C. D., Ribeiro-Dasilva, M. C., et al. (2009). Sex, gender, and pain: a review of recent clinical and experimental findings. *J Pain*, 10(5), 447-485.

14. Hannersla, M., & Kapustin, J. F. (2012). Peripheral neuropathy: evidence-based treatment of a complex disorder. *Nurse Pract*, 37(5):33-39.

15. Herr, K., Bursch, H., Ersek, M., et al. (2010). Use of pain-behavioral assessment tools in the nursing home: expert consensus recommendations for practice. *J Gerontol Nurs*, 36(3), 18-29.

16. Hicks, C. L., von Baeyer, C. L., Spafford, P., et al. (2001). The Faces Pain Scale—revised: toward a common metric in pediatric pain measurement. *Pain*, 93, 173-183.

17. Horgas, A., Elliott, A., & Marsiske, M. (2009). Pain assessment in persons with dementia: relationship between self-report and behavioral observation. *J Am Geriatr Soc*, 57(1), 126-132.

18. International Association for Hospice and palliative care. Available at www.hospicecare.com/resources/pain-research.htm.

19. International Association for the Study of Pain (IASP). Available at http://www.iasp-pain.org/Content/NavigationMenu/GeneralResourceLinks/PainDefinitions/default.htm#Neuropathicpain.

20. Jablonski, A. M., DuPen, A. R., & Ersek, M. (2011). The use of algorithms in assessing and managing persistent pain in older adults. *Am J Nurs* 111(3), 34-45.

21. Krechel, S. W., & Bildner, J. (1995). CRIES: a new neonatal postoperative pain measurement score—initial testing of validity and reliability. *Paediatr Anaesth*, 5(1), 53-61.

22. Knaepen, L., Patijn, J., van Kleef, M. et al. (2013). Neonatal repetitive needle pricking: plasticity of the spinal nociceptive circuit and extended postoperative pain in later life. *Dev Neurobiol*, 73(1), 85-97.

23. Lee, M. C., & Tracey, I. (2010). Unraveling the mystery of pain, suffering, and relief with brain imaging. *Curr Pain Headache Rep*, 14(2), 124-131.

24. Lowery, C. L., Hardman, M. P., Manning, N., et al. (2007). Neurodevelopmental changes of fetal pain. *Semin Perinatol*, 31, 275-282.

25. Mackey, S. C. (2013). Central neuroimaging of pain. *J Pain*, 14(4), 328-331.

26. McCaffery, M., & Pasero, C. (1999). *Pain: clinical manual* (2nd ed.). St. Louis: Mosby.

27. Melzack, R. (1987). The short-form McGill Pain Questionnaire. *Pain*, 30, 191-197.

28. Merkel, S. I., Voepel-Lewis, T., Shayevitz, J. R., et al. (1997). The FLACC: a behavioral scale for scoring postoperative pain in young children. *Pediatr Nurs*, 23, 293-297.

29. Mogil, J. S. (2012). Pain genetics: past, present and future. *Trends Genet*, 28(6), 258-266.

30. Narayan, M.C. (2010). Culture's effects on pain assessment and management. *Am J Nurs*, 110(4), 38-47.

31. National Institute of Health Pain Consortium. Available at http://painconsortium.nih.gov/pain_scales/index.html.

32. Passero, C., & McCaffery, M. (2010). *Pain assessment and pharmacologic management*. St. Louis: Mosby.

33. Powell, R. A., Downing, J., Ddungu, H., et al. (2010). Pain history and pain assessment. In *Guide to pain management in low resource settings*. Seattle: IASP.

34. Quinlan-Colwell, A. (2012). *Compact clinical guide to geriatric pain management: an evidence-based approach for nurses*. New York: Springer Publishing.

35. Spencer, C., & Burke, P. (2011). The impact of culture on pain management. *Acad Med Surg Nurses*, 20(4), 12-15.

36. Todd, A. J. (2010). Neuronal circuitry for pain processing in the dorsal horn. *Nature Rev Neurosci*, 11(12), 823-826.

37. Voepel-Lewis, T., Zanotti, J., Dammeyer, J. A., et al. (2010). Reliability and validity of the face, legs, activity, cry, consolability behavioral tool in assessing acute pain in critically ill patients. *Am J Crit Care Nurses*, 19(1), 55-61.

38. Wager, T. D., Atlas, L. Y., Lindquist, M. A., et al. (2013). An fMRI-based neurologic signature of physical pain. *N Engl J Med*, 368(15), 1388-1397.

39. Warden, V., Hurley, A. C., & Volicer, L. (2003). Development and psychometric evaluation of the Pain Assessment in Advanced Dementia (PAINAD) scale. *J Am Med Dir Assoc*, 4(1), 9-15.

CHAPTER 11

Nutritional Assessment

STRUCTURE AND FUNCTION

11-1   (© Cavan Images.)

DEFINING NUTRITIONAL STATUS

Nutritional status is the balance between nutrient intake and nutrient requirements. This balance is affected by physiologic, psychosocial, developmental, cultural, and economic factors.

Optimal nutritional status is achieved when sufficient nutrients are consumed to support day-to-day body needs and any increased metabolic demands caused by growth, pregnancy, or illness (Fig. 11-1). People having optimal nutritional status are more active, have fewer physical illnesses, and live longer than people who are malnourished.

Undernutrition occurs when nutritional reserves are depleted and/or when nutrient intake is inadequate to meet day-to-day needs or added metabolic demands. Vulnerable groups (i.e., infants, children, pregnant women, recent immigrants, people with low incomes, hospitalized people, and aging adults) are at risk for impaired growth and development, lowered resistance to infection and disease, delayed wound healing, longer hospital stays, and higher health care costs.

Overnutrition is caused by the consumption of nutrients, especially calories, sodium, and fat, in excess of body needs. A major nutritional problem today, overnutrition can lead to obesity and is a risk factor for heart disease, type 2 diabetes, hypertension, stroke, gallbladder disease, sleep apnea, certain cancers, and osteoarthritis.[24]

An estimated one third of children and adolescents (ages 2 to 19 years) in the United States are overweight or obese,

and nearly one sixth (17%) are obese. Approximately two thirds of adults in the United States are either overweight or obese, and more than one third are obese.[5,10,27] For children overweight is a body mass index (BMI) at or above the 85th percentile based on age- and gender-specific BMI charts, and obesity is a BMI equal to or greater than the 95th percentile. For adults overweight is a BMI of 25 or greater, and obesity is a BMI of 30 or greater.[5] Although obesity rates in both children and adults seem to be leveling off after several years of increases, these data are alarming. Being overweight during childhood and adolescence is associated with an increased risk for becoming overweight during adulthood.[24]

If childhood overweight or obesity continues until adulthood, there is an increased risk for type 2 diabetes, hypertension, dyslipidemia, and carotid artery atherosclerosis.[17] However, if these children become nonobese by adulthood, these disease risks are similar to those who were never obese. Thus it behooves nurses and other health care professionals to implement childhood obesity interventions.

❖ DEVELOPMENTAL COMPETENCE

Infants and Children

The time from birth to 4 months of age is the most rapid period of growth in the life cycle. Although infants lose weight during the first few days of life, they usually regain birth weight by the 7th to 10th day after birth. Thereafter infants double their birth weight by 4 months and triple it by 1 year of age.

Breastfeeding is recommended for full-term infants for the first year of life because breast milk is ideally formulated to promote normal infant growth and development and natural immunity. Other advantages of breastfeeding are (1) fewer food allergies and intolerances, (2) reduced likelihood of overfeeding, (3) less cost than commercial infant formulas, and (4) increased mother-infant interaction time. Because cow's milk may cause gastrointestinal (GI) and kidney problems and is a poor source of iron and vitamins C and E, it is not recommended for infants until 1 year of age.

Infants increase their length by 50% during the first year of life and double it by 4 years of age. Brain size also increases very rapidly during infancy and childhood. By 2 years of age the brain has reached 50% of its adult size; by age 4, 75%; and by age 8, 100%. For this reason infants and children younger than 2 years should not drink skim or low-fat milk

181

Structure and Function

or be placed on low-fat diets; fat (calories and essential fatty acids) is required for proper growth and central nervous system development.

Adolescence

After a period of slow growth in late childhood, adolescence presents rapid physical growth and endocrine and hormonal changes. Caloric and protein requirements increase to meet this demand, and because of bone growth and increasing muscle mass (and in girls the onset of menarche), calcium and iron requirements also increase. Typically these increased requirements cannot be met by three meals per day; therefore nutritious snacks play an important role. Consider the following factors when working with adolescents to select healthier food choices: skipped meals, excessive fast food and sweetened beverage consumption, limited fruit and vegetable intake, peer pressure, alternative dietary patterns, eating disorders, hectic schedules, and possible experimentation with drugs and alcohol. New research shows that one of these factors, drinking sugar-sweetened beverages, interacts with the genes that affect weight and increases a person's risk of obesity beyond what heredity alone would have done.[29]

In general boys grow taller and have less body fat than girls. The percentage of body fat increases in females to about 25% and decreases in males (replaced by muscle mass) to about 12%. Typically girls double their body weight between the ages of 8 and 14 years; boys double their body weight between the ages of 10 and 17 years.

Childhood has been the most active period in the lifespan, with levels of physical activity decreasing in following decades. However, evidence shows that 32.5% of U.S. high school students watch television ≥3 hours per day on an average school day.[17a] More alarming is the surge in the number of students (41.3%) who play video or computer games for ≥3 hours per day on a school day. In addition, only 47.3% of students had been physically active in a heart rate–increasing activity for 60 minutes for 5 out of 7 days before the survey.[17a]

This inactivity contributes to development of overweight and obesity. The health-related outcomes of childhood and adolescent obesity include high blood pressure (BP), dyslipidemia, metabolic syndrome, type 2 diabetes, orthopedic problems, sleep apnea, asthma, and fatty liver disease.[28] Of further concern are the psychosocial and behavioral outcomes related to obesity: problems with body image and self-esteem, social isolation and discrimination, depression, and decreased quality of life.[28]

Pregnancy and Lactation

To support the synthesis of maternal and fetal tissues, sufficient calories, protein, vitamins, and minerals must be consumed during pregnancy. In particular, iron, folate, and zinc are essential for fetal growth, and vitamin and mineral supplements are often required. The National Academy of Sciences (NAS) recommends a weight gain of 25 to 35 lbs during pregnancy for women of normal weight, 28 to 40 lbs for

underweight women, 15 to 25 lbs for overweight women, and 11 to 20 lbs for obese women, a new weight gain category.

Adulthood

During adulthood growth and nutrient needs stabilize (Fig. 11-2). Most adults are in relatively good health. However, lifestyle factors such as cigarette smoking; stress; lack of exercise; excessive alcohol intake; and diets high in saturated fat, cholesterol, salt, and sugar and low in fiber can be factors in the development of hypertension, obesity, atherosclerosis, cancer, osteoporosis, and diabetes mellitus. Therefore the adult years are an important time for education to preserve health and prevent or delay the onset of chronic disease.

These lifestyle factors contribute toward obesity, which is a cardinal sign in the adult emergence of **metabolic syndrome.** This syndrome carries increased cardiac risk and is diagnosed when a person has 3 of the following 5 biomarkers: elevated BP, increased fasting plasma glucose, elevated triglycerides, increased waist circumference, and low high-density lipoprotein (HDL) cholesterol (see exact parameters in Table 11-5 on p. 197). The Framingham Offspring Study evidence showed that the combination of high BP, increased waist circumference, and hyperglycemia have the greatest risk for cardiac disease and death.[12]

The Aging Adult

Older adults have increased risk for undernutrition or overnutrition. Poor physical or mental health, social isolation, alcoholism, limited functional ability, poverty, and polypharmacy are the major risk factors for malnutrition in older adults.[20]

Normal physiologic changes in aging adults that directly affect nutritional status include poor dentition, decreased visual acuity, decreased saliva production, slowed GI motility, decreased GI absorption, and diminished olfactory and taste sensitivity. Important nutritional features of the older years are a decrease in energy requirements caused by loss of lean body mass (the most metabolically active tissue) and an increase in fat mass. Because protein and vitamin and mineral

11-2   (Agricultural Research Service, 2012.)

needs remain the same or increase (e.g., vitamin D and calcium), nutrient-dense food choices (e.g., milk, eggs, cheese, and peanut butter) are important to offset lower energy/calorie needs.

Socioeconomic conditions frequently affect the nutritional status of the aging adult. The decline of extended families and increased mobility of families reduce available support systems. Facilities for meal preparation and eating, transportation to grocery stores, physical limitations, reduced income, and social isolation are frequent problems that interfere with acquiring a balanced diet. Medications must also be considered because aging adults frequently take multiple medications that have a potential for interaction with nutrients and with one another.

The age-related loss of muscle mass is termed **sarcopenia.** It is **sarcopenic obesity** when combined with an increase in body fat. It is attributed to a decrease in physical activity and a decreased protein intake with aging.[3] Sarcopenic obesity results in a loss of muscle strength and function, decreased quality of life, physical frailty, and increased mortality rates.[3] Aerobic exercise plays its part for cardiac fitness, but resistance training is needed to treat weakened muscles. A resistance training program uses free weights, machines, or elastic bands; two to three sessions per week are recommended. Obviously financial resources and access to safe exercise gyms are factors in meeting this need.

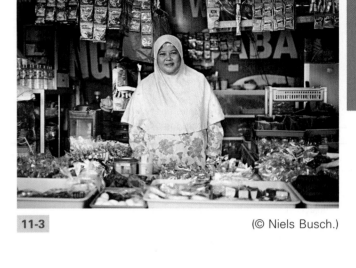

11-3 (© Niels Busch.)

CULTURE AND GENETICS

Because foods and eating customs are culturally distinct, each person has a unique cultural heritage that may affect nutritional status. Immigrants commonly maintain traditional eating customs long after the language and manner of dress of an adopted country become routine (especially for holidays and observance of religious customs) (Fig. 11-3). Occupation, class, religion, gender, and health awareness also have a great bearing on eating customs. Within the past decade, hundreds of thousands of individuals from Mexico, the Caribbean, Central and South America, Asia, Africa, and the Middle East have immigrated to the United States. Their food habits not only change to accommodate their new cultures but also influence their adoptive country. The popularity of tortillas, salsa, plantains, tofu, pita bread, hummus, and curry are examples of these influences on American eating habits.

Newly arriving immigrants may be at nutritional risk because they frequently come from countries with limited food supplies resulting from poverty, poor sanitation, war, or political strife. General undernutrition, hypertension, diarrhea, lactose intolerance, osteomalacia (soft bones), scurvy, and dental caries are among the more common nutrition-related problems of new immigrants from developing countries.

When immigrants arrive in the United States, other factors such as unfamiliar foods, food storage, food preparation, and food-buying habits contribute to their nutritional problems.

Foods from the native country are difficult to obtain, and low income limits the access to familiar foods. When traditional food habits are disrupted by a new culture, borderline deficiencies or adverse nutritional consequences may result. As an example, Latino immigrants to the United States have an increased risk of becoming overweight and obese as they adapt to a diet in the United States that is higher in saturated fats and calories.[24]

The cultural factors to consider are the cultural definition of food, frequency and number of meals eaten away from home, form and content of ceremonial meals, amount and types of foods eaten, and regularity of food consumption. The 24-hour dietary recalls or 3-day food records used traditionally for assessment may be inadequate when dealing with people from culturally diverse backgrounds. Standard dietary handbooks may not provide culture-specific diet information because nutritional content and exchange tables are generally based on Western diets. Another source of error may be cultural patterns of eating. For example, some ethnic groups eat sparingly or moderately during the week (i.e., simple rice or bean dishes), whereas weekend meals are markedly more elaborate (i.e., meats, fruits, vegetables, and sweets are added).

Dietary Practices of Selected Cultural Groups

Cultural food preferences are often interrelated with religious dietary beliefs and practices. Many religions use foods as symbols in celebrations and rituals. Knowing the person's religious practices related to food enables you to suggest improvements or modifications that do not conflict with dietary laws. Table 11-1 summarizes dietary practices for selected religious groups.

Other issues are fasting and other religious observations that may limit a person's food or liquid intake during specified times (e.g., many Catholics fast and abstain from meat on Ash Wednesday and the Fridays of Lent; Muslims fast from dawn to sunset during the month of Ramadan in the Islamic calendar and eat only twice a day—before dawn and after sunset; Jews observe a 24-hour fast on Yom Kippur).

Structure and Function

TABLE 11-1   Religious Dietary Practices

RELIGIOUS GROUP	FOOD RESTRICTIONS
Buddhism	All meat
Catholicism	Meat by some denominations on Ash Wednesday, Good Friday, and other holy days
	Alcoholic beverages by some denominations
Hinduism	Beef, pork, and some fowl
	Alcohol
	Garlic and onions by some
	Red-colored foods (e.g., tomatoes) by some
Islam	All pork and pork products
	Meat not slaughtered according to ritual
	Alcoholic beverages and alcohol products (e.g., vanilla extract), coffee, and tea
	Food and beverages before sunset during Ramadan
Mormon	Alcoholic beverages
	Caffeinated beverages (e.g., coffee, tea, sodas) and medicines containing caffeine, stimulants, or alcohol (e.g., Anacin, NoDoz, Nyquil)
	Food and beverages on first Sunday of each month
Orthodox Judaism	All pork and pork products
	Meat not slaughtered according to ritual
	All shellfish (e.g., crab, lobster, shrimp, oysters)
	Dairy products and meat at the same meal
	Leavened bread and cake during Passover
	Food and beverages on Yom Kippur
Seventh-Day Adventist	All pork and pork products
	Shellfish
	Meat, dairy products, and eggs by some
	Alcoholic beverages, coffee, and tea
	Highly seasoned foods

TYPES OF NUTRITIONAL ASSESSMENT

Nutritional assessment techniques are noninvasive, inexpensive, and easy to perform. **Nutrition screening** is the first step in assessing nutritional status. Based on easily obtained data, nutrition screening is a quick and easy way to identify individuals at nutrition risk such as those with weight loss, inadequate food intake, or recent illness. Parameters used for nutrition screening typically include weight and weight history, conditions associated with increased nutritional risk, diet information, and routine laboratory data. A variety of valid tools are available for screening different populations. For example, the Malnutrition Screening Tool[9,31] was validated for use in adult acute-care patients, and the Mini Nutritional Assessment (MNA®) was designed and validated for use in older adults in long-term care and community settings.[31,35]

Malnutrition is estimated to occur in one third of hospitalized patients and is associated with adverse outcomes:

impaired wound healing, increased infection risk, suppression of immune system, functional loss with increased falls risk, increased risk of pressure ulcers, longer hospital stay, and increased mortality.[2,31a] Individuals identified to be at nutritional risk during screening should undergo a **comprehensive nutritional assessment,** which includes dietary history and clinical information, physical examination for clinical signs, anthropometric measures, and laboratory tests. The skills needed to collect the clinical and dietary history and to perform the physical examination are described in the Subjective and Objective Data sections that follow. Various methods for collecting current dietary intake information are available: 24-hour recall, food frequency questionnaire, and food diary. During hospitalization documentation of nutritional intake is achieved through calorie counts of nutrients consumed and/or infused.

The easiest and most popular method for obtaining information about dietary intake is the **24-hour recall.** The individual or family member completes a questionnaire or is interviewed and asked to recall everything eaten within the last 24 hours. An advantage is that the 24-hour recall can elicit specific information about dietary intake over a specific period of time. However, there are several significant sources of error: (1) the individual or family member may not be able to recall the type or amount of food eaten; (2) intake within the last 24 hours may be atypical of usual intake; (3) the individual or family member may alter the truth for a variety of reasons; and (4) snack items and use of gravies, sauces, and condiments may be underreported.

To counter some of the difficulties inherent in the 24-hour recall method, you can use a **food frequency questionnaire.** With this tool information is collected on how many times per day, week, or month the individual eats particular foods, providing an estimate of usual intake. Drawbacks to the use of the food frequency questionnaire are: (1) it does not always quantify amount of intake, and (2) like the 24-hour recall, it relies on the individual's or family member's memory for how often a food was eaten.

Food diaries or records ask the individual or family member to write down everything consumed for a certain period of time. Three days (i.e., two weekdays and one weekend day) are customarily used. A food diary is most complete and accurate if you teach the individual to record information immediately after eating. Potential problems with the food diary include (1) noncompliance, (2) inaccurate recording, (3) atypical intake on the recording days, and (4) conscious alteration of diet during the recording period.

Direct observation of the feeding and eating process can detect problems not readily identified through standard nutrition interviews. For example, observing the typical feeding techniques used by a parent or caregiver and the interaction between the individual and caregiver can help when assessing failure to thrive in children or unintentional weight loss in older adults. Increasingly mobile devices and applications are being used to assess and monitor intake, including taking photos of meals and tracking weight changes and dietary adherence. Because these technologies are so new, their validity is as yet unclear.[16,19]

ChooseMyPlate, Dietary Guidelines, and the Dietary Reference Intakes (DRIs) are three guides commonly used to determine an adequate diet. Please access the websites ChooseMyPlate.gov and Dietaryguidelines.gov for additional information plus interactive features, such as SuperTracker, that allow you and your patients to create individualized nutrition and health plans. The DRIs are recommended amounts of nutrients to prevent deficiencies and reduce the risk for chronic diseases. In addition to recommending adequate intakes, they also specify upper limits of nutrients to avoid toxicity. With increased use of dietary supplements, the risk for nutrient toxicities is on the rise. Examples of specific DRIs and interactive tools can be found at fnic.nal.usda.gov/dietary-guidance/dietary-reference-intakes.

SUBJECTIVE DATA

Subjective Data

1. Eating patterns
2. Usual weight
3. Changes in appetite, taste, smell, chewing, swallowing
4. Recent surgery, trauma, burns, infection
5. Chronic illnesses
6. Nausea, vomiting, diarrhea, constipation
7. Food allergies or intolerances
8. Medications and/or nutritional supplements
9. Patient-centered care
10. Alcohol or illegal drug use
11. Exercise and activity patterns
12. Family history

Examiner Asks	Rationale
1. Eating patterns • Number of meals/snacks per day? • Kind and amount of food eaten? • Fad, special, or alternative diets? • Where is food eaten? • Food preferences and dislikes? • Religious or cultural restrictions? • Able to feed self?	Most individuals know about or are interested in the foods they consume. If misconceptions are present, begin gradual instruction to build self-care of healthy eating patterns. Many alternative diets are not supported by scientific safety or efficacy data.
2. Usual weight. What is your usual weight? • 20% below or above desirable weight? • Recent weight change? How much lost or gained? Over what time period? • Reason for loss or gain?	People with a recent weight loss or who are obese are at risk. Underweight individuals are vulnerable because their fuel reserves are depleted. Excess weight carries risk of hypertension, diabetes, heart disease, and cancer.
3. Changes in appetite, taste, smell, chewing, swallowing • Type of change? • When did change occur?	These changes interfere with adequate nutrient intake.
4. Recent surgery, trauma, burns, infection • When? Type? How treated? • Conditions that increase nutrient loss (e.g., draining wounds, effusions, blood loss, dialysis)?	These conditions have caloric and nutrient needs that are 2 or 3 times greater than normal.
5. Chronic illnesses • Type? When diagnosed? How treated? • Dietary modifications? • Recent cancer chemotherapy or radiation therapy?	Cancer treatment or chronic illnesses that affect nutrient use (e.g., diabetes mellitus, pancreatitis, or malabsorption) carry twice the risk for nutritional deficits.
6. Nausea, vomiting, diarrhea, constipation • Any problems? Caused by? How long?	GI symptoms interfere with nutrient intake or absorption.
7. Food allergies or intolerances • Any problematic foods? Type of reaction? How long?	Food allergies, especially peanut allergies, are on the rise and are a major health concern.

Examiner Asks	Rationale

Subjective Data

	Intolerances such as gluten and lactose may cause nutrient deficiencies (e.g., diarrhea).
8. Medications and/or nutritional supplements • Prescription medications? • Nonprescription? • Use over a 24-hour period?	Analgesics, antacids, anticonvulsants, antibiotics, diuretics, laxatives, antineoplastic drugs, steroids, and oral contraceptives are drugs that interact with nutrients, impairing their digestion, absorption, metabolism, or use.
• Type of vitamin/mineral supplement? Amount? Duration of use?	Vitamin/mineral supplements have harmful side effects if taken in large amounts.
• Herbal and botanical products? Functional foods or foods enhanced with nutrients? Specific type/brand and where obtained? How often used? Who recommended? How does it help you? Any problems?	Use of herbal/botanical supplements is often not reported; therefore ask and discuss proper use and potential adverse effects. Refer to www.nccam.nih.gov.
9. Patient-centered care • Meal preparation facilities? • Transportation for travel to market? • Adequate income for food purchase? • Who prepares meals and does shopping? • Environment during mealtimes?	Poverty and lack of access to nutritious groceries interfere with ingestion of adequate amounts of food or usual diet.
10. Alcohol or illegal drug use • When was last drink of alcohol? • Amount taken that episode? • Amount alcohol each day? Each week? • Duration of use? • (Repeat question for each drug used.)	Alcohol is "empty calories" devoid of nutrients. Alcohol and drugs block absorption of some nutrients. Pregnant women who smoke, drink alcohol, or use illegal drugs give birth to infants with low birth weights, failure to thrive, and other serious complications.
11. Exercise and activity patterns • Amount? • Type?	Caloric and nutrient needs increase with competitive sports and manual labor. Inactive or sedentary lifestyles lead to excess weight gain.
12. Family history. Heart disease, osteoporosis, cancer, gout, GI disorders, obesity, or diabetes? • Effect of each on eating patterns? • Effect on activity patterns?	Long-term nutritional deficiencies or excesses may first appear as diseases such as these. Early identification permits dietary and activity modifications when the body can recover.

Additional History for Infants and Children

Dietary histories of infants and children are obtained from the parents, caregiver, or daycare center. Usually the person responsible for food preparation provides a fairly accurate dietary history. Having the caregivers keep a thorough daily food diary and occasionally requesting 24-hour recalls during clinic visits are the usual techniques.

1. Gestational nutrition • Maternal history of alcohol or illegal drug use? • Any diet-related complications during gestation?	Low birth weight (<2500 g) is a major factor in infant morbidity and mortality. Poor gestational nutrition, low maternal

Examiner Asks	Rationale

- Infant's birth weight?
- Any evidence of delayed physical or mental growth?

weight gain, and maternal alcohol and drug use—all factors in low birth weight—can lead to birth defects and delayed growth and development.

2. Infant breastfed or bottle fed
- Type, frequency, amount, and duration of feeding?
- Any difficulties encountered?
- Timing and method of weaning?

Well-nourished infants have appropriate physical and social growth and development. Inexperienced mothers may have problems with feeding or questions about whether the infant is receiving adequate food.

3. Child's willingness to eat what you prepare
- Any special likes or dislikes?
- How much will child eat?
- How do you control non-nutritious snack foods?
- How do you avoid food aspiration?

The preschooler has increasing growth. Lifelong food habits form. Use of small portions, finger foods, simple meals, and nutritious snacks improve dietary intake. Avoid foods likely to be aspirated (e.g., hot dogs, nuts, grapes, round candies, popcorn).

4. Overweight and obesity risk factors
- Overweight or obese parent?
- Low-income family?
- Maternal smoking during pregnancy?
- Large-for-gestational-age birth weight?
- Rapid weight gain from birth to 5 months?

Risk factors for overweight and obesity may be present during gestation, at birth, or during infancy, progressing to obesity in childhood, adolescence, and adulthood.[32]

Additional History for the Adolescent

1. Your present weight
- What would you like to weigh?
- How do you feel about your present weight?
- On any special diet to lose weight?
- On other diets to lose weight? If so, were they successful?
- Constantly think about "feeling fat?" Constantly exercising?
- Intentionally vomit or use laxatives or diuretics after eating?

Obesity, particularly in girls, may precipitate fad dieting and malnutrition. Adolescents' increased body awareness and self-consciousness may cause eating disorders (anorexia nervosa or bulimia) when the real or perceived body image does not compare favorably to an ideal image in advertisements or pictures of fashion models.

2. Use of anabolic steroids or other agents to increase muscle size and physical performance
- When?
- How much?
- Any problems?

Once confined to male professional athletes, the use of performance-enhancing agents now extends to junior high, high school, and college. Adverse effects include personality disorders (aggressiveness) and liver and other organ damage.

- Use of caffeinated, energy-boosting drinks? When? Type? Duration?

Energy-boosting drinks such as Red Bull and Sprint contain large amounts of caffeine, stimulants, and/or herbal products. Side effects include dehydration, high BP and heart rate, and sleep problems.

3. Overweight and obesity risk factors
- Are large amounts of food eaten in a short period of time or for hours on end?
- Which meals do you skip? How often? Which snacks, fast foods, and sweetened beverages do you like? How often do you eat them?

Binge eating is now the most common eating disorder across all age-groups. Skipping meals and consuming fast foods and sweetened beverages are associated with increased weight gain from adolescence to adulthood.[26,34]

Subjective Data

Examiner Asks	Rationale
4. Age first started menstruating • What is your menstrual flow like?	Malnutrition delays menarche. Likewise amenorrhea or scant menstrual flow occurs with nutritional deficiency.

Additional History for the Pregnant Woman

1. Number of pregnancies
- How many times have you been pregnant?
- When?
- Any problems encountered during previous pregnancies?
- Problems this pregnancy?
- Do you take prenatal vitamins or supplements?

A multiparous mother with pregnancies less than 1 year apart has risk for depleted nutritional reserves. Note previous complications of pregnancy (excessive vomiting, anemia, or gestational diabetes). Slower GI motility and pressure from the fetus may cause constipation, hemorrhoids, and indigestion. A history of a low-birth-weight infant suggests past nutritional problems. Giving birth to an infant weighing 4.5 kg (10 lbs) or more may signal *latent* diabetes in the mother.

2. Food preferences when pregnant
- What foods do you avoid?
- Crave any particular foods?

The expectant mother is vulnerable to familial, cultural, and traditional influences for food choices. Cravings for or aversions to particular foods are common; evaluate their contribution to, or interference with, dietary intake.

- How much fish do you eat each week?

Large amounts of fish consumption may be associated with maternal, fetal, and newborn mercury toxicity.

Additional History for the Aging Adult

1. Any diet differences from when you were in your 40s and 50s?
- Why?
- Which factors affect the way you eat?
- Adequate vitamin D and calcium intake?

Note any physiologic or psychological changes of aging or socioeconomic changes that affect nutritional status.

Vitamin D and calcium can help prevent osteoporosis.

OBJECTIVE DATA

CLINICAL SIGNS

The general appearance (i.e., obese, cachectic [fat and muscle wasting], or edematous) can provide clues to overall nutritional status. More specific clinical signs of nutritional deficiencies can be detected through a physical examination. Because clinical signs are late manifestations of malnutrition, only in areas of rapid turnover of epithelial tissue (i.e., skin, hair, mouth, lips, and eyes) are the deficiencies readily detectable. These signs may also be non-nutritional in origin. Therefore laboratory testing is required to make an accurate diagnosis. Clinical signs of various nutritional deficiencies are summarized in Table 11-2 and depicted in the section on abnormalities at the end of this chapter (see Tables 11-3 to 11-4).

EQUIPMENT NEEDED

Lange or Harpenden skinfold calipers
Ross insertion tape or other
    measurement tape
Anthropometer
Pen or pencil
Nutritional assessment data form

TABLE 11-2	Clinical Signs of Malnutrition		
AREA OF EXAMINATION	**NORMAL APPEARANCE**	**SIGNS ASSOCIATED WITH MALNUTRITION**	**NUTRIENT DEFICIENCY**
Skin	Smooth, no signs of rashes, bruises, flaking	Dry, flaking, scaly	Vitamin A, vitamin B–complex, linoleic acid
		Petechiae/ecchymoses	Vitamins C and K
		Follicular hyperkeratosis (dry, bumpy skin)	Vitamin A, linoleic acid
		Cracks in skin; lesions on hands, legs, face, or neck	Niacin, tryptophan
		Eczema	Linoleic acid
		Xanthomas (excessive deposits of cholesterol)	Excessive serum levels of LDLs or VLDLs
Hair	Shiny, firm, does not fall out easily; healthy scalp	Dull, dry, sparse	Protein, zinc, linoleic acid
		Color changes	Copper or protein
		Corkscrew hair	Copper
Eyes	Corneas are clear, shiny; membranes are pink and moist; no sores at corners of eyelids	Foamy plaques (Bitot spots)	Vitamin A
		Dryness (xerophthalmia)	Vitamin A
		Softening (keratomalacia)	Vitamin A
		Pale conjunctivae	Iron, vitamins B_6, B_{12}
		Red conjunctivae	Riboflavin
		Blepharitis	Vitamin B–complex, biotin
Lips	Smooth, not chapped or swollen	Cheilosis (vertical cracks in lips)	Riboflavin, niacin
		Angular stomatitis (red cracks at sides of mouth)	Riboflavin, niacin, iron, vitamin B_6
Tongue	Red in appearance, not swollen or smooth, no lesions	Glossitis (beefy red)	Vitamin B–complex
		Pale	Iron
		Papillary atrophy	Niacin
		Papillary hypertrophy	Multiple nutrients
		Magenta or purplish-colored	Riboflavin
Gums	Reddish-pink, firm, no swelling or bleeding	Bleeding	Vitamin C
Nails	Smooth, pink	Brittle, ridged, or spoon-shaped (koilonychia)	Iron
		Splinter hemorrhages	Vitamin C
Musculoskeletal	Erect posture, no malformations, good muscle tone, can walk or run without pain	Pain in calves, thighs	Thiamine
		Osteomalacia	Vitamin D, calcium
		Rickets	Vitamin D, calcium
		Joint pain	Vitamin C
		Muscle wasting	Protein, carbohydrate, fat
Neurologic	Normal reflexes, appropriate affect	Peripheral neuropathy	Thiamine, vitamin B_6
		Hyporeflexia	Thiamine
		Disorientation or irritability	Vitamin B_{12}

LDL, Low-density lipoprotein; *VLDL,* very low–density lipoprotein.

Normal Range of Findings

Anthropometric Measures

Derived Weight Measures

The **percent usual body weight** is calculated as follows:

$$\text{Percent usual body weight} = \frac{\text{Current weight}}{\text{Usual weight}} \times 100$$

Abnormal Findings

A current weight of 85% to 95% of usual body weight indicates mild malnutrition; 75% to 84%, moderate malnutrition; and <75%, severe malnutrition.

Normal Range of Findings

Recent weight change is calculated using the following formula:

$$\frac{\text{Usual weight} - \text{Current weight}}{\text{Usual weight}} \times 100$$

Body Mass Index

BMI is a practical marker of optimal weight for height and an indicator of obesity or undernutrition (see p. 130 in Chapter 9). It is calculated by:

$$\text{Body mass index} = \frac{\text{Weight (kilograms)}}{\text{Height (meters)}^2}$$

$$\text{Or} \quad \frac{\text{Weight (pounds)}}{\text{Height (inches)}^2} \times 703$$

Waist-to-Hip Ratio

The waist-to-hip ratio assesses body fat distribution as an indicator of health risk. Obese people with a greater proportion of fat in the upper body, especially in the abdomen, have android obesity; obese people with most of their fat in the hips and thighs have gynoid obesity. The equation is:

$$\text{Waist-to-hip ratio} = \frac{\text{Waist circumference}}{\text{Hip circumference}}$$

where waist circumference is measured in inches just above the iliac crests of the hips, and hip circumference is measured in inches at the largest circumference of the buttocks. In addition, **waist circumference (WC)** alone can be used to predict greater health risk (Fig. 11-4).

11-4

Skinfold Thickness

Skinfold thickness measurements estimate the body fat stores or the extent of obesity or undernutrition. Although other sites can be used (biceps, subcapsular, or suprailiac skinfolds), the triceps skinfold (TSF) is most easily accessible, and standards and techniques are most developed for this site. To measure TSF thickness:

1. Have the ambulatory person stand with arms hanging freely at the sides and back to the examiner. (Nonambulatory people should lie on one side. The

Abnormal Findings

An unintentional loss of >5% of body weight over 1 month, >7.5% of body weight over 3 months, or >10% of body weight over 6 months is clinically significant.

BMI interpretation for adults[24]:

<18.5	Underweight
18.5-24.9	Normal weight
25-29.9	Overweight
30-39.9	Obesity
≥40	Extreme obesity

BMI interpretation for children ages 2 to 20 years[5]:

<5th percentile	Underweight
5th-85th percentile	Healthy weight
85th-95th percentile	Overweight
≥95th percentile	Obese

A waist-to-hip ratio of 1.0 or greater in men or 0.8 or greater in women indicates android (upper body) obesity and increasing risk for obesity-related diseases and early mortality.

A WC >35 inches in women and >40 inches in men increases risk for heart disease, type 2 diabetes, and metabolic syndrome.

Normal Range of Findings	Abnormal Findings

uppermost arm should be fully extended, with the palm of the hand resting on the thigh.)

2. Using the thumb and forefinger of your left hand, gently grasp a fold of skin and fat on the back of the person's left upper arm, midway between the acromion process of the scapula and the olecranon process (the tip of the elbow). Gently pull the skinfold away from the underlying muscle.

3. While grasping the skinfold, pick up the calipers with your right hand and depress the spring-loaded lever. Apply caliper jaws horizontally to the fat fold. Release the lever of the calipers while holding the skinfold. Wait 3 seconds and then take a reading. Repeat 3 times and average the three skinfold measurements (Fig. 11-5).

TSF values 10% below or above standard suggest undernutrition and overnutrition, respectively.

11-5

4. Record measurements to the nearest 5 mm (0.5 cm) on the nutritional assessment data form. Compare the person's measurements with standards by age, gender, and body frame size (see tables at www.cdc.gov/nchs/data/series/sr_11/sr11_252).

Two newer techniques to measure body composition are **bioelectrical impedance analysis (BIA)** and **dual-energy x-ray absorptiometry (DEXA)**. Both BIA and DEXA measure fat and lean body mass; in addition, DEXA measures bone mineral density.

Nonreproducible readings may be caused by instrument malfunctions, use of plastic calipers (which are less accurate), or examiner error. Edema may produce falsely high readings.

Arm Span or Total Arm Length

Measurement of arm span is useful for situations in which height is difficult to measure such as in children with cerebral palsy or scoliosis or aging persons with spinal curvature. Arm span, which is nearly equivalent to height, is sometimes used clinically instead of height. Measure the distance from the sternal notch to the longest finger on the dominant hand and multiply the number by 2.8.[6]

❖ DEVELOPMENTAL COMPETENCE

Infants, Children, and Adolescents

Skinfold Thickness and Body Mass Index. Determine skinfold thickness and/or BMI to evaluate childhood and teenage overnutrition.

About 33% of children and adolescents in the United States are overweight or obese.

Normal Range of Findings	Abnormal Findings

The Pregnant Woman

Weight. Measure weight monthly up to 30 weeks' gestation and then every 2 weeks until the last month of pregnancy, when weight should be measured weekly. See Chapter 30 for a discussion of expected weight gain during pregnancy.

Consider the expectant mother at nutritional risk if her weight is 10% or more below ideal or 20% or more above the norm for her height and age-group.

The Aging Adult

Height. With age, height declines in both men and women very slowly from the early 30s, leading to an average 2.9-cm loss in men and 4.9-cm loss in women.[15,30] Height measures may not be accurate in individuals confined to a bed or wheelchair or those older than 60 years (because of osteoporotic changes). Therefore arm span, which is correlated with height, may be a better measure.

Other Measurements. TSF measures are difficult to obtain in older adults (because of sagging skin, changes in fat distribution, and declining muscle mass). (See Frisancho[13] for data on weight and TSF thickness by height in U.S. men and women ages 55 to 74 years.) BMI and waist-to-hip ratio are better indicators of obesity in this age-group.

Serial Assessment

To monitor nutritional status in malnourished individuals or individuals at risk for malnutrition, serial measurements are made at routine intervals. At a minimum, weight and dietary intake should be evaluated weekly. Because the other nutritional assessment parameters change more slowly, data on these indicators may be collected biweekly or monthly.

Based on the findings of the nutritional assessment, the type of malnutrition can be diagnosed. The four major types of malnutrition are obesity, marasmus, kwashiorkor, and marasmus-kwashiorkor mix (see Table 11-3). Each type of malnutrition has characteristic clinical and laboratory findings and a distinct cause.

Approaches to weight loss for overweight and obesity must be tailored to the individual, be culturally sensitive, and consider the patient's readiness to lose weight and his or her health care and self-care beliefs. Weight-loss programs that provide less than 1000 to 1200 calories may not provide adequate nutrients. Regardless of macronutrient composition, any diet that reduces caloric intake or contains 1400 to 1500 calories per day results in weight loss. In other words, it is not eating too much of any particular nutrient such as carbohydrate or fat that makes us gain weight but rather the overall number of calories ingested. The **cardinal features** of a successful long-term weight loss plan are (1) getting regular physical exercise (i.e., 4 to 5 times/week for 30 minutes); (2) eating a low-calorie ($\approx$1400 to 1500 kcal/day), low-fat (20% to 25% of total calories) diet; and (3) monitoring daily food intake (e.g., food diary, portion size) and weight.

Documentation and Critical Thinking

DOCUMENTATION AND CRITICAL THINKING

Sample Charting

SUBJECTIVE

A.J. is a 70-year-old retired teacher with no history of diseases or surgery that would alter intake/requirements; no recent weight changes; no appetite changes. Socioeconomic history is noncontributory. Does not smoke; drink alcohol; or use illegal, prescription, or over-the-counter drugs. No food allergies. Sedentary lifestyle; plays golf twice per week using riding cart. Reports losing 40 lbs during past 6 months through monitored commercial weight-loss program.

OBJECTIVE

Dietary intake is adequate to meet protein and energy needs. No clinical signs of nutrient deficiencies. Height 70", weight 209 lbs, BMI 30, and screening laboratory tests within normal ranges.

ASSESSMENT

Obesity, improving through monitored program
Sedentary lifestyle

Case Study 1

K.L. is a 44-year-old African-American female who has been overweight most of her life. Recently diagnosed with hypertension and type 2 diabetes. Comes to the clinic today for a nutritional assessment.

SUBJECTIVE

K.L. reports a lifelong struggle with obesity. Multiple failed diet attempts. Daily calorie intake approximately 3000 calories/day. Typical day: pastry or doughnut with coffee for breakfast, fast-food meal with soft drink for lunch, and "whatever I can find" for dinner. Lives in a low-income neighborhood. Nearest grocery store with fresh produce approximately 25 minutes by car. Few safe places in neighborhood for outdoor exercise.

OBJECTIVE

Inspection: General appearance is obese for age and height.
Anthropometric: Height 157.5 cm (62 in). Weight 120 kg (265 lbs). BMI 48.5 (obese).
Laboratory: Hemoglobin, hematocrit, and albumin within normal limits. Hemoglobin A1c 12%. Fasting glucose 213 mg/dL.

ASSESSMENT

Morbid obesity; uncontrolled type 2 diabetes
Altered nutrition: more than body requirements R/T high-fat, high-calorie diet
Impaired physical mobility R/T morbid obesity

Case Study 2

S.A. is a 14-year-old Caucasian girl who has been overweight most of her life. She now has a weight gain of 12 pounds since starting high school 6 months PTA. She lives in a low-income neighborhood where the nearest grocery store with fresh fruits and vegetables is a bus ride away. There are no parks or well-lit areas with sidewalks near her home.

SUBJECTIVE

Based on S.A.'s diet recall, estimated daily calorie intake averages 2500 to 3000 calories/day. States, "I either skip breakfast or eat a doughnut on the way to school. At lunch, I eat what they give me that I don't have to pay for." Dinner is usually items from a fast-food restaurant such as a double cheeseburger, fries, and soft drink. Enjoys snacking on toaster pastries, instant ramen noodles, potato chips, and macaroni and cheese at home and consumes fruit punch and sweet tea throughout the day.

OBJECTIVE

Vital signs: Temp 98.6° F (37° C) (oral); BP 118/68 mm Hg (sitting); Pulse 82 bpm (resting); Resp 18/min.
Anthropometric: Height 162.6 cm (64 in). Weight 68.6 kg (151 lbs). BMI 26.
General appearance: Appears overweight for age and height; moderate amount of open and closed comedones and acne lesions generalized to face, neck, and back.

ASSESSMENT

Overweight with BMI of 26
Risk for disturbed body image R/T excess weight
Risk-prone health behavior R/T negative attitude toward health care

ABNORMAL FINDINGS

TABLE 11-3 Classification of Malnutrition

Type/Etiology	Clinical Features	Anthropometric Measures	Laboratory Findings
Obesity caused by caloric excess refers to weight more than 20% above ideal body weight or body mass index (BMI) of 30.0-39.9. The causes are complex and multifaceted—genetic, social, cultural, pathologic, psychological, and physiologic factors. In most cases a small caloric surplus over a long period results in the extra pounds. Although visceral protein levels are normal in the obese individual, anthropometric measures are above normal.	Obese appearance	Weight >120% standard for height BMI >30 Triceps skinfold (TSF) >10% above standard Waist-to-hip ratio >1 (men) or >0.8 (women) BMI ≥40 is morbid or extreme obesity (see Table 9-1, p. 131)	Serum cholesterol 200 mg/dL Serum triglycerides >250 mg/dL
Marasmus (protein-calorie malnutrition) is caused by inadequate intake of protein and calories or prolonged starvation. Anorexia, bowel obstruction, cancer cachexia, and chronic illness are among the clinical conditions leading to marasmus. It is characterized by decreased anthropometric measures (i.e., weight loss and subcutaneous fat and muscle wasting). Visceral protein levels may remain within normal ranges.	Starved appearance	Weight ≤80% standard for height TSF <90% standard Mid–upper arm muscle circumference (MAMC) ≤90% standard	
Kwashiorkor (protein malnutrition) is caused by diets high in calories but little or no protein (e.g., low-protein liquid diets, fad diets, and long-term use of dextrose-containing intravenous fluids). In contrast to individuals with marasmus, those with kwashiorkor have decreased visceral protein levels but adequate anthropometric measures. Therefore they may appear well nourished or even obese.	Well-nourished appearance Edematous	Weight ≥100% standard for height TSF ≥100% standard	Serum albumin <3.5 g/dL Serum transferrin <150 mg/dL

TABLE 11-3 Classification of Malnutrition—cont'd

Type/Etiology	Clinical Features	Anthropometric Measures	Laboratory Findings
Marasmus/kwashiorkor mix is caused by prolonged inadequate intake of protein and calories such as severe starvation and severe catabolic states. Nutritional assessment findings include muscle, fat, and visceral protein wasting. Individuals have usually undergone acute catabolic stress such as major surgery, trauma, or burns in combination with prolonged starvation or have AIDS wasting. Without nutritional support, this type of malnutrition is associated with the highest risk for morbidity and mortality.	Emaciated appearance	Weight ≤70% standard TSF ≤80% standard MAMC ≤60% standard	Serum albumin <2.8 g/dL Serum transferrin <100 mg/dL

See Illustration Credits for source information.

TABLE 11-4 Abnormalities Caused by Nutritional Deficiencies

Scorbutic Gums

Deficiency of vitamin C. Gums are swollen, ulcerated, and bleeding because of vitamin C deficiency–induced defects in oral epithelial basement membrane and periodontal collagen fiber synthesis.

Rickets

Sign of vitamin D and calcium deficiencies in children (disorders of cartilage cell growth, enlargement of epiphyseal growth plates) and adults (osteomalacia).

◀ Bitot Spots

Foamy plaques of the cornea that are a sign of vitamin A deficiency. Severe depletion may result in conjunctival xerosis (drying) and progress to corneal ulceration and finally destruction of the eye (keratomalacia).

Continued

TABLE 11-4 Abnormalities Caused by Nutritional Deficiencies—cont'd

Follicular Hyperkeratosis

Dry, bumpy skin associated with vitamin A and/or linoleic acid (essential fatty acid) deficiency. Linoleic acid deficiency may also result in eczematous skin, especially in infants.

Pellagra

Pigmented keratotic scaling lesions resulting from a deficiency of niacin. These lesions are especially prominent in areas exposed to the sun such as hands, forearms, neck, and legs.

Magenta Tongue

A sign of riboflavin deficiency. In contrast, a pale tongue is probably attributable to iron deficiency; a beefy red–colored tongue is caused by vitamin B–complex deficiency.

ABNORMAL FINDINGS
FOR ADVANCED PRACTICE

TABLE 11-5 Metabolic Syndrome (MetS)

Waist circumference

≥102 cm (≥40 inches) in men
≥88 cm (≥35 inches) in women

Glucose

≥100 mg/dL
or
Drug treatment for elevated glucose

MetS

Blood pressure

≥130 mm Hg systolic BP
or
≥85 mm Hg diastolic BP
or
Drug treatment for hypertension

High-density lipoprotein

<40 mg/dL in men
<50 mg/dL in women
or
Drug treatment for reduced HDL-C

Triglyceride (TG)

≥150 mg/dL
or
Drug treatment for elevated TG

Having 3 of these 5 biomarkers signifies MetS. MetS is associated with increased risk for cardiovascular disease, type 2 diabetes mellitus, and mortality. Its prevalence is estimated to be 28% among adolescents and 22% among adults.[11,21]

TABLE 11-6 Nutritional Consequences of Bariatric Surgery*†

Potential Nutritional Consequences	Related Dietary Changes
Malabsorption of protein and calories caused by decreased absorptive surface and availability of digestive enzymes	Eating small, nutrient-dense meals
Malabsorption of vitamins and minerals caused by achlorhydria or loss of site of absorption	Taking vitamin and mineral supplements
Weight regain	Avoiding excessive intake of calorically dense liquids/foods
Obstruction of bypassed sections or pouch	Avoiding chunks of food that could cause blockage

*Vertical and adjustable gastric banding, Roux-en-Y gastric bypass.
†People who are 100% or more above ideal body weight or have a body mass index (BMI) ≥40 are categorized as morbidly or extremely obese and are possible candidates for bariatric or weight-loss surgery, as are people with BMIs ≥35 and comorbid conditions.

Summary Checklist: Nutritional Assessment

1. Obtain a **health history** relevant to nutritional status.
2. Elicit **dietary history** if indicated.
3. **Inspect** skin, hair, eyes, oral cavity, nails, and musculoskeletal and neurologic systems for clinical signs and symptoms suggestive of nutritional deficiencies.
4. **Measure** height, weight, BMI, WC, and other anthropometric parameters as indicated.
5. Review relevant **laboratory tests**.
6. Offer **health promotion** teaching.

Abnormal Findings

BIBLIOGRAPHY

1. Academy of Nutrition and Dietetics: www.eatright.org.
2. Barker, L. A., Gout, B. S., & Crowe, T. C. (2011). Hospital malnutrition: prevalence, identification and impact on patients and the health care system. *Int J Environ Res and Public Health, 8*(2):514-527.
3. Benton, M. J., Whyte, M. D., & Dyal, B. W. (2011). Sarcopenic obesity: strategies for management. *Am J Nurs, 111*(12), 38-46.
4. Bosak, K. (2012). Managing metabolic syndrome in women. *Nurse Pract, 37*(8):14-21.
5. Centers for Disease Control and Prevention. (2013). *Overweight and obesity.* Available at www.cdc.gov/obesity/data/index.html.
6. Charney, P., & Malone, A. M. (2009). *ADA pocket guide to nutrition assessment.* (2nd ed.). Chicago: American Dietetic Association.
7. Chernecky, C. C., & Berger, B. J. (2013). *Laboratory tests and diagnostic procedures.* (6th ed.). St. Louis: Saunders.
7a. Cunningham, S. A., Kramer, M. R., Narayan, K. M. (2014). Incidence of childhood obesity in the United States. *N Engl J Med, 370*(5), 403-411.
8. FDA Food Safety: www.foodsafety.gov.
9. Ferguson, M., Capra, S., Bauer, J., et al. (1999). Development of a valid and reliable malnutrition screening tool for adult acute care hospital patients. *Nutrition, 15,* 458-464.
10. Flegal, K. M., Carroll, M. D., Kit, B. K., et al. (2012). Prevalence of obesity and trends in the distribution of body mass index among US adults, 1999-2010. *JAMA, 307*(5), 491-497.
11. Ford, E. S., Li, C., Zhao, G., et al. (2008). Prevalence of the metabolic syndrome among U.S. adolescents using the definition from the International Diabetes Federation. *Diabetes Care, 31*(3), 587-589.
12. Franco, O. H., Massaro, J. M., Civil, J., et al. (2009). Trajectories of entering the metabolic syndrome: the Framingham Heart Study. *Circulation, 120*(20), 1943-1950.
13. Frisancho, A. R. (1984). New standards of weight and body composition by frame size and height for assessment of nutritional status of adults and the elderly. *Am J Clin Nutr, 40,* 808-819.
14. Reference deleted in proofs.
15. Gabriella, S. E., & Sinclair, A. J. (1997). Diagnosing undernutrition in elderly people. *Rev Clin Gerontol, 7,* 367-371.
16. Illner, A. K., Freisling, H., Boeing, H., et al. (2012). Review and evaluation of innovative technologies for measuring diet in nutritional epidemiology. *Int J Epidemiol, 41*(4), 1187-1203.
17. Juonala, M., Magnussen, C. G., Berenson, G. S., et al. (2011). Childhood adiposity, adult adiposity, and cardiovascular risk factors. *N Engl J Med, 365*(20), 1876-1885.
17a. Kann, L., Kinchen, S., Shanklin, S. L., et al. (2014). Youth risk behavior surveillance—United States, 2013. *MMWR, 63*(4), 1-172. Available at: www.cdc.gov/mmwr/pdf/ss/ss6304.pdf.
18. Lee, R. D., & Nieman, D. C. (2012). *Nutritional assessment.* (6th ed.). New York: McGraw-Hill.
19. Lieffers, J. R. L, & Hanning, R. M. (2012). Dietary assessment and self-monitoring with nutrition applications for mobile devices. *Can J Diet Pract Res, 73*(3), e253-e260.
20. Morley, J. E. (2012). Undernutrition in older adults. *Fam Pract, 29* (Suppl 1), i89-i93.
21. Mozumdar, A., & Liguori, G. (2011). Persistent increase in prevalence of metabolic syndrome among U.S. adults: NHANES III to NHANES 1999-2006. *Diabetes Care, 34*(1), 216-219.
22. National Academy of Sciences, Committee to Reexamine IOM Pregnancy Weight Guidelines, Institute of Medicine, National Research Council. Rasmussen, K. M., & Yaktine, A. L. (Eds.), (2009). *Weight gain during pregnancy: reexamining the guidelines.* Washington, DC: National Academies Press.
23. National Eating Disorders Organization: www.edap.org.
24. National Heart, Lung, and Blood Institute, National Institutes of Health, Department of Health and Human Services. (2013). *Overweight and obesity.* Available at www.nhlbi.nih.gov/guidelines/obesity/ob_home.htm.
25. National Institutes of Health. *Guidelines for obesity.* www.nhlbi.nih.gov/guidelines/obesity/ob_gdlns.htm.
26. Niemeier, H. M., Raynor, H. A., Lloyd-Richardson, E. E., et al. (2006). Fast food consumption and breakfast skipping: predictors of weight gain from adolescence to adulthood in a nationally representative sample. *J Adolesc Health, 29,* 842-849.
27. Ogden, C. L., Carroll, M. D., Kit, B. K., et al. (2012). Prevalence of obesity and trends in body mass index for age among U.S. children and adolescents, 1999-2010. *JAMA, 307*(5), 483-490.
28. Pulgaron, E. R. (2013). Childhood obesity: a review of increased risk for physical and psychological comorbidities. *Clin Ther, 35*(1), A18-A32.
29. Qi, Q., Chu, A. Y., Kang, J. H., et al. (2012). Sugar-sweetened beverages and genetic risk of obesity. *N Engl J Med, 367*(15), 1387-1396.
30. Reuben, D. B., Greendale, G. A., & Harrison, G. G. (1995). Nutrition screening in older persons. *J Am Geriatr Soc, 43*(4), 415-425.
31. Skipper, A., Ferguson, M., Thompson, K., et al. (2012). Nutrition screening tools: an analysis of evidence. *J Parenter Enter Nutr, 36*(3), 292-298.
31a. Tappenden K.A., Quatrara B., Parkhurst M.L., et al. (2013). Critical role of nutrition in improving quality of care: an interdisciplinary call to action to address adult hospital malnutrition. *J Parenter Enter Nutr, 37*(4), 482-497.
32. Trapp, L. W., Ryan, A. A., Ariza, A. J., et al. (2009). Primary care identification of infants at high risk for overweight and obesity. *Clin Pediatr, 48*(3), 313-316.
33. USDA Food and Nutrition Information Center: www.nutrition.govwww.usda.gov.
34. Vartanian, L. R., Schwartz, M. B., & Brownell, K. D. (2007). Effects of soft drink consumption on nutrition and health: a systematic review and meta-analysis. *Am J Public Health, 97,* 667-675.
35. Vellas, B., Vellars, H., Abellan, G., et al. (2006). Overview of the MNA®: its history and challenges. *J Nutr Health Aging, 10*(6), 456-465.

CHAPTER 12

Skin, Hair, and Nails

STRUCTURE AND FUNCTION

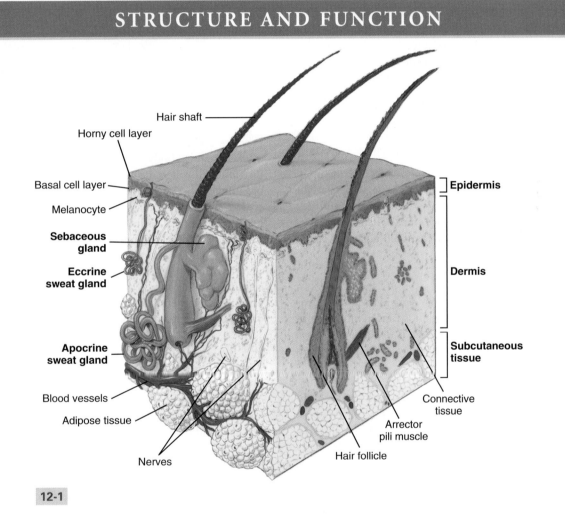

Hair shaft

Horny cell layer

Basal cell layer

Melanocyte

Sebaceous gland

Eccrine sweat gland

Apocrine sweat gland

Blood vessels

Adipose tissue

Nerves

Epidermis

Dermis

Subcutaneous tissue

Connective tissue

Arrector pili muscle

Hair follicle

12-1

SKIN

Think of the skin as the largest organ system in the body—it covers 20 square feet of surface area in the average adult. The skin is the sentry that guards the body from environmental stresses (e.g., trauma, pathogens, dirt) and adapts it to other environmental influences (e.g., heat, cold). The skin has two layers: the outer, highly differentiated *epidermis* and the inner, supportive *dermis* (Fig. 12-1). Beneath these is the *subcutaneous* layer of adipose tissue.

Epidermis

The **epidermis** is thin but tough. Its cells are bound tightly together into sheets that form a rugged protective barrier. It is stratified into several zones. The inner **basal cell layer** forms

new skin cells. Their major ingredient is the tough, fibrous protein *keratin*. The melanocytes interspersed along this layer produce the pigment *melanin*, which gives brown tones to the skin and hair. People of all skin colors have the same number of melanocytes; however, the amount of melanin they produce varies with genetic, hormonal, and environmental influences.

From the basal layer the new cells migrate up and flatten into the outer **horny cell layer.** This consists of dead keratinized cells that are interwoven and closely packed. The cells are constantly being shed, or desquamated, and are replaced with new cells from below. The epidermis is completely replaced every 4 weeks.

On the palms and soles skin is thicker because of work and weight bearing. The epidermis is avascular; it is nourished by blood vessels in the dermis below.

Skin color is derived from three sources: (1) mainly from the brown pigment *melanin*, (2) from the yellow-orange tones of the pigment *carotene*, and (3) from the red-purple tones in the underlying vascular bed. All people have skin of varying shades of brown, yellow, and red; the relative proportion of these shades affects the prevailing color. Skin color is further modified by the thickness of the skin and the presence of edema.

Dermis

The **dermis** is the inner supportive layer consisting mostly of connective tissue, or *collagen*. This is the tough, fibrous protein that enables the skin to resist tearing. The dermis also has resilient elastic tissue that allows the skin to stretch with body movements. The nerves, sensory receptors, blood vessels, and lymphatics lie in the dermis. In addition, appendages from the epidermis such as the hair follicles, sebaceous glands, and sweat glands are embedded in the dermis.

Subcutaneous Layer

The *subcutaneous layer* is adipose tissue, which is made up of lobules of fat cells. The subcutaneous tissue stores fat for energy, provides insulation for temperature control, and aids in protection by its soft cushioning effect. The loose subcutaneous layer also gives skin its increased mobility over structures underneath.

Hair

Hairs are threads of keratin. The hair *shaft* is the visible projecting part, and the *root* is below the surface embedded in the follicle. At the root the *bulb matrix* is the expanded area where new cells are produced at a high rate. Hair growth is cyclical, with active and resting phases. Each follicle functions independently; thus while some hairs are resting, others are growing. Around the hair follicle are the muscular *arrector pili*, which contract and elevate the hair so it resembles "goose flesh" when the skin is exposed to cold or in emotional states.

People have two types of hair. Fine, faint **vellus hair** covers most of the body (except the palms and soles, the dorsa of the distal parts of the fingers, the umbilicus, the glans penis, and inside the labia). The other type is **terminal hair,** the darker, thicker hair that grows on the scalp and eyebrows and, after puberty, on the axillae, the pubic area, and the face and chest in the male.

Sebaceous Glands

These glands produce a protective lipid substance, *sebum,* which is secreted through the hair follicles. Sebum oils and lubricates the skin and hair and forms an emulsion with water that retards water loss from the skin. (Dry skin results from loss of water, not directly from loss of oil.) Sebaceous glands are everywhere except on the palms and soles. They are most abundant in the scalp, forehead, face, and chin.

Sweat Glands

There are two types of sweat glands. The **eccrine** glands are coiled tubules that open directly onto the skin surface and

12-2

produce a dilute saline solution called *sweat*. The evaporation of sweat reduces body temperature. Eccrine glands are widely distributed through the body and are mature in the 2-month-old infant.

The **apocrine** glands produce a thick, milky secretion and open into the hair follicles. They are located mainly in the axillae, anogenital area, nipples, and navel and are vestigial in humans. They become active during puberty, and secretion occurs with emotional and sexual stimulation. Bacterial flora residing on the skin surface react with apocrine sweat to produce a characteristic musky body odor. The functioning of apocrine glands decreases in the aging adult.

Nails

The nails are hard plates of keratin on the dorsal edges of the fingers and toes (Fig. 12-2). The nail plate is clear, with fine longitudinal ridges that become prominent in aging. Nails take their pink color from the underlying nail bed of highly vascular epithelial cells. The lunula is the white, opaque, semi-lunar area at the proximal end of the nail. It lies over the nail matrix where new keratinized cells are formed. The nail folds overlap the posterior and lateral borders. The cuticle works like a gasket to cover and protect the nail matrix.

FUNCTION OF THE SKIN

The skin is a waterproof, almost indestructible covering that has protective and adaptive properties:

- **Protection.** Skin minimizes injury from physical, chemical, thermal, and light-wave sources.
- **Prevents penetration.** Skin is a barrier that stops invasion of microorganisms and loss of water and electrolytes from within the body.
- **Perception.** Skin is a vast sensory surface holding the neurosensory end-organs for touch, pain, temperature, and pressure.
- **Temperature regulation.** Skin allows heat dissipation through sweat glands and heat storage through subcutaneous insulation.

- **Identification.** People identify one another by unique combinations of facial characteristics, hair, skin color, and even fingerprints. Self-image is often enhanced or deterred by the way society standards of beauty measure up to each person's perceived characteristics.
- **Communication.** Emotions are expressed in the sign language of the face and body posture. Vascular mechanisms such as blushing or blanching also signal emotional states.
- **Wound repair.** Skin allows cell replacement of surface wounds.
- **Absorption and excretion.** Skin allows limited excretion of some metabolic wastes, by-products of cellular decomposition such as minerals, sugars, amino acids, cholesterol, uric acid, and urea.
- **Production of vitamin D.** The skin is the surface on which ultraviolet (UV) light converts cholesterol into vitamin D.

❖ DEVELOPMENTAL COMPETENCE

Infants and Children

The hair follicles develop in the fetus at 3 months' gestation; by midgestation most of the skin is covered with **lanugo,** the fine downy hair of the newborn infant. In the first few months after birth, this is replaced by fine vellus hair. If terminal hair on the scalp is present at birth, it tends to be soft and suffer a patchy loss, especially at the temples and occiput. Also present at birth is **vernix caseosa,** the thick, cheesy substance made up of sebum and shed epithelial cells.

The newborn's skin is similar in structure to the adult's, but many of its functions are not fully developed. The newborn's skin is thin, smooth, and elastic and is relatively more permeable than that of the adult; thus the infant is at greater risk for fluid loss. Sebum, which holds water in the skin, is present for the first few weeks of life, producing milia (see p. 218) and cradle cap in some babies. Then sebaceous glands decrease in size and production and do not resume functioning until puberty. Temperature regulation is ineffective. Eccrine sweat glands do not secrete in response to heat until the first few months of life and then only minimally throughout childhood. The skin cannot protect much against cold because it cannot contract and shiver and because the subcutaneous layer is inefficient. In addition, the pigment system is inefficient at birth.

As the child grows, the epidermis thickens, toughens, and darkens, and the skin becomes better lubricated. Hair growth accelerates. At puberty secretion from apocrine sweat glands increases in response to heat and emotional stimuli, producing body odor. Sebaceous glands become more active; the skin looks oily, and acne develops. Subcutaneous fat deposits increase, especially in females.

Secondary sex characteristics that appear during adolescence are evident in the skin. In the female the diameter of the areola enlarges and darkens, and breast tissue develops. Coarse pubic hair develops in males and females, then axillary hair, and then coarse facial hair in males.

The Pregnant Woman

The change in hormone levels results in increased pigment in the areolae and nipples, vulva, and sometimes in the midline of the abdomen (**linea nigra**) or in the face (**chloasma**). Hyperestrogenemia probably also causes the common vascular spiders and palmar erythema. Connective tissue develops increased fragility, resulting in **striae gravidarum** (stretch marks), which may develop in the skin of the abdomen, breasts, or thighs. Metabolism is increased in pregnancy; as a way to dissipate heat, the peripheral vasculature dilates, and the sweat and sebaceous glands increase secretion. Fat deposits are laid down, particularly in the buttocks and hips, as maternal reserves for the nursing baby.

The Aging Adult

The skin is a mirror that reflects aging changes that proceed in *all* our organ systems; it just happens to be the one organ that we can view directly. The aging process carries a slow atrophy of skin structures. The aging skin loses its elasticity; it folds and sags. By the 70s to 80s, it looks parchment thin, lax, dry, and wrinkled.

The outer layer of the epidermis thins and flattens. This allows chemicals easier access into the body. Wrinkling occurs because the underlying dermis thins and flattens. A loss of elastin, collagen, and subcutaneous fat and reduction in muscle tone occur. The loss of collagen increases the risk for shearing, tearing injuries.

Sweat and sebaceous glands decrease in number and function, leaving dry skin. Decreased response of the sweat glands to thermoregulatory demand also puts the aging person at greater risk for heat stroke. The vascularity of the skin diminishes while the vascular fragility increases; a minor trauma may produce dark red discolored areas, or **senile purpura.**

Sun exposure and cigarette smoking further accentuate aging changes in the skin. Coarse wrinkling, decreased elasticity, atrophy, speckled and uneven coloring, more pigment changes, and a yellowed, leathery texture occur. Chronic sun damage is even more prominent in pale or light-skinned persons.

An accumulation of factors places the aging person at risk for skin disease and breakdown: the thinning of the skin, the decrease in vascularity and nutrients, the loss of protective cushioning of the subcutaneous layer, a lifetime of environmental trauma to skin, the social changes of aging (e.g., less nutrition, limited financial resources), the increasingly sedentary lifestyle, and the chance of immobility. When skin breakdown does occur, subsequent cell replacement is slower, and wound healing is delayed.

In the aging hair matrix, the number of functioning melanocytes decreases; therefore the hair looks gray or white and feels thin and fine. A person's genetic script determines the onset of graying and the number of gray hairs. Hair distribution changes. Males may have a symmetric W-shaped balding in the frontal areas. Some testosterone is present in both males and females; as it decreases with age, axillary and pubic hair decrease. As the female's estrogen also decreases, testosterone is unopposed, and the female may have some bristly facial hairs. Nails grow more slowly. Their surface is lusterless and characterized by longitudinal ridges resulting from local trauma at the nail matrix.

Because the aging changes in the skin and hair can be viewed directly, they carry a profound psychological impact. For many people self-esteem is linked to a youthful appearance. This view is compounded by media advertising in Western society. Although sagging and wrinkling skin and graying and thinning hair are normal processes of aging, they prompt a loss of self-esteem for many adults.

CULTURE AND GENETICS

Skin of color includes people of African, Asian, American Indian, Hispanic, and Middle Eastern descent.[16] As described earlier, melanin is responsible for the various colors and tones of skin observed among people. Melanin protects the skin against harmful UV rays, a genetic advantage accounting for the lower incidence of skin cancer among darkly pigmented African Americans and American Indians. The incidence of melanoma is 20 times higher among Whites than among African Americans and 5 times higher among Whites than among Hispanics.[1] The incidence of skin cancer increases with age, but it is also common in young people. Several genes are responsible for increased chromosomal sensitivity to sun damage. Thus a history of melanoma in first-degree relatives increases one's risk for melanoma.

The most important environmental risk factor for skin cancer is exposure to UV radiation from the sun; however, indoor tanning also is a source of UV exposure.[18] The popularity of indoor tanning with adolescents and young people increases their risk of skin cancer, including deadly melanoma. Artificial tanning rates approach 40% for older teens in some regions. California, Vermont, and Illinois have passed laws banning indoor tanning for minors under age 18 years.[2] Sunburn is another risk factor for melanoma; risk increases with increasing numbers of sunburn during all age-groups.[8]

Several skin conditions are found among Blacks:
1. Keloids—Scars that form at the site of a wound and grow beyond the normal boundaries of the wound (see p. 232). African Americans have very compact bundles of collagen just below the epidermis, which may affect keloid production.[11]
2. Areas of postinflammatory hypopigmentation or hyperpigmentation that appear as dark or light spots
3. Pseudofolliculitis—"Razor bumps" or "ingrown hairs" caused by shaving too closely with an electric or straight razor
4. Melasma—The "mask of pregnancy," a patchy tan-to–dark brown discoloration of the face.

The incidence of systemic lupus erythematosus (SLE) is higher in African-American women than in Whites, and they tend to have more severe levels of disease.[32a] Although SLE is an autoimmune disorder, it has manifestations on the skin that lead to diagnosis.

The hair of African Americans varies widely in texture. It may be fragile and ranges from long and straight to short, spiraled, thick, and kinky. The hair and scalp have a natural tendency to be dry and require daily combing, gentle brushing, and the application of oil. Hair care products designed to care specifically for kinky hair should be available in clinical settings. In comparison, people of Asian backgrounds generally have straight, silky hair.

SUBJECTIVE DATA

1. Past history of skin disease (allergies, hives, psoriasis, eczema)
2. Change in pigmentation
3. Change in mole (size or color)
4. Excessive dryness or moisture
5. Pruritus
6. Excessive bruising
7. Rash or lesion
8. Medications
9. Hair loss
10. Change in nails
11. Environmental or occupational hazards
12. Patient-centered care

Examiner Asks	Rationale
1. Past history of skin disease. Any past skin disease or problem? • How was this treated? • Any family history of allergies or allergic skin problem? • Any known allergies to drugs, plants, animals? • Any birthmarks, tattoos?	Significant familial predisposition: allergies, hay fever, psoriasis, atopic dermatitis (eczema), acne. Identify offending allergen. Use of nonsterile equipment to apply tattoos increases risk for hepatitis C. Stock bottles of tattoo ink may contain pathogenic bacteria, especially if ink was diluted with nonsterile water.[15]

Examiner Asks	Rationale

2. Change in pigmentation. Any **change** in skin color or **pigmentation**?

- A generalized color change (all over) or localized?

Hypopigmentation (loss of color); hyperpigmentation (increase in color).
Generalized change suggests systemic illness: pallor, jaundice, cyanosis.

3. Change in mole. Any **change in a mole:** color, size, shape, sudden appearance of tenderness, bleeding, itching?
- Any "sores" that do not heal?

Signs suggest neoplasm in pigmented nevus. May be unaware of change in nevus on back or buttocks that he or she cannot see.

4. Excessive dryness or moisture. Any change in the feel of your skin: temperature, **moisture**, texture?
- Any excess **dryness?** Is it seasonal or constant?

Seborrhea—Oily.
Xerosis—Dry.

5. Pruritus. Any skin itching? Is it mild (prickling, tingling) or intense (intolerable)?
- Does it awaken you from sleep?

- Where is the itching? When did it start?

- Any other skin pain or soreness? Where?

Pruritus is the most common skin symptom; occurs with dry skin, aging, drug reactions, allergy, obstructive jaundice, uremia, lice.
Presence or absence of pruritus helps diagnosis. Scratching causes excoriation of primary lesion.

6. Excessive bruising. Any excess **bruising?** Where on the body?
- How did this happen?
- How long have you had it?

Multiple cuts and bruises, bruises in various stages of healing, bruises above knees and elbows, and illogical explanation—consider physical abuse. Frequent falls may be caused by dizziness of neurologic or cardiovascular origin. Frequent minor trauma may be a side effect of alcoholism or other drug abuse.

7. Rash or lesion. Any skin **rash** or **lesion**?
- Onset. When did you first notice it?

- Location. Where did it start?

- Where did it spread?
- Character or quality. Describe the color.
- Is it raised or flat? Any crust, odor? Does it feel tender, warm?
- Duration. How long have you had it?
- Setting. Anyone at home or work with a similar rash? Have you been camping, acquired a new pet, tried a new food, drug? Does the rash seem to come with stress?
- Alleviating and aggravating factors. What home care have you tried? Bath, lotions, heat? Do they help or make it worse?
- Associated symptoms. Any itching, fever?
- What do you think rash/lesion means?

- Coping strategies. How has rash/lesion affected your self-care, hygiene, ability to function at work/home/socially?

- Any new or increased stress in your life?

Rashes are a common cause of seeking health care. A careful history is important; it may predict the type of lesion you will see in the examination and its cause.
Identify the primary site; it may give clue to cause.
Migration pattern, evolution.

Identify new or relevant exposure, any household or social contacts with similar symptoms.
Myriad over-the-counter remedies are available. People try them and seek professional help only when they do not work.
Assess person's perception of cause: fear of cancer, tickborne illnesses, or sexually transmitted infections.
Assess effectiveness of coping strategies. Chronic skin diseases may increase risk for loss of self-esteem, social isolation, and anxiety.
Stress can exacerbate chronic skin illness.

Subjective Data

8. **Medications.** Which **medications** do you take?
   • Prescription and over-the-counter?
   • Recent change?

   Drugs may cause allergic skin eruption: aspirin, antibiotics, barbiturates, some tonics. Drugs may increase sunlight sensitivity and give burn response: sulfonamides, thiazide diuretics, oral hypoglycemic agents, and tetracycline. Drugs can cause hyperpigmentation: antimalarials, antineoplastic agents, hormones, metals, and tetracycline.

   • How long on medication?

   Even after a long time on medication, a person may develop sensitivity.

9. **Hair loss.** Any recent **hair loss?**
   • A gradual or sudden onset? Symmetric? Associated with fever, illness, increased stress?

   Alopecia is a significant loss. A full head of hair equates with vitality in many cultures. If treated as a trivial problem, the person may seek alternative, unproven methods of treatment.

   • Any unusual hair growth?
   • Any recent change in texture, appearance?

   Hirsutism is shaggy or excessive hair.

10. **Change in nails.** Any **change in nails:** shape, color, brittleness? Do you tend to bite or chew nails?

11. **Environmental or occupational hazards.** Any **environmental** or **occupational** hazards?
    • With your occupation such as dyes, toxic chemicals, radiation?
    • How about hobbies? Do you perform any household or furniture repair work?
    • How much sun exposure do you get from outdoor work, leisure activities, sunbathing, tanning salons?

    Majority of skin neoplasms result from occupational or environmental agents.

    People at risk: outdoor sports enthusiasts, farmers, sailors, outdoor workers; also creosote workers, roofers, coal workers.

    Unprotected sun exposure accelerates aging and produces lesions. At more risk: light-skinned people, light eye and hair color, freckles, and those regularly in sun.

    • Recently been bitten by insect: bee, tick, mosquito?

    Identify contactants that produce lesions or contact dermatitis.

    • Any recent exposure to plants, animals in yard work, camping?

    Tell people with chronic recurrent urticaria (hives) to keep diary of meals and environment to identify precipitating factors.

12. **Patient-centered care.** What do you do to care for your skin, hair, nails? Which cosmetics, soaps, chemicals do you use?
    • Clip cuticles on nails, use adhesive for false fingernails?

    Assess **self-care** and influence on self-concept—may be important with the media emphasis in this society on high norms of beauty. Many over-the-counter remedies are costly and exacerbate skin problems.

    • If you have allergies, how do you control your environment to minimize exposure?
    • Do you perform a skin self-examination?

Additional History for Infants and Children

1. Does the child have any birthmarks?

2. Was there any change in skin color as a newborn?
   • Any jaundice? Which day after birth?
   • Any cyanosis? What were the circumstances?

   Physiologic jaundice, see p. 218.

Examiner Asks	Rationale
3. Have you noted any rash or sores? What seems to bring it on? • Have you introduced a new food or formula? When? Does your child eat chocolate, cow's milk, eggs?	Generalized rash—consider allergic reaction to new food. Irritability and general fussiness may indicate the presence of pruritus.
4. Does the child have any diaper rash? How do you care for this? How do you wash diapers? How often do you change diapers? How do you clean skin?	Occlusive diapers or infrequent changing may cause rash. Infant may be allergic to certain detergent or disposable wipes.
5. Does the child have any burns or bruises? Where? How did it happen?	A careful history can distinguish expected childhood bumps and bruises from any lesion that indicates child abuse or neglect: cigarette burns; excessive bruising, especially above knees or elbows; linear whip marks. With abuse the history often does not coincide with the physical appearance and location of lesion.
6. Has the child had any exposure to contagious skin conditions: scabies, impetigo, lice? Or to communicable diseases: measles, chickenpox, scarlet fever? Or to toxic plants: poison ivy? • Are the child's vaccinations up-to-date?	
7. Does the child have any habits or habitual movements such as nail-biting, twisting hair, rubbing head on mattress?	
8. Which steps are taken to protect the child from sun exposure? What about sunscreens and sunblocks? How do you treat sunburn?	Excessive sun exposure, especially severe or blistering sunburns in childhood, increases risk for melanoma in later life.[24]

Additional History for the Adolescent

1. Have you noticed any skin problems such as pimples, blackheads? • How long have you had them? • How do you treat them? • How do you feel about it?	Over 90% of males and 80% of females will have acne by age 21[43]; the psychological effect is more significant than the physical effect. Self-treatment is common. Causes are increased sebum production and epithelial cells that do not desquamate normally.[43]

Additional History for the Aging Adult

1. Which changes have you noticed in your skin in the past few years?	Assess impact of aging on self-concept. Normal aging changes may cause distress. Many "aging" changes, including skin cancers, are the result of chronic sun damage.
2. Any delay in wound healing? • Any skin itching?	Pruritus is common with aging. Consider side effects of medicine or systemic disease (e.g., liver or kidney disease, cancer, lymphoma), but senile pruritus is usually caused by dry skin (**xerosis**). It is exacerbated by too-frequent bathing or use of soap. Scratching with dirty, jagged fingernails produces excoriations.

Objective Data

Examiner Asks	Rationale
3. Any other skin pain?	Some diseases such as herpes zoster (shingles) produce more intense sensations of pain, itching in aging people. Other diseases (e.g., diabetes) may reduce pain sensation in extremities. In addition, some aging people tolerate chronic pain as "part of growing old" and hesitate to "complain."
4. Any change in feet, toenails? Any bunions? Is it possible to wear shoes?	Some aging people cannot reach down to their feet to give self-care.
5. Have you had any falls this year? How many?	Multiple bruises, trauma from falls.
6. Any history of diabetes, peripheral vascular disease?	Risk for skin lesions in feet or ankles.
7. What do you do to care for your skin?	A bland lotion is important to retain moisture in aging skin. Dermatitis may ensue from certain cosmetics, creams, ointments, and dyes applied to achieve a youthful appearance. Aging skin has a delayed inflammatory response when exposed to irritants. If the person is not alerted by warning signs (e.g., pruritus, redness), exposure may continue, and dermatitis may ensue.

OBJECTIVE DATA

PREPARATION

Try to control external variables that change skin color and confuse your findings (Table 12-1).

Learn to consciously attend to skin characteristics. You grow so accustomed to seeing the skin that you are likely to ignore it as you assess the organ systems underneath. Yet the skin holds information about body circulation, nutritional status, signs of systemic diseases, and topical data on the integument itself.

Know the person's normal skin coloring. Baseline knowledge is important to assess color or pigment changes. If this is the first time you are examining the person, ask about his or her usual skin color and any self-monitoring practices.

The Complete Physical Examination. Although it is presented alone in this chapter, skin assessment is integrated throughout the complete examination; it is not a separate step. At the beginning of the examination, assessing the person's hands and fingernails is a nonthreatening way to accustom him or her to your touch. As you move through the examination, scrutinize the outer skin surface first before you concentrate on the underlying structures. Separate intertriginous areas (areas with skinfolds) such as under large breasts, obese abdomen, and the groin and inspect them thoroughly. These areas are dark, warm, and moist and provide the perfect conditions for irritation or infection. Finally always remove the person's socks and inspect the feet, the toenails, and the folds between the toes.

EQUIPMENT NEEDED

Strong direct lighting (natural daylight is ideal to evaluate skin characteristics, but halogen light will suffice)
Small centimeter ruler
Penlight
Gloves
Needed for special procedures:
Wood's light (filtered UV light)
Magnifying glass for minute lesions

TABLE 12-1	**External Variables Influencing Skin Color**				
VARIABLE		**CAUSES**		**MISLEADING OUTCOME**	
Emotions					
Fear, anger	→	Peripheral vasoconstriction	→	False pallor	
Embarrassment	→	Flushing in face and neck	→	False erythema	
Environment					
Hot room	→	Vasodilation	→	False erythema	
Chilly or air-conditioned room	→	Vasoconstriction	→	False pallor, coolness	
Cigarette smoking	→	Vasoconstriction	→	False pallor	
Physical					
Prolonged elevation	→	Decreased arterial perfusion	→	Pallor, coolness	
Dependent position	→	Venous pooling	→	Redness, warmth, distended veins	
Immobilization, prolonged inactivity	→	Slowed circulation	→	Pallor, coolness, pale nail beds, prolonged capillary filling time	

PREPARATION

The Regional Examination. Help the person remove clothing and assess the skin as one entity. Stand back at first to get an overall impression; this helps reveal distribution patterns. Then inspect lesions carefully. With a skin rash, check all areas of the body because the person cannot see some locations. Inspect mucous membranes, too, because some disorders have characteristic lesions here.

EQUIPMENT NEEDED

Normal Range of Findings

Inspect and Palpate the Skin

Color

General Pigmentation. Observe the skin tone. Normally it is even and consistent with genetic background. It varies from pinkish tan to ruddy dark tan or from light to dark brown and may have yellow or olive overtones. Dark-skinned people normally have areas of lighter pigmentation on the palms, nail beds, and lips (Fig. 12-3, *A*).

12-3 **A,** Even skin tone.

Abnormal Findings

An acquired condition is **vitiligo**, the complete absence of melanin pigment in patchy areas of white or light skin on the face, neck, hands, feet, and body folds and around orifices (Fig. 12-3, *B*). Vitiligo occurs in all people, although dark-skinned people are more severely affected and potentially suffer a greater threat to their body image.

12-3 **B,** Vitiligo. (Lookingbill, 1993.)

<table>
<tr><td>

Normal Range of Findings

</td><td>

Abnormal Findings

</td></tr>
</table>

General pigmentation is darker in sun-exposed areas. Common (benign) pigmented areas also occur:

- **Freckles** (ephelides)—Small, flat macules of brown melanin pigment that occur on sun-exposed skin (Fig. 12-4, *A*).
- **Mole** (nevus)—A clump of melanocytes, tan-to-brown color, flat or raised. Acquired nevi have symmetry, small size (6 mm or less), smooth borders, and single uniform pigmentation. The **junctional nevus** (Fig. 12-4, *B*) is macular only and occurs in children and adolescents. In young adults it progresses to the **compound nevus** (Fig. 12-4, *C*), which is macular and papular. The intradermal nevus (mainly in older age) has nevus cells in only the dermis.

- **Birthmarks**—May be tan to brown in color.

12-4 **A,** Freckles. **B,** Junctional nevus. **C,** Compound nevus. (Hurwitz, 1993.)

Danger signs: abnormal characteristics of pigmented lesions are summarized in the mnemonic **ABCDE**:

Asymmetry (*not* regularly round or oval, two halves of lesion do not look the same)

Border irregularity (notching, scalloping, ragged edges, poorly defined margins)

Color variation (areas of brown, tan, black, blue, red, white, or combination)

Diameter greater than 6 mm (i.e., the size of a pencil eraser), although early melanomas may be diagnosed at a smaller size.

Elevation or **E**volution

Additional symptoms: rapidly changing lesion; a new pigmented lesion; and development of itching, burning, or bleeding in a mole. These signs should raise suspicion of malignant melanoma and warrant referral.

The "ugly duckling" sign is a new technique to help screen for malignant melanoma; the suspicious lesion stands out as looking different compared with neighboring nevi (see Table 12-11, Malignant Skin Lesions, p. 243).[34]

Objective Data

Widespread Color Change. Note any color change over the entire body such as pallor (white), erythema (red), cyanosis (blue), and jaundice (yellow). Note whether the color change is transient and expected or the result of pathology.

In dark-skinned people the amount of normal pigment may mask color changes. Lips and nail beds show some color change, but they vary with the person's skin color and may not always be accurate signs. The more reliable sites are those with the least pigmentation such as under the tongue, the buccal mucosa, the palpebral conjunctiva, and the sclera. See Table 12-2 for specific clues to assessment.

Pallor. When the red-pink tones from the oxygenated hemoglobin in the blood are lost, the skin takes on the color of connective tissue (collagen), which is mostly white. Pallor is common in acute high-stress states such as anxiety or fear because of the powerful peripheral vasoconstriction from sympathetic nervous system stimulation. The skin also looks pale with vasoconstriction from exposure to cold and from cigarette smoking and in the presence of edema.

Look for pallor in dark-skinned people by the absence of the underlying red tones that normally give brown or black skin its luster. The brown-skinned individual shows yellowish-brown color, and the black-skinned person appears

Ashen gray color in dark skin or marked pallor in light skin occurs with anemia, shock, and arterial insufficiency (see Table 12-2, Detecting Color Changes in Light and Dark Skin, p. 226).

The pallor of shock presents with rapid pulse rate, oliguria, apprehension, and restlessness.

Normal Range of Findings

Abnormal Findings

ashen or gray. Generalized pallor can be observed in the mucous membranes, lips, and nail beds. Look for the pallor of anemia in the palpebral conjunctiva and nail beds. Inspect the conjunctiva near the *outer* and inner canthi. The coloration is often lighter near the inner canthus.

Erythema. Intense redness of the skin is from excess blood (hyperemia) in the dilated superficial capillaries. This sign is *expected* with fever, local inflammation, or emotional reactions such as blushing in vascular flush areas (cheeks, neck, and upper chest).

The erythema with fever or localized inflammation has an increased skin temperature from the increased rate of blood flow. Because you cannot see inflammation in dark-skinned people, you must palpate the skin for increased warmth or taut or tightly pulled surfaces that may indicate edema and hardening of deep tissues or blood vessels.

Cyanosis. This is a bluish mottled color from decreased perfusion (Fig. 12-5); the tissues have high levels of deoxygenated blood. This is best seen in the lips, nose, cheeks, ears, and oral mucous membranes and in artificial fluorescent light. Do not confuse cyanosis with the common and normal bluish tone on the lips of dark-skinned persons of Mediterranean origin.

Chronic iron deficiency anemia may show "spoon" nails, with a concave shape. Fatigue, exertional dyspnea, rapid pulse, dizziness, and impaired mental function accompany most severe anemias.

Erythema occurs with polycythemia, venous stasis, carbon monoxide poisoning, and the extravascular presence of red blood cells (petechiae, ecchymosis, hematoma) (see Table 12-2 and Table 12-8, Vascular Lesions, p. 236).

12-5 Cyanosis, especially in fingertips. (Patton, 2012.)

Be aware that cyanosis can be a nonspecific sign. A person who is anemic could have hypoxemia without ever looking blue, because not enough hemoglobin is present (either oxygenated or reduced) to color the skin. On the other hand, a person with polycythemia (an increase in the number of red blood cells) looks ruddy blue at all times and may not necessarily be hypoxemic. This person just cannot fully oxygenate the massive numbers of red blood cells.

Cyanosis is difficult to observe in darkly pigmented people (see Table 12-2). Given that most conditions causing cyanosis also cause decreased oxygenation of the brain, other clinical signs such as changes in level of consciousness and signs of respiratory distress are evident.

Jaundice. A yellowish skin color indicates rising amounts of bilirubin in the blood. Except for physiologic jaundice in the newborn (p. 218), jaundice does not occur normally. It is *first* noted in the junction of the hard and soft palate in the mouth and in the sclera. But do not confuse scleral jaundice with the normal yellow subconjunctival fatty deposits that are common in the outer sclera of dark-skinned persons. The scleral yellow of jaundice extends up to the edge of the iris.

As levels of serum bilirubin rise, jaundice is evident in the skin over the rest of the body. This is best assessed in direct natural daylight. Common calluses on palms and soles often look yellow; do not interpret these as jaundice.

Cyanosis indicates hypoxemia and occurs with shock, cardiac arrest, heart failure, chronic bronchitis, and congenital heart disease.

Jaundice occurs with hepatitis, cirrhosis, sickle-cell disease, transfusion reaction, and hemolytic disease of the newborn.

Light or clay-colored stools and dark golden urine often accompany jaundice in both light- and dark-skinned people.

Normal Range of Findings	Abnormal Findings

Temperature

Note the temperature of your own hands. Then use the backs (dorsa) of your hands to palpate the person and check bilaterally. The skin should be warm, and the temperature should be equal bilaterally; warmth suggests normal circulatory status. Hands and feet may be slightly cooler in a cool environment.

Hypothermia. Generalized coolness may be induced such as in hypothermia used for surgery or high fever. Localized coolness is expected with an immobilized extremity, as when a limb is in a cast or with an intravenous infusion.

> General hypothermia accompanies shock, cardiac arrest.
> Localized hypothermia occurs in peripheral arterial insufficiency and Raynaud disease.
> Hyperthyroidism has an increased metabolic rate, causing warm, moist skin.

Hyperthermia. Generalized hyperthermia occurs with an increased metabolic rate such as in fever or after heavy exercise. A localized area feels hyperthermic with trauma, infection, or sunburn.

Moisture

Perspiration appears normally on the face, hands, axillae, and skinfolds in response to activity, a warm environment, or anxiety. **Diaphoresis,** or profuse perspiration, accompanies an increased metabolic rate such as occurs in heavy activity or fever.

> Diaphoresis occurs with thyrotoxicosis, heart attack, anxiety, or pain.

Look for **dehydration** in the oral mucous membranes. Normally there is none, and the mucous membranes look smooth and moist. Be aware that dark skin may normally look dry and flaky but this does not necessarily indicate systemic dehydration.

> With dehydration, mucous membranes are dry, and lips look parched and cracked. With extreme dryness the skin is fissured, resembling cracks in a dry lake bed.

Texture

Normal skin feels smooth and firm, with an even surface.

> Hyperthyroidism—skin feels smoother and softer, like velvet.
> Hypothyroidism—skin feels rough, dry, and flaky.

Thickness

The epidermis is uniformly thin over most of the body, although thickened callus areas are normal on palms and soles. A callus is a circumscribed overgrowth of epidermis and is an adaptation to excessive pressure from the friction of work and weight bearing.

> Very thin, shiny skin (atrophic) occurs with arterial insufficiency.

Edema

Edema is fluid accumulating in the interstitial spaces; it is not present normally. To check for edema, imprint your thumbs firmly for 3 to 4 seconds against the ankle malleolus or the tibia. Normally the skin surface stays smooth. If your pressure leaves a dent in the skin, "pitting" edema is present. Its presence is graded on a four-point scale:

  1+ Mild pitting; slight indentation; no perceptible swelling of the leg
  2+ Moderate pitting; indentation subsides rapidly
  3+ Deep pitting; indentation remains for a short time; leg looks swollen
  4+ Very deep pitting; indentation lasts a long time; leg is very swollen

This scale is subjective; outcomes vary among examiners (see further content on grading scale in Chapter 20).

Edema masks normal skin color and obscures pathologic conditions such as jaundice or cyanosis because the fluid lies *between* the surface and the pigmented and vascular layers. It makes dark skin look lighter.

> Edema shows in dependent body parts (feet, ankles, and sacral areas), where the skin looks puffy and tight. It makes the hair follicles more prominent; thus you note a pigskin or orange-peel look (called **peau d'orange.**)
> Unilateral edema—consider a local or peripheral cause.
> Bilateral edema or edema that is generalized over the whole body (**anasarca**)—consider a central problem such as heart failure or kidney failure.

Normal Range of Findings	**Abnormal Findings**

Mobility and Turgor

Pinch up a large fold of skin on the anterior chest under the clavicle (Fig. 12-6). Mobility is the ease of skin to rise, and turgor is its ability to return to place promptly when released. This reflects the elasticity of the skin.

12-6

Mobility is decreased with edema.

Poor turgor is evident in severe dehydration or extreme weight loss; the pinched skin recedes slowly or "tents" and stands by itself.

Scleroderma, literally "hard skin," is a chronic connective tissue disorder associated with decreased mobility.

Vascularity or Bruising

Cherry (senile) angiomas are small (1 to 5 mm), smooth, slightly raised bright red dots that commonly appear on the trunk in all adults older than 30 years (Fig. 12-7). They normally increase in size and number with aging and are not significant.

12-7   Cherry angioma.   (Lemmi & Lemmi, 2011.)

Any bruising (contusion) should be consistent with the expected trauma of life. Normally there are no venous dilations or varicosities.

Multiple bruises at different stages of healing and excessive bruises above knees or elbows raise concern about physical abuse (see Table 12-7, Lesions Caused by Trauma or Abuse, p. 234).

Document the presence of any tattoos (a permanent skin design from indelible pigment) on the person's chart. Advise the person that the use of tattoo needles, equipment, and ink of doubtful sterility increases the risk for hepatitis C.

Needle marks from intravenous street drugs may be visible on the antecubital fossae, forearms, or on any available vein.

Objective Data

Normal Range of Findings	Abnormal Findings

Lesions

If any lesions are present, note the:

1. Color.
2. Elevation: flat, raised, or pedunculated.
3. Pattern or shape: the grouping or distinctness of each lesion (e.g., annular, grouped, confluent, linear). The pattern may be characteristic of a certain disease.
4. Size, in centimeters: Use a ruler to measure. Avoid household descriptions such as "quarter size" or "pea size."
5. Location and distribution on body: Is it generalized or localized to area of a specific irritant; around jewelry, watchband, eyes?
6. Any exudate. Note its color and any odor.

Palpate lesions. Wear a glove if you anticipate contact with blood, mucosa, any body fluid, or skin lesion. Roll a nodule between the thumb and index finger to assess depth. Gently scrape a scale to see if it comes off. Note the nature of its base or whether it bleeds when the scale comes off. Note the surrounding skin temperature. However, the erythema associated with rashes is not always accompanied by noticeable increases in skin temperature.

Does the lesion blanch with pressure or stretch? Stretching the area of skin between your thumb and index finger decreases (blanches) the normal underlying red tones, thus providing more contrast and brightening the macules. Red macules from dilated blood vessels *will* blanch momentarily, whereas those from extravasated blood (petechiae) do not. Blanching also helps identify a macular rash in dark-skinned people.

Use a magnifier and light for closer inspection of the lesion (Fig. 12-8). Use a Wood's light (i.e., a UV light filtered through a special glass) to detect fluorescing lesions. With the room darkened, shine the Wood's light on the area.

Abnormal Findings

Lesions are traumatic or pathologic changes in previously normal structures. When a lesion develops on previously unaltered skin, it is **primary**. However, when a lesion changes over time or changes because of scratching or infection, it is **secondary**. Study Table 12-3 for the shapes and Tables 12-4 and 12-5 for the characteristics of primary and secondary skin lesions. The terms used (e.g., *macule, papule*) are helpful to describe any lesion you encounter.

Note the pattern and characteristics of common skin lesions (see Table 12-10, p. 241) and malignant skin lesions (Table 12-11, p. 243).

Under the Wood's light, lesions with blue-green fluorescence indicate fungal infection (e.g., tinea capitis [scalp ringworm]).

12-8

Inspect and Palpate the Hair

Color

Hair color comes from melanin production and may vary from pale blonde to total black. Graying begins as early as the 30s because of reduced melanin production in the follicles. Genetic factors affect the onset of graying.

Normal Range of Findings	Abnormal Findings

Texture

Scalp hair may be fine or thick and may look straight, curly, or kinky. It should look shiny, although this characteristic may be lost with the use of some beauty products such as dyes, rinses, or permanents.

Note dull, coarse, or brittle scalp hair. Gray, scaly, well-defined areas with broken hairs accompany tinea capitis, a ringworm infection found mostly in school-age children (see Table 12-12, Abnormal Conditions of Hair, p. 244).

Distribution

Fine vellus hair coats the body, whereas coarser terminal hairs grow at the eyebrows, eyelashes, and scalp. During puberty distribution conforms to normal male and female patterns. At first coarse curly hairs develop in the pubic area, then in the axillae, and last in the facial area in boys. In the genital area the female pattern is an inverted triangle; the male pattern is an upright triangle with pubic hair extending up to the umbilicus. In Asians body hair may be diminished.

Absent or sparse genital hair suggests endocrine abnormalities.

Hirsutism—excess body hair. In females this forms a male pattern on the face and chest and indicates endocrine abnormalities (see Table 12-12).

Lesions

Separate the hair into sections and lift it, observing the scalp. With a history of itching, inspect the hair behind the ears and in the occipital area as well. All areas should be clean and free of any lesions or pest inhabitants. Many people normally have seborrhea (dandruff), which is indicated by loose white flakes.

Head or pubic lice. Distinguish dandruff from nits (eggs) of lice, which are oval and adherent to hair shaft and cause intense itching (see Table 12-12).

Inspect and Palpate the Nails

Shape and Contour

The nail surface is normally slightly curved or flat, and the posterior and lateral nail folds are smooth and rounded. Nail edges are smooth, rounded, and clean, suggesting adequate self-care.

Jagged nails, bitten to the quick, or traumatized nail folds suggest nervous picking habits.

Chronically dirty nails suggest poor self-care or the chronic staining of some occupations.

Clubbing of nails occurs with congenital cyanotic heart disease, lung cancer, and pulmonary diseases.

The Profile Sign. View the index finger at its profile and note the angle of the nail base; it should be about 160 degrees (Fig. 12-9). The nail base is firm to palpation. Curved nails are a variation of normal with a convex profile. They may look like clubbed nails, but notice that the angle between nail base and nail is normal (i.e., 160 degrees or less).

In early clubbing the angle straightens out to 180 degrees, and the nail base feels spongy to palpation. Then the nail becomes convex as the digit grows (see Late Clubbing, p. 248).

Objective Data

Normal   160°
Curved nail   160° or less
Early clubbing   180°

12-9

TABLE 12-8 Vascular Lesions—cont'd

Purpuric Lesions

Caused by blood flowing out of breaks in the vessels. Red blood cells and blood pigments are deposited in the tissues (extravascular). Difficult to see in dark-skinned people.

◀ Petechiae

Tiny punctate hemorrhages, 1 to 3 mm, round and discrete; dark red, purple, or brown in color. Caused by bleeding from superficial capillaries; will not blanch. May indicate abnormal clotting factors. In dark-skinned people petechiae are best visualized in the areas of lighter melanization (e.g., the abdomen, buttocks, and volar surface of the forearm). When the skin is black or very dark brown, petechiae cannot be seen in the skin.

Most of the diseases that cause bleeding and microembolism formation such as thrombocytopenia, subacute bacterial endocarditis, and other septicemias are characterized by petechiae in the mucous membranes and on the skin. Thus you should inspect for petechiae in the mouth, particularly the buccal mucosa, and in the conjunctivae.

Ecchymosis

A purplish patch resulting from extravasation of blood into the skin, >3 mm in diameter.

Purpura

Confluent and extensive patch of petechiae and ecchymoses; >3 mm, flat, red to purple, macular hemorrhage. Seen in generalized disorders such as thrombocytopenia and scurvy. Also occurs in old age as blood leaks from capillaries in response to minor trauma and diffuses through dermis.

See Illustration Credits for source information.

TABLE 12-9 Common Skin Lesions in Children

Diaper Dermatitis

Red, moist, maculopapular patch with poorly defined borders in diaper area, extending along inguinal and gluteal folds. History of infrequent diaper changes or occlusive coverings. Inflammatory disease caused by skin irritation from ammonia, heat, moisture, occlusive diapers.

Intertrigo (Candidiasis)

Scalding red, moist patches with sharply demarcated borders, some loose scales. Usually in genital area extending along inguinal and gluteal folds. Aggravated by urine, feces, heat, and moisture; the *Candida* fungus infects the superficial skin layers.

Impetigo

Moist, thin-roofed vesicles with thin, erythematous base. Rupture to form thick, honey-colored crusts. Highly contagious bacterial infection of skin; most common in infants and children. Infection can spread to other body areas and other children and adults by direct contact.

Atopic Dermatitis (Eczema)

Erythematous papules and vesicles, with weeping, oozing, and crusts. Lesions usually on scalp, forehead, cheeks, forearms and wrists, elbows, backs of knees. Paroxysmal and severe pruritus. Family history of allergies.

Continued

TABLE 12-9 Common Skin Lesions in Children—cont'd

Measles (Rubeola) in Dark Skin

Measles (Rubeola) in Light Skin

Red-purple maculopapular blotchy rash in dark skin *(on left)* and light skin *(on right)* appears on third or fourth day of illness. Rash appears first behind ears and spreads over face and then over neck, trunk, arms, and legs; looks "coppery" and does not blanch. Also characterized by Koplik spots in mouth—bluish white, red-based elevations of 1 to 3 mm (see Table 16-4, p. 380). Laxity in vaccination has repatriated measles in the United States.

German Measles (Rubella)

Pink, papular rash (similar to measles but paler) first appears on face, then spreads. Distinguished from measles by presence of neck lymphadenopathy and absence of Koplik spots.

Chickenpox (Varicella)

Small, tight vesicles first appear on trunk and spread to face, arms, and legs (not palms or soles). Shiny vesicles on an erythematous base are commonly described as the "dewdrop on a rose petal." Vesicles erupt in succeeding crops over several days; they become pustules and then crusts. Intensely pruritic.

TABLE 12-10 Common Skin Lesions

Primary Contact Dermatitis

Local inflammatory reaction to an irritant in the environment or an allergy. Characteristic location of lesions often gives clue. Often erythema shows first, followed by swelling, wheals (or urticaria), or maculopapular vesicles, scales. Frequently accompanied by intense pruritus. Example here: poison ivy.

Allergic Drug Reaction

Erythematous and symmetric rash, usually generalized. Some drugs produce urticarial rash or vesicles and bullae. History of drug ingestion.

Tinea Corporis (Ringworm of the Body)

Scales—hyperpigmented in whites, depigmented in dark-skinned people; on chest, abdomen, back of arms forming multiple circular lesions with clear centers.

Tinea Pedis (Ringworm of the Foot)

"Athlete's foot," a fungal infection, first appears as small vesicles between toes, on sides of feet, and on soles; grows scaly and hard. Found in chronically warm, moist feet: children after gymnasium activities, athletes, aging adults who cannot dry their feet well.

Continued

TABLE 12-10   Common Skin Lesions—cont'd

Labial Herpes Simplex (Cold Sores)

Herpes simplex virus (HSV) infection has a prodrome of skin tingling and sensitivity. Lesion then erupts with tight vesicles followed by pustules and produces acute gingivostomatitis with many shallow, painful ulcers. Common location is upper lip; also in oral mucosa and tongue.

Tinea Versicolor

Fine, scaling, round patches of pink, tan, or white (thus the name) that do not tan in sunlight, caused by a superficial fungal infection. Usual distribution is on neck, trunk, and upper arms—a short-sleeved turtleneck sweater area. Most common in otherwise healthy young adults. Responds to oral antifungal medication.

Herpes Zoster (Shingles)

Small, grouped vesicles emerge along route of cutaneous sensory nerve, then pustules, then crusts. Caused by the varicella zoster virus (VZV), a reactivation of the dormant virus of chickenpox. Acute appearance, unilateral, does not cross midline. Commonly on trunk; can be anywhere. If on ophthalmic branch of cranial nerve V, it poses risk to eye. Most common in adults older than 50 years. Pain is often severe and long lasting in aging adults, called *postherpetic neuralgia.*

    Note: Be observant! The photo above is *not* genital herpes. This is herpes zoster with a linear lesion on only one side.

Erythema Migrans of Lyme Disease

Lyme disease (LD) is not fatal but may have serious arthritic, cardiac, or neurologic sequelae. It is caused by a spirochete bacterium carried by the black or dark brown deer tick. Deer ticks are common in the Northeast, upper Midwest, and California (with cases occurring in people who spend time outdoors) in May through September.

    The first stage (early localized LD) has the distinctive bull's eye, red macular or papular rash (shown above) in 50% of cases. The rash radiates from the site of the tick bite (5 cm or larger) with some central clearing; it is usually located in axillae, midriff, inguina, or behind knees, with regional lymphadenopathy. Rash fades in 4 weeks; untreated individual then may have disseminated disease with fatigue, anorexia, fever, chills, or joint or muscle aches. Antibiotic treatment shortens symptoms and decreases risk for sequelae.

TABLE 12-10   Common Skin Lesions—cont'd

◀ **Psoriasis**

Scaly, erythematous patch, with silvery scales on top. Usually on scalp, outside of elbows and knees, low back, and anogenital area.

See Illustration Credits for source information.

TABLE 12-11   Malignant Skin Lesions

The link between ultraviolet (UV) radiation and skin cancer is well known; the UV radiation in sunlight promotes all three forms of skin cancer shown below. More than half a person's lifetime sun damage occurs before adulthood.

Basal Cell Carcinoma ▶

Usually starts as a skin-colored papule (may be deeply pigmented) with a pearly translucent top and overlying telangiectasia (broken blood vessel). Then develops rounded, pearly borders with central red ulcer or looks like large open pore with central yellowing. Most common form of skin cancer; slow but inexorable growth. Basal cell cancers occur on sun-exposed areas of face, ears, scalp, shoulders.

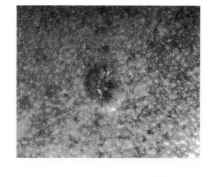

Squamous Cell Carcinoma ▶

Squamous cell cancers arise from actinic keratoses or de novo. Erythematous scaly patch with sharp margins, 1 cm or more. Develops central ulcer and surrounding erythema. Usually on hands or head, areas exposed to UV radiation; *at right*, on habitually sun-exposed bald scalp. Less common than basal cell carcinoma but grows rapidly.

Continued

Abnormal Findings

TABLE 12-11   Malignant Skin Lesions—cont'd

Malignant Melanoma

Metastatic Malignant Melanoma

Potentially lethal lesions that are the malignant transformation of melanocytes.[36] May arise from preexisting nevus or de novo. Usually brown; can be tan, black, pink-red, purple, or mixed pigmentation. Often irregular or notched borders. May have scaling, flaking, oozing texture. Common locations: trunk and back; legs in women; and palms, soles of feet, and nails in Blacks. Risk factors are UV radiation from sun exposure and indoor tanning and family history. Rates are increasing in White men over 55 years and White women of all ages. Melanoma is the most common cancer in women ages 25-29 years and 2nd most common (after breast cancer) in women ages 30-34 years.[36]

TABLE 12-12   Abnormal Conditions of Hair

AIDS-related Kaposi Sarcoma: Patch stage

Kaposi sarcoma (KS) is a vascular tumor and is the most common tumor in HIV-infected persons. Considered an AIDS-defining illness, KS can occur at any stage of HIV infection. Here multiple patch-stage early lesions are faint pink on the temple and beard area. They easily could be mistaken for bruises or nevi and be ignored.

Toxic Alopecia

Patchy, asymmetric balding that accompanies severe illness or use of chemotherapy in which growing hairs are lost and resting hairs are spared. Regrowth occurs after illness or discontinuation of toxin.

TABLE 12-12   Abnormal Conditions of Hair—cont'd

◀ Tinea Capitis (Scalp Ringworm)

Rounded, patchy hair loss on scalp, leaving broken-off hairs, pustules, and scales on skin. Caused by fungal infection; lesions may fluoresce blue-green under Wood's light. Usually seen in children and farmers; highly contagious; may be transmitted by another person, by domestic animals, or from soil.

◀ Alopecia Areata

Sudden appearance of a sharply circumscribed, round or oval balding patch, usually with smooth, soft, hairless skin underneath. Unknown cause; when limited to a few patches, person usually has complete regrowth.

◀ Traumatic Alopecia: Traction Alopecia

Linear or oval patch of hair loss along hair line, a part, or scattered distribution; caused by trauma from hair rollers, tight braiding, tight ponytail, barrettes. In Black girls up to 15 years of age, hair care practices of cornrows and using chemical relaxers are associated with traction alopecia, perhaps because cornrows pull the hair at the roots and chemical relaxers weaken the strength of the hair shaft.[44a]

Continued

TABLE 12-12   Abnormal Conditions of Hair—cont'd

Seborrheic Dermatitis (Cradle Cap)

Thick, yellow-to-white, greasy, adherent scales with mild erythema on scalp and forehead; very common in early infancy. Resembles eczema lesions, except that cradle cap is distinguished by absence of pruritus, presence of "greasy" yellow-pink lesions, and negative family history of allergy.

Folliculitis ("razor bumps")

Superficial inflammatory infection of hair follicles. Multiple pustules, "whiteheads," with hair visible at center and erythematous base. Usually involves face and neck and is common in Black men (45%-85% prevalence) and Hispanic men. Occurs after shaving when growing out hairs curl in on themselves and pierce the skin, making a foreign-body inflammatory reaction.[16]

Pediculosis Capitis (Head Lice)

History includes intense itching of the scalp, especially the occiput. The nits (eggs) of lice are easier to see in the occipital area and around the ears, appearing as 2- to 3-mm oval translucent bodies, adherent to the hair shafts. Common among school-age children. Over-the-counter pediculicide shampoos are available; however, nit removal by daily combing of wet hair with a fine-tooth metal comb is especially important.

Trichotillomania

Traumatic self-induced hair loss usually the result of compulsive twisting or plucking. Forms irregularly shaped patch, with broken-off, stublike hairs of varying lengths; person is never completely bald. Occurs as child rubs or twists area absently while falling asleep, reading, or watching television. In adults it can be automatic or associated with a compulsive disorder, leading to distress and social problems.

TABLE 12-12 Abnormal Conditions of Hair—cont'd

Hirsutism

Excess body hair in females forming a male sexual pattern (upper lip, face, chest, abdomen, arms, legs); caused by endocrine or metabolic dysfunction, or occasionally is idiopathic.

Furuncle and Abscess

Red, swollen, hard, tender, pus-filled lesion caused by acute, localized bacterial (usually staphylococcal) infection; usually on back of neck, buttocks, occasionally on wrists or ankles. Furuncles are caused by infected hair follicles, whereas abscesses are caused by traumatic introduction of bacteria into skin. Abscesses are usually larger and deeper than furuncles.

See Illustration Credits for source information.

TABLE 12-13 Abnormal Conditions of the Nails

Scabies

An intensely pruritic contagion caused by the scabies mite. Mites form a linear or curved elevated burrow on the fingers, web spaces of hands, and wrists. Other family members are usually infected. The patient cannot stop scratching.

Paronychia

Red, swollen, tender inflammation of the nail folds. Acute paronychia is usually a bacterial infection with pus in the proximal nail fold, pain, and throbbing. Chronic paronychia is most often a fungal infection from a break in the cuticle in those who perform "wet" work.

Continued

TABLE 12-13 Abnormal Conditions of the Nails—cont'd

Beau Line

Transverse furrow or groove. A depression across the nail that extends down to the nail bed. Occurs with any trauma that temporarily impairs nail formation such as acute illness, toxic reaction, or local trauma. Dent appears first at cuticle and moves forward as nail grows.

Splinter Hemorrhages

Red-brown linear streaks from damage to nail bed capillaries. They occur with systemic diseases (vasculitis) and with trauma or sports-related injuries (soccer).

Onychomycosis

This is a slow, persistent fungal infection of fingernails and, more often, toenails, common in older adults. Fungus causes change in color (green where nail plate separated from bed), texture, and thickness, with nail crumbling or breaking and loosening of the nail plate, usually beginning at the distal edge and progressing proximally.

Late Clubbing

Inner edge of nail elevates; nail bed angle is greater than 180 degrees. Distal phalanx looks rounder, wider, and shiny. Clubbing may result from increased platelet-derived growth factor.[38] Diseases that disrupt normal pulmonary circulation (chronic lung inflammation, bronchial tumors, heart defects with right-to-left shunts) cause fragmented platelets to become trapped in the fingertip vasculature, releasing platelet-derived growth factor and promoting growth of vessels. Clubbing usually develops slowly over years; if the primary disease is treated, clubbing can reverse.

TABLE 12-13   Abnormal Conditions of the Nails—cont'd

Pitting

Sharply defined pitting and crumbling of nails with distal detachment often occurs with psoriasis.

Habit-Tic Dystrophy

Depression down middle of nail or multiple horizontal ridges, caused by continuous picking of cuticle by another finger of same hand, which causes injury to nail base and nail matrix.

See Illustration Credits for source information.

Summary Checklist: Skin, Hair, and Nails Examination

1. **Inspect the skin:**
   Color
   General pigmentation
   Areas of hypopigmentation or hyperpigmentation
   Abnormal color changes
2. **Palpate the skin:**
   Temperature
   Moisture
   Texture
   Thickness
   Edema
   Mobility and turgor
   Hygiene
   Vascularity or bruising
3. **Note any lesions:**
   Color
   Shape and configuration
   Size
   Location and distribution on body
4. **Inspect and palpate the hair:**
   Texture
   Distribution
   Any scalp lesions
5. **Inspect and palpate the nails:**
   Shape and contour
   Consistency
   Color
6. **Teach skin self-examination**

BIBLIOGRAPHY

1. American Cancer Society (ACS). (2012). *Cancer facts & figures 2012.* No. 500812. Altanta, GA: The Society.
2. Balk, S. J., Fisher, D. E., & Geller, A. C. (2013). Teens and indoor tanning: a cancer prevention opportunity for pediatricians. *Pediatrics, 131*(4), 772-785.
3. Beshara, M. A. (2010). Hidradenitis suppurativa. *Nurse Pract, 35*(5), 25-28.
4. Bower, M. G. (2001). Managing dog, cat, and human bite wounds. *Nurse Pract, 26*(4), 36-47.
5. Reference deleted in proofs.
6. Calianno, C. (2012). Bedbugs (Cimexlectularius). *Nurse Pract, 37*(6), 6-10.
7. Calianno, C., & O'Shea, S. (2013). Herpes zoster in older adults. *Nurse Pract, 38*(8), 10-14.
8. Centers for Disease Control and Prevention. (2012). Sunburn and sun protective behaviors among adults aged 18-29 years—United States, 2000-2010. *MMWR Morb Mortal Wkly Rep, 61*, 317-322.
9. Coenraads, P. J. (2012). Hand eczema. *New Engl J Med, 367*(19), 1829-1837.
10. Cohen, J. I. (2013). Herpes zoster. *New Engl J Med, 369*(3), 255-263.
11. Czerkasij, V. (2013). Skin of color: a basic outline of unique differences. *Nurse Pract, 38*(5), 34-40.
12. Firnhaber, J. M. (2012). Diagnosis and treatment of basal cell and squamous cell carcinoma. *Am Fam Physician, 86*(2), 161-168.
13. Gilhar, A., Etzioni, A., & Paus, R. (2012). Alopecia areata. *New Engl J Med, 366*(16), 1515-1525.
14. Gordon, R. (2014). Skin cancer: increasing awareness and screening in primary care. *Nurse Pract, 39*(5), 49-54.
15. Kennedy, B. S., Bedard, B., Younge, M., et al. (2012). Outbreak of *Mycobacterium chelonae* infection associated with tattoo ink. *New Engl J Med, 367*(11), 1020-1024.
16. Kundu, R. V., & Patterson, S. (2013). Dermatologic conditions in skin of color: Part I. Special considerations for common

skin disorders. *Am Fam Physician, 87*(12), 850-856. Part II. Disorders occurring predominantly in skin of color. *Am Fam Physician, 87*(12), 859-865.

17. Le Cleach, L., & Chosidow, O. (2012). Lichen planus. *New Engl J Med, 366*(8), 723-732.

18. Lin, J. S., Eder, M., Weinmann, S., et al. (2011). *Behavioral counseling to prevent skin cancer.* Evidence Synthesis No. 82. AHRQ Publication No. 11-05152-EF-1. Rockville, MD: Agency for Healthcare Research and Quality.

19. Reference deleted in proofs.

20. Madan, V., Lear, J. T., & Szeimies, R. M. (2010). Non-melanoma skin cancer. *Lancet, 375*(9715), 673-685.

20a. Mayo, T.T., Cantrell, W. (2014). Putting onychomycosis under the microscope. *Nurse Pract, 39*(5), 8-11.

21. McMullen, S. M., & Patrick, W. (2013). Cyanosis. *Am J Med, 126*(3), 210-212.

22. Mendyk, M. K. (2008). Community-associated MRSA. *Nurse Pract, 33*(3), 26-32.

23. Miteva, M., & Tosti, A. (2012). Dermatoscopy of hair shaft disorders. *J Am Acad Dermatol, 68*(3), 473-481.

24. Moyer, V. A. (2012). Behavioral counseling to prevent skin cancer: US Preventive Services Task Force recommendation statement. *Ann Intern Med, 157*(1), 59-65.

25. Mulholland, E. K., Griffiths, U. K., & Biellik, R. (2012). Measles in the 21st century. *New Engl J Med, 366*(19), 1755-7.

26. Napierkowski, D. (2013). Uncovering common bacterial skin infections. *Nurse Pract, 38*(3), 30-37.

27. Nash, K. R., & Sheridan, D. J. (2009). Can one accurately date a bruise? State of the science. *J Forensic Nurs, 5,* 31-37.

28. National Pressure Ulcer Advisory Panel (NPUAP). (2013). *Pressure ulcer staging.* Available at www.npaup.org/pr2.htm.

29. Nevas, J. (2012). Tinea versicolor. *Nurse Pract, 37*(1), 11-13.

30. Richert, B., & André, J. (2011). Nail disorders in children. *Am J Clin Dermatol, 12*(2), 101-112.

31. Roebuck, H. (2011). Treatment options for rosacea with concomitant conditions. *Nurse Pract, 36*(2), 25-31.

32. Rucker Wright, D., Gathers, R., Kapke, A., et al. (2011). Hair care practices and their association with scalp and hair disorders in African American girls. *J Am Acad Dermatol, 64*(2), 253-262.

32a. Ruiz-Narvaez, E. A., Fraser, P. A., Palmer, J. R., et al. (2011). MHC region and risk of systemic lupus erythematosus in African American women. *Human Genetics, 130*(6), 807-815.

33. Schmidt, J. A. (2011). Seborrheic dermatitis. *Nurse Pract, 36*(8), 32-37.

34. Scope, A., & Marghoob, A. A. (2014). *The "ugly duckling" sign: an early melanoma recognition tool for clinicians and the public.* Available at http://www.skincancer.org/skin-cancer-information/melanoma/melanoma-warning-signs-and-images/the-ugly-duckling-sign.

35. Shah, K. N., & Rubin, A. I. (2012). Nail disorders as signs of pediatric systemic disease. *Curr Probl Pediatr Adolesc Health Care, 42*(8), 204-211.

35a. Shapiro, E. D. (2014). Lyme disease. *N Engl J Med, 370*(18), 1724-1730.

36. Shenenberger, D. W. (2012). Cutaneous malignant melanoma. *Am Fam Physician, 85*(2), 161-168.

37. Specter, M. (2013, July 1). The Lyme wars. *The New Yorker,* 24-29.

38. Spicknall, K. E., Zirwas, M. J., & English, J. C. (2005). Clubbing: an update on diagnosis, differential diagnosis, pathophysiology, and clinical relevance. *J Am Acad Dermatol, 52,* 1020-1028.

39. Stern, R. S. (2012). Exanthematous drug eruptions. *New Engl J Med, 366*(26), 2492-2501.

40. Reference deleted in proofs.

41. van Rijswijk, L. (2013). Measuring wounds to improve outcomes. *Am J Nurs, 113*(8), 60-61.

42. Weinstein, P. K. (2012). The face of lupus. *Nurse Pract, 37*(12), 38-45.

43. Well, D. (2013). Acne vulgaris: a review of causes and treatment options. *Nurse Pract, 38*(10), 22-31.

43a. Wilson, D. D. (2014). Herpes zoster. *Nurse Pract, 39*(5), 30-37.

44. Winland-Brown, J. E., & Allen, S. (2010). Foreign bodies in the skin. *Nurse Pract, 35*(6), 43-47.

44a. Wright, D. R., Gathers, R., Kapke, A., et al. (2011). Hair care practices and their association with scalp and hair disorders in African American girls. *J Am Acad Dermatol, 64,* 253-262.

45. Yosipovitch, G. & Bernhard, J. D. (2013).Chronic pruritus. *New Engl J Med, 368*(17), 1625-1634.

CHAPTER 13

Head, Face, and Neck, Including Regional Lymphatics

http://evolve.elsevier.com/Jarvis/

STRUCTURE AND FUNCTION

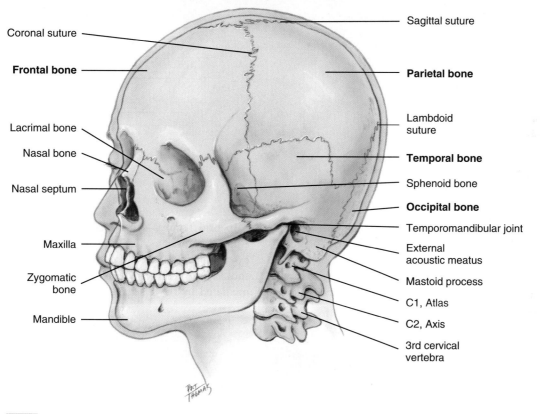

Coronal suture

Frontal bone

Lacrimal bone

Nasal bone

Nasal septum

Maxilla

Zygomatic bone

Mandible

Sagittal suture

Parietal bone

Lambdoid suture

Temporal bone

Sphenoid bone

Occipital bone

Temporomandibular joint

External acoustic meatus

Mastoid process

C1, Atlas

C2, Axis

3rd cervical vertebra

13-1

THE HEAD

The **skull** is a rigid bony box that protects the brain and special sense organs, and it includes the bones of the cranium and the face (Fig. 13-1). Note the location of these **cranial bones:** frontal, parietal, occipital, and temporal. Use these names to describe any of your clinical findings in the corresponding areas.

The adjacent cranial bones unite at meshed immovable joints called the **sutures.** The bones are not firmly joined at birth; this allows for the mobility and change in shape needed for the birth process. The sutures gradually ossify during early childhood. The **coronal** suture *crowns* the head from ear to ear at the union of the frontal and parietal bones. The **sagittal**

suture *separates* the head lengthwise between the two parietal bones. The **lambdoid** suture separates the parietal bones crosswise from the occipital bone.

The 14 **facial bones** also articulate at sutures (note the nasal bone, zygomatic bone, and maxilla), except for the mandible (the lower jaw). It moves up, down, and sideways from the temporomandibular joint, which is anterior to each ear.

The cranium is supported by the cervical vertebrae: C1, the "atlas"; C2, the "axis"; and down to C7. The C7 vertebra has a long spinous process that is palpable when the head is flexed. Feel this useful landmark, the **vertebra prominens,** on your own neck.

The human **face** has many appearances and expressions that reflect mood. The expressions are formed by the facial

251

Frontalis

Galea aponeurotica

Temporalis

Orbicularis oculi

Palpebral fissure

Nasolabial fold

Orbicularis oris

Zygomaticus

Masseter

Buccinator

Sternomastoid

Trapezius

13-2 Facial muscles.

muscles (Fig. 13-2), which are mediated by cranial nerve VII, the facial nerve. Facial muscle function is symmetric bilaterally, except for an occasional quirk or wry expression.

Facial structures are symmetric; the eyebrows, eyes, ears, nose, and mouth appear about the same on both sides. The palpebral fissures—the openings between the eyelids—are equal bilaterally. Also the nasolabial folds—the creases extending from the nose to each corner of the mouth— should look symmetric. Facial sensations of pain or touch are mediated by the 3 sensory branches of cranial nerve V, the

Sternomastoid muscle

Internal jugular vein

External jugular vein

Clavicle

Temporal artery

Parotid gland

Submandibular gland

Sublingual gland

External carotid artery

Internal carotid artery

Common carotid artery

13-3

Sternomastoid muscle

Trapezius muscle

Omohyoid muscle

Clavicle

Anterior triangle

Posterior triangle

13-4

trigeminal nerve. (Testing for sensory function is described in Chapter 23.)

Two pairs of **salivary glands** are accessible to examination on the face (Fig. 13-3). The **parotid** glands are in the cheeks over the mandible, anterior to and below the ear. They are the largest of the salivary glands but are not normally palpable. The **submandibular** glands are beneath the mandible at the angle of the jaw. A third pair, the **sublingual** glands, lie in the floor of the mouth. (Salivary gland function follows in Chapter 16.) The **temporal artery** lies superior to the temporalis muscle; its pulsation is palpable anterior to the ear.

THE NECK

The **neck** is delimited by the base of the skull and inferior border of the mandible above and by the manubrium sterni, the clavicle, the first rib, and the first thoracic vertebra below. Think of the neck as a *conduit* for the passage of many structures that are lying in close proximity: blood vessels, muscles, nerves, lymphatics, and viscera of the respiratory and digestive systems. Blood vessels include the common and internal carotid arteries and their associated veins (see Fig. 13-3). The internal carotid artery branches off the common carotid and runs inward and upward to supply the brain; the external carotid artery supplies the face, salivary glands, and superficial temporal area. The carotid artery and internal jugular vein lie beneath the sternomastoid muscle. The external jugular vein runs diagonally across the sternomastoid muscle. (See assessment of the neck vessels in Chapter 19.)

The major **neck muscles** are the **sternomastoid** and **trapezius** (Fig. 13-4); they are innervated by cranial nerve

XI, the spinal accessory. The sternomastoid muscle arises from the sternum and the clavicle and extends diagonally across the neck to the mastoid process behind the ear. It accomplishes head rotation and flexion. The two trapezius muscles on the upper back arise from the occipital bone and the vertebrae and extend fanning out to the scapula and clavicle. The trapezius muscles move the shoulders and extend and turn the head.

The sternomastoid muscle divides each side of the neck into two triangles. The **anterior triangle** lies in front, between the sternomastoid and the midline of the body, with its base up along the lower border of the mandible and its apex down at the suprasternal notch. The **posterior triangle** is behind the sternomastoid muscle, with the trapezius muscle on the other side and its base along the clavicle below. It contains the posterior belly of the omohyoid muscle. These triangles are helpful guidelines when describing findings in the neck.

The **thyroid gland** is an important endocrine gland with a rich blood supply. It straddles the trachea in the middle of the neck (Fig. 13-5). This highly vascular endocrine gland synthesizes and secretes thyroxine (T_4) and triiodothyronine (T_3), hormones that stimulate the rate of cellular metabolism. The gland has two lobes, both conical in shape, each curving posteriorly between the trachea and the sternomastoid muscle. The lobes are connected in the middle by a thin isthmus lying over the second and third tracheal rings.

Just above the thyroid isthmus, within about 1 cm, is the **cricoid** cartilage or upper tracheal ring. The **thyroid** cartilage is above that, with a small, palpable notch in its upper edge. This is the prominent "Adam's apple" in males. The highest is the **hyoid** bone, palpated high in the neck at the level of the floor of the mouth.

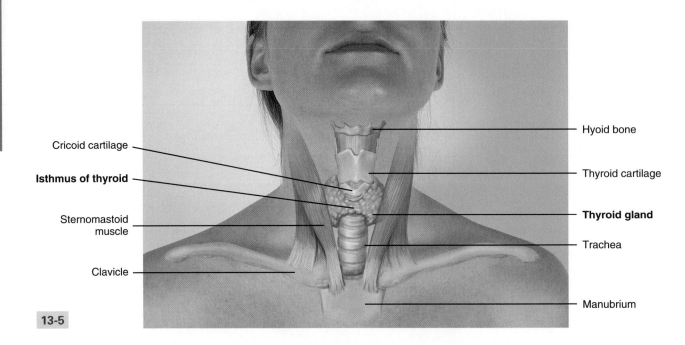

Cricoid cartilage

Isthmus of thyroid

Sternomastoid muscle

Clavicle

Hyoid bone

Thyroid cartilage

Thyroid gland

Trachea

Manubrium

13-5

LYMPHATICS

The lymphatic system is developed more fully in Chapter 20. However, the head and neck have a rich supply of 60 to 70 **lymph nodes** (Fig. 13-6). Note that their labels correspond to adjacent structures.

- *Preauricular,* in front of the ear
- *Posterior auricular* (mastoid), superficial to the mastoid process
- *Occipital,* at the base of the skull
- *Submental,* midline, behind the tip of the mandible

- *Submandibular,* halfway between the angle and the tip of the mandible
- *Jugulodigastric (tonsillar),* under the angle of the mandible
- *Superficial cervical,* overlying the sternomastoid muscle
- *Deep cervical,* deep under the sternomastoid muscle
- *Posterior cervical,* in the posterior triangle along the edge of the trapezius muscle
- *Supraclavicular,* just above and behind the clavicle, at the sternomastoid muscle

Posterior auricular

Occipital

Jugulodigastric

Superficial cervical

Posterior cervical

Supraclavicular

Preauricular

Submandibular

Submental

Deep cervical chain

13-6

13-7

You also should be familiar with the direction of the **drainage patterns** of the lymph nodes (Fig. 13-7). When nodes are enlarged, check the area they drain for the source of the problem. Explore the area proximal (upstream) to the enlarged node. All head and neck structures eventually drain into the deep cervical chain.

The lymphatic system is a separate vessel system from the cardiovascular system and a major part of the immune system, whose job it is to detect and eliminate foreign substances from the body. The vessels gather the clear, watery fluid (lymph) from the tissue spaces into the circulation. Lymph nodes are small, oval clusters of lymphatic tissue that are set at intervals along the lymph vessels like beads on a string. The nodes slowly filter the lymph and engulf pathogens, preventing harmful substances from entering the circulation. Nodes are located throughout the body but are accessible to examination only in four areas: head and neck, arms, axillae, and inguinal region. The greatest supply is in the head and neck.

❖ DEVELOPMENTAL COMPETENCE

Infants and Children

The bones of the neonatal skull are separated by sutures and **fontanels,** the spaces where the sutures intersect (Fig. 13-8). These membrane-covered "soft spots" allow for growth of the brain during the 1st year. They gradually ossify; the triangle-shaped posterior fontanel is closed by 1 to 2 months, and the diamond-shaped anterior fontanel closes between 9 months and 2 years.

During the fetal period head growth predominates. Head size is greater than chest circumference at birth. The head size grows during childhood, reaching 90% of its final size when the child is 6 years old. But during infancy, trunk growth predominates, so head size changes in proportion to body height. Facial bones grow at varying rates, especially nasal and jaw bones. In the toddler the mandible and maxilla are small, and the nasal bridge is low; thus the whole face seems small compared with the skull.

Lymphoid tissue is well developed at birth and grows to adult size when the child is 6 years old. The child's lymphatic tissue continues to grow rapidly until age 10 or 11 years, actually exceeding its adult size before puberty. Then the lymphatic tissue slowly atrophies.

In adolescence facial hair appears on boys, first above the lip, then on cheeks and below the lip, and last on the chin. A noticeable enlargement of the thyroid cartilage occurs, and with it the voice deepens.

The Pregnant Woman

The thyroid gland enlarges slightly during pregnancy as a result of hyperplasia of the tissue and increased vascularity.

The Aging Adult

The facial bones and orbits appear more prominent, and the facial skin sags as a result of decreased elasticity, decreased subcutaneous fat, and decreased moisture in the skin. The lower face may look smaller if teeth have been lost.

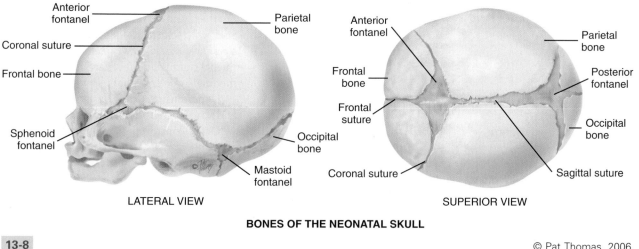

LATERAL VIEW

Anterior fontanel
Coronal suture
Frontal bone
Sphenoid fontanel
Parietal bone
Occipital bone
Mastoid fontanel

SUPERIOR VIEW

Anterior fontanel
Frontal bone
Frontal suture
Coronal suture
Parietal bone
Posterior fontanel
Occipital bone
Sagittal suture

BONES OF THE NEONATAL SKULL

13-8

© Pat Thomas, 2006.

SUBJECTIVE DATA

1. Headache	3. Dizziness	5. Lumps or swelling
2. Head injury	4. Neck pain, limitation of motion	6. History of head or neck surgery

Examiner Asks	Rationale
1. Headache. Any unusually frequent or unusually severe **headaches?**	This is a more meaningful question than "Do you ever have headaches?" because most people have had at least one headache. Because many conditions have a headache, a detailed history is important.
• Onset. When did *this kind* of headache start?	
• Gradual, over hours or a day?	
• Or suddenly, over minutes or less than 1 hour?	
• Ever had *this kind* of headache before?	A red flag is a severe headache in an adult or child who has never had one before.
• Location. Where do you feel it: frontal, temporal, behind your eyes, like a band around the head, in the sinus area, or in the occipital area?	Tension headaches tend to be occipital, frontal, or with bandlike tightness; migraines (vascular) tend to be supraorbital, retro-orbital, or frontotemporal; cluster headaches (vascular) produce pain around the eye, temple, forehead, cheek.
• Is pain localized on one side or all over?	Unilateral or bilateral (e.g., with cluster headaches, pain is always unilateral and always on the same side of the head).
• Character. Throbbing (pounding, shooting) or aching (viselike, constant pressure, dull)?	Character is viselike with tension headache, throbbing with migraine or temporal arteritis (see Table 13-1, p. 271).
• Is it mild, moderate, or severe?	Pain is often severe with migraine or excruciating with cluster headache.
• Course and duration. What time of day do the headaches occur: morning, evening, awaken you from sleep? How long do they last? Hours, days? Have you noted any daily headaches or several within a time period?	Migraines occur about twice per month, each lasting 1 to 3 days; cluster headaches occur once or twice per day, each lasting $\frac{1}{2}$ to 2 hours for 1 to 2 months, and remission may last for months or years.
• Precipitating factors. What brings it on: activity or exercise, work environment, emotional upset, anxiety, alcohol? (Also note signs of depression.)	Alcohol ingestion and daytime napping typically precipitate cluster headaches, whereas alcohol, stress, menstruation, and eating chocolate or cheese precipitate migraines.
• Associated factors. Any relation to other symptoms: any nausea and vomiting? (Note which came first, headache or nausea.) Any vision changes, pain with bright lights, neck pain or stiffness, fever, weakness, moodiness, stomach problems?	Nausea, vomiting, and visual disturbances are associated with migraines; eye reddening and tearing, eyelid drooping, rhinorrhea, and nasal congestion are associated with cluster headaches; anxiety and stress are associated with tension headaches; nuchal rigidity and fever are associated with meningitis or encephalitis.
• Do you have any other illness?	Hypertension, fever, hypothyroidism, and vasculitis produce headaches.
• Do you take any medications?	Oral contraceptives, bronchodilators, alcohol, nitrates, and carbon monoxide inhalation produce headaches.
• What makes it worse: movement, coughing, straining, exercise?	
• Pattern. Any family history of headache?	Migraines are associated with family history of migraine.

Examiner Asks	Rationale
• What is the frequency of your headaches: once a week? Are your headaches occurring closer together? • Are they getting worse? Or are they getting better? • (For females) When do they occur in relation to your menstrual periods? • Effort to treat. What seems to help: going to sleep, medications, positions, rubbing the area? • Patient-centered care. How have these headaches affected your self-care or your ability to function at work, home, and socially? What do you need to help you cope?	See Table 13-1, Primary Headaches, p. 271. With migraines people lie down to feel better, whereas with cluster headaches they need to move—even to pace the floor—to feel better.
2. **Head injury.** Any **head injury** or blow to your head? • Onset. When? Please describe exactly what happened. • Setting. Any hazardous conditions? Were you wearing a helmet or hard hat? • How did you feel just before injury: dizzy, light-headed, had a blackout, had a seizure? • Lose consciousness and then fall? (Note which came first.) • Knocked unconscious? Or did you fall and lose consciousness a few minutes later? • Any history of illness (e.g., heart trouble, diabetes, epilepsy)? • Location. Exactly where did you hit your head? • Duration. How long were you unconscious? Any symptoms afterward—headache, vomiting, projectile vomiting? Any change in level of consciousness *after* injury: dazed or sleepy? • Associated symptoms. Any pain in the head or neck, vision change, discharge from ear or nose—is it bloody or watery? Are you able to move all extremities? Any tremors, staggered walk, numbness, and tingling? • Pattern. Are symptoms worse, better, unchanged since injury? • Effort to treat. Emergency department or hospitalized? Any medications?	Loss of consciousness *before* a fall may have a cardiac cause (e.g., heart block). A change in level of consciousness is most important in evaluating a neurologic deficit.
3. **Dizziness.** Experienced any **dizziness**? Tell me what you mean by dizziness. Describe it for me. ("Dizziness" is a vague, general term, related to multiple causes. Try not to prompt the person by suggesting descriptors such as "spinning," but note words offered. "I feel like I'm going to faint" suggests presyncope; "I feel like I'm spinning" suggests vertigo; "I feel like I'm going to fall down" suggests disequilibrium.)[16] • Onset. Abrupt or gradual? After a change in position such as sudden standing? • Associated factors. Any nausea and vomiting, pallor, immobility, decreased hearing acuity, or tinnitus along with the dizziness? Any palpitations or shortness of breath?	Dizziness includes: **Presyncope,** a light-headed, swimming sensation or feeling of fainting or falling caused by decreased blood flow to brain or heart irregularity causing decreased cardiac output. **Vertigo** is true rotational spinning often from labyrinthine-vestibular disorder in inner ear. With *objective* vertigo the person feels like the room is spinning; with *subjective* vertigo the person feels like he or she is spinning. **Disequilibrium** is a shakiness or instability when walking related to musculoskeletal disorder or multisensory deficits.[16]

Examiner Asks	Rationale

Subjective Data

4. **Neck pain.** Any neck pain?
  - Onset. How did the pain start: injury, automobile accident, after lifting, from a fall? Or with fever? Or did it have a gradual onset?

    Acute onset of neck stiffness with headache and fever occurs with meningeal inflammation.

  - Location. Does pain radiate? To the shoulders, arms?
  - Associated symptoms. Any **limitations to range of motion** (ROM), numbness or tingling in shoulders, arms, or hands?
  - Precipitating factors. Which movements cause pain? Do you need to lift or bend at work or home?
  - Does stress seem to bring it on?
  - Patient-centered care. Able to do your work, sleep? What do you need to help you cope?

    Pain creates a vicious circle. Tension increases pain and disability, which produces more anxiety.

5. **Lumps or swelling.** Any **lumps** or **swelling** in the neck?
  Any recent infection? Any tenderness?
  For a lump that persists, how long have you had it? Has it changed in size?

    Tenderness suggests acute infection.
    A persistent lump arouses suspicion of malignancy. For people older than 40 years, suspect malignancy until proven otherwise.
    Increased risk for salivary and thyroid tumors.

  - Any history of prior irradiation of head, neck, upper chest?

  - Any difficulty swallowing?
  - Do you smoke? For how long? How many packs a day? Do you chew tobacco?
  - When was your last alcoholic drink? How much alcohol do you drink a day?
  - Ever had a thyroid problem? Overfunctioning or underfunctioning? How was it treated: surgery, irradiation, any medication?

    Dysphagia.
    Smoking and chewing tobacco increase risk for oral and respiratory cancer.
    Smoking and large alcohol consumption together increase the risk for cancer.

6. **History of head or neck surgery.** Ever had surgery of the head or neck? For what condition? When did the surgery occur? How do you feel about results?

    Surgery for head and neck cancer often is disfiguring and increases risk for body image disturbance.

Additional History for Infants and Children

1. Did the mother use alcohol or street drugs during pregnancy? How often? How much was used per episode?

    Alcohol increases the risk for fetal alcohol syndrome, with distinctive facial features (see Table 13-2, Pediatric Abnormalities, p. 274). Cocaine use causes neurologic, developmental, and emotional problems.

2. Was delivery vaginal or by cesarean section? Any difficulty? Use of forceps?

    Forceps may increase the risk for caput succedaneum, cephalhematoma, and Bell palsy.

3. What were you told about the baby's growth? Was it on schedule? Did the head seem to grow and fontanels close on schedule? At what age (in months) did the baby achieve head control?

Additional History for the Aging Adult

1. Patient-centered care. If dizziness is a problem, how does this affect your daily activities? Are you able to drive safely, maneuver about the house safely?

    Assess self-care. Assess potential for injury.

2. If neck pain is a problem, how does this affect your daily activities? Are you able to drive, perform at work, do housework, sleep, look down when using stairs?

OBJECTIVE DATA

Normal Range of Findings	Abnormal Findings

The Head

Inspect and Palpate the Skull
Size and Shape

Note the general size and shape. **Normocephalic** is the term that denotes a round symmetric skull that is appropriately related to body size. Be aware that "normal" includes a wide range of sizes.

To assess shape, place your fingers in the person's hair and palpate the scalp. The skull normally feels symmetric and smooth. Cranial bones that have normal protrusions are the forehead, the side of each parietal bone, the occipital bone, and the mastoid process behind each ear. There is no tenderness to palpation.

Deformities: microcephaly, abnormally small head; macrocephaly, abnormally large head (hydrocephaly, acromegaly), (see Table 13-2, p. 272).

Note lumps, depressions, or abnormal protrusions.

Temporal Area

Palpate the temporal artery above the zygomatic (cheek) bone between the eye and top of the ear.

The temporomandibular joint is just below the temporal artery and anterior to the tragus. Palpate the joint as the person opens the mouth and note normally smooth movement with no limitation or tenderness.

The artery looks tortuous, feels hardened, and is tender with temporal arteritis.

Crepitation, limited ROM, or tenderness.

Inspect the Face
Facial Structures

Inspect the face, noting the facial expression and its appropriateness to behavior or reported mood. Anxiety is common in the hospitalized or ill person.

Although the shape of facial structures may vary somewhat depending on ancestry, features always should be symmetric. Expect symmetry of eyebrows, palpebral fissures, nasolabial folds, and sides of the mouth.

Note any abnormal facial structures (coarse facial features, exophthalmos, changes in skin color or pigmentation) or any abnormal swelling. Also note any involuntary movements (tics) in the facial muscles. Normally none occur.

Hostility or aggression.
Tense, rigid muscles may indicate anxiety or pain; a flat affect may indicate depression.
Marked asymmetry with central brain lesion (e.g., stroke) or peripheral cranial nerve VII damage (Bell palsy). See Table 13-5, Abnormal Facies with Chronic Illness, p. 278.
Edema in the face occurs first around the eyes (periorbital) and the cheeks where the subcutaneous tissue is relatively loose.
Note grinding of jaws, tics, fasciculations, or excessive blinking.

The Neck

Inspect and Palpate the Neck
Symmetry

Head position is centered in the midline, and the accessory neck muscles should be symmetric. The head should be held erect and still.

Head tilt occurs with muscle spasm. Rigid head and neck occur with arthritis.

Range of Motion (ROM)

Note any limitation of movement during active motion. Ask the person to touch the chin to the chest, turn the head to the right and left, try to touch each ear to the shoulder (without elevating shoulders), and extend the head backward. When the neck is supple, motion is smooth and controlled.

Note pain at any particular movement.
Note ratchety or limited movement from cervical arthritis or inflammation of neck muscles. The arthritic neck is rigid; the person turns at the shoulders rather than at the neck.

Objective Data

Normal Range of Findings	Abnormal Findings

Normal Range of Findings

Test muscle strength and the status of cranial nerve XI by trying to resist the person's movements with your hands as the person shrugs the shoulders and turns the head to each side.

As the person moves the head, note enlargement of the salivary and lymph glands. Normally, no enlargement is present. Note a swollen parotid gland when the head is extended; look for swelling below the angle of the jaw. Also note thyroid gland enlargement. Normally, none is present.

Also note any obvious pulsations. The carotid artery runs medial to the ster-nomastoid muscle, and it creates a brisk localized pulsation just below the angle of the jaw. Normally, there are no other pulsations while the person is in the sitting position (see Chapter 19).

Lymph Nodes

Using a gentle circular motion of your finger pads, palpate the lymph nodes (Fig. 13-9). (Normally, the salivary glands are not palpable. When symptoms warrant, check for parotid tenderness by palpating in a line from the outer corner of the eye to the lobule of the ear.) Beginning with the preauricular lymph nodes in front of the ear, palpate the 10 groups of lymph nodes in a routine order. Many nodes are closely packed, so you must be systematic and thorough in your examination. Once you establish your sequence, do not vary or you may miss some small nodes.

Posterior auricular
Occipital
Jugulodigastric
Superficial cervical
Posterior cervical
Supraclavicular

Preauricular
Submandibular
Submental
Deep cervical chain

13-9

Use gentle pressure because strong pressure could push the nodes into the neck muscles. It is usually most efficient to palpate with both hands, comparing the two sides symmetrically. However, the submental gland under the tip of the chin is easier to explore with one hand. When you palpate with one hand, use your other hand to position the person's head. For the deep cervical chain, tip

Abnormal Findings

Thyroid enlargement may be a unilateral lump, or it may be diffuse and look like a doughnut lying across the lower neck (see Table 13-3, Swellings on the Head or Neck, p. 275).

The parotid is swollen with mumps (see Table 13-3, p. 276).

Parotid enlargement has been found with AIDS.

Normal Range of Findings	**Abnormal Findings**

13-10   Palpate the deep cervical chain.

the person's head toward the side being examined to relax the ipsilateral muscle (Fig. 13-10). Then you can press your fingers under the muscle. Search for the supraclavicular node by having the person hunch the shoulders and elbows forward (Fig. 13-11); this relaxes the skin. The inferior belly of the omohyoid muscle crosses the posterior triangle here; do not mistake it for a lymph node.

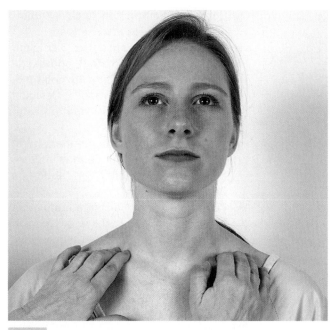

13-11   Palpate supraclavicular nodes.

Objective Data

Normal Range of Findings

If any nodes are palpable, note their location, size, shape, delimitation (discrete or matted together), mobility, consistency, and tenderness. Cervical nodes often are palpable in healthy persons, although this palpability decreases with age (Fig. 13-12, A). Normal nodes feel movable, discrete, soft, and nontender.

13-12, A

If nodes are enlarged or tender, check the area they drain for the source of the problem. For example, those in the upper cervical or submandibular area often relate to inflammation or a neoplasm in the head and neck. Follow up on or refer your findings. An enlarged lymph node, particularly when you cannot find the source of the problem, deserves prompt attention.

Abnormal Findings

Lymphadenopathy means enlargement of the lymph nodes (>1 cm) from infection, allergy, or neoplasm. (See Fig. 13-12, *B*, due to infectious mononucleosis.)

B

13-12, B   (Dean, Garrett, and Tyrrell, 2008.)

The following criteria are common clues but are not definitive in all cases:

- Acute infection—acute onset, <14 days' duration; nodes are bilateral, enlarged, warm, tender, and firm but freely movable.
- Chronic inflammation (e.g., in tuberculosis the nodes are clumped).
- Cancerous nodes are hard, >3 cm, unilateral, nontender, matted, and fixed.
- Nodes with HIV infection are enlarged, firm, nontender, and mobile. Occipital node enlargement is common with HIV infection.
- A single enlarged, nontender, hard, left supraclavicular node may indicate neoplasm in thorax or abdomen (Virchow node).
- Painless, rubbery, discrete nodes that gradually appear occur with Hodgkin lymphoma, commonly in the cervical region.

Trachea

Normally, the trachea is midline; palpate for any tracheal shift. Place your index finger on the trachea in the sternal notch and slip it off to each side (Fig. 13-13). The space should be symmetric on both sides. Note any deviation from the midline.

Normal Range of Findings

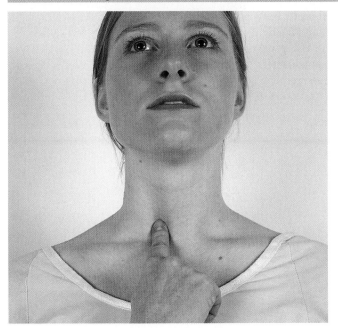

13-13

Thyroid Gland

The thyroid gland is difficult to palpate; arrange your setting to maximize your likelihood of success. Position a standing lamp to shine tangentially across the neck to highlight any possible swelling. Tilt the head back to stretch the skin against the thyroid. Supply the person with a glass of water and first inspect the neck as the person takes a sip and swallows. Thyroid tissue moves up with a swallow and then falls into its resting position.

Posterior Approach.   To palpate, move behind the person (Fig. 13-14, *A*). Ask the person to sit up very straight and then to bend the head slightly forward and to the right. This relaxes the neck muscles on the right side. Use the fingers of your left hand to push the trachea slightly to the right.

Curve your right fingers between the trachea and the sternomastoid muscle, retracting it slightly, and ask the person to take a sip of water. The thyroid moves up under your palpating fingers with the trachea and larynx as the person swallows. Reverse the procedure for the left side.

Usually you cannot palpate the normal adult thyroid. If the person has a long, thin neck, you sometimes feel the isthmus over the tracheal rings. The lateral lobes usually are not palpable; palpable lobes feel rubbery but smooth. Check them for enlargement, consistency, symmetry, and the presence of nodules.

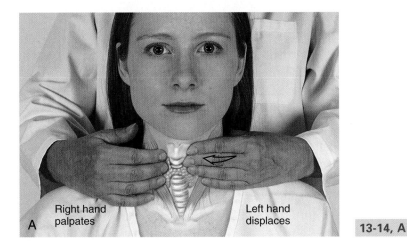

Right hand palpates

Left hand displaces

A   13-14, A

Abnormal Findings

Conditions of tracheal shift:
- The trachea is *pushed to the unaffected* (or healthy) side with an aortic aneurysm, a tumor, unilateral thyroid lobe enlargement, and pneumothorax.
- The trachea is *pulled toward the affected* (diseased) side with large atelectasis, pleural adhesions, or fibrosis.
- Tracheal tug is a rhythmic downward pull that is synchronous with systole and occurs with aortic arch aneurysm.

Look for diffuse enlargement or a nodular lump.

Abnormalities: enlarged lobes that are easily palpated before swallowing or are tender to palpation (see large goiter in Fig. 13-14, *B*) or the presence of nodules or lumps. See Table 13-4, Thyroid Hormone Disorders, p. 277.

B

13-14, B   (Lemmi & Lemmi, 2011.)

Objective Data

Normal Range of Findings	Abnormal Findings

Anterior Approach. This is an alternate method of palpating the thyroid, but it is more awkward to perform, especially for a beginning examiner. Stand facing the person. Ask him or her to tip the head forward and to the right. Use your right thumb to displace the trachea slightly to the person's right. Hook your left thumb and fingers around the sternomastoid muscle. Feel for lobe enlargement as the person swallows (Fig. 13-15).

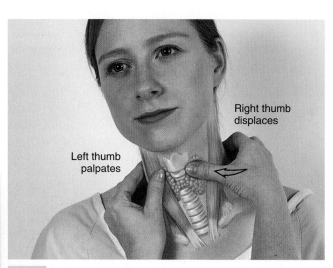

Left thumb
palpates

Right thumb
displaces

13-15

Auscultate the Thyroid

If the thyroid gland is enlarged, auscultate it for the presence of a **bruit.** This is a soft, pulsatile, whooshing, blowing sound heard best with the bell of the stethoscope. The bruit is not present normally.

A bruit occurs with accelerated or turbulent blood flow, indicating hyperplasia of the thyroid (e.g., hyperthyroidism).

❖ DEVELOPMENTAL COMPETENCE

Infants and Children
Skull

Measure an infant's **head size** with measuring tape at each visit up to age 2 years, then annually up to age 6 years. (Measurement of head circumference is presented in detail in Chapter 9.)

The newborn's head measures about 32 to 38 cm (average around 34 cm) and is 2 cm larger than chest circumference. At age 2 years both measurements are the same. During childhood the chest circumference grows to exceed head circumference by 5 to 7 cm.

Observe the infant's head from all angles, not just the front. The contour should be symmetric. Some racial variation occurs in normal head shapes.

Two common variations in the newborn cause the shape of the skull to look markedly asymmetric. A **caput succedaneum** is edematous swelling and ecchymosis of the presenting part of the head caused by birth trauma (Fig. 13-16). It feels soft, and it may extend across suture lines. It gradually resolves during the first few days of life and needs no treatment.

Note an abnormal increase in head size or failure to grow.

Microcephalic—head size below norms for age. Macrocephalic—an enlarged head or head rapidly increasing in size (e.g., hydrocephalus [increased cerebrospinal fluid]).

Frontal bulges, or "bossing," occur with prematurity or rickets.

Normal Range of Findings	Abnormal Findings

13-16   Caput succedaneum. (Murray and McKinney, 2014.)

A **cephalhematoma** is a subperiosteal hemorrhage, which is also a result of birth trauma (Fig. 13-17, *A*). It is soft, fluctuant, and well defined over one cranial bone because the periosteum (i.e., the covering over each bone) holds the bleeding in place. It appears several hours after birth and gradually increases in size. No discoloration is present, but it looks bizarre; parents need reassurance that it will be resorbed during the first few weeks of life without treatment. Rarely a large hematoma may persist to 3 months.

As you palpate the newborn's head, the suture lines feel like ridges. By 5 to 6 months they are smooth and not palpable.

An infant with cephalhematoma is at greater risk for jaundice as the red blood cells within the hematoma are broken down and resorbed (Fig. 13-17, *B*).

Sutures palpable when the child is older than 6 months.

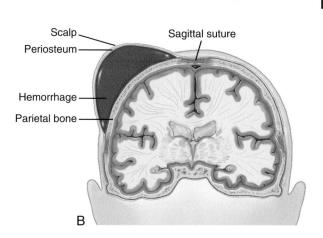

Scalp
Periosteum
Hemorrhage
Parietal bone
Sagittal suture

13-17   **A,** Cephalhematoma. (Murray and McKinney, 2014.)

A newborn's head may feel asymmetric, and the involved ridges more prominent because of *molding* of the cranial bones during engagement and passage through the birth canal. Molding is overriding of the cranial bones; usually the parietal bone overrides the frontal or occipital bone. Reassure parents that this lasts only a few days or a week. Babies delivered by cesarean section are noted for their evenly round heads.

Marked asymmetry, as in *craniosynostosis,* a severe deformity caused by premature closure of the sutures. This causes a distinctive head shape (see Table 13-2, p. 273) that correlates with the specific closed suture.

Normal Range of Findings	Abnormal Findings

Also, *positional molding* (**positional plagiocephaly**) may occur if the infant continually sleeps in the recommended position on the back to decrease the incidence of sudden infant death syndrome (SIDS). This is a flattening of the dependent cranial bone, the occiput, in an infant who did not have occipital flatness at birth. Inspection from behind shows a normal-appearing head shape with even horizontally placed ears. Inspection from the top shows a flat side of the occiput with the ear on that side displaced anteriorly, and the ear may fold forward. Head circumference is normal. Teach parents to reposition the baby's head to avoid further deformity.

Gently palpate the skull and **fontanels** while the infant is calm and somewhat in a sitting position (crying, lying down, or vomiting may cause the anterior fontanel to look full and bulging). The skull should feel smooth and fused except at the fontanels. The fontanels feel firm, slightly concave, and well defined against the edges of the cranial bones. You may see slight arterial pulsations in the anterior fontanel.

The posterior fontanel may not be palpable at birth. If it is, it measures 1 cm and closes by 1 to 2 months. The anterior fontanel may be small at birth and enlarge to 2.5 cm × 2.5 cm. A large diameter of 4 to 5 cm occasionally may be normal under 6 months. A small fontanel usually is normal. The anterior fontanel closes between 9 months and 2 years. Early closure may be insignificant if head growth proceeds normally.

Abnormal Findings:

Marked plagiocephaly (see Table 13-2) requires a custom-shaped helmet to afford room for brain growth in the flattened area while moderating growth in other areas. Used before sutures fuse.

Flattening also occurs with rickets.

A true tense or bulging fontanel occurs with acute increased intracranial pressure.

Depressed and sunken fontanels occur with dehydration or malnutrition.

Marked pulsations occur with increased intracranial pressure.

Delayed closure or larger-than-normal fontanel size occurs with hydrocephalus, Down syndrome, hypothyroidism, or rickets.

A small fontanel is a sign of microcephaly, as is early closure.

13-18 Tonic neck reflex.

Note the infant's **head posture** and **head control.** The infant can turn the head side to side by 2 weeks and shows the **tonic neck reflex** when supine and the head is turned to one side (extension of same arm and leg, flexion of opposite arm and leg) (Fig. 13-18). The tonic neck reflex disappears between 3 and 4 months, and then the head is maintained in the midline. Head control is achieved by 4 months, when the baby can hold the head erect and steady when pulled to a vertical position. (See Chapters 22 and 23 for further details.)

Tonic neck reflex beyond 5 months may indicate brain damage.

In children head tilt occurs with habit spasm, poor vision, and brain tumor.

Head lag after 4 months may indicate mental or motor retardation.

Face

Check **facial features** for symmetry, appearance, and presence of swelling. Note symmetry of wrinkling when the infant cries or smiles (e.g., both sides of the lips rise, and both sides of forehead wrinkle). Children love to comply when you

Unilateral immobility indicates nerve damage (central or peripheral) (e.g., note angle of mouth droop on paralyzed side).

Normal Range of Findings	Abnormal Findings

ask them to "make a face." Normally, no swelling is evident. Parotid gland enlargement is seen best when the child sits and looks up at the ceiling; the swelling appears below the angle of the jaw.

Some facies are characteristic of congenital abnormalities or chronic allergy. See Table 13-2, p. 273.

Neck

An infant's neck looks short; it lengthens during the first 3 to 4 years. You can see the neck better by supporting the infant's shoulders and tilting the head back a little. This positioning also enhances palpation of the trachea, which is buried deep in the neck. Feel for the row of cartilaginous rings in the midline or just slightly to the right of midline.

A short neck or webbing (loose fanlike folds) may indicate congenital abnormality (e.g., Down or Turner syndrome), or it may occur alone.

Assess muscle development with gentle passive ROM. Cradle the infant's head with your hands and turn it side to side and test forward flexion, extension, and rotation. Note any resistance to movement, especially flexion. Ask a child to actively move through the ROM, as you would an adult.

Head tilt and limited ROM occur with torticollis (wryneck) or from sternomastoid muscle injury during birth or a congenital defect.

Resistance to flexion (nuchal rigidity) and pain on flexion indicate meningeal irritation or meningitis.

During infancy cervical lymph nodes are not palpable normally. But a child's lymph nodes are—they feel more prominent than an adult's until after puberty, when lymphoid tissue begins to atrophy. Palpable nodes less than 3 mm are normal. They may be up to 1 cm in size in the cervical and inguinal areas but are discrete, move easily, and are nontender. Children have a higher incidence of infection, so you can expect a greater incidence of inflammatory adenopathy. No other mass should occur in the neck.

Cervical nodes >1 cm are considered enlarged.

Thyroglossal duct cyst—cystic lump high up in midline, freely movable, and rises up when swallowing.

Supraclavicular nodes enlarge with Hodgkin disease.

The thyroid gland is difficult to palpate in an infant because of the short, thick neck. The child's thyroid may be palpable normally.

Special Procedures

Percussion. With an infant, you may directly percuss with your plexor finger against the head surface. This yields a resonant or "cracked pot" sound, which is normal before closure of the fontanels.

Auscultation. Bruits are common in the skull in children younger than 4 or 5 years or in children with anemia. They are systolic or continuous and are heard over the temporal area.

The sound occurs with hydrocephalus from separation of cranial sutures (Macewen sign).

After 5 years of age, bruits indicate increased intracranial pressure, aneurysm, or arteriovenous shunt.

The Pregnant Woman

During the second trimester chloasma may show on the face. This is a blotchy, hyperpigmented area over the cheeks and forehead that fades after delivery. The thyroid gland may be palpable normally during pregnancy.

The Aging Adult

The temporal arteries may look twisted and prominent. In some aging adults a mild rhythmic tremor of the head may be normal. **Senile tremors** are benign and include head nodding (as if saying yes or no) and tongue protrusion. If some teeth have been lost, the lower face looks unusually small, with the mouth sunken in.

The neck may show an increased anterior cervical (concave or inward) curve when the head and jaw are extended forward to compensate for kyphosis of the spine. During the examination, direct the aging person to perform ROM slowly; he or she may experience dizziness with side movements. An aging person may have prolapse of the submandibular glands, which could be mistaken for a tumor. But drooping submandibular glands feel soft and are present bilaterally.

Objective Data

PROMOTING A HEALTHY LIFESTYLE

Sports Concussion Toolkit

The American Academy of Neurology (AAN) released an updated evidence-based guideline for evaluating and managing athletes with concussion. The updated *Sports Concussion Guideline* and *Toolkit* is available online at: http://www.aan.com/go/practice/concussion. The Toolkit includes a myriad of resources for health care professionals and patients, coaches, and athletic trainers. Of particular note is that anyone can download the Concussion Quick Check Reference Sheet and Quick Check App.

Concussion is a clinical diagnosis, and symptom checklists are available, including the Standardized Assessment of Concussion (SAC) and Balance Error Scoring System; but checklists alone should not be used for making a diagnosis. It is important to remember that loss of consciousness occurs in only 10% of concussions. Signs and symptoms can include:

- Headache or pressure
- Nausea/vomiting
- Sensitivity to light and/or sound
- Changes to reaction time, balance, and/or coordination
- Changes in memory, judgment, and/or speech
- Sleep pattern changes

These symptoms can arise quickly or be delayed, appearing over days. For most individuals all signs and symptoms disappear in 10 days, but symptoms persist in a subgroup of individuals. If an athlete is having any of these symptoms, he or she should be taken out of play immediately and evaluated individually. Currently there is a move away from concussion grading systems that were popular in the past.

One thing to remember is that having one concussion raises the risk for having another, especially in the 10 days following the initial concussion.

The Centers for Disease Control and Prevention (CDC) has created online courses for health care professionals and youth, including parents and coaches, called *HEADS UP: Concussion in Youth Sports*. Both are easily accessed, along with other information about concussion, at: http://www.cdc.gov/CONCUSSION/.

References
American Academy of Neurology (AAN); http://www.aan.com/.
National Institutes of Health—NIH News in Health: A Bang to the Brain: http://newsinhealth.nih.gov/issue/May2013/Feature1.

DOCUMENTATION AND CRITICAL THINKING

Sample Charting

SUBJECTIVE

Denies any unusually frequent or severe headache; no history of head injury, dizziness, or syncope; no neck pain, limitation of motion, lumps, or swelling.

OBJECTIVE

Head: Normocephalic, no lumps, no lesions, no tenderness, no trauma.
Face: Symmetric, no drooping, no weakness, no involuntary movements.
Neck: Supple with full ROM, no pain. Symmetric, no cervical lymphadenopathy or masses. Trachea midline, thyroid not palpable. No bruits.

ASSESSMENT

Normocephalic, atraumatic, and symmetric head and neck

Clinical Case Study 1

F.V. is a 57-year-old insurance executive who is in his 4th postoperative day after a transurethral resection of the prostate gland. He also has chronic hypertension, managed by oral hydrochlorothiazide, exercise, and a low-salt diet.

Documentation and Critical Thinking

SUBJECTIVE

Complaining of dizziness, a light-headed feeling that occurred on standing and cleared on sitting. States, "I'm afraid of falling." No previous episodes of dizziness. Denies palpitations, nausea, or vomiting. States urine pink-tinged as it was yesterday, with no red blood. No pain medications today. On 2nd day of same antihypertensive medication he took before surgery.

OBJECTIVE

Vital signs: BP 142/88 mm Hg RA sitting, 94/58 mm Hg RA standing. Pulse 94 bpm sitting and standing, regular rhythm, no skipped beats. Temp 98.6° F (37° C). Color tannish-pink, no pallor, skin warm and dry.

Neuro: Alert and oriented to person, place, and time. Speech clear and fluent. Moving all extremities, no weakness. No nystagmus, no ataxia, past-pointing test normal. Romberg sign negative (normal). Intake/output in balance. Urine faint pink-tinged, no clots.

Lab: Hematocrit 45%, serum chemistries normal.

ASSESSMENT

Orthostatic hypotension
Presyncope R/T orthostatic hypotension
Risk for injury R/T orthostatic hypotension

Clinical Case Study 2

A.B. is a 33-year-old Caucasian female, civil engineer, with no known health problems, on no medication, taking a multivitamin daily.

SUBJECTIVE

Delivered a healthy baby girl 13 months PTA, not breastfeeding, baby sleeps through the night. A.B.'s menses regular since delivery but reports that the flow is heavy. A.B. reports that she feels depressed, is unable to lose weight despite efforts, has severe fatigue, reporting "some days I feel like I can't even lift my arms," weakness (hard to open a jar). She also reports brittle nails, constipation, and an increased sensitivity to cold.

OBJECTIVE

Vital signs: BP 118/88 mm Hg. Temp 96.9° F (36.1° C); Pulse 62 bpm regular. Resp 12/min.
General appearance: Skin cool, pale, and dry. Nails appear brittle but kempt.
Neck: Thyroid enlarged on palpation but no nodules. No lymphadenopathy.
Lungs: Clear and equal bilaterally.
Heart: S_1 S_2 regular, no murmurs or extra heart sounds.
Lab: TSH 6.29 MIU/mL (range 0.47-4.68 MIU/mL), free T4: 0.9 ng/dL (range 0.8-2.2 ng/dL)

ASSESSMENT

Hypothyroidism by lab results
Fatigue R/T hypothyroidism
Diastolic prehypertension R/T hypothyroidism

Clinical Case Study 3

L.M. is a 36-year-old female auto plant worker here today for mild abdominal pain, hot flashes, palpitations, and anxiety, reporting, "I'm going to jump out of my skin."

SUBJECTIVE

Has been experiencing the previous symptoms for 3 months along with mild hand tremors, increased appetite, weight loss, heat intolerance, poor concentration, and difficulty sleeping. For the past month, L.M. has noticed that her eyes feel dry and irritated. She reports menstrual periods that are "not regular anymore." Last menstrual period 2 weeks PTA, scant flow.

OBJECTIVE

Vital signs: BP 90/60 mm Hg. Temp: 99.5°F (37.5°C). Pulse 145 bpm and irregular. Resp 24/min. Cardiac monitor located in office shows atrial fibrillation.

Eyes: White sclera shows between iris and upper/lower lids. Staring, unblinking appearance.

Skin: Warm, moist, smooth. Perspiration evident.

Neck: Moderately enlarged thyroid with no nodules. No lymphadenopathy.

Heart: S_1 S_2 irregularly irregular with midsystolic murmur grade 2/6 at left lower sternal border.

Lungs: Clear and equal bilaterally.

Abdomen: Soft, no masses or tenderness. Active bowel sounds.

DTRs: Brisk ankle jerk. Other DTRs 2+ and = bilaterally.

Lab: Serum T4 18.5 mcg/dL; TSH undetectable.

ASSESSMENT

Hyperthyroidism—Graves disease

Clinical Case Study 4

A.M. is a 5-year-old Caucasian boy who presents to the clinic with his father. The family adopted a dog from the animal shelter 8 months PTA.

SUBJECTIVE

A.M.'s father reports that A.M. has had "sneezing fits," a runny nose, and coughing for the past few months and that it seems better when A.M. is at school. Father states, "He just won't stop rubbing his nose and eyes."

OBJECTIVE

Vital signs: Temp 98.6° F (37° C). BP 93/60 mm Hg (sitting). Pulse 90 bpm. Resp 24/min (at rest, open-mouthed).

General appearance: Alert and active child who is smiling and talkative.

HEENT: Normocephalic, no lumps, no lesions. Palpable anterior cervical lymph nodes (1 mm), discrete, move easily, nontender. Light-blue areas in skin under eyes, creasing present on palpebrae inferior and superior to the tip of nose. Minimal fluid in middle ear, denies tenderness to palpation of sinus cavities; swollen turbinates bilat, and consistently sniffles and clears throat. Reddened posterior pharynx c̄ exudate present.

Cardiovascular: No murmurs or abnormal heart sounds.

Respiratory: Breath sounds = bilat, expiratory wheezing present bilat that clears with cough.

ASSESSMENT

Allergic rhinitis R/T to newly obtained household pet
Ineffective health maintenance R/T deficient knowledge regarding allergies

Documentation and Critical Thinking

ABNORMAL FINDINGS

TABLE 13-1	**Primary Headaches** (Diagnosed by Patient History with No Abnormal Findings in Physical Examination or Laboratory Testing)		
	Tension	**Migraine**	**Cluster**
	Tension	Migraine	Cluster
Definition	Headache (HA) of musculoskeletal origin; may be a mild-to-moderate, less disabling form of migraine	HA of genetically transmitted vascular origin; headache plus prodrome, aura, other symptoms	HA that is intermittent, excruciating, unilateral, with autonomic signs
Location	Usually both sides, across frontal, temporal, and/or occipital region of head: forehead, sides, and back of head	Commonly one-sided but may occur on both sides Pain is often behind the eyes, the temples, or forehead	Always one-sided Often behind or around the eye, temple, forehead, cheek
Character	Bandlike tightness, viselike Nonthrobbing, nonpulsatile	Throbbing, pulsating	Continuous, burning, piercing, excruciating
Duration	Gradual onset, lasts 30 minutes to days	Rapid onset, peaks 1-2 hr, lasts 4-72 hr, sometimes longer	Abrupt onset, peaks in minutes, lasts 45-90 min
Quantity and severity	Diffuse, dull aching pain Mild-to-moderate pain	Moderate-to-severe pain	Can occur multiple times a day, in "clusters," lasting weeks Severe, stabbing pain
Timing	Situational, in response to overwork, posture	≈2 per month, last 1-3 days ≈1 in 10 patients have weekly headaches	1-2/day, each lasting $\frac{1}{2}$ to 2 hr for 1 to 2 months; then remission for months or years
Aggravating symptoms or triggers	Stress, anxiety, depression, poor posture Not worsened by physical activity	Hormonal fluctuations (premenstrual) Foods (e.g., alcohol, caffeine, MSG, nitrates, chocolate, cheese) Hunger Letdown after stress Sleep deprivation Sensory stimuli (e.g., flashing lights or perfumes) Changes in weather Physical activity	Exacerbated by alcohol, stress, daytime napping, wind or heat exposure

Continued

TABLE 13-1   Primary Headaches (Diagnosed by Patient History with No Abnormal Findings in Physical Examination or Laboratory Testing)—cont'd

	Tension	Migraine	Cluster
Associated symptoms	Fatigue, anxiety, stress Sensation of a band tightening around head, of being gripped like a vice Sometimes photophobia or phonophobia	Aura (visual changes such as blind spots or flashes of light, tingling in an arm or leg, vertigo) Prodrome (change in mood, behavior, hunger, cravings, yawning) Nausea, vomiting, photophobia, phonophobia, abdominal pain Person looks sick Family history of migraine	Ipsilateral autonomic signs: Nasal congestion or runny nose, watery or reddened eye, eyelid drooping, miosis Feelings of agitation
Relieving factors, efforts to treat	Rest, massaging muscles in area, NSAID medication	Lie down, darken room, use eyeshade, sleep, take NSAID early, try to avoid opioid	Need to move, pace floor

Images © Pat Thomas, 2014.

TABLE 13-2   Pediatric Abnormalities

Hydrocephalus

Obstruction of drainage of cerebrospinal fluid results in excessive accumulation, increasing intracranial pressure, and enlargement of the head. The face looks small compared with the enlarged cranium. The increasing pressure also produces dilated scalp veins, frontal bossing, and downcast or "setting sun" eyes (sclera visible above iris). The cranial bones thin, sutures separate, and percussion yields a "cracked pot" sound (Macewen sign).

Down Syndrome

Chromosomal aberration (trisomy 21). Head and face characteristics may include upslanting eyes with inner epicanthal folds; flat nasal bridge; small, broad, flat nose; protruding, thick tongue; ear dysplasia; short, broad neck with webbing; and small hands with single palmar crease.

TABLE 13-2   Pediatric Abnormalities—cont'd

Plagiocephaly

Positional or deformational plagiocephaly has increased dramatically since the "Back to Sleep" campaign started in 1992 to prevent SIDS. It is asymmetry of the cranium when seen from the top caused by a positional preference. It is not associated with premature closing of cranial sutures, and growth of the brain proceeds normally. This can be mitigated by "tummy time," when the parent places the infant prone for awake playing. Physical therapy and helmet therapy are further treatments.

Craniosynostosis

Premature closing of one or multiple cranial sutures (shown above) results in a malformed head and a cosmetic deformity. Mechanisms involve genetic mutations coding structural proteins or growth factor receptors. Severe deformities cannot contain the brain, eyes and optic nerves inside the cranial vault, and hypoplasia of the face results, warranting surgery.

Atopic (Allergic) Facies

Children with chronic allergies such as atopic dermatitis often develop characteristic facial features. These include exhausted face, blue shadows below the eyes ("allergic shiners") from sluggish venous return; a double or single crease on the lower eyelids (Morgan lines); central facial pallor; and open-mouth breathing (allergic gaping), which can lead to malocclusion of the teeth and malformed jaw because the child's bones are still forming.

▶

Continued

TABLE 13-2 **Pediatric Abnormalities—cont'd**

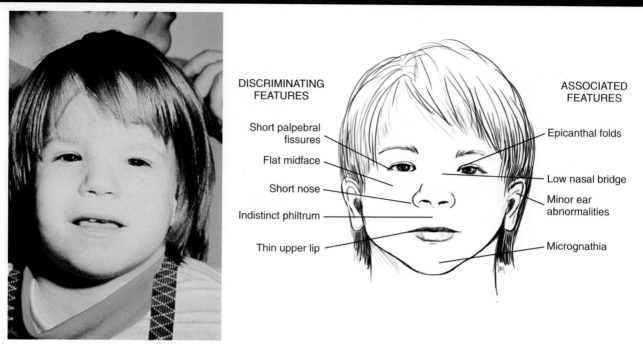

DISCRIMINATING FEATURES
- Short palpebral fissures
- Flat midface
- Short nose
- Indistinct philtrum
- Thin upper lip

ASSOCIATED FEATURES
- Epicanthal folds
- Low nasal bridge
- Minor ear abnormalities
- Micrognathia

Fetal Alcohol Syndrome (FAS)

Alcohol is teratogenic to the developing fetus, resulting in severe cognitive and psychosocial impairment and changes in facial and brain structure. The incidence is increasing in the United States, even with public warnings to avoid alcohol during pregnancy. Characteristic facies include narrow palpebral fissures, epicanthal folds, and midfacial hypoplasia. These malformations may be recognizable at birth but more so during childhood. Fetal alcohol spectrum disorders (FASDs) include a wide range of neurologic and behavioral deficits, even without facial malformations. The risk of FASDs increases with the amount of alcohol the pregnant woman drinks.

◀ Allergic Salute and Crease

The transverse line on the nose is also a feature of chronic allergies. It is formed when the child chronically uses the hand to push the nose up and back (the "allergic salute") to relieve itching and free swollen turbinates, which allow air passage.

See Illustration Credits for source information.

TABLE 13-3   Swellings on the Head or Neck

Torticollis (Wryneck)

A hematoma in one sternomastoid muscle, probably injured by intrauterine malposition, results in head tilt to one side and limited neck ROM to the opposite side. You feel a firm, discrete, nontender mass in mid-muscle on the involved side. This requires treatment, or the muscle can become fibrotic and permanently shortened with permanent limitation of ROM, asymmetry of the head and face, and visual problems from a nonhorizontal position of the eyes.

Simple Diffuse Goiter (SDG)

Goiter, a chronic enlargement of the thyroid gland, is common in wide regions of the world (especially mountainous regions) where the soil is low in iodine. Iodine is an essential element in the formation of thyroid hormones.

◀ Thyroid—Multinodular Goiter (MNG)

Multiple nodules usually indicate inflammation or a multinodular goiter rather than a neoplasm. However, suspect any rapidly enlarging or firm nodule. Refer all patients with a nodule for ultrasonography.

Single Nodule (not illustrated): Thyroid nodules are palpable in 1% to 5% of ambulatory care patients but can be identified in 50% of ultrasound studies.[8] Over 95% of these are benign. Suspect any painless, rapidly growing nodule, especially a single nodule in a young person. Cancerous nodules usually are hard and fixed to surrounding structures. At increased risk are males ages <15 years and >45 years; size >4 cm; and history of radiation exposure, especially in childhood.

Continued

TABLE 13-3   Swellings on the Head or Neck—cont'd

◄ Pilar Cyst (Wen)

This is a smooth, firm, fluctuant swelling on the scalp that contains sebum and keratin. Tense pressure of the contents causes overlying skin to be shiny and taut. It is a benign growth.

◄ Parotid Gland Enlargement

Rapid painful inflammation of the parotid occurs with mumps. Parotid swelling also occurs with blockage of a duct, abscess, or tumor. Note swelling anterior to lower ear lobe. Stensen duct obstruction can occur in aging adults dehydrated from diuretics or anticholinergics.

ROM, Range of motion.
See Illustration Credits for source information.

TABLE 13-4   Thyroid Hormone Disorders

© Pat Thomas, 2014.

The hypothalamic-pituitary-thyroid axis regulates the production of thyroid hormones by a negative feedback system, much like the thermostat that guides your household furnace. (1) The hypothalamus secretes thyrotropin-releasing hormone (TRH), which (2) acts on the anterior pituitary to secrete thyroid-stimulating hormone (TSH), which (3) directs the thyroid gland to produce T_3 and T_4 hormones. When T_3 and T_4 hormones are high in the bloodstream ("hot" like a furnace), they (4) direct the pituitary and hypothalamus to shut off their signaling hormones. That is the negative feedback. When T_3 and T_4 hormone levels are low (thyroid is like a cold furnace), the pituitary sends out TSH to stimulate new production of T_3 and T_4 hormones. Your body metabolism is most comfortable in a healthy balance of hormone levels.

Graves Disease (Hyperthyroidism)

Increased production of thyroid hormones causes an increased metabolic rate, just like ramping up the furnace. This is manifested by goiter and exophthalmos (bulging eyeballs). Symptoms include nervousness, fatigue, weight loss, muscle cramps, and heat intolerance. Signs include forceful tachycardia; shortness of breath; excessive sweating; fine muscle tremor; thin silky hair; warm, moist skin; infrequent blinking; and a staring appearance.

Myxedema (Hypothyroidism)

A deficiency of thyroid hormone means that the thyroid furnace is cold. This reduces the metabolic rate and, when severe, causes a nonpitting edema or myxedema. Usual cause is Hashimoto thyroiditis. Symptoms include fatigue and cold intolerance. Signs include puffy, edematous face, especially around eyes (periorbital edema); puffy hands and feet; coarse facial features; cool, dry skin; and dry, coarse hair and eyebrows.

See Illustration Credits for source information.

10. Moloney, M. F., & Cranwell-Bruce, L. A. (2010). Migraine headaches. *Nurse Pract, 35*(9), 17-22.

11. Reference deleted in proofs.

12. National Stroke Association. (2013). What is stroke? www.stroke.org/site/PageServer?pagename=stroke.

13. Nuñez, S. C., Roussotte, F., & Sowell, E. R. (2011). Focus on: structural and functional brain abnormalities in fetal alcohol spectrum disorders. *Alcohol Res Health, 34*(1), 121-131.

14. Papaleontiou, M., & Haymart, M. R. (2012). Approach to and treatment of thyroid disorders in the elderly. *Med Clin North Am, 96*(2), 297-310.

15. Rekate, H. L. (2009). A contemporary definition and classification of hydrocephalus. *Semin Pediatr Neurol, 16*(1), 9-15.

16. Saccomano, S. J. (2012). Dizziness, vertigo, and presyncope: what's the difference? *Nurse Pract, 37*(12), 46-52.

17. Sandhaus, S. (2002). Stop the spinning: diagnosing and managing vertigo. *Nurse Pract, 27*(8), 11-25.

18. Simmons, S. (2010). A delicate balance: detecting thyroid disease. *Nursing, 40*(7), 22-30.

19. Steefel, L., & Novak, D. (2012). When tension headaches become chronic. *Nurse Pract, 37*(11), 25-29.

20. Woodhouse, K. N. (2012). Thyrotoxicosis: evaluation and treatment of a multinodular goiter. *Nurse Pract, 37*(7), 6-10.

CHAPTER 14

Eyes

STRUCTURE AND FUNCTION

Pupil
Iris
Upper eyelid
Sclera
Palpebral fissure
Medial canthus
Lateral canthus
Caruncle
Lower eyelid
Limbus
(border between
cornea and sclera)

14-1   © Pat Thomas, 2006.

EXTERNAL ANATOMY

About 1 inch in diameter, the eye is the sensory organ of vision. Humans are very visual beings. The eyes carry visual data that are crucial for our survival, education, and pleasure. More than half of our neocortex is involved with processing visual information.

Because this sense is so important to humans, the eye is well protected by the bony orbital cavity, surrounded with a cushion of fat. The **eyelids** are like two rapid window shades that further protect the eye from injury, strong light, and dust. The upper eyelid is the larger and more mobile one. The eyelashes are short hairs in double or triple rows that curve outward from the lid margins, filtering out dust and dirt.

The **palpebral fissure** is the elliptical open space between the eyelids (Fig. 14-1). When closed, the lid margins approximate completely. When open, the upper lid covers part of the iris. The lower lid margin is just at the **limbus,** the border between the cornea and sclera. The **canthus** is the corner of the eye, the angle where the lids meet. At the inner canthus the **caruncle** is a small, fleshy mass containing sebaceous glands.

Within the upper lid, **tarsal plates** are strips of connective tissue that give it shape (Fig. 14-2). The tarsal plates contain the **meibomian glands,** modified sebaceous glands that

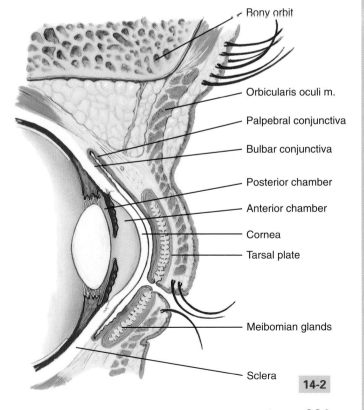

Bony orbit
Orbicularis oculi m.
Palpebral conjunctiva
Bulbar conjunctiva
Posterior chamber
Anterior chamber
Cornea
Tarsal plate
Meibomian glands
Sclera

14-2

281

14-3 Lacrimal apparatus.   © Pat Thomas, 2006.

secrete an oily lubricating material onto the lids. This stops the tears from overflowing and helps form an airtight seal when the lids are closed.

The exposed part of the eye has a transparent protective covering, the **conjunctiva.** The conjunctiva is a thin mucous membrane folded like an envelope between the eyelids and the eyeball. The *palpebral* conjunctiva lines the lids and is clear, with many small blood vessels. It forms a deep recess and then folds back over the eye. The *bulbar* conjunctiva overlays the eyeball, with the white sclera showing through. At the limbus, the conjunctiva merges with the cornea. The cornea covers and protects the iris and pupil.

The **lacrimal apparatus** provides constant irrigation to keep the conjunctiva and cornea moist and lubricated (Fig. 14-3). The lacrimal gland, in the upper outer corner over the eye, secretes tears. The tears wash across the eye and are drawn up evenly as the lid blinks. They drain into the **puncta,** visible on the upper and lower lids at the inner canthus. They then drain into the nasolacrimal sac, through the ½ inch–long nasolacrimal duct, and empty into the inferior meatus inside the nose. A tiny fold of mucous membrane prevents air from being forced up the nasolacrimal duct when the nose is blown.

Extraocular Muscles

Six muscles attach the eyeball to its orbit (Fig. 14-4, *A*) and serve to direct our eyes to points of our interest. These **extraocular muscles** (EOMs) give the eye both straight and rotary

MUSCLE ATTACHMENTS

A

B   DIRECTION OF MOVEMENT

14-4   © Pat Thomas, 2006.

movement. The four straight, or *rectus,* muscles are the superior, inferior, lateral, and medial rectus muscles. The two slanting, or *oblique,* muscles are the superior and inferior muscles.

Each muscle is coordinated, or yoked, with one in the other eye. This ensures that when the two eyes move, their axes always remain parallel (called *conjugate movement).* Parallel axes are important because the human brain can tolerate seeing only one image. Although some animals can perceive two different pictures through each eye, humans have a binocular, single-image visual system. This occurs because our eyes move as a pair. For example, the two yoked muscles that allow looking to the far right are the right lateral rectus and the left medial rectus.

Movement of the EOMs (Fig. 14-4, *B*) is stimulated by three **cranial nerves** (CNs). The abducens nerve (CN VI) innervates the lateral rectus muscle (which abducts the eye); the trochlear nerve (CN IV) innervates the superior oblique muscle; and the oculomotor nerve (CN III) innervates all the rest—the superior, inferior, and medial rectus and the inferior oblique muscles. Note that the superior oblique muscle is located on the superior aspect of the eyeball; but, when it contracts, it enables the person to look downward and inward.

INTERNAL ANATOMY

The eye is an asymmetric sphere composed of three concentric coats: (1) the outer fibrous **sclera,** (2) the middle vascular **choroid,** and (3) the inner nervous **retina** (Fig. 14-5). Inside the retina is the transparent vitreous body. The only parts accessible to examination are the sclera anteriorly and the retina through the ophthalmoscope.

The Outer Layer. The **sclera** is a tough, protective, white covering. It is continuous anteriorly with the smooth, transparent cornea, which covers the iris and pupil. The cornea is part of the refracting media of the eye, bending incoming light rays to focus them on the inner retina.

The **cornea** is thin, transparent, and very sensitive to touch; contact with a wisp of cotton stimulates a blink in both eyes, called the *corneal reflex.* The trigeminal nerve (CN V) carries the afferent sensation into the brain, and the facial nerve (CN VII) carries the efferent message that stimulates the blink.

The Middle Layer. The **choroid** has dark pigmentation to prevent light from reflecting internally and is heavily vascularized to deliver blood to the retina. Anteriorly the choroid is continuous with the ciliary body and the iris. The muscles of the ciliary body control the thickness of the lens. The iris functions as a diaphragm, varying the opening at its center, the pupil. This controls the amount of light admitted into the retina. The muscle fibers of the iris contract the pupil in bright light and accommodate for near vision; they dilate the pupil in dim light and accommodate for far vision. The color of the iris varies from person to person.

The **pupil** is round and regular. Its size is determined by a balance between the parasympathetic and sympathetic chains of the autonomic nervous system. Stimulation of the parasympathetic branch, through CN III, causes constriction of the pupil. Stimulation of the sympathetic branch dilates the pupil and elevates the eyelid. As mentioned earlier, the pupil size also reacts to the amount of ambient light and accommodation, or focusing an object on the retina.

The **lens** is a biconvex disc located just posterior to the pupil. The transparent lens serves as a refracting medium,

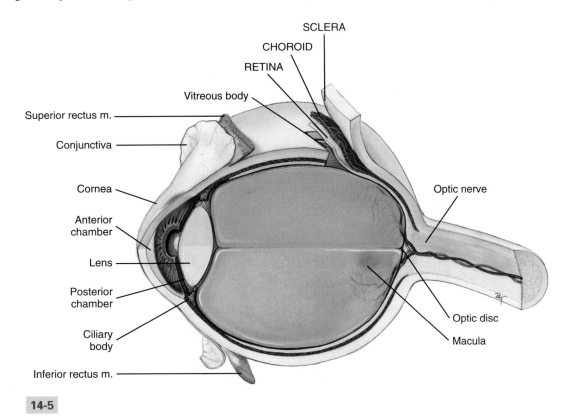

SCLERA
CHOROID
RETINA
Vitreous body
Superior rectus m.
Conjunctiva
Cornea
Anterior chamber
Lens
Posterior chamber
Ciliary body
Inferior rectus m.
Optic nerve
Optic disc
Macula

14-5

keeping a viewed object in continual focus on the retina. Its thickness is controlled by the ciliary body; the lens bulges for focusing on near objects and flattens for far objects.

The **anterior chamber** is posterior to the cornea and in front of the iris and lens. The **posterior chamber** lies behind the iris to the sides of the lens. These contain the clear, watery aqueous humor that is produced continually by the ciliary body. The continuous flow of fluid serves to deliver nutrients to the surrounding tissues and drain metabolic wastes. Intraocular pressure is determined by a balance between the amount of aqueous produced and resistance to its outflow at the angle of the anterior chamber.

The Inner Layer. The **retina** is the visual receptive layer of the eye in which light waves are changed into nerve impulses. It surrounds the soft, gelatinous vitreous humor. The retinal structures viewed through the ophthalmoscope are the optic disc, the retinal vessels, the general background, and the macula (Fig. 14-6).

The **optic disc** (or optic papilla) is the area in which fibers from the retina converge to form the optic nerve. Located toward the nasal side of the retina, it has these characteristics: a color that varies from creamy yellow-orange to pink; a round or oval shape; margins that are distinct and sharply demarcated, especially on the temporal side; and a physiologic cup, the smaller circular area inside the disc where the blood vessels exit and enter.

The **retinal vessels** normally include a paired artery and vein extending to each quadrant, growing progressively smaller in caliber as they reach the periphery. The arteries appear brighter red and narrower than the veins, and they have a thin sliver of light on them (the arterial light reflex). The general background of the fundus varies in color, depending on the person's skin color. The **macula** is located on the temporal side of the fundus. It is a slightly darker pigmented region surrounding the **fovea centralis,** the area of sharpest and keenest vision. The macula receives and transduces light from the center of the visual field.

VISUAL PATHWAYS AND VISUAL FIELDS

Objects reflect light. The light rays are refracted through the transparent media (cornea, aqueous humor, lens, and vitreous body) and strike the retina. The retina transforms the light stimulus into nerve impulses that are conducted through the optic nerve and the optic tract to the visual cortex of the occipital lobe.

The image formed on the retina is upside down and reversed from its actual appearance in the outside world (Fig. 14-7) (i.e., an object in the upper temporal visual field of the right eye reflects its image onto the lower nasal area of the retina). All retinal fibers collect to form the optic nerve; but they maintain this same spatial arrangement, with nasal fibers running medially and temporal fibers running laterally.

At the optic chiasm nasal fibers (from both temporal visual fields) cross over. The left optic tract now has fibers from the left half of each retina, and the right optic tract contains fibers only from the right. Thus the right side of the brain looks at the left side of the world.

VISUAL REFLEXES

Pupillary Light Reflex. The pupillary light reflex is the normal constriction of the pupils when bright light shines on

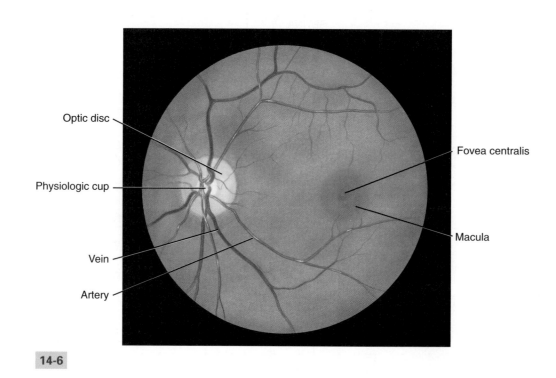

Optic disc

Physiologic cup

Vein

Artery

Fovea centralis

Macula

14-6

LEFT VISUAL FIELD   RIGHT VISUAL FIELD
Temporal   Nasal   Nasal   Temporal

Optic nerve

Optic chiasm

Optic tract

Occipital cortex

14-7   Visual pathways (viewed from above).

the retina (Fig. 14-8). It is a subcortical reflex arc (i.e., we have no conscious control over it); the sensory afferent link is CN II (the optic nerve), and the motor efferent path is CN III (the oculomotor nerve).

When one eye is exposed to bright light, a *direct light reflex* (constriction of that pupil) and a *consensual light reflex* (simultaneous constriction of the other pupil) occur. This happens because the optic nerve carries the sensory afferent message in and then synapses with both sides of the brain. For example, consider the light reflex in a person who is blind in one eye. Stimulation of the normal eye produces both a direct and a consensual light reflex. Stimulation of the blind eye causes no response because the sensory afferent in CN II is destroyed.

Fixation. Fixation is a reflex direction of the eye toward an object attracting our attention. The image is fixed in the center of the visual field, the fovea centralis. This consists of very rapid ocular movements to put the target back on the fovea and somewhat slower (smooth pursuit) movements to track the target and keep its image on the fovea. These ocular movements are impaired by drugs, alcohol, fatigue, and inattention.

Accommodation. Accommodation is adaptation of the eye for near vision. It is accomplished by increasing the curvature of the lens through the muscles of the ciliary body. Although the lens cannot be observed directly, the components of accommodation that can be observed are convergence (motion toward) of the axes of the eyeballs and pupillary constriction.

CONSENSUAL LIGHT REFLEX
constricts pupil, opposite eye

c.n. III

c.n. II

Afferent nerve

Optic nerve c.n. II

Optic chiasm

Midbrain

c.n. III

DIRECT LIGHT REFLEX
efferent nerve constricts
pupil, same eye

Key
━ Sensory afferent into brain
━ Motor efferent out to iris

14-8

Structure and Function

✦ DEVELOPMENTAL COMPETENCE

Infants and Children

At birth eye function is limited, but it matures fully during the early years. Peripheral vision is intact in the newborn infant. The macula, the area of keenest vision, is absent at birth but is developing by 4 months and is mature by 8 months. Eye movements may be poorly coordinated at birth. By 3 to 4 months of age the infant establishes binocularity and can fixate on a single image with both eyes simultaneously. Most babies (80%) are born farsighted; this gradually decreases after 7 to 8 years of age.

In structure the eyeball reaches adult size by 8 years. At birth the iris shows little pigment, and the pupils are small. The lens is nearly spherical at birth, growing flatter throughout life. Its consistency changes from that of soft plastic at birth to rigid glass in old age.

The Aging Adult

Changes in eye structure cause distinct facial changes of the aging person. Loss of skin elasticity causes wrinkling and drooping; fat tissues and muscles atrophy; and the external eye structures appear as on p. 307. Lacrimal glands involute, causing decreased tear production and a feeling of dryness and burning.

On the globe itself an infiltration of degenerative lipid material shows around the limbus (see discussion of *arcus senilis,* p. 308). Pupil size decreases. The lens loses elasticity, becoming hard and glasslike. This glasslike quality decreases the ability of the lens to change shape to accommodate for near vision, a condition termed **presbyopia.** By 40 years of age 50% of people have presbyopia and need printed images magnified.[5] By 70 years of age the normally transparent fibers of the lens begin to thicken and yellow; this is the beginning of a cataract.

Inside the globe the vitreous is not renewed as continuously as the aqueous humor. Thus *floaters* appear from debris that accumulates. Visual acuity diminishes gradually after 50 years and even more so after 70 years. Near vision is commonly affected because of the decreased power of accommodation in the lens (presbyopia). In the early 40s a person may have blurred vision and difficulty reading. The aging person also needs more light to see because of a decreased adaptation to darkness, and this condition may affect the function of night driving. All of these changes affect **safety**, increase the risk of falls and other accidental injuries, and challenge the ability to live independently.

In older adults the most common causes of decreased visual functioning are:

1. **Cataract** formation—a clouding of the crystalline lens from a clumping of proteins. This is curable with lens-replacement surgery. Age is the primary risk factor; about 17.2% of Americans over 40 years of age have cataracts, and by age 80 more than half of adults have cataracts.[1] Women also have a 37% higher risk than men.[24]

2. **Glaucoma**—an optic nerve neuropathy characterized by loss of peripheral vision, caused by increased intraocular pressure. Age is the primary risk; over 2.2 million adults over 40 years of age have the disease, and another 2 million do not know that they have it.[1] Newer evidence shows a higher risk for women.[24]

3. **Age-related macular degeneration (AMD)**—a loss of central vision caused by yellow deposits (drusen) and neovascularity in the macula. AMD risk rises sharply with older age, and women have a slightly greater risk.[24] With AMD the person is unable to read books or papers, sew, or do fine work and has difficulty distinguishing faces. When the lifestyle is oriented around these activities, loss of central vision causes great distress. Peripheral vision is not affected; for a while the person can manage self-care and not become completely disabled.

4. **Diabetic retinopathy**—the leading cause of blindness in working-age adults 25 to 74 years of age.[14] This results in vision impairment with difficulty driving, reading, managing diabetes treatment, and other self-care. In the United States the prevalence has decreased as a result of improved management of hyperglycemia, hypertension, and lipid levels. However, worldwide the prevalence will grow because of increasing obesity rates, increasing life span, and improved detection of diabetes[2] (see Table 14-10, Retinal Vessel and Background Abnormalities, p. 323).

🌐 CULTURE AND GENETICS

Racial differences are evident in the palpebral fissures. People of Asian origin are often identified by their characteristic eyes, whereas the presence of narrowed palpebral fissures in non-Asian individuals may be diagnostic of a serious congenital disorder, Down syndrome.

Culturally based variability exists in the color of the iris and retinal pigmentation, with darker irides having darker retinas behind them. Individuals with light retinas generally have better night vision but can have pain in an environment that has too much light.

Racial Variations in Disease

Cataracts occur at higher prevalence among Whites compared to Blacks and Hispanics; however, a greater prevalence exists among younger Black females compared with younger White females.[24] The prevalence of primary open-angle glaucoma is 3 times higher in Blacks, with Whites and Hispanics having similar rates. Other evidence shows Hispanics having rates similar to those of Blacks.[24] AMD is more prevalent among Whites, especially among the very old over 75 years of age, and causes the leading form of blindness in Whites.[24] Diabetic retinopathy is a complication of diabetes mellitus caused by damage to blood vessels in the retina. There is a slightly elevated prevalence rate among Blacks and Hispanics compared to Whites.

Visual impairment is not being able to see letters on the line 20/50 or below on the eye chart. The prevalence rates are 50% higher for those living below the poverty level than among other adults. Differences among racial groups occurred when asked two questions: "Do you have any trouble seeing, even when wearing glasses or contact lenses?" and "Are you blind or unable to see at all?" Among middle adults (45 to 64 years), Native Americans, Puerto Ricans, Dominicans, and people of mixed race reported higher prevalence of visual impairment than did Whites. Among older adults over 65 years of age, prevalence of visual impairment was highest among Native Americans, Chinese Americans, Puerto Ricans, Dominicans, and Central and South Americans.[13] Thus racial disparities exist among major eye diseases and in visual impairment. In summary, Blacks and Hispanics have higher levels of vision loss and less access to health care than do Whites.

SUBJECTIVE DATA

1. Vision difficulty (decreased acuity, blurring, blind spots)
2. Pain
3. Strabismus, diplopia
4. Redness, swelling
5. Watering, discharge
6. History of ocular problems
7. Glaucoma
8. Use of glasses or contact lenses
9. Patient-centered care

Examiner Asks	Rationale
1. Vision difficulty. Any **difficulty seeing** or any blurring? Any blind spots? Come on suddenly or progress slowly? In one eye or both? • Constant or does it come and go? • Do objects appear out of focus, or does it feel like a clouding over objects? Does it feel like "grayness" of vision? • Do spots move in front of your eyes? One or many? In one or both eyes? • Any halos/rainbows around objects? Or rings around lights? • Any blind spot? Does it move as you shift your gaze? Any loss of peripheral vision? • Any night blindness?	 Floaters are common with myopia or after middle age as a result of condensed vitreous fibers. Usually not significant, but acute onset of floaters ("shade" or "cobwebs") occurs with retinal detachment. Halos around lights occur with acute narrow-angle glaucoma. **Scotoma,** a blind spot surrounded by an area of normal or decreased vision, occurs with glaucoma and optic nerve disorders. Night blindness occurs with optic atrophy, glaucoma, vitamin A deficiency.
2. Pain. Any eye pain? Please describe. • Come on suddenly? • Quality—Burning or itching? Or sharp, stabbing pain? Pain with bright light? • A foreign body sensation? Or deep aching? Or headache in brow area?	*Sudden onset* of eye symptoms (pain, floaters, blind spot, loss of peripheral vision) requires emergency referral. Quality is valuable in diagnosis. **Photophobia** is the inability to tolerate light. **NOTE:** Some common eye diseases cause no pain (e.g., cataract, glaucoma).
3. Strabismus, diplopia. Any history of crossed eyes? Now or in the past? Does this occur with eye fatigue? • Ever see double? Constant, or does it come and go? Does your double vision go away if you cover one eye or the other?	Strabismus is a deviation in the axis of the eye. **Diplopia** is the perception of two images of a single object. Diplopia in one eye is caused by eye problem: dry eyes, uncorrected refractive error, cataract. Binocular diplopia seen only when both eyes open occurs with misalignment of axes of eyes.

Subjective Data

Examiner Asks	Rationale
4. Redness, swelling. Any **redness** or **swelling** in the eyes? • Any infections? Now or in the past? When do these occur? In a particular time of year? Anyone else in home with same condition?	Redness occurs with conjunctivitis and other "red-eye" conditions (see Table 14-6, p. 319).
5. Watering, discharge. Any **watering** or excessive tearing?	Lacrimation (tearing) and epiphora (excessive tearing) are caused by irritants or obstruction in drainage of tears.
• Any **discharge?** Any matter in the eyes? Is it hard to open your eyes in the morning? What color is the discharge? • How do you remove matter from your eyes?	Purulent discharge is thick and yellow. Crusts form at night. Assess hygiene practices and how to avoid cross-contamination.
6. History of ocular problems. Any **history** of injury or surgery to eye? Or any history of allergies?	Allergens (e.g., makeup, contact lens solution) cause irritation of conjunctiva or cornea.
7. Glaucoma. Ever been tested for **glaucoma?** Results? • Any family history of glaucoma?	Glaucoma is characterized by increased intraocular pressure.
8. Use of glasses or contact lenses. Do you wear **glasses** or **contact lenses?** How do they work for you? • Last time your prescription was checked? Was it changed? • If you wear contact lenses, are there any problems such as pain, photophobia, watering, or swelling? • How do you care for contacts? How long do you wear them? How do you clean them? Do you remove them for certain activities?	Adults with glasses or contacts need an annual check to keep prescription current; adults without correction need a check every 2 or 3 years. An examination after age 40 should screen for age-related eye diseases. Assess self-care behaviors.
9. Patient-centered care. Last vision test? Ever tested for color vision? • Any environmental conditions at home or at work that may affect your eyes? For example, flying sparks, metal bits, smoke, dust, chemical fumes? If so, do you wear goggles to protect your eyes? • Which medications are you taking? Systemic or topical? Do you take any medication specifically for the eyes? • How about smoking—Do you smoke? • If you have experienced a vision loss, how do you cope? Do you have books with large print, books on audio tape or CD, braille? • Do you maintain your living environment the same? • Do you sometimes fear complete loss of vision?	Self-care behaviors for eyes and vision. Work-related eye disease (e.g., an auto mechanic with a foreign body from metal working or radiation damage from welding). Some medications affect the eyes (e.g., prednisone may cause cataracts or increased intraocular pressure). Cigarette smoking is associated with AMD, cataract, diabetic retinopathy, and eye inflammation. A constant spatial layout eases navigation through the home.

Additional History for Infants and Children

1. Any vaginal infections in the mother at time of delivery?	Genital herpes and gonorrhea have risk of eye disease for the newborn.
2. Considering age of child, which developmental milestones of vision have you (parent) noted?	The parent is most often the one to detect vision problems.
3. Does the child have routine vision testing at school?	
4. Are you (parent) aware of safety measures to protect child's eyes from trauma? Do you inspect toys? • Have you taught the child safe care of sharp objects and how to carry and use them?	

Examiner Asks	Rationale

Additional History for the Aging Adult

1. Have you noticed any visual difficulty with climbing stairs or driving? Any problem with night vision?

Loss of depth perception or central vision may occur.

2. When was the last time you were tested for glaucoma?

At age 60 or 65 years people need annual examination to screen for vision changes and age-related eye diseases.

  - Any aching pain around eyes? Any loss of peripheral vision?
  - If you have glaucoma, how do you manage your eyedrops?

Compliance may be a problem if symptoms are absent. Assess ability to administer eyedrops.

3. Is there a history of cataracts? Any loss or progressive blurring of vision?
4. Do your eyes ever feel dry? Burning? What do you do for this?

Decreased tear production may occur with aging.

5. Any decrease in usual activities such as reading or sewing? Driving?

AMD is a loss of central vision that impairs daily pleasures and activities.

OBJECTIVE DATA

PREPARATION

Position the person standing for vision screening; then sitting up with the head at your eye level.

EQUIPMENT NEEDED

Snellen eye chart
Handheld visual screener
Opaque card or occluder
Penlight
Applicator stick
Ophthalmoscope

Normal Range of Findings	Abnormal Findings

Test Central Visual Acuity

Snellen Eye Chart

The Snellen alphabet chart is the most commonly used and accurate measure of visual acuity. It has lines of letters arranged in decreasing size.

Place the Snellen alphabet chart in a well-lit spot at eye level. Position the person on a mark exactly 20 feet from the chart. Use an opaque card to shield one eye at a time during the test; inadvertent peeking may result when shielding the eye with the person's own fingers (Fig. 14-9). If the person wears glasses or contact lenses, leave them on. Remove only reading glasses because they blur distance vision. Ask the person to read through the chart to the smallest line of letters possible. Encourage trying the next smallest line also. (NOTE: Use a Snellen picture chart for people who cannot read letters. See p. 303.)

Note hesitancy, squinting, leaning forward, misreading letters.

Normal Range of Findings	Abnormal Findings

14-9

Record the result using the numeric fraction at the end of the last successful line read. Indicate whether the person missed any letters or if corrective lenses were worn (e.g., "Right 20/30 −1, with glasses") (i.e., the right eye scored 20/30, missing one letter).

Normal visual acuity is 20/20. Contrary to some people's impression, the numeric fraction is *not* a percentage of normal vision. Instead, the top number (numerator) indicates the distance the person is standing from the chart, and the denominator gives the distance at which a normal eye could have read that particular line. Thus "20/30" means, "You can read at 20 feet what the normal eye can see from 30 feet away."

The larger the denominator, the poorer the vision. If vision is poorer than 20/30, refer to an ophthalmologist or optometrist. Impaired vision results from refractive error, opacity in the media (cornea, lens, vitreous), or disorder in the retina or optic pathway.

If the person is unable to see even the largest letters, shorten the distance to the chart until it is seen and record that distance (e.g., "10/200"). If visual acuity is even lower, assess whether the person can count your fingers when they are spread in front of the eyes or distinguish light perception from your penlight.

Near Vision

For people older than 40 years or those who report increasing difficulty reading, test near vision with a handheld vision screener with various sizes of print (e.g., a Jaeger card) (Fig. 14-10). Hold the card in good light about 35 cm (14 inches) from the eye—this distance equals the print size on the 20-foot chart. Test each eye separately with the person wearing glasses. A normal result is "14/14" in each eye, read without hesitancy and without moving the card closer or farther away. When no vision screening card is available, ask the person to read from a magazine or newspaper.

Presbyopia, the decrease in power of accommodation with aging, is suggested when the person moves the card farther away.

Objective Data

Normal Range of Findings	Abnormal Findings

14-10

Test Visual Fields

Confrontation Test

This test screens for loss of peripheral vision. It compares the person's peripheral vision with your own, assuming that yours is normal. Position yourself at eye level about 2 feet away. Looking straight at you, the person covers one eye with an opaque card (here the right eye) as you cover the opposite eye (here the left) (Fig. 14-11, *A* and *B*). You are testing the uncovered eye. Hold a wiggling finger as a target midline between you and the person and slowly advance it in from the periphery in several directions.

A   B

14-11

Normal Range of Findings

Ask the person to say "now" as the target is first seen; this should be just as you also see the object. For the temporal direction, start your finger somewhat behind the person. Estimate the angle between the anteroposterior axis of the eye and the peripheral axis where the object is first seen. Normal results are about 50 degrees upward, 90 degrees temporally, 70 degrees inferiorly, and 60 degrees nasally (Fig. 14-12).[3]

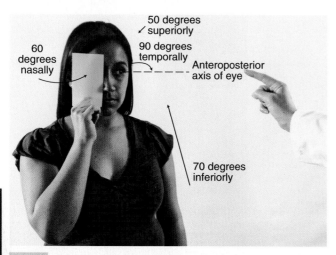

60 degrees nasally

50 degrees superiorly

90 degrees temporally

Anteroposterior axis of eye

70 degrees inferiorly

14-12 Range of peripheral vision.

The sensitivity of confrontation testing can be increased by combining the wiggling finger test with a moving red target.[11] Hold a 5-mm red-topped pin beyond the boundary of each quadrant between the horizontal and vertical axes. Move it inward and ask the person to state when the pin first appears as red.

Inspect Extraocular Muscle Function

Corneal Light Reflex (Hirschberg Test)

Assess the parallel alignment of the eye axes by shining a light toward the person's eyes. Direct the person to stare straight ahead as you hold the light about 30 cm (12 inches) away. Note the reflection of the light on the corneas; it should be in exactly the same spot on each eye. See the bright white dots in Fig. 14-27 for symmetry of the corneal light reflex.

Diagnostic Positions Test

Leading the eyes through the six cardinal positions of gaze elicits any muscle weakness during movement (Fig. 14-13). Ask the person to hold the head steady and follow the movement of your finger only with the eyes. Hold the target back about 30 cm (12 inches) so the person can focus on it comfortably, move it to each of the six positions, hold it momentarily, then back to center. Progress clockwise. A normal response is parallel tracking of the object with both eyes.

Abnormal Findings

If the person is unable to see the object as the examiner does, the test suggests peripheral field loss. In an older adult this screens for glaucoma. Refer to a specialist for more precise testing (see Table 14-5, Visual Field Loss). Acutely diminished visual fields occur with diseases of the retina and with stroke.

Asymmetry of the light reflex indicates deviation in alignment from eye muscle weakness or paralysis. If you see this, perform the cover test described on p. 304.

Eye movement is not parallel. Failure to follow in a certain direction indicates weakness of an EOM or dysfunction of the cranial nerve innervating it.

Normal Range of Findings	Abnormal Findings

14-13 Diagnostic positions test.

In addition to parallel movement, note any **nystagmus**—a fine, oscillating movement best seen around the iris. Mild nystagmus at an extreme lateral gaze is normal; nystagmus at any other position is not.

Nystagmus occurs with disease of the semicircular canals in the ears, a paretic eye muscle, multiple sclerosis, or brain lesions.

Finally note that the upper eyelid continues to overlap the superior part of the iris, even during downward movement. You should not see a white rim of sclera between the lid and the iris. If noted, this is termed *lid lag*.

Lid lag occurs with hyperthyroidism.

Inspect External Ocular Structures

Begin with the most external points and logically work your way inward.

General

Already you will have noted the person's ability to move around the room, with vision functioning well enough to avoid obstacles and to respond to your directions. Also note the facial expression; a relaxed expression accompanies adequate vision.

Groping with hands.

Squinting or craning forward.

Eyebrows

Look for symmetry between the two eyes. Normally the eyebrows are present bilaterally, move symmetrically as the facial expression changes, and have no scaling or lesions (Fig. 14-14).

Unequal or absent movement with nerve damage.
Scaling with seborrhea.

14-14

Objective Data

Normal Range of Findings	Abnormal Findings

Eyelids and Lashes

The upper lids normally overlap the superior part of the iris and approximate completely with the lower lids when closed. The skin is intact without redness, swelling, discharge, or lesions.

The palpebral fissures are horizontal in non-Asians, whereas Asians normally have an upward slant.

> Lid lag with hyperthyroidism.
> Incomplete closure creates risk for corneal damage.
> Ptosis, drooping of upper lid.
> Periorbital edema, lesions (see Tables 14-2, Eyelid Abnormalities, and 14-3, Lesions on the Eyelids).
> Ectropion and entropion (see Table 14-2, p. 314).

Note that the eyelashes are distributed evenly along the lid margins and curve outward.

Eyeballs

The eyeballs are aligned normally in their sockets with no protrusion or sunken appearance. Blacks normally may have a slight protrusion of the eyeball beyond the supraorbital ridge.

> Exophthalmos (protruding eyes) and enophthalmos (sunken eyes) (see Table 14-2).

Conjunctiva and Sclera

Ask the person to look up. Using your thumbs, slide the lower lids down along the bony orbital rim. Take care not to push against the eyeball. Inspect the exposed area (Fig. 14-15). The eyeball looks moist and glossy. Numerous small blood vessels normally show through the transparent conjunctiva. Otherwise the conjunctivae are clear and show the normal color of the structure below—pink over the lower lids and white over the sclera. Note any color change, swelling, or lesions.

> General reddening (see Table 14-6, Red Eye—Vascular Disorders, p. 319).
> Cyanosis of the lower lids.
> Pallor near the outer canthus of the lower lid may indicate anemia (the inner canthus normally contains less pigment).

14-15

The sclera is china white, although Blacks occasionally have a gray-blue or "muddy" color to the sclera. Also in dark-skinned people you normally may see small brown macules (like freckles) on the sclera, which should not be confused with foreign bodies or petechiae. Finally, Blacks may have yellowish fatty deposits beneath the lids away from the cornea. Do not confuse these yellow spots with the overall scleral yellowing that accompanies jaundice.

> **Scleral icterus** is an even yellowing of the sclera extending up to the cornea, indicating jaundice.
> Tenderness, foreign body, discharge, or lesions.

Eversion of the Upper Lid

This maneuver is not part of the normal examination, but it is useful when you must inspect the conjunctiva of the upper lid, as with eye pain or suspicion of a foreign body. Most people are apprehensive of any eye manipulation. Enhance their cooperation by using a calm and gentle, yet deliberate, approach.

Normal Range of Findings	**Abnormal Findings**

1. Ask the person to keep both eyes open and look down. This relaxes the eyelid, whereas closing it would tense the orbicularis muscle.
2. Slide the upper lid up along the bony orbit to lift up the eyelashes.
3. Grasp the lashes between your thumb and forefinger and gently pull down and outward.
4. With your other hand, place the tip of an applicator stick on the upper lid above the level of the internal tarsal plates (Fig. 14-16, *A*).
5. Gently push down with the stick as you lift the lashes. This uses the edge of the tarsal plate as a fulcrum and flips the lid inside out. Take special care not to push in on the eyeball.
6. Secure the everted position by holding the lashes against the bony orbital rim (Fig. 14-16, *B*).
7. Inspect for any color change, swelling, lesion, or foreign body.
8. To return to normal position, gently pull the lashes outward as the person looks up.

A   B   14-16

Lacrimal Apparatus

Ask the person to look down. With your thumbs, slide the outer part of the upper lid up along the bony orbit to expose under the lid. Inspect for any redness or swelling.

Normally the puncta drain the tears into the lacrimal sac. Presence of excessive tearing may indicate blockage of the nasolacrimal duct. Check this by pressing the index finger against the sac, just inside the lower orbital rim, not against the side of the nose (Fig. 14-17). Pressure slightly everts the lower lid, but there should be no other response to pressure.

Swelling of the lacrimal gland may show as a visible bulge in the outer part of the upper lid.

Puncta red, swollen, tender to pressure.

Watch for any regurgitation of fluid out of the puncta, which confirms duct blockage.

14-17

Objective Data

Normal Range of Findings	Abnormal Findings

Inspect Anterior Eyeball Structures

Cornea and Lens

Shine a light from the side across the cornea and check for smoothness and clarity. This oblique view highlights any abnormal irregularities in the corneal surface. There should be no opacities (cloudiness) in the cornea, the anterior chamber, or the lens behind the pupil. Do not confuse an **arcus senilis** with opacity. The arcus senilis is a normal finding in aging persons and is illustrated on p. 308.

A corneal abrasion causes irregular ridges in reflected light, producing a shattered look to light rays (see Table 14-7, Abnormalities on Cornea and Iris, p. 320).

Iris and Pupil

The iris normally appears flat, with a round regular shape and even coloration. Note the size, shape, and equality of the pupils. Normally the pupils appear round, regular, and of equal size in both eyes. In the adult resting size is from 3 to 5 mm. A small number of people (5%) normally have pupils of two different sizes, which is termed **anisocoria.**

To test the **pupillary light reflex,** darken the room and ask the person to gaze into the distance. (This dilates the pupils.) Advance a light in from the side* and note the response. Normally you will see (1) constriction of the same-sided pupil (a *direct light reflex*), and (2) simultaneous constriction of the other pupil (a *consensual light reflex*).

In the acute-care setting, gauge the pupil size in millimeters, both before and after the light reflex. Recording the pupil size in millimeters is more accurate when many nurses and physicians care for the same person or when small changes may be significant signs of increasing intracranial pressure. Normally the resting size is 3, 4, or 5 mm and decreases equally in response to light. A normal response is recorded as:

$$\text{Right } \frac{3}{1} = \frac{3}{1} \text{ Left}$$

This indicates that both pupils measure 3 mm in the resting state and that both constrict to 1 mm in response to light. A graduated scale printed on a handheld vision screener or taped onto a tongue blade facilitates your measurement (see Fig. 23-58).

Test for **accommodation** by asking the person to focus on a distant object (Fig. 14-18). This process dilates the pupils. Then have the person shift the gaze to a near object such as your finger held about 7 to 8 cm (3 inches) from the person's nose. A normal response includes (1) pupillary constriction, and (2) convergence of the axes of the eyes.

Irregular shape.

Although they may be normal, all unequal-size pupils call for a consideration of central nervous system injury.

Dilated pupils.

Dilated and fixed pupils.

Constricted pupils.

Unequal or no response to light (see Table 14-4, Pupil Abnormalities, p. 316).

Absence of constriction or convergence. Asymmetric response.

Far vision - pupils dilate   Near vision - pupils constrict

14-18   © Pat Thomas, 2006.

*Always advance the light in from the *side* to test the light reflex. If you advance from the front, the pupils constrict to accommodate for near vision. Thus you do not know what the pure response to the light would have been.

Normal Range of Findings	Abnormal Findings

Record the normal response to all these maneuvers as PERRLA, or **P**upils **E**qual, **R**ound, **R**eact to **L**ight, and **A**ccommodation.

Inspect the Ocular Fundus

The ophthalmoscope enlarges your view of the eye so you can inspect the **media** (anterior chamber, lens, vitreous) and the **ocular fundus** (the internal surface of the retina). It accomplishes this by directing a beam of light through the pupil to illuminate the inner structures. Thus using the ophthalmoscope is like peering through a keyhole (the pupil) into an interesting room beyond.

The ophthalmoscope should function as an appendage of your own eye. This takes some practice. Practice holding the instrument and focusing at objects around the room before you approach a "real" person. Hold the ophthalmoscope right up to your eye, braced firmly against the cheek and brow. Extend your index finger onto the lens selector dial so you can refocus as needed during the procedure without taking your head away from the ophthalmoscope to look. Now look about the room, moving your head and the instrument together as one unit. Keep both your eyes open; just view the field through the ophthalmoscope.

Recall that the ophthalmoscope contains a set of lenses that control the focus (Fig. 14-19). The unit of strength of each lens is the *diopter*. The black numbers indicate a positive diopter; they focus on objects nearer in space to the ophthalmoscope. The red numbers show a negative diopter and are for focusing on objects farther away.

— Viewing aperture

— Lens selector dial

— Diopter indicator

14-19

To examine a person, darken the room to help dilate the pupils. (Dilating eyedrops are not needed during a screening examination. When indicated, they dilate the pupils for a wider look at the fundus background and macular area. Eyedrops are used only when glaucoma can be ruled out completely because dilating the pupils in the presence of glaucoma can precipitate an acute episode.)

Remove your eyeglasses and those of the other person; they obstruct close movement and you can compensate for their correction by using the diopter setting. Contact lenses may be left in; they pose no problem as long as they are clean.

Objective Data

Normal Range of Findings	Abnormal Findings

Select the large round aperture with the white light for the routine examination. If the pupils are small, use the smaller white light. (Although the instrument has other shape and color apertures, these are rarely used in a screening examination.) The light must have maximum brightness; replace old or dim batteries.

Tell the person, "Please keep looking at that light switch (or mark) on the wall across the room, even though my head will get in the way." Staring at a distant fixed object helps to dilate the pupils and hold the retinal structures still.

Match sides with the person. That is, hold the ophthalmoscope in your *right* hand up to your *right* eye to view the person's *right* eye. You must do this to avoid bumping noses during the procedure. Place your free hand on the person's shoulder or forehead (Fig. 14-20, *A*). This helps orient you in space because, once you have the ophthalmoscope in position, you have only a very narrow range of vision. In addition, your thumb can anchor the upper lid and help prevent blinking.

14-20, A

Begin about 25 cm (10 inches) away from the person at an angle about 15 degrees lateral to the person's line of vision. Note the red glow filling the person's pupil. This is the **red reflex,** caused by the reflection of your ophthalmoscope light off the inner retina. Keep sight of the red reflex and steadily move closer to the eye. If you lose the red reflex, the light has wandered off the pupil and onto the iris or sclera. Adjust your angle to find it again.

As you advance, adjust the lens to +6 and note any opacities in the media. These appear as dark shadows or black dots interrupting the red reflex. Normally none are present. Progress toward the person until your foreheads almost touch (Fig. 14-20, *B*).

Cataracts appear as opaque black areas against the red reflex (see Table 14-8, Lens Opacities, p. 322).

14-20, B

Normal Range of Findings

Adjust the diopter setting to bring the ocular fundus into sharp focus. If you and the person have normal vision, this should be at 0. Moving the diopters compensates for nearsightedness or farsightedness. Use the red lenses for nearsighted eyes and the black for farsighted eyes (Fig. 14-21).

Abnormal Findings

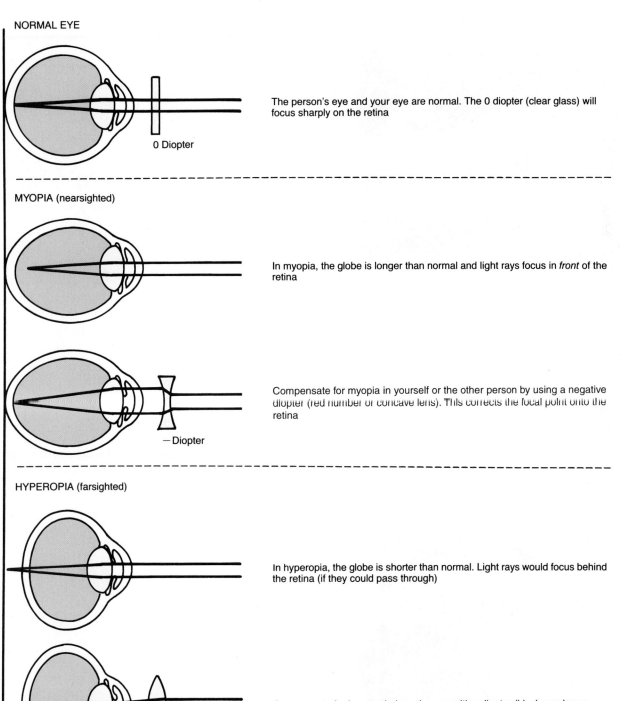

NORMAL EYE

0 Diopter

The person's eye and your eye are normal. The 0 diopter (clear glass) will focus sharply on the retina

MYOPIA (nearsighted)

In myopia, the globe is longer than normal and light rays focus in *front* of the retina

−Diopter

Compensate for myopia in yourself or the other person by using a negative diopter (red number or concave lens). This corrects the focal point onto the retina

HYPEROPIA (farsighted)

In hyperopia, the globe is shorter than normal. Light rays would focus behind the retina (if they could pass through)

+ Diopter

Compensate for hyperopia by using a positive diopter (black number or convex lens). This bends the light rays so the focal point is on the retina

14-21

Objective Data

Normal Range of Findings	Abnormal Findings

Objective Data

Moving in on the 15-degree lateral line should bring your view just to the optic disc. If the disc is not in sight, track a blood vessel as it grows larger, and it will lead you to the disc. Systematically inspect the structures in the ocular fundus: (1) optic disc, (2) retinal vessels, (3) general background, and (4) macula (Fig. 14-22). (NOTE: The illustration here shows a large area of the fundus. Your actual view through the ophthalmoscope is much smaller—slightly larger than 1 disc diameter.)

14-22 Normal ocular fundus. (Heather Boyd-Monk and Wills Eye Hospital.)

Optic Disc

The most prominent landmark is the optic disc, located on the nasal side of the retina. Explore these characteristics:

1. **Color**	Creamy yellow-orange to pink.	Pallor. Hyperemia.
2. **Shape**	Round or oval.	Irregular shape.
3. **Margins**	Distinct and sharply demarcated, although the nasal edge may be slightly fuzzy.	Blurred margins.
4. **Cup-disc ratio**	Distinctness varies. When visible, physiologic cup is a brighter yellow-white than rest of the disc. Its width is not more than one-half the disc diameter (Fig. 14-23).	Cup extending to the disc border (see Table 14-9, Optic Disc Abnormalities, p. 322).

14-23 Normal optic disc.   (Lemmi & Lemmi, 2011.)

| **Normal Range of Findings** | **Abnormal Findings** |

Two normal variations may ring around the disc margins. A **scleral crescent** is a gray-white, new-moon shape. It occurs when pigment is absent in the choroid layer and you are looking directly at the sclera. A **pigment crescent** is black; it is caused by accumulation of pigment in the choroid.

The diameter of the disc, or DD, is a standard of measure for other fundus structures (Fig. 14-24). To describe a finding, note its clock-face position and its relationship to the disc in size and distance (e.g., "... macula at 3:00, 2 DD from the disc").

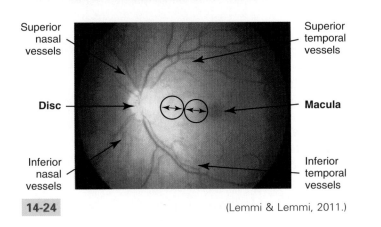

Superior nasal vessels

Disc

Inferior nasal vessels

Superior temporal vessels

Macula

Inferior temporal vessels

14-24   (Lemmi & Lemmi, 2011.)

Retinal Vessels

This is the only place in the body where you can view blood vessels directly. Many systemic diseases that affect the vascular system show signs in the retinal vessels. Follow a paired artery and vein out to the periphery in the four quadrants (see Fig. 14-22), noting these points:

1. **Number**	A paired artery and vein pass to each quadrant. Vessels look straighter at the nasal side.
2. **Color**	Arteries are brighter red than veins. They also have the arterial light reflex, with a thin stripe of light down the middle.
3. **A:V ratio**	The ratio comparing the artery-to-vein width is 2:3 or 4:5.
4. **Caliber**	Arteries and veins show a regular decrease in caliber as they extend to the periphery.
5. **A-V (arteriovenous) crossing**	An artery and vein may cross paths. This is not significant if within 2 DD of disc and if no sign of interruption in blood flow is seen. There should be no indenting or displacing of vessel.
6. **Tortuosity**	Tortuosity is mild vessel twisting; when present in both eyes is usually congenital and not significant.
7. **Pulsations**	Pulsations are present in veins near the disc as their drainage meets the intermittent pressure of arterial systole (often hard to see).

General Background of the Fundus

The color normally varies from light red to dark brown–red, generally corresponding with the person's skin color. Your view of the fundus should be clear; no lesions should obstruct the retinal structures.

Absence of major vessels.

Arteries too constricted.
Veins dilated.
Focal constriction.
Neovascularization (proliferation of new vessels).
Crossings more than 2 DD away from disc.
Nicking or pinching of underlying vessel. Vessel engorged peripheral to crossing (see Table 14-10).
Extreme tortuosity or marked asymmetry in two eyes.
Absent pulsations.

Abnormal lesions: hemorrhages, exudates, microaneurysms.

Normal Range of Findings	Abnormal Findings

Macula

The macula is 1 DD in size and located 2 DD temporal to the disc (Fig. 14-24). Inspect this area last in the funduscopic examination. A bright light on this area of central vision causes some watering and discomfort and pupillary constriction. Note that the normal color of the area is somewhat darker than the rest of the fundus but is even and homogeneous. Clumped pigment may occur with aging.

Within the macula you may note the foveal light reflex. This is a tiny white glistening dot reflecting your ophthalmoscope light.

Clumped pigment occurs with trauma or retinal detachment.

Hemorrhage or exudate in the macula occurs with senile macular degeneration.

❖ DEVELOPMENTAL COMPETENCE

Infants and Children

The eye examination is often deferred at birth because of transient edema of the lids from birth trauma or instillation of silver nitrate at birth. The eyes should be examined within a few days and at every well-child visit thereafter.

Visual Acuity. The child's age determines the screening measures used. With a newborn, test visual reflexes and attending behaviors. Test **light perception** using the blink reflex; the neonate blinks in response to bright light (Fig. 14-25). The pupillary light reflex also shows that the pupils constrict in response to light. These reflexes indicate that the lower portion of the visual apparatus is intact. But you cannot infer that the infant can *see*; this requires later observation to show that the brain has received images and can interpret them.

Absent blinking.
Absent pupillary light reflex, especially after 3 weeks, indicates blindness.

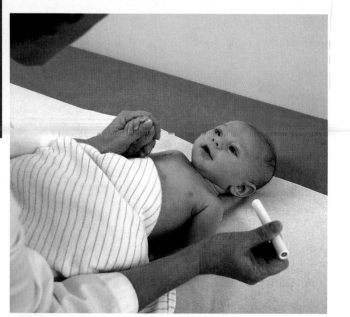

14-25

As you introduce an object to the infant's line of vision, note these attending behaviors:

- **Birth to 2 weeks**—Refusal to reopen eyes after exposure to bright light; increasing alertness to object; infant may fixate on an object.
- **By 2 to 4 weeks**—Infant can fixate on an object.
- **By 1 month**—Infant can fixate and follow a light or bright toy.
- **By 6 weeks**—Infant makes some visual response to your face.
- **By 3 to 4 months**—Infant can fixate, follow, and reach for the toy.
- **By 6 to 10 months**—Infant can fixate and follow the toy in all directions.

Normal Range of Findings

The Allen test (picture cards) screens children from 2½ years to 2 years and 11 months of age and is even reliable with cooperative toddlers as young as 2 years. The test contains seven cards of familiar objects (birthday cake, teddy bear, tree, house, car, telephone, and horse and rider). First show the pictures up close to the child to make sure that the child can identify them. Then present each picture at a distance of 15 feet. Results are normal if the child can name three of seven cards within three to five trials.

Use a picture chart or the Snellen E chart for the preschooler from 3 to 6 years of age. The E chart shows the capital letter E in varying sizes pointing in different directions. The child points his or her fingers in the direction the "table legs" are pointing. By 7 to 8 years of age, when the child is familiar with reading letters, begin to use the standard Snellen alphabet chart. Normally a child achieves 20/20 acuity by 6 to 7 years of age (Fig. 14-26).

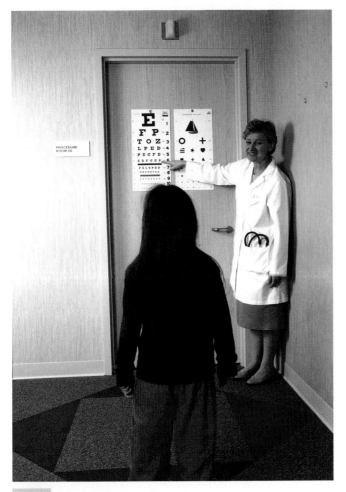

14-26

Visual Fields. Assess peripheral vision with the confrontation test in children older than 3 years when the preschooler is able to stay in position. As with the adult, the child should see the moving target at the same time your normal eyes do. Often a young child forgets to say "now" or "stop" as the moving object is seen. Rather, note the instant the child's eyes deviate or head shifts position to gaze at the moving object. Match this nearly automatic response with your own sighting.

Abnormal Findings

The National Society for Prevention of Blindness states these criteria for referral:
1. Age 3 years—Vision 20/50 or less in either eye.
2. Age 4 years and older—20/40 or less in either eye.
3. Difference between two eyes is one line or more.
4. Child shows other signs of vision impairment, regardless of acuity.

Screen two separate times before referral.

Objective Data

| **Normal Range of Findings** | **Abnormal Findings** |

Objective Data

Color Vision. Color blindness is an inherited recessive X-linked trait affecting about 8% of White males and 4% of Black males. It is rare in females (0.4%). *Color deficient* is a more accurate term because the condition is relative and not disabling. Often it is just a social inconvenience, although it may affect the person's ability to discern traffic lights or school performance in which color is a learning tool.

Test only boys for color vision, once between the ages of 4 and 8 years. Use the Ishihara test, a series of polychromatic cards. Each card has a pattern of dots printed against a background of many colored dots. Ask the child to identify each pattern. A boy with normal color vision can see each pattern. A color-blind person cannot see the letter against the field color.

Extraocular Muscle Function. Testing for **strabismus** (squint, crossed eye) is an important screening measure between ages 3 and 5 years. Strabismus causes disconjugate vision because one eye deviates off the fixation point. To avoid diplopia or unclear images, the brain begins to suppress data from the weak eye (a suppression scotoma), causing visual acuity in this otherwise normal eye to begin to deteriorate from disuse. Early recognition and treatment are essential to restore binocular vision. Diagnosis after 6 years of age has a poor prognosis. Test malalignment by the corneal light reflex and the cover test.

Check the **corneal light reflex** by shining a light toward the child's eyes. The light should be reflected at exactly the same spot in the two corneas (Fig. 14-27).

Some asymmetry (where one light falls off center) under 6 months of age is normal.

Untreated strabismus can lead to permanent visual damage. The resulting loss of vision from disuse is amblyopia ex anopsia. About 2% to 4% of preschool children have this.[22]

Asymmetry in the corneal light reflex after 6 months is abnormal and must be referred.

14-27

Perform the **cover test** on all children. This test detects small degrees of deviated alignment by interrupting the fusion reflex that normally keeps the two eyes parallel. Ask the child to stare straight ahead at your nose or at a familiar puppet.

Normal Range of Findings

With an opaque card, cover one eye. As it is covered, note the uncovered eye. A normal response is a steady, fixed gaze.

Meanwhile the macular image has been suppressed on the covered eye. If muscle weakness exists, the covered eye drifts into a relaxed position.

Now uncover the eye and observe it for movement. It should stare straight ahead. If it jumps to re-establish fixation, eye muscle weakness exists. Repeat with the other eye.

Function of the extraocular muscles during movement can be assessed during the early weeks by the child's following a brightly colored toy as a target. An older infant can sit on the parent's lap as you move the toy in all directions. After 2 years of age, direct the child's gaze through the six cardinal positions of gaze. You may stabilize the child's chin with your hand to prevent him or her from moving the entire head.

External Eye Structures. Inspect the ocular structures as described in the earlier section. A neonate usually holds the eyes tightly shut. Do not attempt to pry them open; that just increases contraction of the orbicularis oculi muscle. Hold the newborn supine and gently lower the head; the eyes will open. The eyes will also open when you hold the infant at arm's length and slowly turn him or her in one direction (Fig. 14-28). In addition to inspecting the ocular structures, this also tests the vestibular function reflex. The baby's eyes look in the same direction as the body is being turned. When the turning stops, the eyes shift to the opposite direction after a few quick beats of nystagmus. Also termed *doll's eyes,* this reflex disappears by 2 months of age.

14-28

Eyelids and Lashes. Normally the upper lids overlie the superior part of the iris. In newborns the *setting-sun sign* is common. The eyes appear to deviate down, and you see a white rim of sclera over the iris. It may show as you rapidly change the neonate from a sitting to a supine position.

Abnormal Findings

If the eye jumps to fixate on the designated point, it was out of alignment before.

A **phoria** is a mild weakness noted only when fusion is blocked. **Tropia** is more severe—a constant malalignment of the eyes (see Table 14-1, Extraocular Muscle Dysfunction, p. 312)

The setting-sun sign also occurs with hydrocephalus as the globes protrude.
Blank sunken eyes accompany malnutrition, dehydration, and a severe illness.

Normal Range of Findings	Abnormal Findings

Many infants have an *epicanthal fold,* an excess skinfold extending over the inner corner of the eye, partly or totally overlapping the inner canthus. It occurs frequently in Asian children and in 20% of Whites. In non-Asians, it disappears as the child grows, usually by 10 years of age. While they are present, epicanthal folds give a false appearance of malalignment, termed **pseudostrabismus** (Fig. 14-29). Yet the corneal light reflex is normal.

14-29 Pseudostrabismus.　(Zitelli, 2007.)

Asian infants normally have an upward slant of the palpebral fissures. Entropion, a turning inward of the eyelid, is found normally in some Asian children. If the lashes do not abrade the corneas, it is not significant.

Conjunctiva and Sclera. A newborn may have a transient chemical conjunctivitis from the instillation of silver nitrate. This appears within 1 hour and lasts not more than 24 hours after birth. The sclera should be white and clear, although it may have a blue tint as a result of thinness at birth. The lacrimal glands are not functional at birth.

Iris and Pupils. The iris normally is blue or slate gray in light-skinned newborns and brown in dark-skinned infants. By 6 to 9 months the permanent color is differentiated. Brushfield spots, or white specks around the edge of the iris, occasionally may be normal.

A searching nystagmus is common just after birth. The pupils are small but constrict to light.

The Ocular Fundus. The amount of data gathered during the funduscopic examination depends on the child's ability to hold the eyes still and on your ability to glean as much data as possible in a brief period of time.

A complete funduscopic examination is difficult to perform on an infant, but at least check the red reflex when the infant fixates at the bright light for a few seconds. Note any interruption.

Perform a funduscopic examination on an infant between 2 and 6 months of age. Position the infant (up to 18 months) lying on the table. The fundus appears pale, and the vessels are not fully developed. There is no foveal light reflection because the macula area will not be mature until 1 year.

Inspect the fundus of the young child and school-age child as described in the preceding section on the adult. Allow the child to handle the equipment. Explain why you are darkening the room and that you will leave a small light on. Assure the child that the procedure will not hurt. Direct the young child to look at an appealing picture, perhaps a toy or an animal, during the examination.

Abnormal Findings

An upward lateral slope together with epicanthal folds and hypertelorism (large spacing between eyes) occurs with Down syndrome.

Ophthalmia neonatorum (conjunctivitis of the newborn) is a purulent discharge caused by a chemical irritant or a bacterial or viral agent from the birth canal.

Absence of iris color occurs with albinism.

Brushfield spots usually suggest Down syndrome.

Constant nystagmus, prolonged setting-sun sign, marked strabismus, and slow lateral movements suggest vision loss.

An interruption in the red reflex indicates opacity in the cornea or lens. An absent red reflex occurs with congenital cataracts or retinal disorders.

Papilledema is rare in the infant because the fontanels and open sutures absorb any increased intracranial pressure if it occurs.

Normal Range of Findings	Abnormal Findings

The Aging Adult

Visual Acuity. Perform the same examination as described in the adult section. Central acuity may decrease, particularly after 70 years of age. Peripheral vision may be diminished.

Ocular Structures. The eyebrows may show a loss of the outer one third to one half of hair because of a decrease in hair follicles. The remaining brow hair is coarse (Fig. 14-30). As a result of atrophy of elastic tissues, the skin around the eyes may show wrinkles or crow's feet. The upper lid may be so elongated as to rest on the lashes, resulting in a pseudoptosis.

In older adults an increased risk of falls and fractures occurs with a distance visual acuity of 20/25 or greater.[17]

14-30 Pseudoptosis. (Albert and Jakobiec, 1994.)

The eyes may appear sunken from atrophy of the orbital fat. In addition, the orbital fat may herniate, causing bulging at the lower lids and inner third of the upper lids.

The lacrimal apparatus may decrease tear production, causing the eyes to look dry and lusterless and the person to report a burning sensation. **Pingueculae** commonly show on the sclera (Fig. 14-31). These yellowish elevated nodules are caused by a thickening of the bulbar conjunctiva from prolonged exposure to sun, wind, and dust. Pingueculae appear at the 3 and 9 o'clock positions—first on the nasal side and then on the temporal side.

Ectropion (lower lid dropping away) and entropion (lower lid turning in) (see Table 14-2).

Distinguish pinguecula from the abnormal **pterygium,** also an opacity on the bulbar conjunctiva, but one that grows over the cornea (see Table 14-7).

14-31 Pinguecula. (Lemmi & Lemmi, 2011.)

Objective Data

Normal Range of Findings	Abnormal Findings

The cornea may look cloudy with age. An **arcus senilis** is commonly seen around the cornea (Fig. 14-32). This is a gray-white arc or circle around the limbus; it is caused by deposition of lipid material. As more lipid accumulates, the cornea may look thickened and raised, but the arcus has no effect on vision.

14-32 Arcus senilis. (Swartz, 2005.)

Xanthelasma are soft, raised yellow plaques occurring on the lids at the inner canthus (Fig. 14-33). They commonly occur around the 50s and more frequently in women. They occur with both high and normal blood levels of cholesterol and have no pathologic significance.

14-33 Xanthelasma. (Lemmi & Lemmi, 2011.)

Pupils are small in old age, and the pupillary light reflex may be slowed. The lens loses transparency and looks opaque.

The Ocular Fundus. Retinal structures generally have less shine. The blood vessels look paler, narrower, and attenuated. Arterioles appear paler and straighter, with a narrower light reflex. More arteriovenous crossing defects occur.

A normal development on the retinal surface are **drusen,** or benign degenerative hyaline deposits (Fig. 14-34). They are small, round, yellow dots that are scattered haphazardly on the retina. Although they do not occur in a pattern, they are usually symmetrically placed in the two eyes. They have no effect on vision.

Drusen are easily confused with the abnormal finding *hard exudates,* which occur with a more circular or linear pattern (see Table 14-10, p. 323). Also, drusen in the macular area occur with macular degeneration.

(side margin) Objective Data

Normal Range of Findings	Abnormal Findings

14-34 Drusen. (Friedman, N., & Pineda, R., 1998.)

PROMOTING A HEALTHY LIFESTYLE

Glaucoma Screening

According to the National Eye Institute (NEI), the National Institutes of Health (NIH) lead agency for vision research, glaucoma is a leading cause of blindness in the United States, especially among African Americans and Hispanics. Of particular concern is that among African Americans between the ages of 45 and 64, glaucoma is 15 times more likely to cause blindness.

Over 2 million Americans have been diagnosed with glaucoma, and it is estimated that an additional 2 million have the disease but don't know it. Glaucoma is a condition that most often involves optic nerve damage and visual field changes. The problem is that glaucoma can reduce peripheral vision without harming central vision. Of note is that people with advanced glaucoma were able to pass their driver's visual acuity test because it checks only straight-ahead distance vision. A visual field test could identify these individuals earlier, prevent those with severe peripheral vision loss from renewing their licenses, or trigger a requirement for special mirrors to be installed on the individual's vehicle.

The risk of glaucoma increases with age, but it can occur in anyone in any age- group. While there is no cure for glaucoma, there has been progress in understanding the genetics of glaucoma that holds promise for the future. Medication, laser trabeculoplasty, and/or surgery can slow or prevent further vision loss. Unfortunately treatments do not improve sight already lost from glaucoma. Therefore early detection is critical to stopping the progress of the disease. The American Academy of Ophthalmology (AAO) recommends screening for glaucoma as a part of the comprehensive eye examination starting at age 20 years. Subsequent screening schedules depend on individual risk factors.

There are many forms of glaucoma, but most fall into one of two categories: open-angle or closed-angle glaucoma. Open-angle glaucoma is more common. In *open-angle glaucoma* the drainage canals of the eye gradually become clogged over time. As a result, intraocular pressure builds up slowly, as fluids continue to be produced at normal rates. The entrance to the drainage canals of the eye is clear, or open, and working correctly. The clogging occurs farther inside the canals. The process is gradual, painless, and causes no early symptoms. Vision loss begins with the peripheral vision, which often goes unnoticed because individuals learn to compensate intuitively by turning their heads. As the condition progresses, individuals have a decreasing field of peripheral vision until eventually they may not be able to see anything to either side, which is called *tunnel vision.*

In *closed-angle glaucoma* the drainage canals are blocked or covered over by the outer edge of the iris when the pupil enlarges too much or too quickly. The blockage most often occurs suddenly (acute) but can develop slowly (chronic). In *acute closed-angle glaucoma*, there is an abrupt onset of symptoms, including eye pain; headaches; nausea and/or vomiting; blurred or sudden loss of vision; and rainbow-colored halos around lights, especially at night. If left untreated, individuals can lose their vision within 2 to 3 hours.

Resources

EyeSmart™: Know your Risk, Save your Sight *is a public-awareness campaign sponsored by the AAO. Health care providers can access patient-friendly information sheets on various eye diseases or refer the public to their website, http://www .geteyesmart.org/eyesmart/.*

American Academy of Ophthalmology (AAO): http://www.aao .org/aao/.

National Eye Institute: Facts About Glaucoma: *http://www.nei .nih.gov/health/glaucoma/glaucoma_facts.asp.*

NEI educational division, NEHEP, provides health care professionals with information to educate patients and the public about eye health and the importance of comprehensive dilated eye examinations. Of particular note is the Keep Vision in Your Future: Glaucoma Toolkit *(http://www.nei.nih.gov/nehep/programs/ glaucoma/toolkit.asp) and its Spanish counterpart* ¡Ojo con su vision! *(http://www.nei.nih.gov/nehep/programs/ojo/index.asp).*

Objective Data

DOCUMENTATION AND CRITICAL THINKING

SUBJECTIVE

Vision reported "good" with no recent change. No eye pain, no inflammation, no discharge, no lesions. Wears no corrective lenses, vision last tested 1 year PTA; test for glaucoma at that time was normal.

OBJECTIVE

Snellen chart: Right 20/20, Left 20/20 −1. Fields normal by confrontation. Corneal light reflex symmetric bilaterally. Diagnostic positions test shows EOMs intact. Brows and lashes present. No ptosis. Conjunctiva clear. Sclera white. No lesions. PERRLA.
Fundi: Red reflex present bilaterally. Discs flat with sharp margins. Vessels present in all quadrants without crossing defects. Retinal background has even color with no hemorrhages or exudates. Macula has even color.

ASSESSMENT

Healthy vision function
Healthy eye structures

Clinical Case Study 1

E.K. is a 34-year-old married, White female homemaker brought to the emergency department by police after a reported domestic quarrel.

SUBJECTIVE

States husband struck her about the face and eyes with his fists about 1 hour PTA. "When he's drunk, he goes crazy." Pain in left cheek and both eyes felt immediately and continues. Alarmed at "bright red blood on eyeball." No bleeding from eye area or cheek. Vision intact just after trauma. Now reports difficulty opening lids.

OBJECTIVE

Sitting quietly and hunched over, hands over eyes. Voice tired and flat. L cheek swollen and discolored; no laceration. Lids edematous and discolored both eyes. No skin laceration. L lid swollen almost shut. L eye—Round 1-mm bright red patch over lateral aspect of globe. No active bleeding out of eye, iris intact, anterior chamber clear. R eye—Conjunctiva clear, sclera white, cornea and iris intact, anterior chamber clear. PERRLA. Pupils R 4/1 = 4/1 L. Vision 14/14 both eyes by Jaeger card.

ASSESSMENT

Ecchymoses L cheek and both eyes
Subconjunctival hemorrhage L eye
Pain R/T inflammation
Chronic low self-esteem R/T effects of domestic violence

Clinical Case Study 2

S.T. is a 63-year-old married, White male postal carrier admitted to the medical center for surgery for suspected brain tumor. After postanesthesia recovery, S.T. is admitted to the neurology ICU, awake, lethargic with slowed but correct verbal responses, oriented × 3, moving all four extremities, vital signs stable. Pupils R 4/2 = 4/2 L with sluggish response. Assessments are made q 15 minutes.

SUBJECTIVE

No response now to verbal stimuli.

OBJECTIVE

Semicomatose—No response to verbal stimuli, does withdraw R arm and leg purposefully to painful stimuli. No movement L arm or leg. Pupils R 5/5 ≠ L 4/2. Vitals remain stable as noted on graphic sheet.

ASSESSMENT

Unilateral dilated and fixed R pupil
Clouding of consciousness
Focal motor deficit—No movement L side
Ineffective tissue perfusion R/T interruption of cerebral flow

Clinical Case Study 3

N.T. is a 14-year-old Caucasian teen who presents to your office with "eye pain × 1 day."

SUBJECTIVE

"My eyes itch so bad. It feels like something is in there; and this morning when I woke up, I couldn't open my eyes. They were matted shut." Reports that yesterday his left eye felt "dry and itchy even though it kept watering," but now reports same symptoms in both eyes.

OBJECTIVE

Vital signs: Temp 97.8° F (36.6° C). BP 100/68 mm Hg (sitting). Pulse 78 bpm. Resp 14/min.
Vision: 20/20 both eyes without correction by Snellen chart.
General appearance: Anxious, consistently rubbing eyes and dabbing with the sleeve of his shirt.
HEENT: Normocephalic, preauricular nodes palpable (1 mm); purulent yellow discharge from both eyes, conjunctivae bright red bilat.; external canals clear w/o redness, bilat tympanic membranes pearly gray with visible landmarks; no exudate to throat.
Respiratory: Breath sounds clear in all fields; no adventitious sounds.

ASSESSMENT

Conjunctivitis, both eyes R/T bacterial infection
Acute pain R/T inflammatory process

Clinical Case Study 4

V.K. is an 87-year-old widowed, Black female homemaker living independently who is admitted to hospital for observation and adjustment of digitalis medication. Cardiac status has been stable during hospital stay.

SUBJECTIVE

Reports desire to monitor own medication at home but fears problems because of blurred vision. First noted distant vision blurred 5 years ago, but near vision seemed to improve at that time. "I started to read better without my glasses!" Since then, blurring at distant vision has increased; near vision now blurred also.

Able to navigate home environment without difficulty. Fixes simple meals with cold foods. Receives hot meal from "Meals on Wheels" at lunch. Enjoys TV, though it looks somewhat blurred. Unable to write letters, sew, or read paper, which she regrets.

OBJECTIVE

Vision by Jaeger card Right 20/200, Left 20/400 −1, with glasses on. Fields intact by confrontation. EOMs intact. Brow hair absent lateral third. Upper lids have folds of redundant skin, but lids do not droop. Lower lids and lashes intact. Xanthelasma present both inner canthi. Conjunctiva clear, sclera white, iris intact, L pupil looks cloudy, PERRLA, pupils R 3/2 = 3/2 L.
Fundi: Red reflex has central dark spot both eyes. Discs flat, with sharp margins. Observed vessels normal. Unable to see in all four quadrants or macular area because of small pupils.

ASSESSMENT

Central opacity, both eyes
Central visual acuity deficit, both eyes
Deficient diversional activity R/T poor vision

Documentation
and Critical Thinking

ABNORMAL FINDINGS

TABLE 14-1 Extraocular Muscle Dysfunction

Note: Pseudostrabismus has the appearance of strabismus because of epicanthic fold but is normal for a young child (see Fig. 14-29 on p. 306).

Asymmetric Corneal Light Reflex

Strabismus is true disparity of the eye axes. This constant malalignment is also termed *tropia* and is likely to cause amblyopia.
A. Esotropia—Inward turning of the eye.
B. Exotropia—Outward turning of the eyes.

A, Left esotropia.

B, Exotropia.

Cover Test

C. Uncovered eye—If it jumps to fixate on designated point, it was out of alignment before (i.e., when you cover the stronger eye [C1], the weaker eye now tries to fixate [C2]).

Phoria—Mild weakness, apparent only with the cover test and less likely to cause amblyopia than a tropia but still possible.

D. Covered eye—If this is the weaker eye, once macular image is suppressed, it will drift to relaxed position (D1).

As eye is uncovered—If it jumps to reestablish fixation (D2), weakness exists.

Esophoria—Nasal (inward) drift.
Exophoria—Temporal (outward) drift.

C, Right, or uncovered eye, is weaker.

D, Left, or covered eye, is weaker.

TABLE 14-1   Extraocular Muscle Dysfunction—cont'd

Diagnostic Positions Test

(Paralysis apparent during movement through six cardinal positions of gaze.)

If eye will not turn:	Indicates dysfunction in cranial nerve
Straight nasal	III
Up and nasal	III
Up and temporal	III
Straight temporal	VI
Down and temporal	III
Down and nasal	IV

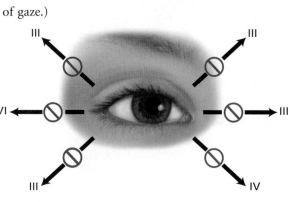

See Illustration Credits for source information.

TABLE 14-2   Eyelid Abnormalities

Periorbital Edema

Lids are swollen and puffy. Lid tissues are loosely connected, so excess fluid is easily apparent. This occurs with local infections; crying; and systemic conditions such as congestive heart failure, renal failure, allergy, hypothyroidism (myxedema).

Exophthalmos (Protruding Eyes)

Exophthalmos is a forward displacement of the eyeballs and widened palpebral fissures. Note "lid lag," in which the upper lid rests well above the limbus and white sclera is visible. Acquired bilateral exophthalmos is associated with thyrotoxicosis.

Enophthalmos (Sunken Eyes) (not illustrated)

A look of narrowed palpebral fissures shows with enophthalmos, in which the eyeballs are recessed. Bilateral enophthalmos is caused by loss of fat in the orbits and occurs with dehydration and chronic wasting illnesses. For illustration, see Cachectic Appearance in Table 13-5, p. 279.

Continued

TABLE 14-2   Eyelid Abnormalities—cont'd

Ptosis (Drooping Upper Lid)

Ptosis occurs from neuromuscular weakness (e.g., myasthenia gravis with bilateral fatigue as the day progresses), oculomotor cranial nerve III damage, or sympathetic nerve damage (e.g., Horner syndrome) or is congenital as in this example. It is a positional defect that gives the person a sleepy appearance and impairs vision.

Upward Palpebral Slant

Although normal in many children, when combined with epicanthal folds, hypertelorism (large spacing between the eyes), and Brushfield spots (light-colored areas in outer iris), it indicates Down syndrome.

Ectropion

The lower lid is loose and rolling out, does not approximate to eyeball. Puncta cannot siphon tears effectively; thus excess tearing results. The eyes feel dry and itchy because the tears do not drain correctly over the corner and toward the medial canthus. Exposed palpebral conjunctiva increases risk for inflammation. It occurs in aging as a result of atrophy of elastic and fibrous tissues but may result from trauma.

Entropion

The lower lid rolls in because of spasm of lids or scar tissue contracting. Constant rubbing of lashes may irritate cornea. The person feels a "foreign body" sensation.

See Illustration Credits for source information.

TABLE 14-3 Lesions on the Eyelids

Blepharitis (Inflammation of the Eyelids)

Red, scaly, greasy flakes and thickened, crusted lid margins occur with staphylococcal infection or seborrheic dermatitis of the lid edge. Symptoms include burning, itching, tearing, foreign body sensation, and some pain.

Chalazion

A beady nodule protruding on the lid, chalazion is an infection or retention cyst of a meibomian gland. If chronic, it is a nontender, firm, discrete swelling with freely movable skin overlying the nodule. If acutely inflamed, it is tender, warm, and red and points inside and not on lid margin (in contrast with stye).

Hordeolum (Stye)

Hordeolum is an acute localized staphylococcal infection of the hair follicles at the lid margin. It is painful, red, and swollen—a superficial, elevated pustule at the lid margin. Rubbing the eyes can cause cross-contamination and development of another stye.

Dacryocystitis (Inflammation of the Lacrimal Sac)

Dacryocystitis is infection and blockage of sac and duct. Pain, warmth, redness, and swelling occur below the inner canthus toward the nose. Tearing is present. Pressure on sac yields purulent discharge from puncta.

Dacryoadenitis is an infection of the lacrimal gland (not illustrated). Pain, swelling, and redness occur in the outer third of the upper lid. It occurs with mumps, measles, and infectious mononucleosis or from trauma.

Continued

TABLE 14-3   Lesions on the Eyelids—cont'd

Central ulceration   Basal cell carcinoma

◀ Basal Cell Carcinoma

It is most often on the lower lid and presents as a small, painless nodule with central ulceration and sharp, rolled-out pearly edges. It occurs in older adults; associated with ultraviolet exposure and light skin. It is locally invasive, but metastasis is rare.

See Illustration Credits for source information.

TABLE 14-4   Pupil Abnormalities

Red lines indicate the location of a lesion that stops the transmission of vision.

A. Unequal Pupil Size—Anisocoria

Although this exists normally in 5% of the population, consider central nervous system disease.

B. Monocular Blindness

When light is directed to the blind eye, no response occurs in either eye. When light is directed to the normal eye, both pupils constrict (direct and consensual response to light) as long as the oculomotor nerve is intact.

TABLE 14-4   Pupil Abnormalities—cont'd

C. Dilated and Fixed Pupils—Mydriasis

Enlarged pupils occur with stimulation of the sympathetic nervous system, reaction to sympathomimetic drugs, use of dilating drops, acute glaucoma, or past or recent trauma. They also herald central nervous system injury, circulatory arrest, or deep anesthesia.

D. Constricted and Fixed Pupils—Miosis

Miosis occurs with the use of pilocarpine drops for glaucoma treatment, the use of narcotics, with iritis, and with brain damage of pons.

E. Argyll Robertson Pupil

There is no reaction to light; pupil does constrict with accommodation. Small and irregular bilaterally. Argyll Robertson pupil occurs with central nervous system syphilis, brain tumor, meningitis, and chronic alcoholism.

F. Tonic Pupil (Adie's Pupil)

Reaction to light and accommodation is sluggish. Tonic pupil is usually unilateral, a large regular pupil that does react, but sluggishly after long latent time. There is no pathologic significance.

G. Horner Syndrome

A unilateral, small, regular pupil does react to light and accommodation. Occurs with Horner syndrome, a lesion of the sympathetic nerve. Also note ptosis and absence of sweat (anhidrosis) on same side.

H. Cranial Nerve III Damage

Unilateral dilated pupil has no reaction to light or accommodation and occurs with oculomotor nerve damage. Ptosis with eye deviating down and laterally may be present.

Abnormal Findings

ABNORMAL FINDINGS
FOR ADVANCED PRACTICE

TABLE 14-5 **Visual Field Loss**

Red lines indicate the location of a lesion that interrupts the transmission of vision.

1. Retinal damage
   - Macula—Central blind area (e.g., diabetes):

   - Localized damage—Blind spot (scotoma) corresponding to particular area:

   - Increasing intraocular pressure—Decrease in peripheral vision (e.g., glaucoma). Starts with paracentral scotoma in early stage:

   - Retinal detachment—A shadow or diminished vision in one quadrant or one half of visual field:

2. Lesion in globe or optic nerve
   Injury here yields one blind eye, or unilateral blindness:

3. Lesion at optic chiasm (e.g., pituitary tumor)—injury to crossing fibers only yields loss of nasal part of each retina and loss of both temporal visual fields. Bitemporal (heteronymous) hemianopsia:

4. Lesion of outer uncrossed fibers at optic chiasm (e.g., aneurysm of left internal carotid artery exerts pressure on uncrossed fibers). Injury yields left nasal hemianopsia:

5. Lesion R optic tract or R optic radiation
   Visual field loss in R nasal and L temporal fields
   Loss of same half of visual field in both eyes is homonymous hemianopsia:

TABLE 14-6   Red Eye—Vascular Disorders

NOTE: Always check visual acuity with any eye disorder. The following warrant emergency referral to ophthalmologist: sudden vision loss, trauma, herpes zoster infection (shingles) on face, corneal damage, distorted pupil, and severe pain.

Conjunctivitis

Infection of the conjunctiva, "pink eye," has red, beefy-looking vessels at periphery but is usually clearer around iris, commonly from viral or bacterial infection, allergy, or chemical irritation. Purulent discharge accompanies bacterial infection. Preauricular lymph node is often swollen and painful, with a history of upper respiratory infection. Symptoms include itching, burning, foreign body sensation, and eyelids stuck together on awakening. Person has normal vision, normal pupil size, and reaction to light.

Allergic Conjunctivitis

Note the upper lid, conjunctiva, and cornea are inflamed from seasonal allergen (e.g., pollen, spores) or persistent allergen (e.g., house dust mite, animal dander). Symptoms include eye itching (not present in nonallergic conditions), redness, watering, discomfort. It does not obscure vision. Signs are diffuse redness of conjunctivae, lid swelling, upper tarsal surface that shows velvety thickening, redness, small papillae (shown above).[9]

Iritis (Circumcorneal Redness)

There is a deep, dull red halo around the iris and cornea. Note that redness is around the iris, in contrast with conjunctivitis, in which redness is more prominent at the periphery. Pupil shape may be irregular from swelling of iris. Person also has marked photophobia, constricted pupil, blurred vision, and throbbing pain. Warrants immediate referral.

Primary Angle-Closure Glaucoma

Acute narrow-angle glaucoma shows circumcorneal redness around the iris, with a dilated pupil. Pupil is oval, dilated; cornea looks "steamy"; and anterior chamber is shallow. Acute glaucoma occurs with sudden increase in intraocular pressure from blocked outflow from anterior chamber. The person experiences a sudden clouding of vision, sudden eye pain, and halos around lights. This requires emergency treatment to avoid permanent vision loss.

Continued

TABLE 14-6 Red Eye—Vascular Disorders—cont'd

Seropurulent vesicles due to HSV

Subconjunctival Hemorrhage

A red patch on the sclera, subconjunctival hemorrhage looks alarming but is usually not serious. The red patch has sharp edges like a spot of paint, although here it is extensive. It occurs from increased intraocular pressure from coughing, vomiting, weight lifting, labor during childbirth, straining at stool, or trauma.

Herpes Simplex Virus

Lid vesicles from primary HSV, associated with fever, pre-auricular lymphadenopathy. **Herpes zoster ophthalmicus** is a serious presentation of "shingles" involving the ophthalmic nerve. May have prodrome: numbness and tingling or burning along nerve route, fever, headache, malaise. Signs are acute, painful reddened conjunctivae; unilateral maculopapular rash with vesicles and ulcers; and ocular signs that threaten vision. Severity increases with older age.

See Illustration Credits for source information.

TABLE 14-7 Abnormalities on Cornea and Iris

Pterygium

A triangular opaque wing of bulbar conjunctiva overgrows toward the center of the cornea. It looks membranous, translucent, and yellow to white; usually invades from nasal side; and may obstruct vision as it covers pupil. It occurs usually from chronic exposure to hot, dry, sandy climate, which stimulates the growth of a pinguecula (see p. 307) into a pterygium.

Corneal Abrasion

This is the most common result of a blunt eye injury, but irregular ridges are usually visible only when fluorescein stain reveals yellow-green branching. Top layer of corneal epithelium is removed, from scratches or poorly fitting or overworn contact lenses. Because the area is rich in nerve endings, the person feels intense pain; a foreign body sensation; and lacrimation, redness, and photophobia.

TABLE 14-7 Abnormalities on Cornea and Iris—cont'd

Normal Anterior Chamber (for Contrast)

A light directed across the eye from the temporal side illuminates the entire iris evenly because the normal iris is flat and creates no shadow.

Shallow Anterior Chamber

The iris is pushed anteriorly because of increased intraocular pressure. Because direct light is received from the temporal side, only the temporal part of the iris is illuminated; the nasal side is shadowed, the "shadow sign." This may be a sign of acute angle-closure glaucoma; the iris looks bulging because aqueous humor cannot circulate.

Hyphema

Blood in the anterior chamber is a serious result of herpes zoster infection. Also occurs with blunt trauma (a fist or a baseball) or spontaneous hemorrhage. Suspect scleral rupture or major intraocular trauma. Note that gravity settles blood in front of iris.

Hypopyon

Purulent matter in anterior chamber occurs with iritis and with inflammation in the anterior chamber.

See Illustration Credits for source information.

TABLE 14-8 **Lens Opacities**

Cataracts

Central Gray Opacity—Nuclear Cataract

Nuclear cataract shows as an opaque gray surrounded by a black background as it forms in the center of lens nucleus. Through the ophthalmoscope it looks like a black center against the red reflex. It begins after age 40 years and develops slowly, gradually obstructing vision.

Star-Shaped Opacity—Cortical Cataract

Cortical cataract shows as asymmetric, radial, white spokes with black center. Through ophthalmoscope, black spokes are evident against the red reflex (not shown here). This forms in the outer cortex of lens, progressing faster than nuclear cataract.

See Illustration Credits for source information.

TABLE 14-9 **Optic Disc Abnormalities**

Papilledema   Retinal hemorrhages

Optic Atrophy (Disc Pallor)

Optic atrophy is a white or gray color of the disc as a result of partial or complete death of the optic nerve. This results in decreased visual acuity, decreased color vision, and decreased contrast sensitivity.

Papilledema (Choked Disc)

Increased intracranial pressure causes venous stasis in the globe, showing redness, congestion, and elevation of the disc; blurred margins; hemorrhages; and absent venous pulsations. This is a serious sign of intracranial pressure, usually caused by a space-occupying mass (e.g., a brain tumor or hematoma). Visual acuity is not affected.

◄ **Excessive Cup-Disc Ratio**

With primary open-angle glaucoma, the increased intraocular pressure decreases blood supply to retinal structures. The physiologic cup enlarges to more than half of the disc diameter, vessels appear to plunge over edge of cup, and vessels are displaced nasally. This is asymptomatic, although the person may have decreased vision or visual field defects in the late stages of glaucoma.

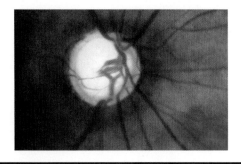

See Illustration Credits for source information.

TABLE 14-10 Retinal Vessel and Background Abnormalities

Macular star   Retinal folds   Disc edema

Age: 14 Yrs   Age: 61 Yrs

Arteriovenous Crossing (Nicking)

Inset shows arteriovenous crossing with interruption of blood flow. When vein is occluded, it dilates distal to crossing. This person also has disc edema and hard exudates in a macular star pattern that occur with acutely elevated (malignant) hypertension. With hypertension, the arteriole wall thickens and becomes opaque so that no blood is seen inside it (silver-wire arteries).

Narrowed (Attenuated) Arteries

This is a generalized decrease in arteriole diameter. The light reflex also narrows. It occurs with severe hypertension (shown above on the right) and with occlusion of the central retinal artery and retinitis pigmentosa.

Diabetic Retinopathy

Findings are nonproliferative changes that occur *within* the retina (microaneurysms, dot hemorrhages, blot hemorrhages, lipid exudates), and proliferative changes on the inner surface of the retina or vitreous. Proliferative changes are new vessel formations or neovascularization, which increase risk of retinal detachment or vitreous hemorrhage.[14]

Lipid   Dot hemorrhage   Micro-
exudate   aneurysm

◀ **Moderate nonproliferative diabetic retinopathy.** Microaneurysms are round, punctate red dots that are localized dilations of a small vessel. Their edges are smooth and discrete. The vessel itself is too small to view with the ophthalmoscope; only the isolated red dots are seen. Dot hemorrhages are deep intraretinal hemorrhages that look splattered on. They are distinguished from microaneurysms by the blurred irregular edges. Lipid (hard) exudates are small, yellow-white spots with distinct edges and a smooth, solid-looking surface. They often form a circular or linear pattern. (This is in contrast with drusen, which have a scattered haphazard location [see Fig. 14-34].)

Lipid exudate   Intraretinal hemorrhages

◀ **Severe nonproliferative diabetic retinopathy.** Note lipid exudates as described and larger flame-shaped hemorrhages that look linear or spindle shaped.

Proliferative diabetic retinopathy (not shown). Neovascularization is new vessel formation that looks like radiating spokes.

See Illustration Credits for source information.

Abnormal Findings

Summary Checklist: Eye Examination

1. **Test visual acuity**
   Snellen eye chart
   Near vision (those older than 40 years or having difficulty reading)
2. **Test visual fields—Confrontation test**
3. **Inspect extraocular muscle function**
   Corneal light reflex (Hirschberg test)
   Cover test (if indicated)
   Diagnostics positions test

4. **Inspect external eye structures**
   General
   Eyebrows
   Eyelids and lashes
   Eyeball alignment
   Conjunctiva and sclera
   Lacrimal apparatus
5. **Inspect anterior eyeball structures**
   Cornea and lens
   Iris and pupil
   Size, shape, and equality
   Pupillary light reflex
   Accommodation

6. **Inspect ocular fundus**
   Optic disc (color, shape, margins, cup-disc ratio)
   Retinal vessels (number, color, artery-vein [A:V] ratio, caliber, arteriovenous crossings, tortuosity, pulsations)
   General background (color, integrity)
   Macula

BIBLIOGRAPHY

1. American Academy of Ophthalmology. (n.d.). *Eye health statistics at a glance.* www.aao.org/newsroom/press_kit/upload/Eye_Stats_3-5-07.
2. Antonetti, D. A., Klein, R., & Gardner, T. W. (2012). Diabetic retinopathy. *N Engl J Med, 366*(13), 1227-1239.
3. Bartalena, L., & Tanda, M. L. (2009). Graves' ophthalmopathy. *N Engl J Med, 360*(10), 994-1001.
4. Cronau, H., Kankanala, R. R., & Mauger, T. (2010). Diagnosis and management of red eye in primary care. *Am Fam Physician, 81*(2), 137-144.
5. Friedman, N. J., Kaiser, P. K., & Pineda, R. (2009). *The Massachusetts eye and ear infirmary illustrated manual of ophthalmology.* (3rd ed.). Philadelphia: Saunders.
6. Friedman, D. I. (2010). Pearls: diplopia. *Semin Neurol, 30*(1), 54-65.
7. Galor, A., & Lee, D. J. (2011). Effects of smoking on ocular health. *Curr Opin Ophthalmol, 22*(6), 477-482.
8. Hered, R. W. (2011). Effective vision screening of young children in the pediatric office. *Pediatr Ann, 40*(2), 76-82.
9. Holgate, S. T., Church, M. K., Broide, D. H., et al. (2012). *Allergy.* (4th ed.). Philadelphia: Saunders.
10. Kane, R. T., Ouslander, J. G., & Abrass, I. B. (2009). *Essentials of clinical geriatrics* (6th ed.). New York: McGraw-Hill.
11. Kerr, N. M., Chew, S. S., Eady, E. K., et al. (2010). Diagnostic accuracy of confrontation visual field tests. *Neurol, 74,* 1184-1190.
12. Koch, J., & Sikes, K. (2009). Getting the red out: primary angle-closure glaucoma. *Nurse Pract, 34*(5), 6-9.
13. Lam, B. L., Lee, D. J., Zheng, D. D., et al. (2009). Disparity in prevalence of self-reported visual impairment in older adults among U.S. race-ethnic subgroups. *Ophthal Epidemiol, 16*(3), 144-150.
14. McGee, S. (2012). *Evidence-based physical diagnosis.* (3rd ed.). Philadelphia: Elsevier.
15. Paulus, Y. M., & Gariano, R. F. (2009). Diabetic retinopathy: a growing concern in an aging population. *Geriatrics, 64*(2), 16-26.
16. Rosenbaum, J. T. (2012). Eyeing macular degeneration—a few inflammatory remarks. *N Engl J Med, 367*(8), 768-770.
17. Rowe, S., & MacLean, C. H. (2007). Quality indicators for the care of vision impairment in vulnerable elders. *Am Geriatr Soc 55*(Suppl 2), S450-456.
18. Rucker, J. C., Kennard, C., & Leigh, R. J. (2011). Chapter 3: The neuro-ophthalmological examination. In M. J. Aminoff, F. Boller, & D. F. Swaab (Eds.), *Neuro-Ophthalmol, 102,* (71-94).
19. Sharts-Hopko, N. C, & Glynn-Milley, C. (2009). Primary open-angle glaucoma. *Am J Nurs, 109*(2), 40-48.
20. Smith, G. (2010). Differential diagnosis of red eye. *Pediatr Nurs, 36*(4), 213-215.
21. Tingley, D. (2010). Vision screening essentials: screening today for eye disorders in the pediatric patient. *Pediatr Rev, 28*(2), 53-61.
22. U.S. Preventive Services Task Force. (2011). Vision screening for children 1 to 5 years of age. *Pediatrics, 127*(2), 340-346.
23. Vajaranant, T. S., Nayak, S., Wilensky, J. T., et al. (2010). Gender and glaucoma: what we know and what we need to know. *Curr Opin Ophthalmol, 21*(2), 91-99.
24. Zambelli-Weiner, A., Crews, J. E., et al. (2012). Disparities in adult vision health in the United States. *Am J Ophthalmol, 20*(10), 1-8.

Ears

STRUCTURE AND FUNCTION

15-1 © Pat Thomas, 2010.

EXTERNAL EAR

The ear is the sensory organ for hearing and maintaining equilibrium. It has three parts: the external ear, the middle ear, and the inner ear. The external ear is called the **auricle** or **pinna** and consists of movable cartilage and skin (Fig. 15-1).

Its characteristic shape serves to funnel sound waves into its opening, the **external auditory canal**. The canal is a cul-de-sac 2.5 to 3 cm long in the adult and terminates at the **eardrum**, or **tympanic membrane (TM)**. The canal is lined with glands that secrete cerumen, a yellow, waxy material that lubricates and protects the ear. The wax forms a sticky barrier that helps keep foreign bodies from entering and reaching the sensitive tympanic membrane. Cerumen migrates out to the meatus by the movements of chewing and talking.

The outer one third of the canal is cartilage; the inner two thirds tunnels through the temporal bone and is covered by thin, sensitive skin. The canal has a slight S-curve in the adult.

325

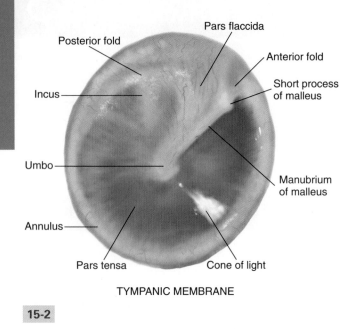

TYMPANIC MEMBRANE

15-2

The outer one third curves up and toward the back of the head, whereas the inner two thirds angles down and forward toward the nose.

The TM separates the external and middle ear and is tilted obliquely to the ear canal, facing downward and somewhat forward. It is translucent with a pearly gray color and a prominent cone of light in the anteroinferior quadrant, which is the reflection of the otoscope light (Fig. 15-2). The drum is oval and slightly concave, pulled in at its center by one of the middle ear ossicles, the **malleus.** The parts of the malleus show through the translucent drum; these are the **umbo,** the **manubrium** (handle), and the **short process.** The small, slack, superior section of the TM is called the **pars flaccida.** The remainder of the drum, which is thicker and more taut, is the **pars tensa.** The **annulus** is the outer fibrous rim of the drum.

Lymphatic drainage of the external ear flows to the parotid, mastoid, and superficial cervical nodes.

MIDDLE EAR

The middle ear is a tiny air-filled cavity inside the temporal bone (see Fig. 15-1). It contains tiny ear bones, or auditory ossicles: the **malleus, incus,** and **stapes.** It has several openings. Its opening to the outer ear is covered by the tympanic membrane. The openings to the inner ear are the oval window at the end of the stapes and the round window. Another opening is the **eustachian tube,** which connects the middle ear with the nasopharynx and allows passage of air. The tube is normally closed, but it opens with swallowing or yawning.

The middle ear has three functions: (1) it conducts sound vibrations from the outer ear to the central hearing apparatus in the inner ear; (2) it protects the inner ear by reducing the amplitude of loud sounds; and (3) its eustachian tube allows equalization of air pressure on each side of the tympanic membrane so the membrane does not rupture (e.g., during altitude changes in an airplane).

INNER EAR

The inner ear is embedded in bone. It contains the **bony labyrinth,** which holds the sensory organs for equilibrium and hearing. Within the bony labyrinth, the **vestibule** and the **semicircular canals** compose the vestibular apparatus, and the **cochlea** (Latin for "snail shell") contains the central hearing apparatus. Although the inner ear is not accessible to direct examination, you can assess its functions.

HEARING

Note the landmarks of the auricle, and use these terms to describe your findings (Fig. 15-3). The mastoid process, the bony prominence behind the lobule, is not part of the ear but is an important landmark.

The function of hearing involves the auditory system at three levels: peripheral, brainstem, and cerebral cortex. At the peripheral level the ear transmits sound and converts its vibrations into electrical impulses, which can be analyzed by the brain. For example, you hear an alarm bell ringing in the hall. Its sound waves travel instantly to your ears. The *amplitude* is how loud the alarm is; its *frequency* is the pitch (in this case, high) or the number of cycles per second. The sound waves produce vibrations on your tympanic membrane. These vibrations are carried by the middle ear ossicles to your oval window. Then the sound waves travel through your cochlea, which is coiled like a snail shell, and are dissipated against the round window. Along the way the **basilar membrane** vibrates at a point specific to the frequency of the sound. In this case the high frequency of the alarm stimulates the basilar membrane at its base near the stapes (Fig. 15-4). The numerous fibers along the basilar membrane are the receptor hair cells of the **organ of Corti,** the sensory organ of hearing. As the hair cells bend, they mediate the

15-3

Bone conduction pathway

Uncoiled cochlea

Cochlear nerve

②

③

Apex

Base

①

High frequency

Medium frequency

Low frequency

Air conduction pathway

① Tympanic membrane
② Stapes embedded in oval window
③ Basilar membrane of cochlea
   contains organ of Corti hair cells

PATHWAYS OF HEARING

15-4

©Pat Thomas, 2006.

vibrations into electric impulses. The electrical impulses are conducted by the auditory portion of cranial nerve VIII to the brainstem.

The function at the brainstem level is *binaural interaction,* which permits locating the direction of a sound in space and identifying the sound. How does this work? Each ear is actually one half of the total sensory organ. The ears are located on each side of a movable head. Cranial nerve VIII from each ear sends signals to both sides of the brainstem. Areas in the brainstem are sensitive to differences in intensity and timing of the messages from the two ears, depending on the way the head is turned.

Finally the function of the cortex is to interpret the meaning of the sound and begin the appropriate response. All this happens in the split second that it takes you to react to the alarm.

Pathways of Hearing. The normal pathway of hearing is air conduction (AC), described earlier; it is the most efficient. An alternate route of hearing is by bone conduction (BC). Here the bones of the skull vibrate. These vibrations are transmitted directly to the inner ear and to cranial nerve VIII.

Hearing Loss. Anything that obstructs the transmission of sound impairs hearing. A **conductive** hearing loss involves a mechanical dysfunction of the external or middle ear. It is a partial loss because the person is able to hear if the sound amplitude is increased enough to reach normal nerve elements in the inner ear. Conductive hearing loss may be caused

by impacted cerumen, foreign bodies, a perforated tympanic membrane, pus or serum in the middle ear, and otosclerosis (a decrease in mobility of the ossicles).

Sensorineural (or perceptive) loss signifies pathology of the inner ear, cranial nerve VIII, or the auditory areas of the cerebral cortex. A simple increase in amplitude may not enable the person to understand words. Sensorineural hearing loss may be caused by *presbycusis,* a gradual nerve degeneration that occurs with aging, and by ototoxic drugs, which affect the hair cells in the cochlea. A **mixed** loss is a combination of conductive and sensorineural types in the same ear.

Equilibrium. The 3 semicircular canals, or labyrinth, in the inner ear constantly feed information to your brain about the position of your body in space. They work like plumb lines to determine verticality or depth. The plumb lines of the ear register the angle of your head in relation to gravity. If the labyrinth ever becomes inflamed, it feeds the wrong information to the brain, creating a staggering gait and a strong, spinning, whirling sensation called *vertigo.*

❖ DEVELOPMENTAL COMPETENCE

Infants and Children

The inner ear starts to develop early in the fifth week of gestation. In early development the ear is posteriorly rotated and low set; later it ascends to its normal placement around eye level. If maternal rubella infection occurs during the first trimester, it can damage the organ of Corti and impair hearing.

The infant's eustachian tube is relatively shorter and wider, and its position is more horizontal than the adult's; thus it is easier for pathogens from the nasopharynx to migrate through to the middle ear (Fig. 15-5). The lumen is surrounded by lymphoid tissue, which increases during childhood; thus the lumen is easily occluded. These factors place the infant at greater risk for middle ear infections than the adult. The infant's and the young child's external ear canals are shorter and have a slope opposite to that of the adult's.

The Adult

Otosclerosis is a common cause of conductive hearing loss in young adults between the ages of 20 and 40 years. It is a gradual bone formation that causes the footplate of the stapes to become fixed in the oval window, impeding the transmission of sound and causing progressive deafness.

The Aging Adult

In the aging person, cilia lining the ear canal become coarse and stiff. This may cause cerumen to accumulate and oxidize, which greatly reduces hearing. The cerumen itself is drier because of atrophy of the apocrine glands. A life history of frequent ear infections also may result in scarring on the drum.

Impacted cerumen is common in aging adults (up to 57%) and other at-risk groups (e.g., institutionalized and mentally disabled), who may underreport the associated hearing loss. Cerumen impaction also blocks conduction in those wearing hearing aids. Cerumen should be removed when it leads to conductive hearing loss or interferes with full assessment of the ear. Ceruminolytics are wax-softening agents that expedite removal with electric or manual irriga-

tors. After removal, over half of those with impaction passed the whispered voice test.[15]

A person living or working in a noise-polluted area has a greater risk for sensorineural hearing loss. But **presbycusis** is a type of hearing loss that occurs with 60% of those older than 65 years, even in people living in a quiet environment. It is a gradual sensorineural loss caused by nerve degeneration in the inner ear that slowly progresses after the fifth decade.[7,10] The person first notices a high-frequency tone loss; it is harder to hear consonants than vowels. Much speech information is lost, and words sound garbled. The ability to localize sound is impaired also. This communication dysfunction is accentuated when unfavorable background noise is present (e.g., with music, with dishes clattering, or at a large, noisy party).

CULTURE AND GENETICS

Otitis media, or OM (middle ear infection), occurs because of obstruction of the eustachian tube or passage of nasopharyngeal secretions into the middle ear. This creates a ripe environment for bacteria to grow. OM is so common in childhood that 90% of all children younger than 2 years of age have had at least one episode.[9a] The incidence and severity are increased in indigenous children from North America, Australia, New Zealand, and Northern Europe, although genetic factors have not been determined. Rather, the most important cause is environmental; children in high-risk groups usually have multiple pathogens, and the total bacterial load is high.[8]

Besides the anatomy of the infant eustachian tube, the following risk factors predispose to acute OM: absence of breastfeeding in the first 3 months of age, exposure to secondhand tobacco smoke (SHS), daycare attendance, male sex, pacifier use, seasonality (fall and winter), and bottle feeding in the supine position.[9a] But there is a new trend in the United States—ambulatory visits for acute OM have decreased by

INFANT
Horizontal eustachian tube

ADULT
Sloped eustachian tube

15-5

40% from 1993 to 2006.[1] This decrease is best explained by a concurrent increase in the number of smoke-free households (up by 89% during the same time period). Public awareness of the dangers of SHS on child health together with the surge in no-smoking rules in households and vehicles may be responsible for the reversal in pediatric visits for OM in the United States.

The most important side effect of acute OM is the persistence of fluid in the middle ear after treatment. This middle ear effusion can impair hearing, placing the child at risk for delayed cognitive development.

Genetic variations. Cerumen is genetically determined to be of two major types: (1) dry cerumen, which is gray and flaky and frequently forms a thin mass in the ear canal; and (2) wet cerumen, which is honey brown to dark brown and moist. Chromosome 16 holds one gene trait determining the wet or dry phenotype.[13] The wet cerumen phenotype occurs more often in Caucasians and African Americans, whereas the dry cerumen is more frequent in Asians and American Indians.[4] The presence and composition of cerumen are not related to poor hygiene. Take caution to avoid mistaking the flaky, dry cerumen for eczematous lesions.

SUBJECTIVE DATA

1. Earache
2. Infections
3. Discharge
4. Hearing loss
5. Environmental noise
6. Tinnitus
7. Vertigo
8. Patient-centered care

Examiner Asks	Rationale
1. Earache. Any **earache** or other pain in ears? • Location—Feel close to the surface or deep in the head? • Does it hurt when you push on the ear? • Character—Dull, aching or sharp, stabbing? Constant or come and go? Is it affected by changing position of head? • Any accompanying cold symptoms or sore throat? Any problems with sinuses or teeth? • Ever been hit on the ear or the side of the head or had any sport injury? Ever had any trauma from a foreign body? • What have you tried to relieve pain?	**Otalgia** may be caused directly by ear disease or may be referred pain from a problem in teeth or oropharynx. Virus/bacteria from upper respiratory infection (URI) may migrate up the eustachian tube to involve the middle ear. Trauma may rupture the TM. Assess effect of coping strategies.
2. Infections. Any ear **infections?** As an adult or in childhood? • How frequent were they? How were they treated?	A history of chronic ear problems suggests possible sequelae.
3. Discharge. Any **discharge** from your ears? • Does it look like pus, or is it bloody? • Any odor to the discharge? • Any relation between the discharge and the ear pain?	**Otorrhea** suggests infected canal or perforated eardrum such as: *External otitis*—Purulent, sanguineous, or watery discharge. *Acute OM with perforation*—Purulent discharge. *Cholesteatoma*—Dirty yellow/gray discharge, foul odor. Typically with perforation—Ear pain occurs first, stops with a popping sensation; then drainage occurs.
4. Hearing loss. Do you have any trouble hearing? • Onset—Did the loss come on slowly or all at once?	**Presbycusis** is gradual onset over years, symmetric, mostly high-frequency loss, worse in noisy environments, whereas a trauma hearing loss is often sudden. Refer any sudden loss in one or both ears *not* associated with URI.

Subjective Data

- Character—Has all your hearing decreased or just on hearing certain sounds?
- In which situations do you notice the loss: conversations, using the telephone, listening to TV, at a party?
- Do people seem to shout at you?

Loss shows with competition from background noise, as at a party.

Recruitment—A marked loss when speech is at low intensity, but sound actually becomes painful when speaker repeats in a loud voice.

- Do ordinary sounds seem hollow, as if you are hearing in a barrel or under water?
- Recently traveled by airplane?
- Any family history of hearing loss?
- Effort to treat—Any hearing aid or other device? Anything to help hearing?
- Coping strategies—How does the loss affect your daily life? Any job problems? Feel embarrassed? Frustrated? How do your family, friends react?

This happens when cerumen expands and becomes impacted, as after swimming or showering.

Hearing loss can cause social isolation, decreased quality of life, functional decline, cognitive decline, depression.[10,14]

Note to examiner—During history note these clues from normal conversation that indicate possible hearing loss.
1. Person lip-reads or watches your face and lips closely rather than your eyes
2. Frowns or strains forward to hear
3. Postures head to catch sounds with better ear
4. Misunderstands your questions or frequently asks you to repeat
5. Acts irritable or shows startle reflex when you raise your voice (recruitment)
6. Person's speech sounds garbled, possibly vowel sounds distorted
7. Inappropriately loud voice
8. Flat, monotonous tone of voice

5. Environmental noise. Do you consider the noise level where you are working now to be high? What about your leisure time? Are you regularly exposed to sounds so loud that you have to shout to make yourself heard by someone standing more than one yard away? Regularly exposed to gunfire noise?
- Noise protection—Any steps to protect your ears such as headphones or ear plugs?

Old trauma to hearing initially goes unnoticed but results in further decibel loss in later years.

6. Tinnitus. Ever felt ringing, crackling, or buzzing in your ears? When did this occur?

Tinnitus is a "phantom sound"[11] that originates within the person; it occurs with cerumen impaction, middle ear infection, and other ear disorders.

- Seem louder at night?

Tinnitus seems louder with no competition from environmental noise.

- Are you taking any medications?

Many medications have ototoxic sequelae: aspirin, aminoglycosides (gentamicin, tobramycin, amikacin), ethacrynic acid, furosemide, indomethacin, naproxen, quinine, vancomycin.

- How does tinnitus affect your everyday life? Difficulty concentrating, sleeping, at work, leisure time, time with others?

Severe tinnitus can cause depression or anxiety and be so debilitating that person cannot lead a normal life.[11]

Examiner Asks	Rationale
7. Vertigo. Ever felt **vertigo;** that is, the room spinning around or yourself spinning? (Vertigo is a true twirling motion.)	True rotational spinning occurs with dysfunction of labyrinth. **Objective vertigo**—Feels as if room spins. **Subjective vertigo**—Person feels as if he or she spins. Distinguish true vertigo from dizziness or light-headedness.
• Ever felt dizzy, as if you are not quite steady, like falling or losing your balance? Giddy, light-headed?	
8. Patient-centered care. How do you clean your ears?	Assess potential trauma from invasive instruments. Cotton-tipped applicators can impact cerumen, causing hearing loss.
• Last time you had your hearing checked? • If a hearing loss was noted, did you obtain a hearing aid? How long have you had it? Do you wear it? How does it work? Any trouble with upkeep, cleaning, changing batteries?	Prescribe frequency of hearing assessment according to person's age or risk factors.

Additional History for Infants and Children

Examiner Asks	Rationale
1. Ear infections. At what age was the child's first episode? How many ear infections in the past 6 months? How many total? How were these treated? • Has the child had any surgery such as insertion of ear tubes or removal of tonsils? • Are infections increasing in frequency or severity or staying the same? • Does anyone in the home smoke cigarettes?	A first episode that occurs within 3 months of life increases risk for recurrent OM.[12] Recurrent OM is 3 episodes in past 3 months or 4 within past year.
• Does your child receive child care outside your home? In a daycare center or someone else's home? How many children are in the group?	Passive and gestational smoke are risk factors for OM.[1] Daycare attendance and bottle-feeding (as opposed to breastfeeding) are risk factors for OM.
2. Does the child seem to be hearing well? • Have you noticed that the infant startles with loud noise? Did the infant babble around 6 months? Does he or she talk? At what age did he or she start talking? Was the speech intelligible? • Ever had the child's hearing tested? If there was a hearing loss, did it follow any diseases in the child or mother during pregnancy? (**Note:** It is important to catch any problem early, because a child with hearing loss is at risk for delayed speech and social development and learning deficit.)	Children at risk for hearing deficit include those exposed to maternal rubella or maternal ototoxic drugs in utero; premature infants; low-birth-weight infants; trauma or hypoxia at birth; and infants with congenital liver or kidney disease. In children the incidence of meningitis, measles, mumps, OM, and any illness with persistent high fever may increase risk for hearing deficit.
3. Does the child tend to put objects in the ears? Is the older child or adolescent active in contact sports?	These children are at increased risk for trauma.

OBJECTIVE DATA

PREPARATION

Position the adult sitting up straight with his or her head at your eye level. Occasionally the ear canal is partially filled with cerumen, which obstructs your view of the TM. If the eardrum is intact and no current infection is present, a preferred method of cleaning the adult canal is to soften the cerumen with a warmed solution of mineral oil and hydrogen peroxide. Then the canal is irrigated with warm water (body temperature) with a bulb syringe or a low-pulsatile dental irrigator (Water-Pik). Direct fluid to the posterior wall. Leave space around the irrigator tip for water to escape. Do not irrigate if the history or examination suggests perforation or infection.

EQUIPMENT NEEDED

Otoscope with bright light (fresh batteries give off white—not yellow—light).
Pneumatic bulb attachment, sometimes used with infant or young child.

Objective Data

Normal Range of Findings	Abnormal Findings

Inspect and Palpate the External Ear

Size and Shape

The ears are of equal size bilaterally with no swelling or thickening. Ears of unusual size and shape may be a normal familial trait with no clinical significance.

Microtia—ears smaller than 4 cm vertically; *macrotia*—ears larger than 10 cm. Edema with infection or trauma.

Skin Condition

The skin color is consistent with the person's facial skin color. The skin is intact, with no lumps or lesions. On some people you may note **Darwin's tubercle,** a small, painless nodule at the helix. This is a congenital variation and is not significant (Fig. 15-6).

Reddened, excessively warm skin with inflammation (see Table 15-1, External Ear Abnormalities, p. 342).

Crusts and scaling occur with otitis externa, eczema, contact dermatitis, seborrhea.

Enlarged, tender lymph nodes in the region indicate inflammation of the pinna or mastoid process.

Red-blue discoloration with frostbite.

Tophi, sebaceous cyst, chondrodermatitis, keloid, carcinoma (see Table 15-2, Lumps and Lesions on the Ear, p. 343).

— Darwin's tubercle

15-6

Tenderness

Move the pinna and push on the tragus. They should feel firm, and movement should produce no pain. Palpating the mastoid process should also produce no pain.

Pain with movement occurs with otitis externa and furuncle.

Pain at the mastoid process may indicate mastoiditis or enlarged posterior auricular node.

The External Auditory Meatus

Note the size of the opening to direct your choice of speculum for the otoscope. No swelling, redness, or discharge should be present.

Some cerumen is usually present. The color varies from gray-yellow to light brown and black, and the texture varies from moist and waxy to dry and desiccated. A large amount of cerumen obscures visualization of the canal and drum.

A sticky, yellow discharge accompanies otitis externa or may indicate OM if the drum has ruptured.

Impacted cerumen is a common cause of conductive hearing loss.

Inspect with the Otoscope

As you inspect the external ear, note the size of the auditory meatus. Choose the largest speculum that fits comfortably in the ear canal, and attach it to the otoscope. Tilt the person's head slightly away from you toward the opposite shoulder. This method brings the obliquely sloping eardrum into better view.

Pull the pinna up and back on an adult or older child; this helps straighten the S-shape of the canal (Fig. 15-7). (Pull the pinna down on an infant and a child younger than 3 years [see Fig. 15-13]). Hold the pinna gently but firmly. Do not release traction on the ear until you have finished the examination and the otoscope is removed.

Objective Data

Normal Range of Findings	**Abnormal Findings**

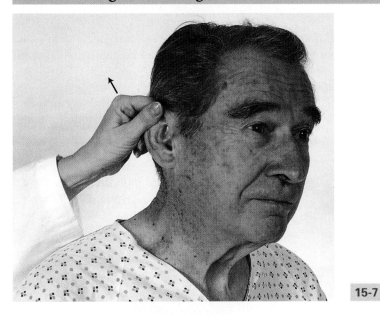

15-7

Hold the otoscope "upside down" along your fingers and have the dorsa (back) of your hand along the person's cheek braced to steady the otoscope (Fig. 15-8). This position feels awkward to you only at first. It soon will feel natural, and you will find it useful to prevent forceful insertion. Your stabilizing hand also acts as a protecting lever if the person suddenly moves the head.

15-8

Insert the speculum slowly and carefully along the axis of the canal. Watch the insertion; then put your eye up to the otoscope. Avoid touching the inner "bony" section of the canal wall, which is covered by a thin epithelial layer and is sensitive to pain. Sometimes you cannot see anything but canal wall. If so, try to reposition the person's head, apply more traction on the pinna, and re-angle the otoscope to look forward toward the person's nose.

Once it is in place, you may need to rotate the otoscope slightly to visualize the entire eardrum; do this gently. Last, perform the otoscopic examination before you test hearing; ear canals with impacted cerumen give the erroneous impression of pathologic hearing loss.

Objective Data

Normal Range of Findings	Abnormal Findings

The External Canal

Note any redness and swelling, lesions, foreign bodies, or discharge. If any discharge is present, note the color and odor. (Clean any discharge from the speculum before examining the other ear to avoid contamination with possibly infectious material.) For a person with a hearing aid, note any irritation on the canal wall from poorly fitting ear molds.

Redness and swelling occur with otitis externa; canal may be completely closed with swelling.

Purulent otorrhea suggests otitis externa or OM if the drum has ruptured.

Frank blood or clear, watery drainage (cerebrospinal fluid [CSF]) after trauma suggests basal skull fracture and warrants immediate referral. CSF feels oily and is positive for glucose on Tes-Tape.

Foreign body, polyp, furuncle, exostosis (see Table 15-4, Ear Canal Abnormalities, p. 345).

The Tympanic Membrane

Color and Characteristics. Systematically explore its landmarks (Fig. 15-9). The normal eardrum is shiny and translucent, with a pearl gray color. The cone-shaped light reflex is prominent in the anteroinferior quadrant (at the 5 o'clock position in the right drum and the 7 o'clock position in the left drum). This is the reflection of your otoscope light. Sections of the malleus are visible through the translucent drum: the umbo, manubrium, and short process. (Infrequently you also may see the incus behind the drum; it shows as a whitish haze in the upper posterior area.) At the periphery the annulus looks whiter and denser.

Yellow-amber drum color occurs with OM with effusion (serous).

Red color with acute OM.

Absent or distorted landmarks.

Air/fluid level or air bubbles behind drum indicate OM with effusion (see Tables 15-5, Abnormal Views Seen on Otoscopy, and 15-6, Abnormal Tympanic Membranes).

15-9 Normal tympanic membrane *(right ear)*.

Position. The eardrum is flat and slightly pulled in at the center.

Retracted drum is caused by vacuum in middle ear with obstructed eustachian tube.

Bulging drum is caused by increased pressure in OM.

Integrity of Membrane. Inspect the eardrum and the entire circumference of the annulus for perforations. The normal TM is intact. Some adults may show scarring, which is a dense white patch on the drum. This is a sequela of repeated ear infections.

Examine the other ear but switch otoscope hands so the hand holding the otoscope braces against the person's cheek.

Perforation shows as a dark oval area or as a larger opening on the drum.

Vesicles on drum (see Table 15-5).

Normal Range of Findings	Abnormal Findings

Test Hearing Acuity

Your screening for a hearing deficit begins during the history; "Do you have difficulty hearing now?" If the answer is *yes*, perform audiometric testing or refer for audiometric testing. If the answer is *no*, screen using the whispered voice test described as follows.

This single question in people over 50 years has an 83% to 90% agreement with hearing loss documented by audiometric testing.[14]

A pure tone audiometer gives a precise quantitative measure of hearing by assessing the person's ability to hear sounds of varying frequency. This is a battery-powered, lightweight, handheld instrument that is available in most outpatient settings. With the patient sitting, prop his or her elbow on the armrest of the chair with the hand making a gentle fist. Tell the patient, "You will hear faint tones of different pitches. Please raise your finger as soon as you hear the tone; then lower your finger as soon as you no longer hear the tone." Choose tones of random loudness in decibels on the audioscope. Each tone is on for 1.5 seconds and off for 1.5 seconds. Test each ear separately and record the results. An audiometer gives a precise quantitative measure of hearing by assessing the person's ability to hear sounds of varying frequency.

Whispered Voice Test

Stand arm's length (2 feet) behind the person. Test one ear at a time while masking hearing in the other ear to prevent sound transmission around the head. This is done by placing one finger on the tragus and pushing it in and out of the auditory meatus. Move your head to 1 to 2 feet from the person's ear. Exhale fully and whisper slowly a set of 3 random numbers and letters, such as "5, B, 6." Normally the person repeats each number/letter correctly after you say it. If the response is not correct, repeat the whispered test using a different combination of 3 numbers and letters. A passing score is correct repetition of at least 3 of a possible 6 numbers/letters.[14] Assess the other ear using yet another set of whispered items "4, K, 2."

The person is unable to hear whispered items. A whisper is a high-frequency sound and is used to detect high-tone loss.

Tuning Fork Tests

Tuning fork tests measure hearing by air conduction (AC) or bone conduction (BC), in which the sound vibrates through the cranial bones to the inner ear. The AC route through the ear canal and middle ear is usually the more sensitive route. Traditionally these tests were taught; yet evidence shows that both the Weber and the Rinne tuning fork tests are inaccurate and do not yield precise or reliable data.[10] Close to 40% of normal hearing people lateralize the Weber test, i.e., hear the tone louder in one ear. Thus these tests should not be used for general screening.

With documented hearing loss, these tests may help distinguish conductive loss from sensorineural loss (see Table 15-7, Tuning Fork Tests, p. 350). But they cannot screen a conductive loss from a mixed conductive/sensorineural loss.[7b]

The Vestibular Apparatus

The **Romberg test** assesses the ability of the vestibular apparatus in the inner ear to help maintain standing balance. Because the Romberg test also assesses intactness of the cerebellum and proprioception, it is discussed in Chapter 23 (see Fig. 23-21).

❖ DEVELOPMENTAL COMPETENCE

Infants and Young Children

Examination of the external ear is similar to that described for the adult, with the addition of examination of position and alignment on head. Note the ear position. The top of the pinna should match an imaginary line extending from the corner of the eye to the occiput. The ear should also be positioned within 10 degrees of vertical (Fig. 15-10).

Low-set ears are found with genetic disorders, including trisomy 21 (Down syndrome). Large prominent ears, misshapen ears, and creases on earlobes are nonspecific but occur with certain.

Normal Range of Findings	Abnormal Findings

syndromes and with underlying ear structure abnormalities.

Preauricular skin tags may occur alone or with other facial anomalies.

Normal alignment

15-10

Low-set ears and deviation in alignment

© Pat Thomas, 2006.

Otoscopic Examination. In addition to its place in the complete examination, eardrum assessment is mandatory for any infant or child requiring care for illness or fever. For the infant or young child, the timing of the otoscopic examination is best toward the end of the complete examination. Many young children protest vigorously during this procedure no matter how well you prepare, and it is difficult to re-establish cooperation afterward. Save the otoscopic examination until last.

To help prepare the child, let him or her hold your funny-looking "flashlight." You may wish to have the child look in the parent's or a toy puppet's ear as you hold the otoscope (Fig. 15-11).

Ear pain and ear rubbing are associated with acute OM, as are a bulging red eardrum and middle ear effusion. Fever is usually present but not always (see Table 15-6).

15-11

Normal Range of Findings	Abnormal Findings

Positioning of the child is important. You need a clear view of the canal. Avoid harsh restraint, but you must protect the eardrum from injury in case of sudden head movement (Fig. 15-12). Enlist the aid of a cooperative parent. Prop an infant upright against the parent's chest or shoulder, with the parent's arm around the upper part of the head. A toddler can be held in the parent's lap with his or her arms gently secured. As you pull down on the pinna, gently push in on the child's tragus as a lead-in to inserting the speculum tip. This sometimes helps avoid the startling poke of the speculum tip.

15-12

Remember to pull the pinna straight down on an infant or a child younger than 3 years. This method matches the slope of the ear canal (Fig. 15-13)

ADULT   YOUNG CHILD

15-13 Adult—pull pinna up and back

Infant/child under 3—pull pinna straight down

At birth the patency of the ear canal is determined, but the otoscopic examination is not performed because the canal is filled with amniotic fluid and vernix caseosa. After a few days the TM is examined. During the first few days it often looks thickened and opaque. It may look "injected" and have a mild redness from increased vascularity. The eardrum also looks injected in infants after crying.

Atresia—Absence or closure of the ear canal.

Objective Data

Normal Range of Findings	Abnormal Findings

The position of the eardrum is more horizontal in the neonate, making it more difficult to see completely and harder to differentiate from the canal wall. By 1 month of age the drum is in the oblique (more vertical) position as in the older child, and examination is a bit easier.

When examining an infant or young child, a pneumatic bulb attachment enables you to direct a light puff of air toward the drum to assess **vibratility** (Fig. 15-14). For a secure seal, choose the largest speculum that fits in the ear canal without causing pain. A rubber tip on the end of the speculum gives a better seal. Give a small pump to the bulb (positive pressure) and release the bulb (negative pressure). Normally the TM moves inward with a slight puff and outward with a slight release.

An abnormal response is no movement. Drum hypomobility indicates effusion or a high vacuum in the middle ear. For the newborn's first 6 weeks, drum immobility is the best indicator of middle ear infection.

15-14

Normally the tympanic membrane is intact. In a child being treated for chronic OM, you may note the presence of a tympanostomy tube in the central part of the eardrum. This is inserted surgically to equalize pressure and drain secretions. Finally, although the condition is not normal, it is not uncommon to note a foreign body in a child's canal such as a small stone or a bead.

Chronic OM relieved by tympanostomy tubes (see Table 15-6).
Foreign body must be removed (see Table 15-4).

Test Hearing Acuity. Use the developmental milestones listed here to assess hearing in an infant. Also attend to the parents' concern over the infant's inability to hear; their assessment is usually well founded.

The room should be silent and the baby contented. Make a loud, sudden noise (hand clap or squeeze toy) out of the baby's peripheral range of vision of about 30 cm (12 in). You may need to repeat a few times, but you should note these responses:

- Newborn—Startle (Moro) reflex, acoustic blink reflex
- 3 to 4 months—Acoustic blink reflex, infant stops movement and appears to "listen," stops sucking, quiets if crying, cries if quiet
- 6 to 8 months—Infant turns head to localize sound, responds to own name
- Preschool and school-age child—Child must be screened with audiometry

Absence of alerting behavior may indicate congenital deafness.

Failure to localize sound.

No intelligible speech by age 2 years.

Note that a young child may be unaware of a hearing loss because the child does not know how one "ought" to hear. Note these behavioral manifestations of hearing loss:
1. The child is inattentive in casual conversation.
2. The child reacts more to movement and facial expression than to sound.

Normal Range of Findings	Abnormal Findings

Normal Range of Findings

3. The child's facial expression is strained or puzzled.
4. The child frequently asks to have statements repeated.
5. The child confuses words that sound alike.
6. The child has an accompanying speech problem: speech is monotonous or garbled; the child mispronounces or omits sounds.
7. The child appears shy and withdrawn and "lives in a world of his or her own."
8. The child frequently complains of earaches.
9. The child hears better at times when the environment is more conducive.

The Aging Adult

An aging adult may have pendulous earlobes with linear wrinkling because of loss of elasticity of the pinna. Coarse, wiry hairs may be present at the opening of the ear canal. During otoscopy the eardrum normally may be whiter in color and more opaque, duller than in the younger adult. It also may look thickened.

A high-tone frequency hearing loss is apparent for those affected with **presbycusis**, the hearing loss that occurs with aging. Note any difficulty hearing in the whispered voice test and hearing consonants during conversational speech. The aging adult thinks that "people are mumbling" and feels isolated in family or friendship groups.

PROMOTING A HEALTHY LIFESTYLE

Early Hearing Detection and Intervention—The "1-3-6" Plan

According to the National Institutes of Health (NIH), up to 3 out of every 1000 children in the United States are born deaf or hard-of-hearing. Because the first 3 years of life represent the most intensive period for speech and language development, identifying hearing loss as early as possible is a high priority. In the past newborns at high risk for hearing loss were the only ones screened. Unfortunately as many as 50% of newborns with hearing loss were sent home undetected and often not identified until they were 3 years of age, long after the critical period for speech. In 1993 the NIH endorsed the screening of all newborns for hearing loss before they leave the hospital, which was supported by the U.S. Congress' passage of the Newborn and Infant Hearing and Screening Act of 1999. Today all states have established Early Hearing Detection and Intervention (EHDI) programs.

EHDI programs routinely collect and report data, focusing on the following three benchmarks, commonly known as the "1-3-6" Plan:

1 = All newborns are screened for hearing loss before they are discharged home or within 1 month of birth.

3 = All infants referred for screening undergo a complete diagnostic audiologic evaluation by 3 months of age.

6 = All infants with diagnosed hearing loss receive appropriate interventions by 6 months of age, including amplification selections and early intervention.

The two screening tests recommended for newborn hearing screening include:

1. Otoacoustic emission (OAE) test. For this test a tiny probe is placed just inside the baby's ear canal to measure the response (echo) when clicks or tones are played into the baby's ears.

2. Brainstem auditory evoked response (BAER) test. For this test clicks/tones are played through soft earphones placed over the newborn's ears while electrodes, placed on the newborn's head, measure how the auditory nerve responds to sound.

Both tests can be completed in about 5 to 10 minutes and/or even when the newborn is asleep, and they are painless. The bottom line is that evidence shows that children with hearing loss who receive early intervention and amplification before 6 months of age do better than those receiving services after 6 months of age; and by the first grade children identified earlier are 1 to 2 years ahead of their later-identified peers in language, cognitive, and social skills.

Resources

American Academy of Pediatrics (AAP) resource for parents about newborn hearing screening, http://patiented.aap.org/content2.aspx?aid=5673&lan=en.

The AAP Position Statement: Principles and guidelines for early hearing detection and intervention programs is available online and includes a helpful algorithm for health care professionals with detailed hearing screening guidelines as Appendix 1, http://pediatrics.aappublications.org/content/120/4/898.full.pdf+html?sid=329d46f7-3df8-49e8-be70-653d449ad810.

Hearing Loss in Children, Centers for Disease Control and Prevention (CDC): www.cdc.gov/ncbddd/ehdi/.

National Center for Hearing Assessment and Management (NCHAM), http://infanthearing.org.

This is the site for NCHAM, which serves as the national resource center for implementation and improvement of comprehensive and effective EHDI systems, including A Resource Guide for Early Hearing Detection and Intervention, which is available as an e-book at http://infanthearing.org/ehdi-ebook/index.html.

NIH Fact Sheet: Newborn Hearing Screening, http://report.nih.gov/nihfactsheets/ViewFactSheet.aspx?csid=104.

DOCUMENTATION AND CRITICAL THINKING

Sample Charting

SUBJECTIVE

States hearing is good, no earaches, infections, discharge, hearing loss, tinnitus, or vertigo.

OBJECTIVE

Pinna: Skin intact with no masses, lesions, tenderness, or discharge.
Otoscope: External canals are clear with no redness, swelling, lesions, foreign body, or discharge. Both TMs are pearly gray in color, with light reflex and landmarks intact; no perforations.
Hearing: Responds appropriately to conversation. Whispered sounds heard bilaterally.

ASSESSMENT

Healthy ear structures
Hearing accurate

Clinical Case Study 1

A 2-month-old Latino male (T.W.) is brought to the clinic by his foster mother because he "won't stop crying and just can't seem to stay asleep."

SUBJECTIVE

Foster mom reports that T.W. has had a cold for the past 7 days but the crying and inability to sleep just started yesterday. Foster mom reports, "He seems to be happier when he's sitting up, which makes it hard to feed him his bottle." She states that she usually lays the child down for naps with a bottle elevated on a blanket so she can "get some work done." Reports giving T.W. infant acetaminophen 2 hours PTA for his apparent discomfort.

OBJECTIVE

Vital signs: Temp 100° F (37.8° C) (rectal). Unable to obtain BP because of infant motion. Pulse 180 bpm. Resp 40/min.
General appearance: Infant appears fussy and unable to get comfortable even in mother's arms.
HEENT: Anterior fontanel open and flat w/ minimal overriding sutures, posterior fontanel closed; conjunctivae clear, sclerae white, visibly tearing; bilat TMs dull red and bulging, no light reflex, no mobility on pneumatic otoscopy; oral mucosa pink, tonsils 1+; no lymphadenopathy.
Cardiovascular: Regular rate and rhythm, no murmurs.
Respiratory: Breath sounds equal with coarseness that clears with cough; unlabored.

ASSESSMENT

Acute otitis media (bilat) R/T infectious process
Acute pain R/T inflammation in tympanic membranes
Deficient knowledge (parents) R/T risk factors for otitis media

Clinical Case Study 2

T.R. is a 15-year-old male Caucasian high school student who comes to the health center to seek care for "cough off and on all winter and earache since last night."

SUBJECTIVE

6 weeks PTA—Nonproductive cough throughout day, no fever, no nasal congestion, no chest soreness. T.R.'s father gave him an over-the-counter decongestant, which helped, but cough continued off/on since. Does not smoke.

1 day PTA—Intermittent cough continues, nasal congestion and thick white mucus. Also earache R ear; treated self with heating pad, pain unrelieved. Pain is moderate, not deep and throbbing. Says R ear feels full, "hollow headed," voices sound muffled and far away, switches telephone to L ear to talk. No sore throat, no fever, no chest congestion or soreness.

OBJECTIVE

Vital signs: Temp 98.6° F (37° C) (oral). Pulse 76 bpm. BP 106/72 mm Hg.

Ears: L ear, canal, TM normal. R ear and canal normal, R TM retracted, with multiple air bubbles; drum color is yellow/amber. No sinus tenderness.

Nose: Turbinates bright red and swollen, mucopurulent discharge.

Throat: Not reddened, tonsils 1+.

Neck: One R anterior cervical node enlarged, firm, movable, tender. All others not palpable.

Lungs: Breath sounds clear to auscultation, resonant to percussion throughout.

ASSESSMENT

Otitis media with effusion, R ear, with mild URI
Transient conductive hearing loss
Disturbed sensory perception (auditory) R/T excessive fluid in middle ear
Pain R/T middle ear pressure

Clinical Case Study 3

E.S. is a 78-year-old Caucasian retired woman with a medical diagnosis of angina pectoris, which has responded to nitroglycerin PRN and periods of rest between activity. She has been independent in her own home and is coping well with activity restrictions through help from neighbors and family. Now hospitalized for evaluation of acute chest pain episode; MI has been ruled out, pain diagnosed as anginal; to be released to own home with a beta-blocking medication and nitroglycerin PRN.

Just before this hospitalization, Mrs. S. received a hearing aid after evaluation by an audiologist at senior center. Mrs. S. was born in Germany, immigrated to United States at age 5 years; considers English her primary language.

SUBJECTIVE

Since this hospitalization, feels "irritable and nervous." Relates this to worry about heart and also, "I get so mixed up in here, this room is so strange, and I just can't hear the nurses. They talk like cavemen, 'oo-i-ee-uou.'" Tried using her new hearing aid but no relief. "It just kept screeching in my ear, and it made the monitor beep so loud it drove me crazy." States no tinnitus, no vertigo.

OBJECTIVE

Ears: Pinna with elongated lobes, but no tenderness to palpation, no discharge, no masses or lesions. Both canals clear of cerumen. Both TM appear gray-white, slightly opaque and dull, although all landmarks visible. No perforation.

Hearing: Difficulty hearing room conversation. Unable to hear whispered voice bilaterally.

ASSESSMENT

Chest pain/angina pectoris
Deficient knowledge R/T lack of teaching on hearing aid
Disturbed sensory perception (auditory) R/T effects of aging
Anxiety R/T change in cardiovascular health status and inability to communicate effectively

Examiner Asks	Rationale
8. Smoking, alcohol consumption. Do you smoke? Pipe or cigarettes? Smokeless tobacco? How many packs per day? For how many years?	Chronic tobacco use leads to tooth loss, coronal and root caries, and periodontal disease in older adults.
• When was your last alcoholic drink? How much alcohol did you drink that time? How much alcohol do you usually drink?	Chronic tobacco use and heavy alcohol consumption highly increase risk for oral and pharyngeal cancers.
9. Patient-centered care. Tell me about your daily dental care. How often do you use a toothbrush and floss?	Assess self-care behaviors for oral hygiene.
• Last dental examination? Do dental problems affect which foods you eat?	Periodic dental screening is necessary to note caries.
• Do you have a dental appliance: braces, bridge, head gear?	
• Wear dentures? All the time? How long have you had this set? How do they fit?	
• Any sores or irritation on the palate or gums?	Lesions may arise from ill-fitting dentures, or the presence of dentures may mask the eruption of new lesions.
• Any problems with talking—Do the dentures whistle or drop? Can you chew all foods with them? How do you clean them?	

Additional History for Infants and Children

1. Does the child have any mouth infections or sores such as thrush or canker sores? How frequently do these occur?

2. Does the child have frequent sore throat or tonsillitis? How often? How are these treated? Have they ever been documented as streptococcal infections?

Children have a higher incidence of GAS pharyngitis than adults do (37% vs. 10%), and signs and symptoms cannot diagnose this. Must confirm with rapid strep test or throat culture.[21]

3. Did the child's teeth erupt about on time?

   Eruption is delayed with Down syndrome, cretinism, rickets.

   • Do the teeth seem straight to you?

   Malocclusion.

   • Is the child using a bottle? How often during the day? Does the child go to sleep with a bottle at night?

   Prolonged bottle use increases risk for tooth decay and middle ear infections.

   • Have you noticed any thumb sucking after the child's secondary teeth came in?

   Prolonged thumb sucking (after ages 6 to 7 years) may affect occlusion.

   • Have you noticed the child grinding his or her teeth? Does this happen at night?

   Bruxism usually occurs in sleep or from dental problems or nervous tension.

4. **Patient-centered care.** How are the child's dental habits? Use a toothbrush regularly? How often does the child see a dentist?

   Evaluate child's self-care. Early self-care has best compliance.

   • Do you use fluoridated water or fluoride supplement?
   • Are vaccinations up to date?

   Pertussis (whooping cough) is on the rise because of lack of adherence to recommended vaccination schedule and waning immunity in adolescents and adults who become carriers to unvaccinated infants.[26]

Additional History for the Aging Adult

1. Any dryness in the mouth? Are you taking any medications? (Note prescribed and over-the-counter medications.)

   Xerostomia (dry mouth) is a side effect of many drugs: antidepressants, anticholinergics, antispasmodics, antihypertensives, antipsychotics, bronchodilators.

2. Have you lost any teeth? Can you chew all types of food?

   Note a decrease in eating meat, fresh vegetables, and cleansing foods such as apples.

Examiner Asks	Rationale
3. Are you able to care for your own teeth or dentures?	Self-care may be decreased by physical disability (arthritis), vision loss, confusion, or depression.
4. Noticed a change in your sense of taste or smell?	Some people add extra salt and sugar to enhance food when taste begins to wane. Diminished smell also may decrease the person's ability to detect food spoilage, natural gas leaks, or smoke from a fire.

OBJECTIVE DATA

PREPARATION

Position the person sitting up straight with his or her head at your eye level. If the person wears dentures, offer a paper towel and ask the person to remove them.

EQUIPMENT NEEDED

Otoscope with short, wide-tipped nasal speculum attachment
Penlight
Two tongue blades
Cotton gauze pad (4 × 4 inches)
Gloves

Normal Range of Findings	Abnormal Findings
Inspect and Palpate the Nose	
External Nose	
Normally the nose is symmetric, in the midline, and in proportion to other facial features (Fig. 16-7). Inspect for any deformity, asymmetry, inflammation, or skin lesions. If an injury is reported or suspected, palpate gently for any pain or break in contour. 16-7	
Test the patency of the nostrils by pushing each nasal wing shut with your finger while asking the person to sniff inward through the other naris. This reveals any obstruction, which later is explored with the nasal speculum. The sense of smell, mediated by cranial nerve I, is not tested in a routine examination. (See cranial nerve testing in Chapter 23.)	Absence of sniff indicates obstruction (e.g., common cold, nasal polyps, rhinitis).

Objective Data

Normal Range of Findings

Nasal Cavity

Attach the short, wide-tipped speculum to the otoscope head, and insert this combined apparatus into the nasal vestibule, avoiding pressure on the nasal septum. Gently lift up the tip of the nose with your finger before inserting.

View each nasal cavity with the person's head erect and then with the head tilted back. Inspect the nasal mucosa, noting its normal red color and smooth, moist surface (Fig. 16-8). Note any swelling, discharge, bleeding, or foreign body.

Abnormal Findings

Rhinitis—Nasal mucosa is swollen and bright red with URI.

Discharge is common with rhinitis and sinusitis, varying from watery and copious to thick, purulent, and green-yellow.

With chronic allergy mucosa looks swollen, boggy, pale, and gray.

Middle turbinate
Inferior turbinate

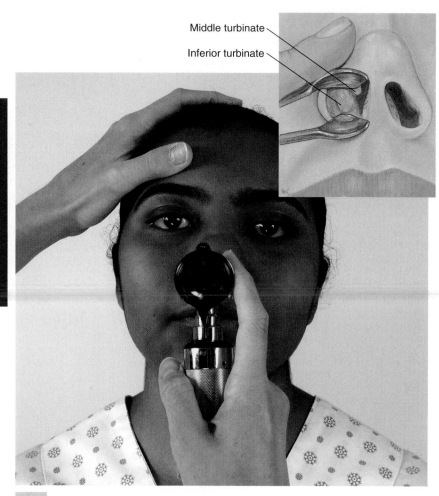

16-8

16-9 Deviated septum. (Fireman, 1996.)

Observe the nasal septum for deviation (Fig. 16-9). A deviated septum is common and is not significant unless air flow is obstructed. (If present in a hospitalized patient, document the deviated septum in the event that the person needs nasal suctioning or a nasogastric tube.) Also note any perforation or bleeding in the septum.

A deviated septum looks like a hump or shelf in one nasal cavity.

Perforation is seen as a spot of light from a penlight shining in the other naris and occurs with cocaine use.

Epistaxis commonly comes from the anterior septum (see Table 16-1, Nose Abnormalities, p. 375).

Normal Range of Findings	Abnormal Findings

Inspect the turbinates (the bony ridges curving down from the lateral walls). The superior turbinate will not be in your view, but the middle and inferior turbinates appear the same light red color as the nasal mucosa. Note any swelling but do not try to push the speculum past it. Turbinates are quite vascular and tender if touched.

Note any polyps (benign growths that accompany chronic allergy), and distinguish them from the normal turbinates.

Polyps are smooth, pale gray, avascular, mobile, nontender (see Table 16-1).

Palpate the Sinus Areas

Using your thumbs, press the frontal sinuses by pressing firmly up and under the eyebrows (Fig. 16-10, *A*) and over the maxillary sinuses below the cheekbones (Fig. 16-10, *B*). Take care not to press directly on the eyeballs.

The person should feel firm pressure but no pain.

Sinus areas are tender to palpation in people with chronic allergies and acute infection (sinusitis).

Another sign of sinusitis is to check for focal pain when the person bends over (if able).

16-10

Transillumination

There is no evidence to support the practice of transillumination of the frontal or maxillary sinuses when you suspect sinus inflammation. The diagnosis requires distinct differences in the illumination of one of the sinus pair. Thus the technique would not help in chronic sinusitis that has diffuse swelling of all sinus mucosa. Although there is more fluid collection with acute sinusitis, the asymmetry of light illumination still is not valid because many healthy sinuses normally do not transilluminate.

Inspect the Mouth

Begin with anterior structures and move posteriorly. Use a tongue blade to retract structures and a bright light for optimal visualization.

Lips

Inspect the lips for color, moisture, cracking, or lesions. Retract the lips and note their inner surface as well (Fig. 16-11). All racial groups have lips that are deeper or pinker than facial skin. However, some African Americans normally may have bluish lips and a dark line on the gingival margin.

In light-skinned people: circumoral pallor occurs with shock and anemia; cyanosis with hypoxemia and chilling; cherry red lips with carbon monoxide poisoning, acidosis from aspirin poisoning, or ketoacidosis.

Normal Range of Findings	Abnormal Findings

16-11

Cheilitis (perlèche)—Cracking at the corners.

Herpes simplex, other lesions (see Table 16-2, Lip Abnormalities, p. 377).

Teeth and Gums

The condition of the teeth is an index of the person's general health. Your examination should not replace the regular dental examination; but you should note any diseased, absent, loose, or abnormally positioned teeth. The teeth normally look white, straight, evenly spaced, and clean and free of debris or decay.

Compare the number of teeth with the number expected for the person's age. Ask the person to bite as if chewing something and note alignment of upper and lower jaw. Normal occlusion in the back is the upper teeth resting directly on the lower teeth; in the front the upper incisors slightly override the lower incisors.

Normally the gums look pink or coral with a stippled (dotted) surface. The gum margins at the teeth are tight and well defined (Fig. 16-12). Check for swelling; retraction of gingival margins; and spongy, bleeding, or discolored gums. Some African Americans normally may have a dark melanotic line along the gingival margin.

Discolored teeth appear brown with excessive fluoride use, yellow with tobacco use.

Grinding down of tooth surface; plaque—soft debris; caries—decay.

Malocclusion (poor biting relationship), protrusion of upper or lower incisors (see Table 16-3, Teeth and Gum Abnormalities, p. 378).

Gingival hyperplasia (see Table 16-3), crevices between teeth and gums, pockets of debris.

Gums bleed with slight pressure, indicating gingivitis.

Dark line on gingival margins occurs with lead and bismuth poisoning.

16-12

Tongue

Check the tongue for color, surface characteristics, and moisture. The color is pink and even. The dorsal surface is normally roughened from the papillae. A thin white coating may be present (Fig. 16-13, *A*). Ask the person to touch the tongue to the roof of the mouth. Its ventral surface looks smooth and glistening and shows veins (Fig. 16-13, *B*). Saliva is present.

Beefy red, swollen tongue. Smooth glossy areas (see Table 16-5, Tongue Abnormalities, p. 381).

Enlarged tongue occurs with mental retardation, hypothyroidism, acromegaly; a small tongue accompanies malnutrition.

Dry mouth occurs with dehydration, fever; tongue has deep vertical fissures.

Normal Range of Findings

16-13

With a glove,* hold the tongue with a cotton gauze pad for traction and swing it out and to each side (Fig. 16-14). Inspect for any white patches or lesions; normally none are present. If any occur, palpate them for induration.

16-14

Inspect carefully the entire U-shaped area under the tongue behind the teeth. Oral malignancies are most likely to develop here. Note any white patches, nodules, or ulcerations. If lesions are present or for any person older than 50 years or with a positive history of smoking or alcohol use, use your gloved hand to palpate the area. Place your other hand under the jaw to stabilize the tissue and to "capture" any abnormality (Fig. 16-15). Note any induration.

*Always wear gloves to examine mucous membranes. This follows Standard Precautions to prevent the spread of communicable disease.

Abnormal Findings

Saliva is decreased when taking anti-cholinergic and other medications.

Excess saliva and drooling occur with gingivostomatitis and neurologic dysfunction.

Oral precancerous and cancerous lesions (see Table 16-5).

Any lesion or ulcer persisting for more than 2 weeks must be investigated.

An indurated area may be a mass or lymphadenopathy, and it must be investigated.

Objective Data

Normal Range of Findings	Abnormal Findings

16-15   Bimanual palpation.

Buccal Mucosa

Hold the cheek open with a wooden tongue blade and check the buccal mucosa for color, nodules, or lesions. It looks pink, smooth, and moist, although patchy hyperpigmentation is common and normal in dark-skinned people.

An expected finding is **Stensen's duct,** the opening of the parotid salivary gland. It looks like a small dimple opposite the upper second molar. You also may see a raised occlusion line on the buccal mucosa parallel with the level the teeth meet. This is caused by the teeth closing against the cheek.

A larger patch also may be present along the buccal mucosa. This is **leukoedema,** a benign, milky, bluish-white, opaque area, more common in Blacks and East Indians. When it is mild, the patch disappears as you stretch the cheeks. It is always bilateral. With age it looks grayish-white and thickened. The cause is unknown. Do not mistake leukoedema for oral infections such as candidiasis (thrush).

Fordyce granules are small, isolated white or yellow papules on the mucosa of cheek, tongue, and lips (Fig. 16-16). These little sebaceous cysts are painless and not significant.

Dappled brown patches are present with Addison's disease (chronic adrenal insufficiency).
Orifice of Stensen's duct looks red with mumps.
Koplik spots—Early prodromal (early warning) sign of measles.

Candida infection usually rubs off, leaving a clear or raw denuded surface.
The chalky white raised patch of **leukoplakia** is abnormal (see Table 16-4, Buccal Mucosa Abnormalities).

16-16   Fordyce granules.   (Ibsen & Phelan, 1996.)

Palate

Shine your light up to the roof of the mouth. The more anterior hard palate is white with irregular transverse rugae. The posterior soft palate is pinker, smooth, and upwardly movable. A normal variation is a nodular bony ridge down the middle of the hard palate, a **torus palatinus** (Fig. 16-17). This benign growth arises after puberty; is more common in American Indians, Inuits, and Asians; and is more common in females than in males.

The hard palate appears yellow with jaundice. In Blacks with jaundice it may look yellow, muddy yellow, or green-brown.

Normal Range of Findings

16-17   Torus palatinus.
(Lemmi & Lemmi, 2011.)

Observe the uvula; it normally looks like a fleshy pendant hanging in the midline (Fig. 16-18). Ask the person to say "ahhh," and note the soft palate and uvula rise in the midline. This tests one function of cranial nerve X, the vagus nerve.

16-18   © Pat Thomas, 2006.

Tonsil   Uvula   Anterior tonsillar pillar

Inspect the Throat

With your light observe the oval, rough-surfaced **tonsils** behind the anterior tonsillar pillar (see Fig. 16-18). Their color is the same pink as the oral mucosa, and their surface is peppered with indentations, or crypts. In some people the crypts collect small plugs of whitish cellular debris. This does not indicate infection. However, there should be no exudate on the tonsils. Tonsils are graded in size as follows:

   1+ Visible
   2+ Halfway between tonsillar pillars and uvula
   3+ Touching the uvula
   4+ Touching one another

Abnormal Findings

Oral Kaposi sarcoma is the most common early lesion in people with AIDS (see Table 16-6, Oropharynx Abnormalities, p. 383).

A *bifid* uvula looks as if it is split in two; more common in American Indians (see Table 16-6).

Any deviation to the side or absent movement indicates nerve damage, which also occurs with poliomyelitis and diphtheria.

With an acute infection tonsils are bright red and swollen and may have exudate or large white spots.

A white membrane covering the tonsils may accompany infectious mononucleosis, leukemia, and diphtheria.

Objective Data

Normal Range of Findings

You may normally see 1+ or 2+ tonsils in healthy people, especially in children, because lymphoid tissue is proportionately enlarged until puberty.

Enlarge your view of the posterior pharyngeal wall by depressing the tongue with a tongue blade (Fig. 16-19). Push down halfway back on the tongue; if you push on its tip, the tongue humps up in back. Press slightly off center to avoid eliciting the gag reflex. You can help the person whose gag reflex is easily triggered by offering a tongue blade to depress his or her own tongue. (Some people can lower their own tongue so the tongue blade is not needed.) Scan the posterior wall for color, exudate, and lesions. When finished, discard the tongue blade.

16-19

Although usually it is not done in the screening examination, touching the posterior wall with the tongue blade elicits the gag reflex. This tests cranial nerves IX and X, the glossopharyngeal and vagus.

Test cranial nerve XII, the hypoglossal nerve, by asking the person to stick out the tongue. It should protrude in the midline. Children enjoy this request! Note any tremor, loss of movement, or deviation to the side.

During the examination notice any breath odor, *halitosis.* This is common and usually has a local cause such as poor oral hygiene and decaying food debris between the teeth. Other common smells are caused by odoriferous foods, alcohol consumption, heavy smoking, or dental infection. Occasionally it may indicate a systemic disease.

✥ DEVELOPMENTAL COMPETENCE

Infants and Children

Because the oral examination is intrusive for the infant or young child, the timing is best toward the end of the complete examination, along with the ear examination. But if any crying episodes occur earlier, seize the opportunity to examine the open mouth and oropharynx.

As with the ear examination, let the parent help position the child. Place the infant supine on the examining table with the arms restrained (Fig. 16-20). The older infant and toddler may be held on the parent's lap with one of the parent's hands holding the arms down and the other hand securing the child's head against the parent's chest.

Abnormal Findings

Tonsils are enlarged to 2+, 3+, or 4+ with an acute infection.

With CN XII damage, the tongue deviates *toward* the paralyzed side.

A fine tremor of the tongue occurs with hyperthyroidism; a coarse tremor occurs with cerebral palsy and alcoholism.

Diabetic ketoacidosis has a sweet, fruity breath odor; this acetone smell also occurs in children with malnutrition or dehydration. Others are an ammonia breath odor with uremia; a musty odor with liver disease; a foul, fetid odor with dental or respiratory infections; an alcohol odor with alcohol ingestion or chemicals; a mouselike smell of the breath with diphtheria.

| **Normal Range of Findings** | **Abnormal Findings** |

16-20

Use a game to help prepare the young child. Encourage the preschool child to use a tongue blade to look into a puppet's mouth. Or place a mirror so the child can look into his or her mouth just as you look. The school-age child is usually cooperative and loves to show off missing or new teeth (Fig. 16-21).

16-21

Be discriminating in your use of the tongue blade. It may be necessary for a full view of oral structures, but it produces a strong gag reflex in the infant. You may avoid the tongue blade completely with a cooperative preschooler and school-age child. Try asking the young child to "Open your mouth as big as a LION." Or say, "Can you stick out your WHOLE TONGUE?" Then ask the child to move the tongue in different directions. To enlarge your view of the oropharynx, ask the child to stick out the tongue and "pant like a dog."

At some point you will encounter an uncooperative young child who clenches the teeth and refuses to open the mouth. If all your other efforts have failed, slide the tongue blade along the buccal mucosa and turn it between the back teeth. Push down to depress the tongue. This stimulates the gag reflex, and the child opens the mouth wide for a few seconds. You will have a *brief* look at the throat. Make the most of it.

Normal Range of Findings	Abnormal Findings

Normal Range of Findings

Nose. The newborn may have milia across the nose. The nasal bridge may be flat in Black and Asian children. There should be no nasal flaring or narrowing with breathing.

It is essential to determine the patency of the nares in the immediate newborn period because most newborns are obligate nose breathers. Nares blocked with amniotic fluid are suctioned gently with a bulb syringe. If obstruction is suspected, a small-lumen (5 to 10 Fr) catheter is passed down each naris to confirm patency.

Avoid the nasal speculum when examining the infant and young child. Instead gently push up the tip of the nose with your thumb while using your other hand to shine the light into the naris. With a toddler be alert for the possible foreign body lodged in the nasal cavity (see Table 16-1, p. 376).

Only in children older than 8 years of age do you need to palpate the sinus areas. In younger children sinus areas are too small for palpation.

Mouth and Throat. A normal finding in infants is the **sucking tubercle,** a small pad in the middle of the upper lip from friction of breastfeeding or bottle-feeding. Note the number of teeth and whether it is appropriate for the child's age. Also note pattern of eruption, position, condition, and hygiene. Use this guide for children younger than 2 years of age: the child's age in months minus the number 6 should equal the expected number of deciduous teeth. Normally all 20 deciduous teeth are in by 2½ years. Saliva is present after 3 months of age and shows in excess with teething children.

Mobility should allow the tongue to extend at least as far as the alveolar ridge.

Note any bruising or laceration on the buccal mucosa or gums of the infant or young child.

On the palate, **Epstein pearls** are a normal finding in newborns and infants (Fig. 16-22). They are small, whitish, glistening, pearly papules along the median raphe of the hard palate and on the gums, where they look like teeth. They are small retention cysts and disappear in the first few weeks.

Abnormal Findings

Nasal flaring in the infant indicates respiratory distress.

A transverse ridge across the nose occurs in a child with chronic allergy from wiping the nose upward with the palm (see Table 13-2, p. 274). Nasal narrowing on inhalation is seen with chronic nasal obstruction and mouth breathing.

Inability to pass catheter through nasal cavity indicates choanal atresia, which needs immediate intervention (see Table 16-1).

No teeth by age 1 year.

Discolored teeth appear yellow or yellow-brown with infants taking tetracycline or who were exposed during the last trimester; appear green or black with excessive iron ingestion (this reverses when the iron is stopped).

Malocclusion: upper or lower dental arches are out of alignment.

Ankyloglossia, a short lingual frenulum, can limit protrusion and impair speech development (see Table 16-5).

Trauma may indicate child abuse from forced feeding of bottle or spoon.

A high-arched palate is usually normal in the newborn, but a very narrow or high arch also occurs with Turner syndrome, Ehlers-Danlos syndrome, Marfan syndrome, and Treacher Collins syndrome or develops in the mouth-breather in chronic allergies.

16-22 Epstein pearls. (Zitelli, 2007.)

Normal Range of Findings	Abnormal Findings

Bednar aphthae are traumatic areas or ulcers on the posterior hard palate on either side of the midline. They result from abrasions while sucking.

The tonsils are not visible in the newborn. They gradually enlarge during childhood, remaining proportionately larger until puberty. Tonsils appear still larger if the infant is crying or gagging. Normally the newborn can produce a strong, lusty cry.

Insert your gloved finger into the baby's mouth and palpate the hard and soft palate as the baby sucks. The sucking reflex can be elicited in infants up to 12 months old.

As teeth begin to erupt in the older infant and child, check age at eruption, sequence, and condition. Teeth should emerge straight up or down from the gums, and enamel should be clear white and smooth. Lift the upper lip to check for dental caries (tooth decay); normally there are none.

Nursing bottle caries are brown discolorations on upper front teeth (see Table 16-3).

The Pregnant Woman

Gum hypertrophy (surface looks smooth, and stippling disappears) may occur normally at puberty or during pregnancy (pregnancy gingivitis) (Fig. 16-23).

16-23 Early gingivitis. (Lemmi & Lemmi, 2011.)

The Aging Adult

The nose may appear more prominent on the face from a loss of subcutaneous fat. In the edentulous person the mouth and lips fold in, giving a "purse-string" appearance. The teeth may look slightly yellowed, although the color is uniform. Yellowing results from the dentin visible through worn enamel. The surface of the incisors may show vertical cracks from a lifetime of exposure to extreme temperatures. The teeth may look longer as the gum margins recede (Fig. 16-24).

16-24 Receded gums. (Lemmi & Lemmi, 2011.)

The surfaces look worn down or abraded. Old dental work deteriorates, especially at the gum margins. The teeth loosen with bone resorption and may move with palpation.

The tongue looks smoother as a result of papillary atrophy. The aging adult's buccal mucosa is thinned and may look shinier, as though it were "varnished."

Smokeless tobacco (SL-T) carries significant health risks, including cancers, fatal myocardial infarction and stroke, dental decay, hypertension, and decreased sperm counts and sterility. The types of SL-T commonly used in the United States include chewing tobacco and snuff. *Chewing tobacco* comes as loose leaf, plug, or twist and, just as the name implies, is chewed. *Snuff* is finely ground tobacco and comes dry, moist, or in packaged sachets like tea bags. Dry snuff can be sniffed through the nose. However, most snuff users put a "pinch" or "dip" between their gingival and buccal mucosa, suck on the tobacco, and spit out the juices, which gives rise to the term *spitting tobacco*. Holding one pinch of SL-T in your mouth ("dipping") for 30 minutes delivers as much nicotine as 3 cigarettes.

Using SL-T carries an even greater risk of oral cavity cancers than smoking. Pain is rarely an early symptom of oral cancer; thus regular examinations are important. The early signs of oral cancer include:

- A sore that does not seem to heal.
- A smooth or leathery white patch or lump.
- A prolonged sore throat or feeling that something is in the throat.
- Difficulty chewing.
- Restricted movement of the tongue or jaw.

SL-T use is higher in young White and American Indian/Alaska native males. There is also increased use of SL-T in sports, primarily baseball; young men often say that they start because they see their idols or heroes participating. Approximately 35% of major league baseball players use SL-T, but at least 50% of these users also report that they are trying to quit. In 1990 major league baseball issued a report on the hazards of SL-T and started efforts to encourage players not to start and to help others to quit. In 1991 minor league baseball banned the use of SL-T at the rookie level, and in 1993 it extended the ban throughout all minor leagues. In 1994 the National Collegiate Athletic Association banned the use of all tobacco products, including SL-T. In addition, the National Institutes of Health (NIH) and the National Institute of Dental and Craniofacial Research (NIDCR), along with the National Cancer Institute, created an informational brochure, "Spit Tobacco: A Guide for Quitting," that targets young men. It can be downloaded directly from: http://www.nidcr.nih.gov/NR/rdonlyres/DF314871-B0A6-4171-B831-C472F543C154/0/SpitTobacco.pdf.

Resources

The Centers for Disease Control and Prevention (CDC)
- *Provides a 5-minute closed-caption video that examines marketing tactics used to sell smokeless tobacco over the past century. Available at http://www.cdc.gov/tobacco/basic_information/tobacco_industry/.*

Office on Smoking and Health (OSH) and National Tobacco Control Program (NTCP): http://www.cdc.gov/tobacco/tobacco_control_programs/ntcp/index.htm.

Oral Health America
- *Developed NSTEP®, the National Spit Tobacco Education Program, http://oralhealthamerica.org/nstep-resources/, which focuses primarily on preventing young people from starting to use SL-T and on helping current users quit; includes a very specific 7-step cessation process. Available at http://oralhealthamerica.org/wp-content/uploads/Quitting-Spit-Tobacco.pdf.*

KidsHealth, which is a popular Internet-based health information site for children and teens, offers information on SL-T at http://kidshealth.org/teen/drug_alcohol/tobacco/smokeless.html.

Alcohol & Drug Abuse Council created an interactive website at: http://www.stopthespit.com/.

DOCUMENTATION AND CRITICAL THINKING

Sample Charting

SUBJECTIVE

Nose: No history of discharge, sinus problems, obstruction, epistaxis, or allergy. Colds 1-2/yr, mild. Fractured nose during high school sports, treated by MD.

Mouth and throat: No pain, lesions, bleeding gums, toothache, dysphagia, or hoarseness. Occasional sore throat with colds. Tonsillectomy, age 8. Smokes cigarettes 1 PPD × 9 years. Alcohol, 1-2 drinks socially about 2×/month. Visits dentist annually, dental hygienist 2×/year, flosses daily. No dental appliance.

OBJECTIVE

Nose: Symmetric, no deformity or skin lesions. Nares patent. Mucosa pink; no discharge, lesions, or polyps; no septal deviation or perforation. Sinuses—no tenderness to palpation.

Mouth: Can clench teeth. Mucosa and gingivae pink, no masses or lesions. Teeth all present, straight, and in good repair. Tongue smooth, pink, no lesions, protrudes in midline, no tremor.

Throat: Mucosa pink, no lesions or exudate. Uvula rises in midline on phonation. Tonsils out. Gag reflex present.

ASSESSMENT

Nose and oral structures intact and appear healthy
Knowledge deficit R/T risks of cigarette smoking

Clinical Case Study 1

B.D., a 34-year-old electrician, seeks care for "sore throat for 2 days."

SUBJECTIVE

2 days PTA—Experienced sudden onset of sore throat, swollen glands, fever 101°F, occasional shaking chills, extreme fatigue.

Today—Symptoms remain. Cough productive of yellow sputum. Treated self with aspirin for minimal relief. Unable to eat past 2 days because "throat on fire." Taking adequate fluids, on bed rest. Not aware of exposure to other sick people. Does not smoke.

OBJECTIVE

Ears: Tympanic membranes pearly gray with landmarks intact.
Nose: No discharge. Mucosa pink, no swelling.
Mouth: Mucosa and gingivae pink, no lesions.
Throat: Tonsils 3+. Pharyngeal wall bright red with yellow-white exudate; exudate also on tonsils.
Neck: Enlarged anterior cervical nodes bilaterally, painful to palpation. No other lymphadenopathy.
Chest: Resonant to percussion throughout. Breath sounds clear anterior and posterior. No adventitious sounds.

ASSESSMENT

Pharyngitis
Pain R/T inflammation
Imbalanced nutrition: less than body requirements R/T dysphagia

Clinical Case Study 2

D.C. is a 67-year-old homeless man who is brought to the emergency department after being found intoxicated in a local park. After 6 hours in the ED, D.C. is awake and cooperative. The nurses notice grimacing as he eats.

SUBJECTIVE

D.C. reports sensitivity when eating and drinking. Does not have medical or dental insurance. Has never been to the dentist. Encouraged to have his teeth cleaned "years ago," but did not have the money.

OBJECTIVE

Vital signs: Temp 98.4° F (36.7° C). Pulse 68 bpm. Resp 14/min, unlabored, in no distress.
Rates pain at 6/10, but only when eating or drinking.
Ears: Pinna intact. TMs pearly gray with landmarks intact. Hearing is good.
Mouth: Oral mucosa pink; uvula rises midline on phonation; tonsils absent. Gums appear red and swollen. Receding gingival margins noted. Brown and black spots noted on all molars bilaterally. All teeth appear yellow.
Chest: Thorax symmetric AP<transverse diameter. Resonant to percussion. Breath sounds clear and = bilat. No adventitious sounds.
Heart: S1 and S2 not accentuated or diminished; no murmurs.

ASSESSMENT

Severe gingivitis
Dental caries
Imbalanced nutrition: less than body requirements R/T dental pain
Acute pain R/T dental caries and gingivitis
Lack of social support R/T homeless situation

Documentation
and Critical Thinking

Clinical Case Study 3

E.V. is a 61-year-old professor who has been admitted to the hospital for chemotherapy for carcinoma of the breast. This is her 5th day in the hospital. She now is worried about "soreness and a white coating" in the mouth.

SUBJECTIVE

Felt soreness on tongue and cheeks during night. Now pain persists, and E.V. can see a "white coating" on tongue and cheeks. "I'm worried. Is this more cancer?"

OBJECTIVE

General appearance: E.V. generally appears restless and overly aware.
Mouth: Oral mucosa pink. Large white, cheesy patches covering most of dorsal surface of tongue and buccal mucosa. Will scrape off with tongue blade, revealing red eroded area beneath.
Bleeds with slight contact. Posterior pharyngeal wall pink, no lesions. Patches soft to palpation. No palpable lymph nodes.

ASSESSMENT

Oral lesion, candidiasis
Impaired oral mucous membrane R/T effects of chemotherapy
Pain R/T infectious process
Anxiety R/T threat to health status

Family-Centered Case Study 4

The mother of a 2½-year-old boy and now of a 10-day-old female presents to the breastfeeding clinic with breast pain. Mother is currently being treated for cracked nipples and plugged milk ducts and appears very frustrated with the breastfeeding process. She insists that you assess her newborn because "something's not right."

SUBJECTIVE

Mom asks, "Can you check her out? I've nursed before, but it didn't hurt like it does this time. Something is different about her suck." Mom reports 6 to 8 wet and "dirty" diapers a day.
Birth history: Full-term pregnancy, spontaneous rupture of membranes (SROM), vaginal birth w/o complications; weight 8 lbs 2 oz (3.6 kg); birth length 20 in (50.8 cm); and head circumference 34 cm.

OBJECTIVE

Vital signs: Temp 99.6° F (37.6° C) (axillary). BP (not available). Pulse 180 bpm (sleeping). Resp 35/min. Weight 7 lbs, 10 oz (3.45 kg). Height 20 in (50.8 cm). Head circumference 34.2 cm.
General appearance: Sleeping in mother's arms; appears well-nourished.
HEENT: Normocephalic w/ anterior and posterior fontanels open; pink skin with milia to chin and nose; mouth has short, thick lingual frenulum.
Cardiovascular: No murmurs or other abnormal heart sounds.
Respiratory: Breath sounds clear; no adventitious sounds.

ASSESSMENT

Ankyloglossia (tongue-tied) in infant
Interrupted breastfeeding R/T short and thick lingual frenulum
Risk for imbalanced nutrition: less than body requirements R/T anatomic abnormality

Documentation and Critical Thinking

ABNORMAL FINDINGS

TABLE 16-1   Nose Abnormalities

Choanal Atresia

Congenital bony septum between the nasal cavity and the pharynx is not common in the newborn; but when bilateral, it is an airway emergency because newborns are obligate nose breathers. Note airway obstruction, stridor, and paradoxical cyanosis (i.e., crying turns the baby pink because now breathing through the mouth).[20] When unilateral, the infant may be asymptomatic until the onset of the first respiratory infection.

Epistaxis

The most common site of a nosebleed is Kiesselbach plexus in the anterior septum. Peak incidence is bimodal, <18 years and >50 years. Causes include nose picking, forceful coughing or sneezing, fracture, foreign body, illicit drug use (cocaine), topical nasal drugs, warfarin (Coumadin), aspirin, or a coagulation disorder. Bleeding from the anterior septum is easily controlled and rarely severe. A posterior hemorrhage is less common (<10%) but more profuse, harder to manage, and more serious.

Sinusitis

Inflamed infected sinus areas following URI are most often viral in origin and do not require antibiotics. Consider bacterial infection when signs last >7-10 days. Major signs are mucopurulent drainage, nasal obstruction, facial pain or pressure, and loss of sense of smell. May also have fever, chills, malaise. Maxillary sinusitis has dull, throbbing pain in cheek and teeth and pain with palpation and when bending over. Frontal sinusitis has pain above supraorbital ridge.

Seasonal Allergic Rhinitis (Hay Fever)

The most common type of rhinitis presents with rhinorrhea, itching of nose and eyes, lacrimation, nasal congestion, and sneezing. Note serous edema and swelling of turbinates to fill the air space. Turbinates are usually pale (although they may appear violet), and their surface looks smooth and glistening. Common allergens are dust mite, animal dander, mold, pollen. When severe, allergic rhinitis produces disordered sleep, obstructive sleep apnea, sinusitis, and poor work performance.[11]

Continued

TABLE 16-1   Nose Abnormalities—cont'd

Furuncle

A small boil located in the skin or mucous membrane; appears red and swollen and is quite painful. Avoid any manipulation or trauma that may spread the infection.

Foreign Body

Children particularly are apt to put an object up the nose (here, yellow plastic foam), producing unilateral mucopurulent drainage and foul odor. Because some risk for aspiration exists, removal should be prompt. Watch out for impaction from a small button battery from an electronic device (watch, video game). Once occluding the nostril, the battery can release voltage or chemicals that cause burns, necrosis, or perforation.

Acute Rhinitis

The first sign is a clear, watery discharge, rhinorrhea, which later becomes purulent. This is accompanied by sneezing, nasal itching, stimulation of cough reflex, and inflamed mucosa, which causes nasal obstruction. Turbinates are dark red and swollen.

Perforated Septum

A hole in the septum, usually in the cartilaginous part, may be caused by snorting cocaine or methamphetamine, chronic infection, trauma from continual picking of crusts, or nasal surgery. It is seen directly or as a spot of light when the penlight is directed into the other naris.

◀ Nasal Polyps

Smooth, pale gray nodules, which are overgrowths of mucosa, are most commonly caused by chronic allergic rhinitis. May be stalked. A common site is protrusion from the middle meatus. Often multiple, they are mobile and nontender in contrast to turbinates. They may obstruct air passageways as they get larger. Symptoms include the absence of a sense of smell and a "valve that moves" in the nose as the person breathes.

TABLE 16-2 Lip Abnormalities

Cleft Lip

Maxillofacial clefts are the most common congenital deformities and are associated with phenytoin (Dilantin), maternal smoking and alcohol use, benzodiazepines, and corticosteroids.[1] Early treatment preserves the functions of speech and language formation and deglutition (swallowing).

Herpes Simplex 1

The cold sores are groups of clear vesicles with a surrounding indurated erythematous base. These evolve into pustules, which rupture, weep, and crust and heal in 4 to 10 days. The most likely site is the lip-skin junction; infection often recurs in the same site. Caused by the herpes simplex virus (HSV-1), the lesion is highly contagious and is spread by direct contact. Recurrent infections may be precipitated by sunlight, fever, colds, and allergy. It is very common, affecting 50% of adults.

Angular Cheilitis (Stomatitis, Perlèche)

Erythema, scaling, and shallow and painful fissures at the corners of the mouth occur with excess salivation and *Candida* infection. It is often seen in edentulous persons and those with poorly fitting dentures, causing folding in of corners of mouth, which creates a warm, moist environment favoring growth of yeast.

Carcinoma

The initial lesion is round and indurated; it becomes crusted and ulcerated with an elevated border. Most occur between the outer and middle thirds of the lip. Any lesion that is still unhealed after 2 weeks should be referred.

◄ Retention "Cyst" (Mucocele)

A round, well-defined, translucent nodule that may be very small or up to 1 to 2 cm. It is a pocket of mucus that forms when a duct of a minor salivary gland ruptures. The benign lesion also may occur on the buccal mucosa, on the floor of the mouth, or under the tip of the tongue.

ABNORMAL FINDINGS
FOR ADVANCED PRACTICE

TABLE 16-3 Teeth and Gum Abnormalities

Baby Bottle Tooth Decay

Destruction of numerous deciduous teeth may occur in infants and toddlers who take a bottle of milk, juice, or sweetened drink to bed and prolong bottle-feeding past the age of 1 year. Liquid pools around the upper front teeth. Mouth bacteria act on carbohydrates in the liquid, especially sucrose, forming metabolic acids. Acids break down tooth enamel and destroy its protein.

Malocclusion

Upper or lower dental arches are not in alignment, and incisors protrude from developmental problem of mandible or maxilla or incompatibility between jaw and tooth size. The condition increases risk for facial deformity, negative body image, chewing problems, or speech dysfluency.

Dental Caries

Progressive destruction of tooth. Decay initially looks chalky white. Later it turns brown or black and forms a cavity. Early decay is apparent only on x-ray image. Susceptible sites are tooth surfaces where food debris, bacterial plaque, and saliva collect.

Epulis

A nontender, fibrous nodule of the gum seen emerging between the teeth; an overgrowth of vascular granulation tissue.

TABLE 16-3   Teeth and Gum Abnormalities—cont'd

Gingival Hyperplasia

Painless enlargement of the gums, sometimes overreaching the teeth. This occurs with puberty, pregnancy, and leukemia and with long therapeutic use of phenytoin (Dilantin).

Gingivitis

Gum margins are red and swollen and bleed easily. This case is severe; gingival tissue has desquamated, exposing roots of teeth. Inflammation is usually caused by poor dental hygiene or vitamin C deficiency. The condition may occur in pregnancy and puberty because of changing hormonal balance.

◄ Meth Mouth

Illicit methamphetamine abuse (crystal meth, meth ice) leads to extensive dental caries, gingivitis, tooth cracking, and edentulism. Methamphetamine causes vasoconstriction and decreased saliva, and its use increases the urge to consume sugars and starches and give up oral hygiene. Absence of the buffering saliva leads to increased acidity in the mouth, and the increased plaque encourages bacterial growth. These conditions and the presence of carbohydrates set up an oral environment prone to caries, cracking of enamel, and the damage seen here.

See Illustration Credits for source information.

TABLE 16-4   Buccal Mucosa Abnormalities

◄ Aphthous Ulcers

A common "canker sore" is a vesicle at first and then a small, round, "punched-out" ulcer with a white base surrounded by a red halo. It is quite painful and lasts for 1 to 2 weeks. The cause is unknown, although it is associated with stress, fatigue, and food allergy.

Continued

TABLE 16-4   Buccal Mucosa Abnormalities—cont'd

Koplik Spots

Small blue-white spots with irregular red halo scattered over mucosa opposite the molars. An early sign, and pathognomonic, of measles.

Leukoplakia

Chalky white, thick, raised patch with well-defined borders. The lesion is firmly attached and does not scrape off. It may occur on the lateral edges of tongue. It is caused by chronic irritation and occurs with heavy smoking and alcohol use. Lesions are precancerous; must refer to specialist. (Here the lesion is associated with squamous carcinoma.)

◄ **Candidiasis or Monilial Infection**

A white, cheesy, curdlike patch on the buccal mucosa and tongue. It scrapes off, leaving a raw, red surface that bleeds easily. Termed *thrush* in the newborn. It is an opportunistic infection that occurs after the use of antibiotics and corticosteroids and in immunosuppressed people.

Candidiasis in Adult

The *Candida* species as normal oral flora is present in 60% of healthy adults. Overgrowth of *Candida* occurs with steroid inhaler use, HIV infection, use of broad-spectrum antibiotics or corticosteroids, leukemia, malnutrition, or reduced immunity.

Herpes Simplex 1

Herpes infection on the hard palate (see discussion in Table 16-2).

See Illustration Credits for source information.

TABLE 16-5   Tongue Abnormalities

Ankyloglossia

A short lingual frenulum, here fixing the tongue tip to the floor of the mouth and gums (tongue-tie). This limits mobility and affects speech (pronunciation of *a, d, n*) if the tongue tip cannot be elevated to the alveolar ridge. A congenital defect.

Geographic Tongue (Migratory Glossitis)

Pattern of normal coating interspersed with bright red, shiny, circular bald areas caused by atrophy of the filiform papillae, with raised pearly borders. Pattern resembles a map and changes with time. Not significant, and its cause is not known.

◀ Smooth, Glossy Tongue (Atrophic Glossitis)

The surface is slick and shiny; the mucosa thins and looks red from decreased papillae. Accompanied by dryness of tongue and burning. Occurs with vitamin B_{12} deficiency (pernicious anemia), folic acid deficiency, and iron deficiency anemia. Here also note angular cheilitis.

◀ Black Hairy Tongue

This is not really hair but rather the elongation of filiform papillae and painless overgrowth of mycelial threads of fungus infection on the tongue. Color varies from black-brown to yellow. It occurs after use of antibiotics, which inhibit normal bacteria and allow proliferation of fungus, and with heavy smoking.

Continued

TABLE 16-5 Tongue Abnormalities—cont'd

Carcinoma

An ulcer with rolled edges; indurated. Occurs particularly at sides, base, and under the tongue. It grows insidiously and may go unnoticed for months. It may have associated leukoplakia. Risk for early metastasis is present because of rich lymphatic drainage. Smoking and heavy alcohol use are associated; the incidence of human papilloma virus (HPV)–related oral pharyngeal cancers also is increased.[8]

Fissured or Scrotal Tongue

Deep furrows divide the papillae into small irregular rows. The condition occurs in 5% of the general population and in Down syndrome. The incidence increases with age. (Vertical, or longitudinal, fissures also occur with dehydration because of reduced tongue volume.)

◄ **Enlarged Tongue (Macroglossia)**

The tongue is enlarged and may protrude from the mouth. The condition is not painful but may impair speech development. Here it occurs with Down syndrome; it also occurs with cretinism, myxedema, and acromegaly. A transient swelling also occurs with local infections.

See Illustration Credits for source information.

TABLE 16-6 Oropharynx Abnormalities

◄ **Bifid Uvula**

The uvula looks partly severed and may indicate a submucous cleft palate, which feels like a notch at the junction of the hard and soft palates. This may affect speech development because it prevents necessary air trapping. The incidence is more common in American Indians.

TABLE 16-6 Oropharynx Abnormalities—cont'd

Oral Kaposi Sarcoma

Bruiselike, dark red or violet, confluent macule, usually on the hard palate, may be on soft palate or gingival margin. Oral lesions may be among the earliest lesions to develop with AIDS.

Peritonsillar Abscess

Untreated acute pharyngitis may cause suppurative complications, peritonsillar abscess, or suppurative thrombophlebitis. Thrombophlebitis is Lemierre syndrome caused by the gram-negative *Fusobacterium necrophorum*. This microbe occurs as often as streptococcal pharyngitis in adolescents and young adults. In this age-group, the two major red flags with this pharyngitis are worsening symptoms or neck swelling.[4,25]

Acute Tonsillitis and Pharyngitis

Bright red throat; swollen tonsils; white or yellow exudate on tonsils and pharynx; swollen uvula; and enlarged, tender anterior cervical and tonsillar nodes. Accompanied by severe sore throat, painful swallowing, fever >101°F of sudden onset. Bacterial infections may have absence of cough.

With severe symptoms (listed above) or sore throat lasting >3-5 days, consider streptococcal infection and confirm with rapid antigen testing or throat culture. Treat positive tests with antibiotics. Untreated GAS pharyngitis may produce peritonsillar abscess, lymphadenitis, or acute rheumatic fever (although this is now rare in the United States).

Cleft Palate

A congenital defect, the failure of fusion of the maxillary processes. Wide variation occurs in the extent of cleft formation, from upper lip only, palate only, uvula only, to cleft of the nostril and the hard and soft palates.

See Illustration Credits for source information.

Summary Checklist: Nose, Mouth, and Throat Examination

Nose
1. Inspect external nose for symmetry, any deformity, or lesions
2. Palpation—Test patency of each nostril
3. Inspect with nasal speculum:
   Color and integrity of nasal mucosa
   Septum—Note any deviation, perforation, or bleeding

Turbinates—Note color, any exudate, swelling, or polyps
4. Palpate the sinus areas—Note any tenderness

Mouth and Throat
1. Inspect with penlight:
   Lips, teeth and gums, tongue, buccal mucosa—Note color; whether structures are intact; any lesions

Palate and uvula—Note integrity and mobility as person phonates
Grade tonsils
Pharyngeal wall—Note color, any exudate, or lesions
2. Palpation:
   When indicated in adults, bimanual palpation of mouth
   In the neonate, palpate for integrity of palate and to assess sucking reflex

---

BIBLIOGRAPHY

1. Basseri, B., Kianmahd, B. D., Roostaeian, J., et al. (2011). Current national incidence, trends, and health care resource utilization of cleft lip–cleft palate. *Plast Reconstruct Surg*, *127*(3), 1255-1262.
2. Beltrán-Aguilar, E.D., Barker, L.K., et al. (2005). Surveillance for dental caries, dental sealants, tooth retention, edentulism, and enamel fluorosis—United States, 1988-1994 and 1999-2002. *MMWR Surveill Summ*, *54*(3), 1-43.
3. Bennett, W. (2013). Torus palatinus. *New Engl J Med*, *368*(15), 1434.
3a. Berger, C., Bachman, J., Casalone, G. G., et al. (2014). An oral health program for children. *Nurse Pract 39*(2), 48-53.
4. Centor, R. M. (2009). Expand the pharyngitis paradigm for adolescents and young adults. *Ann Intern Med*, *151*(11), 812-815.
5. Chawla, M. P. S., & Sundriyal, D. (2012). Burton's line. *N Engl J Med, 367*(10), 937.
6. Chen, A. Y., DeSantis, C., & Jemal, A. (2011). US mortality rates for oral cavity and pharyngeal cancer by educational attainment. *Arch Otolaryngol Head Neck Surg*, *137*(11), 1094-1099.
7. Choby, B. A. (2009). Diagnosis and treatment of streptococcal pharyngitis. *Am Fam Phys*, *79*(5), 383-390.
8. Crozier, E., & Sumer, B. D. (2010). Head and neck cancer. *Medical Clin North Am*, *94*(5), 1031-1043.
9. Curtis, E. K. (2006). Meth mouth: a review of methamphetamine use and its oral manifestations. *Gen Dentist*, *54*(2), 125-129.
10. DeMuri, G. P., & Wald, E. R. (2012). Acute bacterial sinusitis in children. *N Engl J Med*, *367*(12), 1128-1134.
11. Dykewicz, M. S., & Hamilos, D. L. (2010). Rhinitis and sinusitis. *J Allerg Clin Immunol*, *125*, S103-115.
12. Eisenstadt, E. S. (2010). Dysphagia and aspiration pneumonia in older adults. *J Am Acad Nurse Pract*, *22*, 17-22.
13. Gawnde, A. (2002, March 11). Cold comfort. *The New Yorker*, 42-47.
14. Gonsalves, W. C., Chi, A. C., & Neville, B. W. (2007). Common oral lesions: part II. Masses and neoplasia. *Am Fam Phys 75*(4), 509.

15. Kana, A., Markou, L., Arhakis, A., et al. (2013). Natal and neonatal teeth: a systematic review of prevalence and management. *Eur J Paediatr Dent*, *14*(1), 27-32.
16. Kane, R. L., Ouslander, J. G., & Abrass, I. E. (2013). *Essentials of clinical geriatrics* (7th ed.). New York: McGraw-Hill.
16a. Krouse, H. U, Krouse, J. H. (2014). Allergic rhinitis. *Nurse Pract*, *39*(4), 20-29.
17. Manes, R. P. (2010). Evaluating and managing the patient with nosebleeds. *Med Clin North Am*, *94*(5), 903-912.
18. Mehanna, H., Paleri, V., West, C. M., et al. (2010). Head and neck cancer—part 1: epidemiology, presentation, and prevention. *BMJ*, *341*(7774), 663-666.
19. Parthasarathy, P., & Ritamarie, J. (2008). Identification of childhood caries. *Nurse Pract*, *33*(9), 41-48.
20. Ramsden, J. D. (2011). Choanal atresia. *Curr Pediatr Rev*, *7*(1), 9-14.
21. Shaikh, N., Swaminathan, N., & Hooper, E. G. (2012). Accuracy and precision of the signs and symptoms of streptococcal pharyngitis in children: a systematic review. *J Pediatr*, *160*(3), 487-493.
22. Shoup, J. (2011). Management of adult rhinosinusitis. *Nurse Pract*, *36*(11), 22-26.
22a. Sutters, K. A. (2014). Posttonsillectomy pain in children. *Am J Nurs*, *114*(2):36-43.
23. U.S. Department of Health & Human Services, The Office of Minority Health. (2009). *Cleft lip/palate more prevalent in Asians*. Accessed April 25, 2010, from http://minorityhealth.hhs.gov/templates/content.aspx?ID=7590&lvl=3&lvlID=287.
24. Wilson, J. F. (2010). In the clinic: acute sinusitis. *Ann Intern Med*, *153*(5), ITC3-1-17.
25. Young, B. J., & Steele, R. W. (2010). A teenager with sore throat and neck pain. *Clin Pediatr*, *49*(11), 1088-1089.
26. Zastrow, R. L. (2011). Emerging infections: pertussis on the rise. *Am J Nurs*, *111*(6), 51-56.

Breasts and Regional Lymphatics

STRUCTURE AND FUNCTION

Axillary tail of Spence

2nd rib

Montgomery glands

Nipple

Areola

Adipose tissue

Serratus anterior muscle

Pectoralis major muscle

6th rib

17-1

© Pat Thomas, 2010.

The female breasts, or mammary glands, are accessory reproductive organs, and the function is to produce milk for nourishing the newborn. The **breasts** lie anterior to the pectoralis major and serratus anterior muscles (Fig. 17-1). They are located between the second and sixth ribs, extending from the side of the sternum to the midaxillary line. The superior lateral corner of breast tissue, called the axillary **tail of Spence,** projects up and laterally into the axilla.

The **nipple** is just below the center of the breast. It is rough, round, and usually protuberant; its surface looks wrinkled and indented with tiny milk duct openings. The **areola** surrounds the nipple for a 1- to 2-cm radius. In the areola are small elevated sebaceous glands, called *Montgomery glands.* These secrete a protective lipid material during lactation. The areola also has smooth muscle fibers that cause nipple erection when stimulated. Both the nipple and areola are more darkly pigmented than the rest of the breast surface; the color varies from pink to brown, depending on the person's skin color and parity (condition of giving birth). Breasts are present in men too, although rudimentary throughout life.

Lactiferous duct
Lactiferous sinus
Lobule
Lobe

2nd rib
Adipose tissue
Cooper ligaments
Pectoralis major muscle

17-2

© Pat Thomas, 2010.

INTERNAL ANATOMY

The breast is composed of (1) glandular tissue; (2) fibrous tissue, including the suspensory ligaments; and (3) adipose tissue (Fig. 17-2). The **glandular tissue** contains 15 to 20 lobes radiating from the nipple, and these are composed of lobules. Within each lobule are clusters of alveoli that produce milk. Each lobe empties into a lactiferous duct. The 15 to 20 lactiferous ducts form a collecting duct system converging toward the nipple. There the ducts form ampullae, or lactiferous sinuses, behind the nipple, which are reservoirs for storing milk.

The suspensory ligaments, or **Cooper ligaments,** are fibrous connective tissue extending vertically from the skin surface to attach on chest wall muscles. These support the breast tissue. The lobes are embedded in **adipose tissue.** These layers of subcutaneous and retromammary fat actually provide most of the bulk of the breast. The relative proportion of glandular, fibrous, and fatty tissue varies, depending on age, cycle, pregnancy, lactation, and general nutritional state.

The breast may be divided into four quadrants by imaginary horizontal and vertical lines intersecting at the nipple (Fig. 17-3). This makes a convenient map to describe clinical findings. In the upper outer quadrant note the axillary **tail of Spence,** the cone-shaped breast tissue that projects up into the axilla, close to the pectoral group of axillary lymph nodes. The upper outer quadrant is the site of most breast tumors.

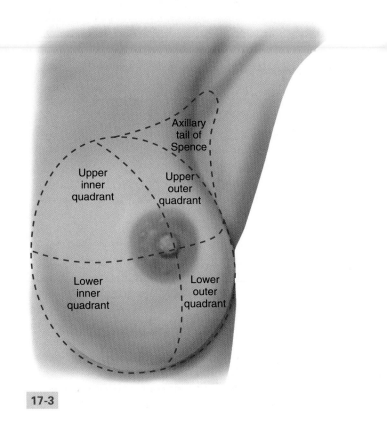

Axillary tail of Spence
Upper inner quadrant
Upper outer quadrant
Lower inner quadrant
Lower outer quadrant

17-3

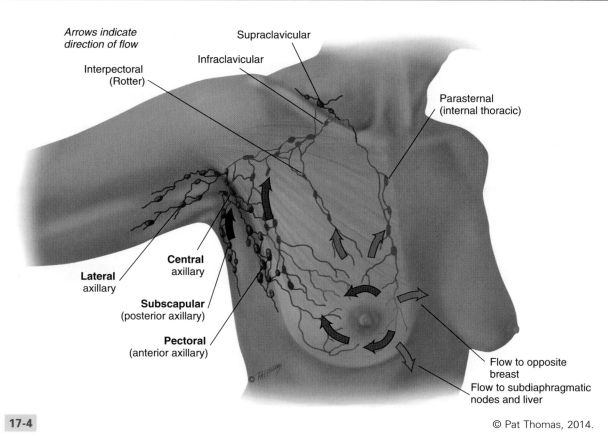

Arrows indicate
direction of flow

Supraclavicular

Infraclavicular

Interpectoral
(Rotter)

Parasternal
(internal thoracic)

Central
axillary

Lateral
axillary

Subscapular
(posterior axillary)

Pectoral
(anterior axillary)

Flow to opposite
breast

Flow to subdiaphragmatic
nodes and liver

17-4

© Pat Thomas, 2014.

LYMPHATICS

The breast has extensive lymphatic drainage. Most of the lymph, more than 75%, drains into the ipsilateral (same side) axillary nodes. Four groups of axillary nodes are present (Fig. 17-4):

1. **Central axillary nodes**—High up in the middle of the axilla, over the ribs and serratus anterior muscle. These receive lymph from the other three groups of nodes.
2. **Pectoral** (anterior)—Along the lateral edge of the pectoralis major muscle, just inside the anterior axillary fold.
3. **Subscapular** (posterior)—Along the lateral edge of the scapula, deep in the posterior axillary fold.
4. **Lateral**—Along the humerus, inside the upper arm.

From the central axillary nodes, drainage flows up to the infraclavicular and supraclavicular nodes.

A smaller amount of lymphatic drainage does not take these channels but instead flows directly up to the infraclavicular group, or deep into the chest, or into the abdomen, or directly across to the opposite breast.

❖ DEVELOPMENTAL COMPETENCE

During embryonic life ventral epidermal ridges, or "milk lines," are present and curve down from the axilla to the groin bilaterally (Fig. 17-5). The breast develops along the ridge over the thorax, and the rest of the ridge atrophies. Occasionally a **supernumerary nipple** (i.e., an extra nipple) persists

and is visible somewhere along the track of the mammary ridge (see Fig. 17-7).

At birth the only breast structures present are the lactiferous ducts within the nipple. No alveoli have developed. Little change occurs until puberty.

Supernumerary
nipple

17-5

The Adolescent

At puberty the estrogen hormones stimulate breast changes. The breasts enlarge, mostly as a result of extensive fat deposition. The duct system also grows and branches; and masses of small, solid cells develop at the duct endings. These are potential alveoli.

The onset of breast development occurs at an average (mean) age between 8 and 9 years for African-American girls and by 10 years for White girls.[21] However, recent evidence shows an earlier onset of breast development in 7-year-olds: 10.4% of White girls, 23.4% of non-Hispanic Black girls, and 15% of Hispanic girls are now developing breasts, compared to 5% of White girls and 15% of Black girls in earlier studies.[6] Early breast development is linked to greater body mass index (BMI) ratings and reflects the rise in obesity in U.S. children.

Occasionally one breast may grow faster than the other, producing a temporary asymmetry. This may cause some distress; reassurance is necessary. Tenderness is common also. Although the age of onset varies widely, the five stages of breast development follow this classic description of sexual maturity rating, or **Tanner staging** (Table 17-1).

Full development from stage 2 to stage 5 takes an average of 3 years, although the range is 1.5 to 6 years. During this

TABLE 17-1	Sexual Maturity Rating in Girls

Stage

1 **Preadolescent:** There is only a small elevated nipple.

2 **Breast bud stage:** A small mound of breast and nipple develops; the areola widens.

3 The breast and areola enlarge; the nipple is flush with the breast surface.

4 The areola and nipple form a secondary mound over the breast.

5 **Mature breast:** Only the nipple protrudes; the areola is flush with the breast contour (the areola may continue as a secondary mound in some normal women).

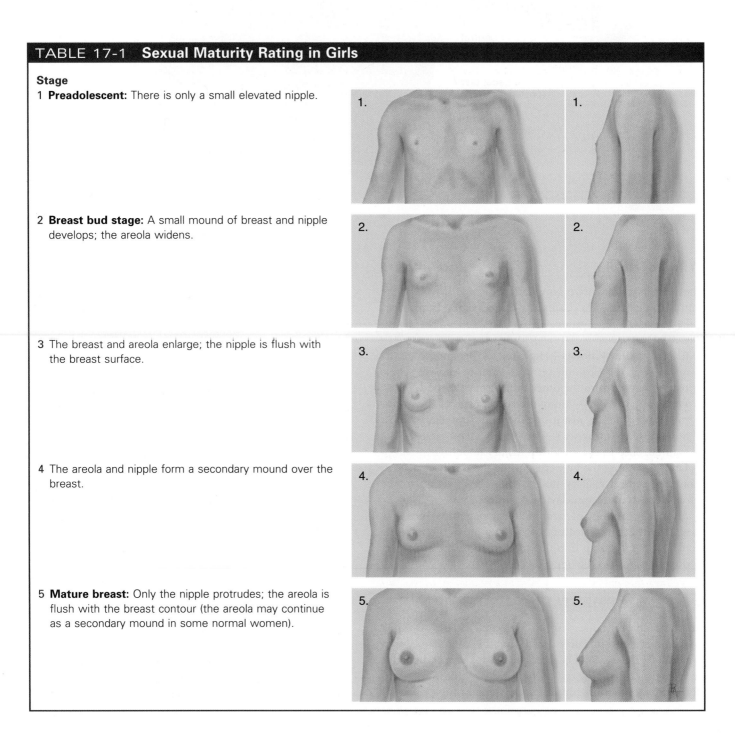

time pubic hair develops, and axillary hair appears 2 years after the onset of pubic hair. The beginning of breast development precedes **menarche** (beginning of menstruation) by about 2 years. Menarche occurs in breast development stage 3 or 4, usually just after the peak of the adolescent growth spurt around 12 years of age. This helps to assess the development of adolescent girls and increases their knowledge about their own development.

Breasts of the nonpregnant woman change with the ebb and flow of hormones during the monthly menstrual cycle. Nodularity increases from midcycle up to menstruation. During the 3 to 4 days before menstruation, the breasts feel full, tight, heavy, and occasionally sore. The breast volume is smallest on days 4 to 7 of the menstrual cycle.

The Pregnant Woman

During pregnancy breast changes start during the second month and are a common early sign of pregnancy. Pregnancy stimulates the expansion of the ductal system and supporting fatty tissue and development of the true secretory alveoli. Thus the breasts enlarge and feel more nodular. The nipples grow larger, darker, and more erectile. The areolae become larger and a darker brown as pregnancy progresses, and the tubercles become more prominent. (The brown color fades after lactation, but the areolae never return to the original color.) A venous pattern is prominent over the skin surface (see Fig. 30-6, p. 816).

After the fourth month **colostrum** may be expressed. This thick, yellow fluid is the precursor for milk, containing the same amount of protein and lactose but practically no fat. The breasts produce colostrum for the first few days after delivery. It is rich with antibodies that protect the newborn against infection; thus breastfeeding is important. Milk production (lactation) begins 1 to 3 days after delivery. The whitish color is from emulsified fat and calcium caseinate.

The Aging Woman

After menopause ovarian secretion of estrogen and progesterone decreases, which causes the breast glandular tissue to atrophy. This is replaced with fibrous connective tissue. The fat envelope atrophies also, beginning in the middle years and becoming marked in the 70s and 80s. These changes decrease breast size and elasticity so the breasts droop and sag, looking flattened and flabby. Drooping is accentuated by kyphosis in some older women.

The decreased breast size makes inner structures more prominent. A breast lump may have been present for years but is suddenly palpable. Around the nipple the lactiferous ducts are more palpable and feel firm and stringy because of fibrosis and calcification. The axillary hair decreases.

THE MALE BREAST

The male breast is a rudimentary structure consisting of a thin disk of undeveloped tissue underlying the nipple. The areola is well developed, although the nipple is relatively very small. During adolescence it is common for the breast tissue to enlarge temporarily, producing **gynecomastia** (see Fig. 17-20, p. 402). This condition is usually temporary, but reassurance is necessary for the adolescent male, whose attention is riveted on his body image. Gynecomastia may reappear in the aging male and may be the result of testosterone deficiency.

CULTURE AND GENETICS

The timing of puberty is influenced by genetic and environmental factors. A 1997 study of 17,077 young girls showed that African-American girls begin puberty about 1 to 1.5 years earlier than White girls and start menstruating about 8.5 months earlier.[21] The onset of breast development occurs at an average age of 8.87 years for African-American girls and 10 years for White girls (Hispanic ethnicity occurs in both groups). Menses begins at an average age of 12.16 years for African-American girls and at almost 13 years for White girls.

As to environmental factors, obesity contributes to early onset of puberty; girls with early onset of breast budding have higher BMI scores than age-matched girls without budding.[21] Among normal-weight girls, signs of puberty occurred before 8 years in fewer than 5% of White girls, 12% of Black girls, and 19% of Mexican-American girls.[33] But girls with overweight or obese BMI levels had a significantly higher occurrence of early breast budding and early menarche. Thus the epidemic of childhood obesity is a major determinant of early-age pubertal milestones.[33]

Breast Cancer

We all have certain tumor suppressor genes termed *BRCA1* and *BRCA2*; women who inherit a mutation on one or both have a significantly increased risk of developing breast or ovarian cancer. Evidence now shows that the prevalence of these mutations is about the same (at 1% to 4%) among breast cancer patients of African, Asian, White, and Hispanic descent.[26] However, worldwide there exists significant racial and ethnic variation among the prevalence of these mutations, the access to genetic testing, and the recommended risk-management interventions.

White women have a higher incidence of breast cancer than African-American women starting at 45 years of age. In contrast, African-American women have a higher incidence before age 45 years, and they are more likely to die of their disease at every age.[2] Women from Asian-American, Hispanic, and American Indian groups have a lower incidence and lower death rates from breast cancer than Whites and African Americans have.

Between 1992 and 2005 U.S. breast cancer rates rose and then started falling, reflecting the trend in hormone replacement therapy in certain perimenopausal women. In July 2002 the results of the Women's Health Initiative (WHI) study confirmed that long-term use of combined estrogen and progestin therapy increased the risk of developing breast cancer. A dramatic reduction in hormone use followed. Since 2006 studies in the United States, Europe, and Australia have shown an annual decline in breast cancer incidence of around

10%.[25] But the decreased incidence in the United States occurred only among White non-Hispanic women living in high-income counties who had estrogen receptor–positive tumors and were 50 years of age and older. The declines did not occur among Black, Hispanic, or Asian women; this may reflect the social pattern of hormone therapy use,[25] i.e., women of color may have had decreased access to hormone replacement therapy, and this may have spared them the increase in breast cancer rates in the 1990s.

Screening mammography can discover small, potentially curable breast cancers, and the American Cancer Society recommends beginning annual screening at 40 years of age. The percentage of women 40 years of age and older who report having a mammogram in the last 2 years was 66.5% in 2010.[2] This included higher rates of cancer screening for women of color in recent years: 67% of non-Hispanic Whites, 66% of African Americans, 64.4% of Hispanics/Latinas, and 62% of Asians reported mammography. However, women least likely to have had a recent mammogram include those with less than a high school education, with no health insurance, or who are recent immigrants.[2] Low-income women have multiple barriers to screening mammography, including lack of insurance coverage, lack of access to care, not having a regular health care provider, and lack of comprehensive breast cancer knowledge, not merely screening awareness.[1]

Lifestyle factors relate to breast cancer risk. Many studies have associated alcohol drinking with breast cancer risk in a dose-dependent measure. Recent evidence using the Nurses' Health Study cohort show that even low levels of drinking (3 to 6 drinks per week) were associated with a small increase in breast cancer risk, although the strongest risks were seen with cumulative consistent alcohol use through adult life.[9] Recreational physical activity at any intensity level may reduce breast cancer risk, especially during the reproductive years and after menopause. However, postmenopausal weight gain may eliminate the profits of regular physical activity.[28] Two dietary patterns have been studied: (1) "alcohol/Western" (meat products, French fries, appetizers, rice/pasta, potatoes, pizza, pies, canned fish, eggs, alcohol, cakes, mayonnaise, butter/cream); and (2) "healthy/Mediterranean" (vegetables, fruits, seafood, olive oil, sunflower oil). The first pattern has a modest positive association with breast cancer risk, especially with estrogen or progesterone receptor–positive tumors. The healthy Mediterranean diet has a modest protective effect.[12,20]

SUBJECTIVE DATA

Breast
1. Pain
2. Lump
3. Discharge
4. Rash
5. Swelling
6. Trauma
7. History of breast disease
8. Surgery or radiation
9. Medications
10. Patient-centered care
    Perform breast self-examination
    Last mammogram

Axilla
1. Tenderness, lump, or swelling
2. Rash

In Western culture the female breasts signify more than their primary purpose of lactation. Women are surrounded by excessive media influence that feminine norms of beauty and desirability are enhanced by and depend on the size of the breasts and their appearance. Women leaders have tried to refocus this attitude, stressing women's self-worth as individual human beings, not as stereotyped sexual objects. The intense cultural emphasis shows that the breasts are crucial to a woman's self-concept and her perception of her femininity. Matters pertaining to the breast affect the body image and generate deep emotional responses.

This emotionality may take strong forms that you observe as you discuss the woman's history. One woman may be acutely embarrassed talking about her breasts, as evidenced by lack of eye contact, minimal response, nervous gestures, or inappropriate humor. Another woman may talk wryly and disparagingly about the size or development of her breasts. A young adolescent is acutely aware of her own development in relation to her peers. Or a woman who has found a breast lump may come to you with fear, high anxiety, and even panic. Although many breast lumps are benign, women initially assume the worst possible outcome (i.e., cancer, disfigurement, and death). While you are collecting the subjective data, tune in to cues for these behaviors that call for a straightforward and reasoned attitude.

Examiner Asks	Rationale

Breast

1. Pain. Any **pain** or tenderness in the breasts? When did you first notice it?
- Where is the pain? Localized or all over?
- Is the painful spot sore to touch? Do you feel a burning or pulling sensation?
- Is the pain cyclic? Any relation to your menstrual period?

- Is the pain brought on by strenuous activity, especially involving one arm; a change in activity; manipulation during sex; part of underwire bra; exercise?

Mastalgia occurs with trauma, inflammation, infection, and benign breast disease.

Cyclic pain is common with normal breasts, oral contraceptives, and benign breast (fibrocystic) disease.
Is pain related to specific cause?

2. Lump. Ever noticed a **lump** or **thickening** in the breast? Where?
- When did you first notice it? Changed at all since then?
- Does the lump have any relation to your menstrual period?
- Noticed any change in the overlying skin: redness, warmth, dimpling, swelling?

Carefully explore the presence of any lump. A lump present for many years and exhibiting no change may not be serious but still should be explored. Approach any recent change or new lump with suspicion.

3. Discharge. Any **discharge** from the nipple?
- When did you first notice this?
- What color is the discharge?
- Consistency—thick or runny?
- Odor?

Galactorrhea. Note medications that may cause clear nipple discharge: oral contraceptives, phenothiazines, diuretics, digitalis, steroids, methyldopa, calcium channel blockers.
Bloody or blood-tinged discharge always is significant. Any discharge with a lump is significant.

4. Rash. Any **rash** on the breast?
- When did you first notice this?
- Where did it start? On the nipple, areola, or surrounding skin?

Paget disease starts with a small crust on the nipple apex and spreads to areola (see Table 17-6, Abnormal Nipple Discharge, p. 410).
Eczema or other dermatitis rarely starts at the nipple unless it is caused by breast-feeding. It usually starts on the areola or surrounding skin and then spreads to the nipple.

5. Swelling. Any **swelling** in the breasts? In one spot or all over?
- Related to your menstrual period, pregnancy, or breastfeeding?
- Any change in bra size?

6. Trauma. Any **trauma** or injury to the breasts?
- Did it result in any swelling, lump, or break in skin?

A lump from an injury (seat belt injury, direct blow) is caused by local hematoma or edema and resolves shortly.

7. History of breast disease. Any history of breast disease yourself?
- What type? How was it diagnosed?
- When did it occur?
- How is it being treated?

- Any breast cancer in your family? Who? Sister, mother, maternal grandmother, maternal aunts, daughter? How about your father's side?
- At what age did this relative have breast cancer?

Past breast cancer increases the risk for recurrent cancer (see Table 17-2, Breast Cancer Risk Factors in Women, p. 393).
The presence of benign breast disease makes the breasts harder to examine; the general lumpiness conceals a new lump.
Breast cancer occurring before menopause in certain family members increases risk for this woman (see Table 17-2).

Subjective Data

Examiner Asks	Rationale

8. Surgery or radiation. Ever had **surgery** on the breasts? Was it a biopsy? What were the biopsy results?
  * Mastectomy? Mammoplasty—augmentation or reduction?
  * Ever had radiation to chest? What was it for? At what age?

Biopsy-confirmed atypical hyperplasia increases breast cancer risk.

Between ages 10 and 30 years, chest radiation exposure has greatest risk of breast cancer later in life.[13]

9. Medications. Have you taken oral contraceptives? For how long?

Oral contraceptives may control symptoms of benign ("fibrocystic") breast disease.

  * Hormone replacement therapy? Estrogen and progestin? Estrogen only? For how long?

Combined hormone therapy after menopause increases risk of breast cancer, even with 2 years' use. Increased risk applies only for current and recent users.[2] Use of estrogen alone does not increase risk of breast cancer.

10. Patient-centered care
  * Have you ever been taught **breast self-examination** (BSE)?
  * How often do you perform it? What helps you remember?
  * Ever had **mammography,** a screening x-ray image of the breasts? When was the last mammogram?
  * The American Cancer Society recommends that women 20 to 39 years of age have a clinical breast examination (CBE) every 3 years; women 40 years of age and older have an annual mammogram and an annual CBE conducted close to the same time.[2]

Awareness that BSE, CBE, and mammograms are complementary screening measures. With good BSE practice, a woman knows how her breasts normally feel and can detect any change more easily. Mammography can reveal cancers too small to be detected by the woman or by the most experienced examiner. However, interval lumps may become palpable between mammograms.

Axilla

1. Tenderness, lump, or swelling. Any **tenderness** or **lump** in the underarm area?
  * Where? When did you first notice it?

Breast tissue extends up into the axilla. The axilla also contains many lymph nodes.

2. Rash. Any axillary **rash?** Please describe it.
  * Seem to be a reaction to deodorant?

Additional History for the Preadolescent

1. Have you noticed your breasts changing?
  * How long has this been happening?
2. Many girls also notice other changes in their bodies that come with growing up. What have you noticed?
  * What do you think about all this?

Developing breasts are the most obvious sign of puberty and the focus of attention for most girls, especially in comparison with peers. Assess each girl's perception of her own development, and provide teaching and reassurance as indicated.

Additional History for the Pregnant Woman

1. Have you noticed any enlargement or fullness in the breasts?
  * Is there any tenderness or tingling?

  * Do you have a history of inverted nipples?

Breast changes are expected and normal during pregnancy. Assess the woman's knowledge and provide reassurance.

Inverted nipples may need special care in preparation for breastfeeding.

Examiner Asks	Rationale
2. Are you planning to breastfeed your baby?	Breastfeeding alone for 6 months provides the perfect food and antibodies for the baby, decreases risk for ear infections, promotes bonding, and provides relaxation. It is also protective against breast cancer.

Additional History for the Menopausal Woman

1. Have you noticed any change in the breast contour, size, or firmness? (NOTE: Change may not be as apparent to obese women or to women whose earlier pregnancies already have produced breast changes.)

Decreased estrogen level causes decreased firmness. Rapid decrease in estrogen level causes actual shrinkage.

Risk Factor Profile for Breast Cancer

Breast cancer is the second major cause of death from cancer in women. However, early detection and improved treatment have increased survival rates. The 5-year survival rate for localized breast cancer has increased from 78% in the 1940s to 98% today. If the cancer has spread regionally, the survival rate is 84%.[2] Note the risk factors listed in Table 17-2.

The best way to detect a person's risk for breast cancer is by asking the right history questions. Table 17-2 highlights risk factors for breast cancer and, from these, you can fashion your questions. Be aware that most breast cancers occur in women with no identifiable risk factors except sex and age. Just because a woman does not report the cited risk factors does not mean that you or she should fail to consider breast cancer seriously.

Subjective Data

TABLE 17-2   Breast Cancer Risk Factors in Women*

Relative Risk	Factor	Relative Risk	Factor
>4.0	• Age (65+ vs. <65 years, although risk increases across all ages until age 80) • Biopsy-confirmed atypical hyperplasia • Certain inherited genetic mutations for breast cancer (BRCA1 and/or BRCA2) • Lobular carcinoma in situ • Mammographically dense breasts • Personal history of early onset (<40 years) breast cancer • Two or more first-degree relatives with breast cancer diagnosed at an early age	1.1-2.0	• Alcohol consumption • Ashkenazi Jewish heritage • Diethylstilbestrol (DES) exposure • Early menarche (<12 years) • Height (tall) • High socioeconomic status • Late age at first full-term pregnancy (>30 years) • Late menopause (>55 years) • Never breastfed a child • No full-term pregnancies • Obesity (postmenopausal)/adult weight gain • Personal history of endometrial, ovarian, or colon cancer • Recent and long-term use of menopausal hormone therapy containing estrogen and progestin • Recent oral contraceptive use
2.1-4.0	• Personal history of breast cancer (40+ years) • High endogenous estrogen or testosterone levels (postmenopausal) • High-dose radiation to chest • One first-degree relative with breast cancer		

From American Cancer Society (2013). *Breast Cancer Facts & Figures 2013-2014.* Atlanta: American Cancer Society.
*Relative risk compares the risk of disease among people with a particular exposure to the risk to the risk among people without that exposure. If the relative risk is above 1.0, risk is higher among exposed than unexposed persons.[2]

OBJECTIVE DATA

PREPARATION

The CBE screens for breast masses and abnormalities, evaluates any presenting symptoms, and presents an opportunity for you to teach breast self-awareness and examination. Some have listed that harms of screening could be false-positive results and overdiagnosis.[29] However, these are mitigated by using proper technique and spending an adequate amount of time. Plan to take a few minutes for a careful examination of the average size breast.[8]

Begin with the woman sitting up and facing you. You may use a short gown, open at the back, and lift it up to the woman's shoulders during inspection. During palpation when the woman is supine, cover one breast with the gown while examining the other. Be aware that many women are embarrassed to have their breasts examined; use a sensitive but matter-of-fact approach.

After your examination be prepared to teach the woman BSE.

EQUIPMENT NEEDED

Small pillow
Ruler marked in centimeters
Pamphlet or teaching aid for BSE

Normal Range of Findings	**Abnormal Findings**

Inspect the Breasts

General Appearance

Note symmetry of size and shape (Fig. 17-6). It is common to have a slight asymmetry in size; often the left breast is slightly larger than the right.

A sudden increase in the size of one breast signifies inflammation or new growth.

17-6

Skin

The skin normally is smooth and of even color. Note any localized areas of redness, bulging, or dimpling. Also note any skin lesions or focal vascular pattern. A fine blue vascular network is visible normally during pregnancy. Pale linear striae, or stretch marks, often follow pregnancy.

Normally no edema is present. Edema exaggerates the hair follicles, giving a "pigskin" or "orange-peel" look (also called *peau d'orange*).

Hyperpigmentation.
Redness and heat with inflammation.
Unilateral dilated superficial veins in a nonpregnant woman.
Edema (see Table 17-3, Signs of Retraction and Inflammation, p. 407).

Lymphatic Drainage Areas

Observe the axillary and supraclavicular regions. Note any bulging, discoloration, or edema.

Normal Range of Findings	Abnormal Findings

Nipple

The nipples should be placed symmetrically on the same plane on the two breasts. Nipples usually protrude, although some are flat and some are inverted. They tend to stay in their original condition. Distinguish a recently retracted nipple from one that has been inverted for many years or since puberty. Normal nipple inversion may be unilateral or bilateral and usually can be pulled out (i.e., it is not fixed).

Note any dry scaling, fissure or ulceration, and bleeding or other discharge.

A **supernumerary nipple** is a normal and common variation (Fig. 17-7). An extra nipple along the embryonic "milk line" on the thorax or abdomen is a congenital finding. Usually it is 5 to 6 cm below the breast near the midline and has no associated glandular tissue. It looks like a mole, although a close look reveals a tiny nipple and areola. It is not significant; merely distinguish it from a mole.

Deviation in pointing (see Table 17-3).

Recent nipple retraction signifies acquired disease (see Table 17-3).

Explore any discharge, especially in the presence of a breast mass.

Rarely additional glandular tissue, called a *supernumerary breast,* is present.

17-7   Supernumerary nipple and areolar complex. (Callen, 1993.)

Maneuver to Screen for Retraction

Direct the woman to change position while you check the breasts for skin retraction signs. First ask her to lift her arms slowly over her head. Both breasts should move up symmetrically (Fig. 17-8).

Retraction signs are caused by fibrosis in the breast tissue, usually caused by growing neoplasms. The fibrosis shortens with time, causing contrasting signs with the normally loose breast tissue.

Note a lag in the movement of one breast.

17-8   Retraction maneuver.

Normal Range of Findings

Next ask her to push her hands onto her hips (Fig. 17-9) and to push her two palms together (Fig. 17-10). These maneuvers contract the pectoralis major muscle. A slight lifting of both breasts occurs.

Abnormal Findings

Note a dimpling or a pucker, which indicates skin retraction (see Table 17-3).

17-9

17-10

Ask the woman with large, pendulous breasts to lean forward while you support her forearms. Note the symmetric free-forward movement of both breasts (Fig. 17-11).

Note fixation to chest wall or skin retraction (see Table 17-3).

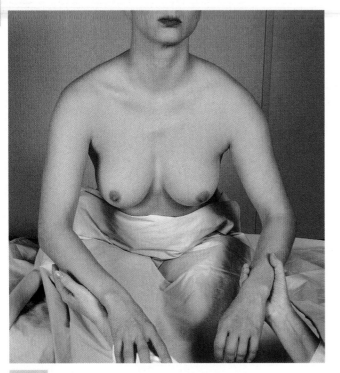

17-11

Normal Range of Findings	**Abnormal Findings**

Inspect and Palpate the Axillae

Examine the axillae while the woman is sitting. Inspect the skin, noting any rash or infection. Lift the woman's arm and support it yourself so her muscles are loose and relaxed. Use your right hand to palpate the left axilla (Fig. 17-12). Reach your fingers high into the axilla. Move them firmly down in four directions: (1) down the chest wall in a line from the middle of the axilla, (2) along the anterior border of the axilla, (3) along the posterior border, and (4) along the inner aspect of the upper arm. Move the woman's arm through range of motion to increase the surface area that you can reach.

Usually nodes are not palpable, although you may feel a small, soft, nontender node in the central group. Expect some tenderness when palpating high in the axilla. Note any enlarged and tender lymph nodes.

Nodes enlarge with any local infection of the breast, arm, or hand and with breast cancer metastases.

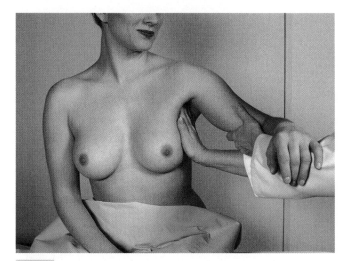

17-12

Palpate the Breasts

Help the woman to a supine position. Tuck a small pad under the side to be palpated and raise her arm over her head. These maneuvers flatten the breast tissue and displace it medially. Any significant lumps then feel more distinct (Fig. 17-13). For pendulous breasts, to distribute the tissue medially across the chest wall, ask the woman to rotate her hips opposite to the side you are palpating.

17-13

Objective Data

Normal Range of Findings	Abnormal Findings

Use the pads of your first 3 fingers and make a gentle rotary motion on the breast. Vary your pressure so you are palpating light, medium, and deep tissue in each location. The vertical strip pattern (Fig. 17-14) is the best way to detect a breast mass, but two other patterns are in common use: from the nipple palpating out to the periphery as if following spokes on a wheel and palpating in concentric circles out to the periphery.

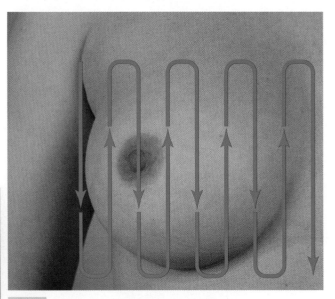

17-14 Vertical strip pattern of palpation.

For the vertical strip pattern, start high in the axilla and palpate down the midaxillary line just lateral to the breast down to the bra line. Proceed medially in overlapping vertical lines ending at the sternal edge. Take care to palpate every square inch of the breast and examine the tail of Spence high into the axilla. This should take a few minutes with each breast. Be consistent and thorough in your approach to each woman.

In nulliparous women normal breast tissue feels firm, smooth, and elastic. After pregnancy the tissue feels softer and looser. Premenstrual engorgement is normal from increasing progesterone. This consists of slight enlargement, tenderness to palpation, and generalized nodularity; the lobes feel prominent, and their margins more distinct.

In addition, normally you may feel a firm transverse ridge of compressed tissue in the lower quadrants (see Fig. 17-13). This is the **inframammary ridge,** and it is especially noticeable in large breasts. Do not confuse it with an abnormal lump.

What about the occasional woman with breast implants? Correctly placed implants are located behind the breast tissue. Therefore follow the same steps for CBE as shown for the woman without implants.

Heat, redness, and swelling in nonlactating and nonpostpartum breasts indicate inflammation.

Objective Data

Normal Range of Findings	**Abnormal Findings**

After palpating over the four breast quadrants, palpate the nipple (Fig. 17-15). Note any induration or subareolar mass. With your thumb and forefinger gently depress the nipple tissue into the well behind the areola. The tissue should move inward easily. If the woman reports spontaneous nipple discharge, press the areola inward with your index finger; repeat from a few different directions. If any discharge appears, note its color and consistency.

Except in pregnancy and lactation, discharge is abnormal (see Table 17-6). Note the number of discharge droplets and the quadrant(s) producing them. Blot the discharge on a white gauze pad to ascertain its color. Test any abnormal discharge for the presence of blood.

17-15

For the woman with large, pendulous breasts, you may palpate by using a bimanual technique (Fig. 17-16). The woman is in a sitting position, leaning forward. Support the inferior part of the breast with one hand. Use your other hand to palpate the breast tissue against your supporting hand.

17-16

Objective Data

| **Normal Range of Findings** | **Abnormal Findings** |

If the woman mentions a breast lump that she has discovered herself, examine the unaffected breast first to learn a baseline of normal consistency for this woman. If you do feel a lump or mass, note the following characteristics (Fig. 17-17):

17-17

1. **Location**—Using the breast as a clock face, describe the distance in centimeters from the nipple (e.g., "7:00, 2 cm from the nipple"). Or diagram the breast in the woman's record and mark in the location of the lump.
2. **Size**—Judge in centimeters in 3 dimensions: width × length × thickness.
3. **Shape**—State whether the lump is oval, round, lobulated, or indistinct.
4. **Consistency**—State whether the lump is soft, firm, or hard.
5. **Movable**—Is the lump freely movable, or is it fixed when you try to slide it over the chest wall?
6. **Distinctness**—Is the lump solitary or multiple?
7. **Nipple**—Is it displaced or retracted?
8. **Note the skin over the lump**—Is it erythematous, dimpled, or retracted?
9. **Tenderness**—Is the lump tender to palpation?
10. **Lymphadenopathy**—Are any regional lymph nodes palpable?

See Table 17-4, Breast Lumps, and Table 17-5, Differentiating Breast Lumps, for a description of common breast lumps with these characteristics.

Screening measures aim to detect breast lumps when small and potentially curable. The acronym BREAST lists physical signs associated with more advanced cancer: *B*reast mass, *R*etraction, *E*dema, *A*xillary mass, *S*caly nipple, *T*ender breast.[34]

Premenopausal women at midcycle often have tissue edema and mastalgia (pain) that make it hard to detect a lesion. If your findings are in question, consider asking this woman to return for a follow-up examination the first week after her menses, when hormone levels are lower and edema is not present.

The woman with a healing or healed **mastectomy** needs special consideration. She may be very concerned about a recurrence of cancer and be anxious for your findings. Inspect and palpate as described previously. Be gentle around the scar area because these tissues are quite sensitive. There should be no inflammation or infection. Lymphedema of the upper arms is a common sequela because of interruption of lymphatic drainage and removal of nodes.

Teach Breast Self-Examination

Finish your own assessment first and then teach breast self-awareness. The goal is that the woman becomes familiar with the look and feel of her breasts so she can detect any change and report it promptly. The American Cancer Society no longer recommends a structured monthly BSE[2] because many women with breast cancer have detected their lumps by chance as when bathing or dressing. Still, use this opportunity to teach the proper technique of BSE, knowing that some women will choose to perform it regularly and some occasionally (Fig. 17-18).

Objective Data

Normal Range of Findings	Abnormal Findings

Breast Self-examination

Lie down. Press the 3 middle fingers in a circular motion and use 3 levels of pressure. Follow an up and down pattern.

Sit up. Examine underarm with arm slightly raised.

Note surface changes with hands pushed on hips, shoulders hunched.

17-18

© Pat Thomas, 2014.

The best time to perform BSE is right after the menstrual period (day 4 to 7) of the cycle), when the breasts are the smallest and least congested. Instruct the woman not having menstrual periods (pregnant or menopausal) to choose a familiar date as a reminder, such as the first of the month. Keep your teaching simple, and give her a pamphlet to reinforce the steps. Tell her what to look for as she inspects her breasts in front of a mirror disrobed to the waist. At home she can palpate while in the shower, where soap and water assist palpation. Or she can lie supine. Watch her palpate her own breasts while you are there to monitor her technique. Correct and encourage her return demonstration.

What are the potential harms of CBE and BSE? Concern exists that these procedures may result in more false-positives, creating anxiety and unnecessary biopsies.[10,37,38] However, the value of early detection of breast cancer is clear. Screening mammography is available for many groups of women in developed countries, and BSE is available to virtually all women. BSE is valuable to women who are younger or older than the ages recommended for screening mammography or who have barriers to access mammography. BSE is cheap and noninvasive, can be accomplished without visits to expert professionals, and enhances self-care action.

The Male Breast

Your examination of the male breast can be abbreviated, but do not omit it. Combine the breast examination with that of the anterior thorax. Inspect the chest wall, noting the skin surface and any lumps or swelling. Palpate the nipple

Objective Data

Normal Range of Findings

area for any lump or tissue enlargement (Fig. 17-19). It should feel even, with no nodules. Palpate the axillary lymph nodes.

17-19

The normal male breast has a flat disk of undeveloped breast tissue beneath the nipple. **Gynecomastia** is a benign growth of this breast tissue, making it distinguishable from the other tissues in the chest wall (Fig. 17-20). It feels like a smooth, firm, movable disk. This occurs in about one half of adolescent boys at 13 or 14 years of age. It can be unilateral or bilateral and is temporary. The adolescent is acutely aware of his body image and feels distressed. Reassure him that this change is normal, common, and temporary.

17-20 Adolescent gynecomastia. (Moore & Persaud, 2008.)

Abnormal Findings

Male breast cancer is rare (see Table 17-8, Male Breast Abnormalities, p. 411) but usually presents with painless, firm, retroareolar lump. Also note less frequent signs: nipple discharge (clear or bloody), ulceration, retraction, axillary lymphadenopathy. Nipple discharge is rare but strongly associated with cancer; thus it demands detailed evaluation.[17]

Gynecomastia also occurs with use of anabolic steroids, some medications, cirrhosis, and other disease states. See Table 17-8.

Normal Range of Findings	Abnormal Findings

❖ DEVELOPMENTAL COMPETENCE

Infants and Children

In the neonate the breasts may be enlarged and visible from maternal estrogen crossing the placenta. They may secrete a clear or white fluid, called *witch's milk*. This is not significant and is resolved within a few days to a few weeks.

Note the position of the nipples on the prepubertal child. They should be symmetric, just lateral to the midclavicular line between the 4th and 5th ribs. The nipple is flat, and the areola is darker pigmented.

Premature thelarche is early breast development with no other hormone-dependent signs (pubic hair, menses).

The Adolescent

Adolescent breast development begins on an average between 8 and 10 years of age. Expect some asymmetry during growth. Record the stage of development using the Tanner staging described on p. 388. Use the chart to teach the adolescent normal developmental stages and to assure her of her own normal progress.

You should consider BMI (derived from weight and height) when evaluating breast budding before age 8 years. With normal BMI levels, breast budding before age 8 is premature in non-Hispanic White girls but may be normal in 7-year-old Black and Mexican-American girls.[33] Note that it is difficult to distinguish breast budding from excess adipose tissue.

With maturing adolescents, palpate the breasts as you would with the adult. The breasts normally feel firm and uniform. Note any mass.

Note precocious development before age 8 years. It is usually normal but also occurs with thyroid dysfunction, stilbestrol ingestion, or ovarian or adrenal tumor.

Note delayed development with hormonal failure, anorexia nervosa, or severe malnutrition.

At this age a mass is almost always a benign fibroadenoma or a cyst (see Table 17-4).

The Pregnant Woman

A delicate blue vascular pattern is visible over the breasts. The breasts increase in size, as do the nipples. Jagged linear stretch marks, or striae, may develop if the breasts have a large increase. The nipples also become darker and more erectile. The areolae widen, grow darker, and contain the small, scattered, elevated Montgomery glands. On palpation the breasts feel more nodular, and thick yellow colostrum can be expressed after the first trimester.

The Lactating Woman

Colostrum changes to milk production around the 3rd postpartum day. At this time the breasts may become engorged, appearing enlarged, reddened, and shiny and feeling warm and hard. Frequent nursing helps drain the ducts and sinuses and stimulate milk production. Nipple soreness is normal, appearing around the 20th nursing, lasting 24 to 48 hours and then disappearing rapidly. The nipples may look red and irritated. They may even crack but heal rapidly if kept dry and exposed to air. Again, frequent nursing is the best treatment for nipple soreness.

One section of the breast surface appearing red and tender indicates a plugged duct (see Table 17-7, Disorders Occurring During Lactation, p. 411).

The Aging Woman

Increasing age is the primary risk factor for developing breast cancer; therefore an annual CBE is important.

On inspection the breasts look pendulous, flattened, and sagging. Nipples may be retracted but can be pulled outward. On palpation the breasts feel more granular, and the terminal ducts around the nipple feel more prominent and stringy. Thickening of the inframammary ridge at the lower breast is normal, and it feels more prominent with age.

Reinforce the value of the BSE. Women older than 50 years have an increased risk for breast cancer. Older women may have problems with arthritis, limited range of motion, or decreased vision that may inhibit self-care. Suggest aids to the self-examination (e.g., talcum powder helps fingers glide over skin).

Because atrophy causes shrinkage of normal glandular tissue, cancer detection is somewhat easier. Any palpable lump that cannot be positively identified as a normal structure should be referred.

Objective Data

PROMOTING A HEALTHY LIFESTYLE

Breast Cancer Risk Assessment Tools

Before a breast examination you have time to review the woman's BSE technique and inquire about scheduled mammogram surveillance. It is also an opportunity to assess the breast cancer risk, including family history.

The use of breast cancer risk-assessment tools in the clinical setting may improve health through cancer prevention and more effective detection of high-risk individuals. A number of tools are available, and new tools are in development that include additional variables such as breast density.

Gail Model. The *Gail Model* is widely used for calculating a woman's risk estimate for breast cancer. This model identifies risk factors, including current age, age at menarche, age at first live birth, and family history of breast cancer in first-degree relatives. It calculates a 5-year and a 30-year or lifetime risk estimate for each individual. It is easy to complete, and many computer-based data programs are available to clinicians. However, this model may underestimate the breast cancer risk in the subgroup of women with family cancer histories suggestive of hereditary breast cancer syndromes such as BRCA1 and BRCA2.

Breast Cancer Risk Assessment Tool. The National Cancer Institute (NCI) created this interactive tool to help health care providers estimate a woman's risk of developing invasive breast cancer based on the Gail Model. It has recently been updated for: (1) African-American women, following the findings from the Contraceptive and Reproductive Experiences (CARE) study; and (2) Asian and Pacific Islander women following findings from the Asian-American Breast Cancer Study (AABCS). It is available on the National Cancer Institute website at: http://www.cancer.gov/bcrisktool/.

Tyrer-Cuzick Model. This model and its associated IBIS Breast Cancer Risk Evaluation Tool incorporate both genetic and nongenetic factors into a computer program that gives a personalized risk estimate. The process begins with a three-generation pedigree and incorporates personal risk factors such as parity, BMI, height, age at menarche and menopause, hormone replacement therapy use, and first live birth. Both genetic and nongenetic factors are then combined to develop a risk estimate. This tool was developed in the United Kingdom and is available at: http://www.ems-trials.org/riskevaluator/.

Resources

For more information about hereditary breast cancer syndromes go to the National Cancer Institute (NCI) website at http://www.cancer.gov/cancertopics/pdq/genetics/breast-and-ovarian/healthprofessional.

Tyrer, J., Duffy, S. W., & Cuzick, J. (2004). A breast cancer prediction model incorporating familial and personal risk factors. *Stat Med, 23(7)*, 1111-1130.

NOTE: Although a tool can estimate a woman's risk of developing breast cancer, it does not accurately predict which woman will actually develop breast cancer.

DOCUMENTATION AND CRITICAL THINKING

Sample Charting

FEMALE

SUBJECTIVE

States no breast pain, lump, discharge, rash, swelling, or trauma. No history of breast disease herself; does have mother with fibrocystic disease. No history of breast surgery. Never been pregnant. Performs BSE monthly.

OBJECTIVE

Inspection: Breasts symmetric. Skin smooth with even color and no rash or lesions. Arm movement shows no dimpling or retractions. No nipple discharge, no lesions.

Palpation: Breast contour and consistency firm and homogeneous. No masses or tenderness. No lymphadenopathy.

ASSESSMENT

Healthy breast structure
Has knowledge of breast self-examination

MALE

SUBJECTIVE

No pain, lump, rash, or swelling.

OBJECTIVE

No masses or tenderness. No lymphadenopathy.

Clinical Case Study 1

L.B. is a 32-year-old Caucasian female, married with a 3-week-old son. Uneventful pregnancy and immediate postpartum period. Successfully breastfeeding. Reports feeding her son every 3 hours during the day and every 4 to 5 hours at night. Alternating breasts as instructed by lactation consultant.

SUBJECTIVE

L.B. reports flulike symptoms for the past 2 days, including extreme fatigue, fever, and chills. Reports "my right breast is hot and really hurts when I nurse. I think maybe I'm doing something wrong." No personal or family history of breast disease.

OBJECTIVE

Vital signs: Temperature 102° F (38.9° C). Pulse 114 bpm. Resp 18/min. BP 110/76 mm Hg.
General appearance: Appears anxious. Grimacing with movement. Dark circles under eyes. Wearing coat over hospital gown.
Breasts: Nipples flat. No lesions. Breast milk discharge from bilateral nipples. Breast movement symmetric bilaterally. No retractions. Upper inner quadrant of right breast red, swollen.
Palpation: Left breast consistency firm and homogenous. No masses or tenderness. Right breast upper inner quadrant warm, hard, and tender. Remainder of breast firm and homogenous. No lymphadenopathy.
Thorax: Symmetric, no lumps or lesions, breath sounds clear and = bilat.
Cardiovascular: S_1 S_2 not accentuated or diminished; no murmurs or extra sounds.

ASSESSMENT

Acute mastitis
Acute pain R/T mastitis
Risk for infection R/T plugged milk duct
Risk for ineffective breastfeeding R/T pain, anxiety
Anxiety R/T acute pain, fear of ineffective breastfeeding

Clinical Case Study 2

D.B. is a 62-year-old African-American female bank comptroller, married, with no children. History of hypertension, managed by diuretic medication and diet. No other health problems until annual company physical exam 3 days PTA, when MD "found a lump in my right breast."

SUBJECTIVE

3 days PTA—MD noted lump in R breast during annual physical exam. MD did not describe lump but told D.B. it was "serious" and needed immediate biopsy. D.B. has not felt it herself. States has noted no skin changes, no nipple discharge. No previous history of breast disease. Mother died age 54 years of breast cancer; no other relative with breast disease. D.B. has had no term pregnancies; two spontaneous abortions, ages 28, 31 years. Menopause completed at age 52 years.
Aware of BSE but has never performed it. "I feel so bad. If only I had been doing it. I should have found this myself." Married 43 years. States husband supportive, but "I just can't talk to him about this. I can't even go near him now."

OBJECTIVE

Inspection—Breasts symmetric when sitting, arms down. Nipples flat. No lesions, no discharge. As lifts arms, left breast elevates, right breast stays fixed. Dimple in right breast, 9 o'clock position, apparent at rest and with muscle contraction. Leaning forward reveals left breast falls free, right breast flattens.

Palpation—Left breast feels soft and granular throughout, no mass. Right breast soft and granular, with large, stony hard mass in outer quadrant. Lump is 5 cm × 4 cm × 2 cm, at 9 o'clock position, 3 cm from nipple. Borders irregular, mass fixed to tissues, no pain with palpation.

One firm, palpable lymph node in center of right axilla. No palpable nodes on the left.

ASSESSMENT

Lump in R breast
Ineffective coping R/T effects of breast lump

Clinical Case Study 3

Father brings a 9-year-old African-American female (B.K.) to the clinic because of complaints of "chest pain." Father has raised her since her mother's death from cancer 7 years ago. He wrings his hands, asks many questions, and at times is tearful as he is present during B.K.'s history intake and physical examination.

SUBJECTIVE

B.K.'s father states, "She's been complaining of her chest hurting for over 3 weeks now. I think it's her breasts, but she's too young for puberty, isn't she? I'm worried something's really wrong. You know, like with what happened to her mother." B.K. doesn't appear concerned but "wonders why it (her breasts) feels this way." Rates pain at a "2" on a 1-to-10 pain scale and describes it as a consistent, dull, aching pain to general breast and nipple area.

OBJECTIVE

Vital signs: Temp 97°.9 F (36.6° C) (orally). BP 96/68 mm Hg (sitting, legs uncrossed). Pulse 70 bpm. Resp 22/min.

General appearance: Good hygiene, dressed appropriate for weather, developmentally appropriate in relation to age, talkative, and appears comfortable except during breast examination.

HEENT: Normocephalic; no lymphadenopathy.

Cardiovascular: No murmurs or other abnormal heart sounds.

Respiratory: Breath sounds clear; no adventitious sounds.

Chest: Visible and palpable elevation of the breast to the left nipple (2.1 cm in width × 0.2 cm in depth) and papillae w/o separation of contour of the breast and areola. Right breast flat w/o detectable elevation. Skin smooth w/even brown color; no rash, lesions or nipple discharge. States tenderness during palpation of breasts. No lymphadenopathy.

Genitourinary: No swelling, lesions or discharge to genitalia and/or urethra. Scant, coarse, pigmented hair to labia.

ASSESSMENT

Age-appropriate breast budding, Tanner stage 2
Acute pain R/T breast tissue growth
Fear (parental) R/T perceived threat to daughter's health status

TABLE 17-3   Signs of Retraction and Inflammation

◀ Dimpling

The shallow dimple (also called a *skin tether)* shown here is a sign of skin retraction. Cancer causes fibrosis, which contracts the suspensory ligaments. The dimple may be apparent at rest, with compression, or with lifting of the arms. Also note the distortion of the areola here as the fibrosis pulls the nipple toward it.

Nipple Retraction. The retracted nipple looks flatter and broader, like an underlying crater. A recent retraction suggests cancer, which causes fibrosis of the whole duct system and pulls in the nipple. It also may occur with benign lesions such as ectasia of the ducts. Do not confuse retraction with the normal long-standing type of nipple inversion, which has no broadening and is not fixed.

◀ Edema (Peau d'Orange)

Lymphatic obstruction produces edema. This thickens the skin and exaggerates the hair follicles, giving a pigskin or orange-peel look. This condition suggests cancer. Edema usually begins in the skin around and beneath the areola, the most dependent area of the breast. Also note nipple infiltration here.

Fixation

Asymmetry, distortion, or decreased mobility with the elevated arm maneuver. As cancer becomes invasive, the fibrosis fixes the breast to the underlying pectoral muscles. Here note that the right breast is held against the chest wall.

Deviation in Nipple Pointing

An underlying cancer causes fibrosis in the mammary ducts, which pulls the nipple angle toward it. Here note the swelling behind the right nipple and that the nipple tilts laterally.

See Illustration Credits for source information.

TABLE 17-4 Breast Lumps

◀ Benign ("Fibrocystic") Breast Disease

Multiple tender masses that occur with numerous symptoms and physical findings:

- Swelling and tenderness (cyclic discomfort)
- Mastalgia (severe pain, both cyclic and noncyclic)
- Nodularity (significant lumpiness, both cyclic and noncyclic)
- Dominant lumps (including cysts and fibroadenomas)
- Nipple discharge (including intraductal papilloma and duct ectasia)
- Infections and inflammations (including subareolar abscess, lactational mastitis, breast abscess, and Mondor disease)

Many women have some form of benign breast disease. Nodularity occurs bilaterally; regular, firm nodules are mobile, well demarcated, and feel rubbery like small water balloons. Pain may be dull, heavy, and cyclic as nodules enlarge. Some women have nodularity but no pain and vice versa. Cysts are discrete, fluid-filled sacs. Dominant lumps and nipple discharge must be investigated carefully. Nodularity itself is not premalignant but produces difficulty in detecting other cancerous lumps.

Cancer

Solitary, unilateral, nontender mass. Single focus in one area, although it may be interspersed with other nodules. Solid, hard, dense, and fixed to underlying tissues or skin as cancer becomes invasive. Borders are irregular and poorly delineated. Grows constantly. Often painless, although the person may have pain. Most common in upper outer quadrant. Found in women 30 to 80 years of age; increased risk across all ages until age 80 years. As cancer advances, signs include firm or hard irregular axillary nodes; skin dimpling; nipple retraction, elevation, and discharge.

Fibroadenoma

Benign tumors; most commonly present as self-detected in late adolescence. Solitary nontender mass that is solid, firm, rubbery, and elastic. Round, oval, or lobulated; 1 to 5 cm. Freely movable, slippery; fingers slide it easily through tissue. Usually no axillary lymphadenopathy. Diagnose by triple test (palpation, ultrasound, and needle biopsy). Because of risk of deformity of surgery to a growing breast, excisional surgery is reserved for masses >5 cm; for continuously enlarging, well-circumscribed, multiple masses; or with suspicious ultrasound findings.[13]

See Illustration Credits for source information.

TABLE 17-5 Differentiating Breast Lumps

	Fibroadenoma	Benign Breast Disease	Cancer
Likely age	15-30 years, can occur up to 55 years	30-55 years; decreases after menopause	30-80 years, risk increases after 50 years
Shape	Round, lobular	Round, lobular	Irregular, star-shaped
Consistency	Usually firm, rubbery	Firm to soft, rubbery	Firm to stony hard
Demarcation	Well demarcated, clear margins	Well demarcated	Poorly defined
Number	Usually single	Usually multiple; may be single	Single
Mobility	Very mobile, slippery	Mobile	Fixed
Tenderness	Usually none	Tender; usually increases before menses; may be noncyclic	Usually none, can be tender
Skin retraction	None	None	Usually
Pattern of growth	Grows quickly and constantly	Size may increase or decrease rapidly; cyclic with menstrual periods	Grows constantly
Risk to health	Benign—Diagnose by ultrasound and biopsy; may spontaneously resolve in women <20 years. Should be resected in women >35 years as it carries a small risk of associated cancer.[30]	Benign, although general lumpiness may mask other cancerous lump	Serious, needs early treatment

ABNORMAL FINDINGS
FOR ADVANCED PRACTICE

TABLE 17-6 Abnormal Nipple Discharge

Mammary Duct Ectasia

Pastelike matter in subareolar ducts produces sticky, purulent discharge that may be white, gray, brown, green, or bloody. A light green, single duct discharge is shown here. Caused by stagnation of cellular debris and secretions in the ducts, leading to obstruction, inflammation, and infection. Usually occurs in perimenopause.

Itching, burning, or drawing pain occurs around nipple. May have subareolar redness and swelling. Ducts are palpable as rubbery, twisted tubules under areola. May have palpable mass, soft or firm, poorly delineated. Not malignant but needs biopsy.

Intraductal Papilloma

These are discrete benign tumors that arise in a single or multiple papillary duct(s). May have serous or serosanguineous discharge. Often there is a palpable nodule in underlying duct (highlighted here). Most common in women ages 40 to 60 years. Most are benign, although multiple papillomas have a higher risk of subsequent cancer than do solitary ones.[30] Requires core needle biopsy and possible excision.

Continued

TABLE 17-6 Abnormal Nipple Discharge—cont'd

Carcinoma

Bloody nipple discharge that is unilateral and from a single duct requires further investigation. Although there was no palpable lump associated with the discharge shown here, mammography revealed a 1-cm, centrally located, ill-defined mass.

Paget Disease (Intraductal Carcinoma)

Early lesion has unilateral, clear, yellow discharge and dry, scaling crusts, friable at nipple apex. Spreads outward to areola with erythematous halo on areola and crusted, eczematous, retracted nipple. Later lesion shows nipple reddened, excoriated, and ulcerated with bloody discharge, and an erythematous plaque surrounding the nipple. Symptoms include tingling, burning, itching. Except for the redness and occasional cracking from initial breastfeeding, any dermatitis of the nipple area must be explored carefully and referred immediately.

See Illustration Credits for source information.

TABLE 17-7 Disorders Occurring During Lactation

Mastitis

This is uncommon; an inflammatory mass before abscess formation. Usually occurs in single quadrant. Area is red, swollen, tender, very hot, and hard, here forming outward from areola upper edge in right breast. The woman also has a headache, malaise, fever, chills, sweating, increased pulse, flulike symptoms. May occur during first 4 months of lactation from infection or from stasis from plugged duct. Treat with rest, local heat to area, antibiotics, and frequent nursing to keep breast as empty as possible. Must not wean now, or the breast will become engorged, and the pain will increase. Mother's antibiotic not harmful to infant. Usually resolves in 2 to 3 days.

Breast Abscess

A rare complication of generalized infection (e.g., mastitis) if untreated. A pocket of pus that feels hard, looks red, and is quite tender accumulates in one local area. Here there is extensive nipple edema, and abscess is "pointing" at 3 o'clock position on areolar margin. May nurse depending on location of abscess, associated pain, and type of medicine. Continue to nurse on unaffected side. Treat with antibiotics, surgical incision, and drainage.

TABLE 17-7   Disorders Occurring During Lactation—cont'd

◄ **Plugged Duct**

This is common when milk is not removed completely because of poor latching, ineffective suckling, infrequent nursing, or switching to second breast too soon.[3] There is a tender lump that may be reddened and warm to touch. No infection. It is important to keep breast as empty as possible and milk flowing. The woman should nurse her baby frequently on affected side first to ensure complete emptying and manually express any remaining milk. A plugged duct usually resolves in less than 1 day.

See Illustration Credits for source information.

TABLE 17-8   Male Breast Abnormalities

Gynecomastia

Benign enlargement of male breast that occurs when estrogen concentration exceeds testosterone levels. It is a mobile disk of tissue located centrally under the nipple-areola. At puberty it is usually mild and transient. In older men it is bilateral, tender, and firm but not as hard as breast cancer. Gynecomastia occurs with Cushing syndrome, liver cirrhosis (because estrogens cannot be metabolized), adrenal disease, hyperthyroidism, and numerous drugs: alcohol and marijuana; estrogen treatment for prostate cancer; antibiotics (metronidazole, isoniazid); spironolactone, digoxin, angiotensin-converting enzyme (ACE) inhibitors; psychoactive drugs (diazepam, tricyclic antidepressants).[14]

Male Breast Cancer

1% of breast cancers occur in men. There is no standard screening mammography; thus it is detected by clinical symptoms. It presents as a painless palpable mass—hard, irregular, nontender, fixed to the area; may have nipple retraction. Nipple discharge, with or without a palpable mass, is a significant warning of early breast cancer.[17] Note retraction and ulceration shown here. Early spread to axillary lymph nodes occurs because of minimal breast tissue. Because of lack of screening and general awareness, men are diagnosed 10 years later than women and at later stages, with the mean age between 60 and 70 years. The stage at diagnosis is the most important indicator for survival.

See Illustration Credits for source information.

Summary Checklist: Breasts and Regional Lymphatics Examination

1. **Inspect breasts** as the woman sits, raises arms overhead, pushes hands on hips, leans forward.
2. **Inspect** the supraclavicular and infraclavicular areas.
3. **Palpate the axillae** and regional lymph nodes.
4. With woman supine, **palpate the breast tissue,** including tail of Spence, the nipples, and areolae.
5. **Teach BSE.**

BIBLIOGRAPHY

1. Ahmed, N. U., Ford, J. G., Fair, A. M., et al. (2009). Breast cancer knowledge and barriers to mammography in a low-income managed care population. *J Cancer Educ, 24*(4), 261-266.
2. American Cancer Society. (2014). *Breast cancer facts and figures 2013-2014.* Atlanta: Author.
3. Balkam, J. J. (2010). Painful breast lumps in nursing mothers. *Am J Nurs, 110*(12), 65-67.
4. Berkey, C. S., Willett, W. C., Frazier, A. L., et al. (2010). Prospective study of adolescent alcohol consumption and risk of benign breast disease in young women. *Pediatrics, 125*(5), e1081-e1087.
5. Berkey, C. S., Willett, W. C., Frazier, A. L., et al. (2011). Prospective study of growth and development in older girls and risk of benign breast disease in young women. *Cancer, 117*(8), 1612-1620.
6. Biro, F. M., Galvez, M. P., Greenspan, L. C., et al. (2010). Pubertal assessment method and baseline characteristics in a mixed longitudinal study of girls. *Pediatrics, 126*(3), e583-e590.
7. Bordini, B., & Rosenfield, R. L. (2011). Normal pubertal development: Part II: Clinical aspects of puberty. *Pediatr Rev, 32*(7), 281-292.
8. Bryan, T., & Snyder, E. (2013). The clinical breast exam: a skill that should not be abandoned. *J Gen Intern Med, 1-4.*
9. Chen, W. Y., Rosner, B., & Hankinson, S. E., et al. (2011). Moderate alcohol consumption during adult life, drinking patterns, and breast cancer risk. *JAMA, 306*(17), 1884-1890.
10. Chiarelli, A. M., Majpruz, V., Brown, P., et al. (2009). The contribution of clinical breast examination to the accuracy of breast screening. *J Nat Cancer Instit, 101*(18), 1236-1243.
11. Costanza, M. E. (2012). Screening mammograms should not be underestimated. *Arch Intern Med, 172*(5), 446.
12. Cottet, V., Touvier, M., Fornier, A., et al. (2009). Postmenopausal breast cancer risk and dietary patterns in the E3N-EPIC Prospective Cohort Study. *Am J Epidemiol, 170*(10), 1257-1267.
13. De Silva, N. (2012). Breast disorders in the female adolescent. *Adolesc Med 23,* 34-52.
14. Dickson, G. (2012). Gynecomastia. *Am Fam Phys, 85*(7), 716-722.
15. Downs-Holmes, C., & Silverman, P. (2011). Breast cancer: overview & updates. *Nurse Pract, 36*(12), 20-26.
16. Dreadin, J., & Mancuso, P. (2010). Diagnostic breast evaluation: when to refer and what the results really mean. *Nurse Pract, 35*(11), 24-30.
17. Farooq, A., & Horgan, K. (2011). Male breast cancer presenting as nipple discharge. *Case Rep Surg,* doi:10.1155/2011/804843.
18. Gómez-Raposo, C., Zambrana Tévar, F., Sereno Moyano, M., et al. (2010). Male breast cancer. *Cancer Treat Rev, 36*(6), 451-457.
19. Hamilton, R. (2012). Being young, female, and BRCA positive. *Am J Nurs, 112*(10), 26-31.
20. Hauner, H., Hauner, D. (2010). The impact of nutrition on the development and prognosis of breast cancer. *Breast Care, 5,* 377-381.
21. Herman-Giddens, M. E., Slora, E. J., Wasserman, R. C., et al. (1997). Secondary sexual characteristics and menses in young girls seen in office practice. *Pediatrics, 99,* 505-512.
22. Johnson, R. E., & Murad, M. H. (2009). Gynecomastia: pathophysiology, evaluation, and management. *Mayo Clin Proceed, 84*(11), 1010-1015.
23. Kass-Wolff, J. H., & Fisher, J. E. (2011). Menopause and the hormone controversy. *Nurse Pract, 36*(7), 22-29.
24. Katz, A. (2011). Breast cancer and women's sexuality. *Am J Nurs, 111*(4), 63-67.
25. Krieger, N., Chen, J. T., & Waterman, P. D. (2010). Decline in U.S. breast cancer rates after the Women's Health Initiative: socioeconomic and racial/ethnic differentials. *Am J Publ Health, 100,* S132-S329.
26. Kurian, A. W. (2010). BRCA1 and BRCA2 mutations across race and ethnicity: distribution and clinical implications. *Curr Opin Obstet Gynecol, 22*(1), 72-78.
27. Lee, C. H., Dershaw, D. D., Kopans, D., et al. (2010). Breast cancer screening with imaging: recommendations on the use of mammography, breast MRI, breast ultrasound, and other technologies for the detection of clinically occult breast cancer. *J Am Coll Radiol, 7*(1), 18-27.
28. McCullough, L. E., Eng, S. M., Bradshaw, P. T., et al. (2012). Fat or fit: the joint effects of physical activity, weight gain, and body size on breast cancer risk. *Cancer, 118*(19), 4860-4868.
29. Miller, A. B., & Baines, C. J. (2011). The role of clinical breast examination and breast self-examination. *Prevent Med, 53*(3), 118-120.
30. Neal, L., Tortorelli, C. L., & Nassar, A. (2010). Clinician's guide to imaging and pathologic findings in benign breast disease. *Mayo Clinic Proceed, 85*(3), 274-279
31. Oliveira, K., Clark, S., Dunn, E., et al. (2011). Spanish as a primary language and its effect on breast cancer presentation. *J Oncol Pract, 7*(3), 165-167.
32. Pandya, S., & Moore, R. G. (2011). Breast development and anatomy. *Clin Obstet Gynecol, 54*(1), 91-95.
33. Rosenfield, R. L., Lipton, R. B., & Drum, M. L. (2009). Thelarche, pubarche, and menarche attainment in children with normal and elevated BMI. *Pediatrics, 123*(1), 84-88.
34. Saslow, D., Hannan, J., Osuch, J., et al. (2004). Clinical breast examination: practical recommendations for optimizing performance and reporting. *CA Cancer J Clin, 54:* 327–344.
35. Tanner, J. M. (1962). *Growth at adolescence* (2nd ed.). Oxford, UK: Blackwell Scientific.
36. Thomas, E. (2010). Men's awareness and knowledge of male breast cancer. *Am J Nurs, 110*(10), 32-37.
37. U.S. Preventive Services Task Force. (2009). Screening for breast cancer. *Ann Intern Med, 151*(10), 716-726.
38. Welch, H. G., & Frankel, B. A. (2011). Likelihood that a woman with screen-detected breast cancer has had her "life saved" by that screening. *Arch Intern Med, 171*(22), 2043-2048.

CHAPTER 18

Thorax and Lungs

ⓔ http://evolve.elsevier.com/Jarvis/

STRUCTURE AND FUNCTION

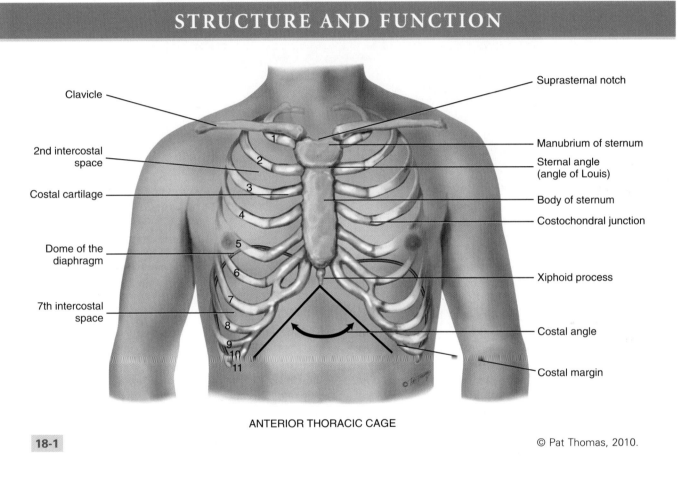

ANTERIOR THORACIC CAGE

18-1

© Pat Thomas, 2010.

POSITION AND SURFACE LANDMARKS

The **thoracic cage** is a bony structure with a conical shape, which is narrower at the top (Fig. 18-1). It is defined by the **sternum,** 12 pairs of **ribs,** and 12 thoracic **vertebrae.** Its "floor" is the **diaphragm,** a musculotendinous septum that separates the thoracic cavity from the abdomen. The first seven ribs attach directly to the sternum via their costal cartilages; ribs 8, 9, and 10 attach to the costal cartilage above, and ribs 11 and 12 are "floating," with free palpable tips. The **costochondral junctions** are the points at which the ribs join their cartilages. They are not palpable.

Anterior Thoracic Landmarks

Surface landmarks on the thorax are signposts for underlying respiratory structures. Knowing landmarks helps you localize

a finding and facilitates communication of your findings to others.

Suprasternal Notch. Feel this hollow U-shaped depression just above the sternum, between the clavicles.

Sternum. The "breastbone" has three parts: the manubrium, the body, and the xiphoid process. Walk your fingers down the manubrium a few centimeters until you feel a distinct bony ridge, the sternal angle.

Sternal Angle. Often called the *angle of Louis,* this is the articulation of the manubrium and body of the sternum, and it is continuous with the second rib. The angle of Louis is a useful place to start counting ribs, which helps localize a respiratory finding horizontally. Identify the angle of Louis, palpate lightly to the second rib, and slide down to the second intercostal space. Each intercostal space is numbered by the rib above it. Continue counting down the ribs in the middle

413

Clavicle

Scapula

Inferior angle of scapula

Vertebra prominens of C7

Spinous process of T3

C7
T1
T12
L1
1
2
3
4
5
6
7
8
9
10
11
12

POSTERIOR THORACIC CAGE

18-2

© Pat Thomas, 2010.

of the hemithorax, not close to the sternum where the costal cartilages lie too close together to count. You can palpate easily down to the tenth rib.

The angle of Louis also marks the site of tracheal bifurcation into the right and left main bronchi; it corresponds with the upper border of the atria of the heart, and it lies above the fourth thoracic vertebra on the back.

Costal Angle. The right and left costal margins form an angle where they meet at the xiphoid process. Usually 90 degrees or less, this angle increases when the rib cage is chronically overinflated, as in emphysema.

Posterior Thoracic Landmarks

Counting ribs and intercostal spaces on the back is a bit harder because of the muscles and soft tissue surrounding the ribs and spinal column (Fig. 18-2).

Vertebra Prominens. Start here. Flex your head and feel for the most prominent bony spur protruding at the base of the neck. This is the spinous process of C7. If two bumps seem equally prominent, the upper one is C7, and the lower one is T1.

Spinous Processes. Count down these knobs on the vertebrae, which stack together to form the spinal column. Note that the spinous processes align with their same numbered ribs only down to T4. After T4 the spinous processes angle downward from their vertebral body and overlie the vertebral body and rib below.

Inferior Border of the Scapula. The scapulae are located symmetrically in each hemithorax. The lower tip is usually at the seventh or eighth rib.

Twelfth Rib. Palpate midway between the spine and the person's side to identify its free tip.

Reference Lines

Use the reference lines to pinpoint a finding vertically on the chest. On the anterior chest note the **midsternal** line and the **midclavicular** line. The midclavicular line bisects the center of each clavicle at a point halfway between the palpated sternoclavicular and acromioclavicular joints (Fig. 18-3).

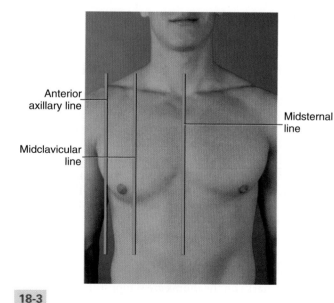

Anterior axillary line

Midclavicular line

Midsternal line

18-3

18-4

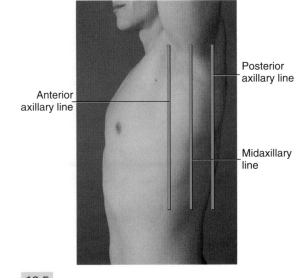

18-5

The posterior chest wall has the **vertebral** (or midspinal) line and the **scapular** line, which extends through the inferior angle of the scapula when the arms are at the sides of the body (Fig. 18-4).

Lift up the person's arm 90 degrees and divide the lateral chest by three lines: the **anterior axillary** line extends down from the anterior axillary fold where the pectoralis major muscle inserts; the **posterior axillary** line continues down from the posterior axillary fold where the latissimus dorsi muscle inserts; and the **midaxillary** line runs down from the apex of the axilla and lies between and parallel to the other two (Fig. 18-5).

THE THORACIC CAVITY

The **mediastinum** is the middle section of the thoracic cavity containing the esophagus, trachea, heart, and great vessels.

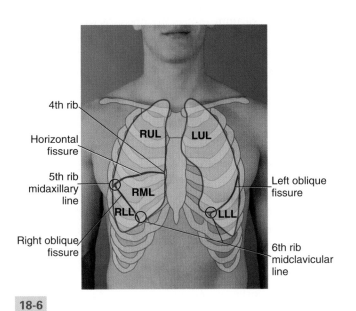

18-6

The right and left **pleural cavities,** on either side of the mediastinum, contain the lungs.

Lung Borders. In the anterior chest the **apex,** or highest point, of lung tissue is 3 to 4 cm above the inner third of the clavicles. The **base,** or lower border, rests on the diaphragm at about the 6th rib in the midclavicular line. Laterally lung tissue extends from the apex of the axilla down to the 7th or 8th rib. Posteriorly the location of C7 marks the apex of lung tissue, and T10 usually corresponds to the base. Deep inspiration expands the lungs, and their lower border drops to the level of T12.

Lobes of the Lungs

The lungs are paired but not precisely symmetric structures (Fig. 18-6). The right lung is shorter than the left lung because of the underlying liver. The left lung is narrower than the right lung because the heart bulges to the left. The right lung has three lobes, and the left lung has two lobes. These lobes are not arranged in horizontal bands like dessert layers in a parfait glass. Rather they stack in diagonal sloping segments and are separated by **fissures** that run obliquely through the chest.

Anterior. On the anterior chest the **oblique** (the major or diagonal) fissure crosses the 5th rib in the midaxillary line and terminates at the 6th rib in the midclavicular line. The right lung also contains the **horizontal** (minor) fissure, which divides the right upper and middle lobes. This fissure extends from the 5th rib in the right midaxillary line to the 3rd intercostal space or 4th rib at the right sternal border.

Posterior. The most remarkable point about the posterior chest is that it is almost all lower lobe (Fig. 18-7). The upper lobes occupy a smaller band of tissue from their apices at T1 down to T3 or T4. At this level the lower lobes begin, and their inferior border reaches down to the level of T10 on expiration and T12 on inspiration. Note that the right middle lobe does not project onto the posterior chest at all. If the person abducts the arms and places the hands on the back of

18-7

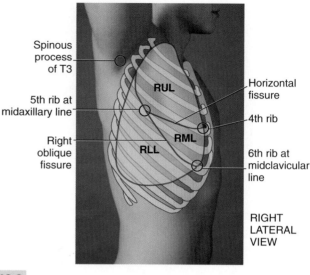

RIGHT
LATERAL
VIEW

18-8

the head, the division between the upper and lower lobes corresponds to the medial border of the scapulae.

Lateral. Laterally lung tissue extends from the apex of the axilla down to the 7th or 8th rib. The right upper lobe extends from the apex of the axilla down to the horizontal fissure at the 5th rib (Fig. 18-8). The right middle lobe extends from the horizontal fissure down and forward to the 6th rib at the midclavicular line. The right lower lobe continues from the 5th rib to the 8th rib in the midaxillary line.

The left lung contains only two lobes, upper and lower (Fig. 18-9). These are seen laterally as two triangular areas separated by the oblique fissure. The left upper lobe extends from the apex of the axilla down to the 5th rib at the midaxillary line. The left lower lobe continues down to the 8th rib in the midaxillary line.

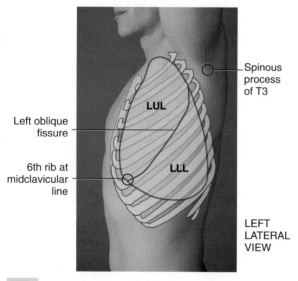

LEFT
LATERAL
VIEW

18-9

Using these landmarks, with a marker try to trace the outline of each lobe on a willing partner. Take special note of the three points that commonly confuse beginning examiners:

1. The left lung has no middle lobe.
2. The anterior chest contains mostly upper and middle lobe with very little lower lobe.
3. The posterior chest contains almost all lower lobe.

Pleurae

The thin, slippery **pleurae** are serous membranes that form an envelope between the lungs and the chest wall (Fig. 18-10). The **visceral** pleura lines the outside of the lungs, dipping down into the fissures. It is continuous with the **parietal** pleura lining the inside of the chest wall and diaphragm.

The inside of the envelope, the pleural cavity, is a potential space filled only with a few milliliters of lubricating fluid. It normally has a vacuum, or negative pressure, which holds the lungs tightly against the chest wall. The lungs slide smoothly and noiselessly up and down during respiration, lubricated by a few milliliters of fluid. Think of this as similar to two glass slides with a drop of water between them; although it is difficult to pull apart the slides, they slide smoothly back and forth. The pleurae extend approximately 3 cm below the level of the lungs, forming the **costodiaphragmatic recess.** This is a potential space; when it abnormally fills with air or fluid, it compromises lung expansion.

Trachea and Bronchial Tree

The **trachea** lies anterior to the esophagus and is 10 to 11 cm long in the adult. It begins at the level of the cricoid cartilage in the neck and bifurcates just below the sternal angle into the right and left main bronchi (Fig. 18-11). Posteriorly tracheal bifurcation is at the level of T4 or T5. The right main bronchus is shorter, wider, and more vertical than the left main bronchus.

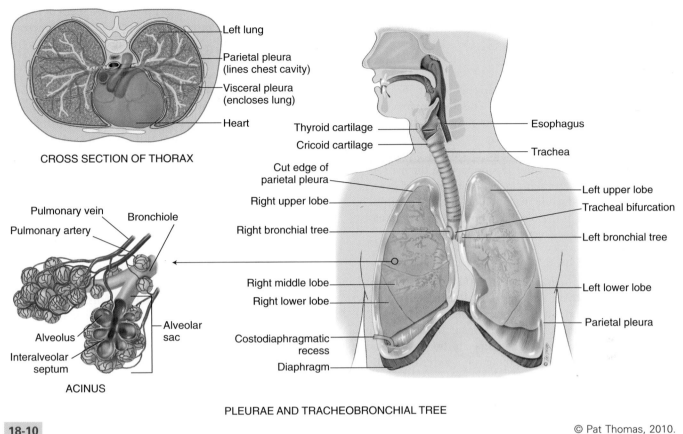

CROSS SECTION OF THORAX

- Left lung
- Parietal pleura (lines chest cavity)
- Visceral pleura (encloses lung)
- Heart

ACINUS

- Pulmonary vein
- Bronchiole
- Pulmonary artery
- Alveolus
- Alveolar sac
- Interalveolar septum

PLEURAE AND TRACHEOBRONCHIAL TREE

- Thyroid cartilage
- Cricoid cartilage
- Cut edge of parietal pleura
- Right upper lobe
- Right bronchial tree
- Right middle lobe
- Right lower lobe
- Costodiaphragmatic recess
- Diaphragm
- Esophagus
- Trachea
- Left upper lobe
- Tracheal bifurcation
- Left bronchial tree
- Left lower lobe
- Parietal pleura

18-10

© Pat Thomas, 2010.

The **trachea** and **bronchi** transport gases between the environment and the lung parenchyma. They constitute the *dead space,* or space that is filled with air but is not available for gaseous exchange. This is about 150 mL in the adult. The bronchial tree also protects alveoli from small particulate matter in the inhaled air. The bronchi are lined with goblet cells, which secrete mucus that entraps the particles, and cilia, which sweep particles upward where they can be swallowed or expelled.

An **acinus** is a functional respiratory unit that consists of the bronchioles, alveolar ducts, alveolar sacs, and the alveoli. Gaseous exchange occurs across the respiratory membrane in the alveolar duct and in the millions of alveoli. Note how the alveoli are clustered like grapes around each alveolar duct. This creates millions of interalveolar septa (walls) that increase tremendously the working space available for gas exchange. This bunched arrangement creates a surface area for gas exchange that is as large as a tennis court.

MECHANICS OF RESPIRATION

There are four major functions of the respiratory system: (1) supplying oxygen to the body for energy production; (2) removing carbon dioxide as a waste product of energy reactions; (3) maintaining homeostasis (acid-base balance) of arterial blood; and (4) maintaining heat exchange (less important in humans).

By supplying oxygen to the blood and eliminating excess carbon dioxide, respiration maintains the pH or the acid-base balance of the blood. The body tissues are bathed by blood that normally has a narrow acceptable range of pH. Although a number of compensatory mechanisms regulate the pH, the lungs help maintain the balance by adjusting the level of carbon dioxide through respiration. Hypoventilation (slow,

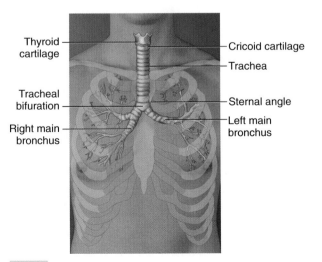

- Thyroid cartilage
- Tracheal bifuration
- Right main bronchus
- Cricoid cartilage
- Trachea
- Sternal angle
- Left main bronchus

18-11

© Pat Thomas, 2010.

shallow breathing) causes carbon dioxide to build up in the blood, and hyperventilation (rapid, deep breathing) causes carbon dioxide to be blown off.

Control of Respirations

Normally our breathing pattern changes without our awareness in response to cellular demands. This involuntary control of respirations is mediated by the respiratory center in the brainstem (pons and medulla). The major feedback loop is humoral regulation, or the change in carbon dioxide and oxygen levels in the blood and, less important, the hydrogen ion level. The *normal stimulus to breathe* for most of us is an increase of carbon dioxide in the blood, or **hypercapnia.** A decrease of oxygen in the blood (**hypoxemia**) also increases respirations but is less effective than hypercapnia.

Changing Chest Size

Respiration is the physical act of breathing; air rushes into the lungs as the chest size increases (inspiration) and is expelled from the lungs as the chest recoils (expiration). The mechanical expansion and contraction of the chest cavity alters the size of the thoracic container in two dimensions: (1) the vertical diameter lengthens or shortens, which is accomplished by downward or upward movement of the diaphragm; and (2) the anteroposterior (AP) diameter increases or decreases, which is accomplished by elevation or depression of the ribs (Fig. 18-12).

In inspiration increasing the size of the thoracic container creates a slightly negative pressure in relation to the atmosphere; therefore air rushes in to fill the partial vacuum. The major muscle responsible for this increase is the diaphragm. During inspiration contraction of the bell-shaped diaphragm causes it to descend and flatten. This lengthens the vertical diameter. Intercostal muscles lift the sternum and elevate the ribs, making them more horizontal. This increases the AP diameter.

Expiration is primarily passive. As the diaphragm relaxes, elastic forces within the lung, chest cage, and abdomen cause it to dome up. All this squeezing creates a relatively positive pressure within the alveoli, and the air flows out.

Forced inspiration such as that after heavy exercise or occurring pathologically with respiratory distress commands the use of the accessory neck muscles to heave up the sternum and rib cage. These neck muscles are the sternomastoids, the scaleni, and the trapezii. In forced expiration the abdominal muscles contract powerfully to push the abdominal viscera

Sternomastoid
(elevate sternum)

Scalenus muscles
(elevate upper ribs)

External intercostals
(elevate ribs)

Diaphragm
descends as it
contracts

Increased
vertical diameter

Increased A-P diameter

INSPIRATION

Internal intercostals
(depress ribs)

External oblique and
abdominal rectus
(depress lower ribs and
compress viscera)

EXPIRATION

18-12

©Pat Thomas, 2006.

forcefully in and up against the diaphragm, making it dome upward and squeeze against the lungs.

◆ DEVELOPMENTAL COMPETENCE

Infants and Children

During the first 5 weeks of fetal life the primitive lung bud emerges; by 16 weeks the conducting airways reach the same number as in the adult; at 32 weeks **surfactant,** the complex lipid substance needed for sustained inflation of the air sacs, is present in adequate amounts; and by birth the lungs have 70 million primitive alveoli ready to start the job of respiration.

Breath is life. When the newborn inhales the first breath, the lusty cry that follows reassures straining parents that their baby is all right (Fig. 18-13). The baby's body systems all develop in utero, but the respiratory system alone does not function until birth. Birth demands its instant performance.

When the cord is cut, blood is cut off from the placenta, and it gushes into the pulmonary circulation. Respiratory development continues throughout childhood, with increases in diameter and length of airways and in size and number of alveoli, reaching the adult range of 300 million by adolescence.

The relatively smaller size and immaturity of children's pulmonary systems and the presence of parents and caregivers who smoke result in enormous vulnerability and increased risks to child health. Prenatal exposure to smoke causes chronic hypoxia, premature delivery, and low birth weight. It also sensitizes the fetal brain to nicotine, which increases risk for addiction when the child is exposed to nicotine at a later age.[3] Prenatal and postnatal exposure to secondhand tobacco smoke leads to sudden infant death syndrome (SIDS), lower respiratory illnesses, acute and chronic otitis media, breathlessness, asthma, and adverse lung function throughout childhood.[3,23] Prenatal nicotine exposure increases risk for attention-deficit/hyperactivity disorder (ADHD) and depression in children and adolescents.[5]

The Pregnant Woman

The enlarging uterus elevates the diaphragm 4 cm during pregnancy. This decreases the vertical diameter of the thoracic cage, but this decrease is compensated for by an increase in the horizontal diameter. The increase in estrogen level relaxes the chest cage ligaments. This allows an increase in the transverse diameter of the chest cage by 2 cm, and the costal angle widens. The total circumference of the chest cage increases by 6 cm. Although the diaphragm is elevated, it is not fixed. It moves with breathing even more during pregnancy, which results in a 40% increase in tidal volume.[19]

The growing fetus increases the oxygen demand on the mother's body. This is met easily by the increasing tidal volume (deeper breathing). Little change occurs in the respiratory rate. An increased awareness of the need to breathe develops early in pregnancy. This **physiologic dyspnea** affects close to 75% of women; does not alter activities of daily living; and is not associated with cough, wheezing, or exercise.[7]

18-13

The Aging Adult

The costal cartilages become calcified; thus the thorax is less mobile. Respiratory muscle strength declines after age 50 years and continues to decrease into the 70s. A more significant change is the decrease in elastic properties within the lungs, making them less distensible and lessening their tendency to collapse and recoil. In all, the aging lung is a more rigid structure that is harder to inflate.

These changes result in an increase in small airway closure, which yields a *decreased vital capacity* (the maximum amount of air that a person can expel from the lungs after first filling the lungs to maximum) and an *increased residual volume* (the amount of air remaining in the lungs even after the most forceful expiration).

With aging, histologic changes (i.e., a gradual loss of intra-alveolar septa and a decreased number of alveoli) also occur; therefore less surface area is available for gas exchange. In addition, the lung bases become less ventilated as a result of closing off of a number of airways. This increases the older person's risk for dyspnea with exertion beyond his or her usual workload.

The histologic changes also increase the older person's risk for postoperative pulmonary complications. He or she has a greater risk for postoperative atelectasis and infection from a decreased ability to cough, a loss of protective airway reflexes, and increased secretions.

◆ CULTURE AND GENETICS

The incidence of **tuberculosis (TB)** has declined for the 20th consecutive year in the United States; however, people who are foreign-born and of racial/ethnic minorities have a disproportionately large burden of TB disease.[12] In 2012 the TB rate was 11.5 times higher in the foreign-born than in people born in the United States. When compared with non-Hispanic Whites, TB rates were 25 times higher in Asians, 6.6 times higher in Hispanics, and 7.3 times higher in Blacks. These data reflect high TB rates in countries of origin for U.S.

Subjective Data

immigrants, as well as barriers to early diagnosis, prevention, and treatment adherence for latent TB infection in some racial groups. The global effects of TB are ravaging, with 8.7 million new cases of active TB worldwide in 2011.[40] The incidence of multidrug-resistant TB also is increasing, especially in China, India, Russia, Pakistan, and South Africa.

The number of people with **asthma** has increased every year in the United States since 2001, to a prevalence of 8.4% in 2011.[11] Prevalence increased in all racial/ethnic groups: in Whites the prevalence increased to 7.8% in 2010; among Blacks it increased to 11.9%; among Hispanics it rose to 7.2%, and it is more prevalent in lower income families. Asthma is the most common chronic disease in childhood, with a prevalence of 9.5% in children ages 0 to 17 years.

Regarding asthma-related problems and medical care use, African Americans, Hispanics, and especially American Indians experience more than do Whites or Asians. When compared with White children, African American and Hispanic children have more indicators of poorly controlled asthma, including more emergency department visits, more daily rescue medication use, and lower use of inhaled corticosteroids.[18] Extrinsic/allergic (or pediatric-onset) asthma involves a complex interaction between genetic susceptibility (bronchial hyperresponsiveness, atopy, elevated immunoglobulin E)[30] and environmental factors (viral respiratory infections, air pollution). Long-term exposure to traffic-related air pollution increases risk for allergic disease in children, as shown from global evidence in China and India.[9]

SUBJECTIVE DATA

1. Cough
2. Shortness of breath
3. Chest pain with breathing

4. History of respiratory infections
5. Smoking history

6. Environmental exposure
7. Patient-centered care

Examiner Asks	Rationale
1. Cough. Do you have a **cough?** When did it start? Gradual or sudden? • How long have you had it? • How often do you cough? At any special time of day or just on arising? Cough wake you up at night?	Acute cough lasts less than 2 or 3 weeks; chronic cough lasts over 2 months. Conditions with characteristic timing of cough: (1) continuous throughout day—acute illness (e.g., respiratory infection); (2) afternoon/evening—may be exposure to irritants at work; (3) night—postnasal drip, sinusitis; (4) early morning—chronic bronchial inflammation of smokers.
• Do you cough up any phlegm or sputum? How much? What color is it?	Chronic bronchitis has a history of productive cough for 3 months of the year for 2 years in a row.
• Cough up any blood? Does it look like streaks or frank blood? Does the sputum have a foul odor?	**Hemoptysis.** Some conditions have characteristic sputum production: (1) white or clear mucoid—colds, bronchitis, viral infections; (2) yellow or green—bacterial infections; (3) rust colored—TB, pneumococcal pneumonia; (4) pink, frothy—pulmonary edema, some sympathomimetic medications have a side effect of pink-tinged mucus.
• How would you describe your cough: hacking, dry, barking, hoarse, congested, bubbling?	Some conditions have a characteristic cough: mycoplasma pneumonia—hacking; early heart failure—dry; croup—barking; colds, bronchitis, pneumonia—congested.
• Does the cough seem to come with anything: activity, position (lying), fever, congestion, talking, anxiety? • Does activity make it better or worse?	

Examiner Asks	Rationale

- Which treatment have you tried? Prescription or over-the-counter medications, vaporizer, rest, position change?
- Does the cough bring on anything: chest pain, ear pain? Is it tiring? Are you concerned about it?

Assess the effectiveness of coping strategies.
Note severity.

2. **Shortness of breath.** Are you having any **shortness of breath** now? Within the last day, have you been short of breath?

In hospitalized patients **dyspnea** is a common symptom and a predictor of adverse outcomes.[1]

- Ever had any shortness of breath or hard-breathing spells? When did it start? What brings it on? How severe is it? How long does it last?

Determine how much activity precipitates the shortness of breath (SOB)—state specific number of blocks walked, number of stairs. Chronic dyspnea is SOB lasting >1 month and may have neurogenic, respiratory, or cardiac origin. It also occurs with anemia, anxiety, and deconditioning[36] (see Table 18-7, p. 448, for the differential diagnosis of dyspnea and its findings).

- Is it affected by position such as lying down?

Orthopnea is difficulty breathing when supine. State number of pillows needed to achieve comfort (e.g., "two-pillow orthopnea").

- Occur at any specific time of day or night?

Paroxysmal nocturnal dyspnea is awakening from sleep with SOB and needing to be upright to achieve comfort.

- SOB episodes associated with night sweats?
- Or cough, chest pain, or bluish color around lips or nails? Wheezing sound?
- Episodes seem to be related to food, pollen, dust, animals, season, emotion, or exercise?

Diaphoresis.
Cyanosis signals hypoxia.

Asthma attacks may occur with a specific allergen or extreme cold, anxiety. Asthma often described as "chest tightness."

- What do you do in a hard-breathing attack? Take a special position or use pursed-lip breathing? Use any oxygen, inhalers, or medications?
- How does the SOB affect your work or home activities? Getting better or worse or staying about the same?

Assess effect of coping strategies and the need for more teaching.
Assess effect on activities of daily living.

Note to examiner: For people with a smoking history, dyspnea, and cough, you can use the short 5-item Lung Function Questionnaire to identify who should be assessed with spirometry for chronic obstructive pulmonary disease (COPD) (see p. 424).

3. **Chest pain with breathing.** Any **chest pain with breathing?** Please point to the exact location.
   - When did it start? Constant, or does it come and go?
   - Describe the pain: burning, stabbing?
   - Brought on by respiratory infection, coughing, or trauma? Is it associated with fever, deep breathing, unequal chest inflation?
   - What have you done to treat it? Medication or heat application?

Chest pain of thoracic origin occurs with muscle soreness from coughing or from inflammation of pleura overlying pneumonia. Distinguish this from chest pain of cardiac origin (see Chapter 19) or heartburn of stomach acid.

4. **History of respiratory infections.** Any **past history** of breathing trouble or lung diseases such as bronchitis, emphysema, asthma, pneumonia?
   - Any unusually frequent or unusually severe colds?

Consider sequelae after these conditions.

Because most people have had some colds, it is more meaningful to ask about excess number or severity.

   - Any family history of allergies, tuberculosis, or asthma?

Assess possible risk factors.

Subjective Data

5. **Smoking history**. Do you **smoke** cigarettes or cigars? At what age did you start? How many packs per day do you smoke now? For how long?

State number of packs per day and number of years smoked.

- Have you ever tried to quit? What helped? Why do you think it did not work? What activities do you associate with smoking?
- Live with someone who smokes?

Note to examiner: Depending on the person's stage of readiness to quit smoking, you can offer counseling and encouragement using the five *As:*[13,32]

Most people already know they should quit smoking. Instead of admonishing, assess smoking behavior and ways to modify daily smoking activities, identify triggers, and how to manage withdrawal.

Ask about his or her tobacco use status at every visit and record the person's response.

Advise Give clear, nonjudgmental, and personalized suggestions for quitting. "I understand that quitting is difficult and challenging, but it is the most important thing you can do for your own health and for your family."

Assess each person's readiness for and interest in quitting. The response will affect the next step. If he or she is willing to quit, you'll offer resources and assistance. If not, you'll help the person determine the barriers to cessation.

Assist each person with a specific cessation plan that includes medications, behavioral modification, exercise programs, or referrals. Encourage to pick a quit date and give support and feedback.

Arrange follow-up visits. If relapse occurs, state that you are there to help start over again. Remind that quitting takes practice and often does not happen in the first attempt.[32]

6. **Environmental exposure**. Are there any **environmental conditions** that may affect your breathing? Where do you work? At a factory, chemical plant, coal mine, farming, outdoors in a heavy traffic area?

Traffic-related air pollution increases risk of allergic rhinitis and asthma.

Farmers may be at risk for grain or pesticide inhalation. People in rural Midwest have risk for histoplasmosis exposure; those in Southwest and Mexico have risk for coccidioidomycosis. Coal miners have risk for pneumoconiosis. Stone cutters, miners, and potters have risk for silicosis. Other irritants: asbestos, radon.

- Do you do anything to protect your lungs such as wear a mask or have the ventilatory system checked at work? Do you do anything to monitor your exposure? Do you have periodic examinations, pulmonary function tests, x-ray image?
- Do you know which specific symptoms to note that may signal breathing problems?

Assess **self-care** measures.

General symptoms: cough, SOB. Some gases produce specific symptoms: carbon monoxide—dizziness, headache, fatigue; sulfur dioxide—cough, congestion.

7. **Patient-centered care**. Last TB skin test, chest x-ray study, pneumonia vaccine or influenza immunization?

"Flu" vaccine is modified annually. The CDC recommends annual flu vaccine for everyone age 6 months or older, especially important for those at high risk of flu complications, including pregnant women, older adults and young children, those with chronic medical conditions, residents of nursing homes and group care, health care workers, and those who are immunosuppressed.

Examiner Asks	Rationale

Additional History for Infants and Children

1. Has the child had any frequent or very severe colds?

Limit of 4 to 6 uncomplicated upper respiratory infections per year is expected in early childhood.

2. Is there any history of allergy in the family?
   - For child younger than 2 years: At what age were new foods introduced? Was the child breastfed or bottle-fed?

Consider new foods or formula as possible allergens. Full breastfeeding for ≥6 months reduces risk for respiratory tract infection and otitis media.[14]

3. Does the child have a cough? Seem congested? Have noisy breathing or wheezing? (Further questions similar to those listed in the section on adults.)

Screen for onset and follow course of childhood chronic respiratory problems: asthma, bronchitis.

4. Which measures have you taken to child-proof your home? Yard? Is there any possibility of the child inhaling or swallowing toxic substances? Has anyone reviewed with you the small things that are choking hazards (e.g., nuts, pins, seed, beans, corn, pen cover, toy pieces, hard candy, paper clip)?
   - Has anyone taught you emergency care measures in case of accidental choking or a hard-breathing spell?

Young child especially <3 years is at risk for foreign body aspiration, poisoning, and injury.

Assess knowledge level of parent and caregivers.

5. Any smokers in the home or in the car with child?

Environmental smoke increases the risk for acute and chronic ear and respiratory infections in children.[3,23]

Additional History for the Aging Adult

1. Have you noticed any shortness of breath or fatigue with your daily activities?

Older adults have a less efficient respiratory system (decreased vital capacity, less surface area for gas exchange); thus they have less tolerance for activity.

2. Tell me about your usual amount of physical activity.

May have reduced exercise capacity because of pulmonary function deficits.
Sedentary or bedridden people are at risk for respiratory dysfunction.

3. For those with a history of COPD, lung cancer, or TB: How are you getting along each day? Any weight change in the past 3 months? How much?
   - How about energy level? Do you tire more easily? How does your illness affect you at home? At work?

Assess coping strategies.

Activities may decrease because of increasing shortness of breath or pain.

4. Do you have any chest pain with breathing?
   - Any chest pain after a bout of coughing? After a fall?

Some older adults feel pleuritic pain less intensely than younger adults.
Precisely localized sharp pain (points to it with one finger)—consider fractured rib or muscle injury.

For people with a frequent productive cough and/or a long smoking history, use the following questionnaire. This is a simple, short tool to identify persons who will need spirometry testing to confirm the diagnosis of COPD.[24]

Examiner Asks	Rationale

Lung Function Questionnaire

Do you suffer from breathing problems and/or frequent cough?

These questions ask about your breathing problems and/or frequent cough. As you answer these questions, think about how you feel physically when you experience these symptoms. For each question, choose the one answer that best describes your symptoms. Share the answers with your healthcare provider.

Step 1: Answer each question and write the score in the box next to it.
Step 2: Add together the scores in each box to get your total score.
Step 3: Take the test to your provider to talk about your score.

1. How often do you cough up mucus?

| Never | (5) | Rarely | (4) | Sometimes | (3) | Often | (2) | Very often | (1) | SCORE |

2. How often does your chest sound noisy (wheezy, whistling, rattling) when you breathe?

| Never | (5) | Rarely | (4) | Sometimes | (3) | Often | (2) | Very often | (1) | |

3. How often do you experience shortness of breath during physical activity (walking up a flight of stairs or walking up an incline without stopping to rest)?

| Never | (5) | Rarely | (4) | Sometimes | (3) | Often | (2) | Very often | (1) | |

4. How many years have you smoked?

| Never smoked | (5) | 10 years or less | (4) | 11-20 years | (3) | 21-30 years | (2) | More than 30 years | (1) | |

5. What is your age?

| Less than 40 years | (5) | 40-49 years | (4) | 50-59 years | (3) | 60-69 years | (2) | 70 years or older | (1) | |

Step 4: If your score is 18 or less, you may be at risk for Chronic Obstructive Pulmonary Disease (COPD). COPD includes chronic bronchitis, emphysema, or both. TOTAL

OBJECTIVE DATA

PREPARATION

Ask the person to sit upright. Ask a man to disrobe to the waist. Ask a woman to leave the gown on and open at the back; when examining the anterior chest, lift up the gown and drape it on her shoulders rather than removing it completely. This promotes comfort by giving her the feeling of being somewhat clothed. These provisions ensure further comfort: a warm room, a warm diaphragm endpiece, and a private examination time with no interruptions.

For smooth choreography in a complete examination, begin the respiratory examination just after palpating the thyroid gland when you are standing behind the person. Perform the inspection, palpation, percussion, and auscultation on the posterior and lateral thorax. Then move to face the person and repeat the four maneuvers on the anterior chest. This avoids repetitiously moving front to back around the person.

Finally clean your stethoscope endpiece with an alcohol wipe. Because your stethoscope touches many people, it is a possible vector for both aerobic and anaerobic bacteria. Cleaning with an alcohol wipe is very effective.

EQUIPMENT NEEDED

Stethoscope
Small ruler, marked in centimeters
Marking pen
Alcohol wipe

Normal Range of Findings	Abnormal Findings

Inspect the Posterior Chest

Thoracic Cage

Note the **shape and configuration** of the chest wall. The spinous processes should appear in a straight line. The thorax is symmetric, in an elliptical shape, with downward sloping ribs, about 45 degrees relative to the spine. The scapulae are placed symmetrically in each hemithorax.

Skeletal deformities may limit thoracic cage excursion: scoliosis, kyphosis (see Table 18-3, Configurations of the Thorax, p. 442).

Normal Range of Findings	Abnormal Findings

The anteroposterior (AP) diameter should be less than the transverse diameter. The ratio of AP to transverse diameter is about 0.70 to 0.75 in adults, and it increases with age.

AP = transverse diameter, or "barrel chest." Ribs are horizontal, chest appears as if held in continuous inspiration. This occurs in COPD from hyperinflation of the lungs (see Table 18-3).

The neck and trapezius muscles should be developed normally for age and occupation.

Neck muscles are hypertrophied in COPD from aiding in forced respirations across the obstructed airways.

Note the **position** the person takes to breathe. This includes a relaxed posture and the ability to support one's own weight with arms comfortably at the sides or in the lap.

People with COPD often sit in a tripod position, leaning forward with arms braced against their knees, chair, or bed. This gives them leverage so the abdominal, intercostal, and neck muscles all can aid in expiration.

Assess the **skin color** and **condition.** Color should be consistent with person's genetic background, with allowance for sun-exposed areas on the chest and the back. No cyanosis or pallor should be present. Note any lesions. Inquire about any change in a nevus on the back (e.g., where the person may have difficulty monitoring) (see Chapter 12).

Cyanosis occurs with tissue hypoxia.

Palpate the Posterior Chest

Symmetric Expansion

Confirm **symmetric chest expansion** by placing your warmed hands sideways on the posterolateral chest wall with thumbs pointing together at the level of T9 or T10. Slide your hands medially to pinch up a small fold of skin between your thumbs (Fig. 18-14).

Ask the person to take a deep breath. Your hands serve as mechanical amplifiers; as the person inhales deeply, your thumbs should move apart symmetrically. Note any lag in expansion.

Unequal chest expansion occurs with marked atelectasis, lobar pneumonia, pleural effusion, thoracic trauma such as fractured ribs, or pneumothorax.

Pain accompanies deep breathing when the pleurae are inflamed.

18-14

Normal Range of Findings	Abnormal Findings

Tactile Fremitus

Assess **tactile** (or **vocal**) **fremitus.** Fremitus is a palpable vibration. Sounds generated from the larynx are transmitted through patent bronchi and the lung parenchyma to the chest wall, where you feel them as vibrations.

Use either the palmar base (the ball) of the fingers or the ulnar edge of one hand and touch the person's chest while he or she repeats the words "ninety-nine" or "blue moon." These are resonant phrases that generate strong vibrations. Start over the lung apices and palpate from one side to another (Fig. 18-15).

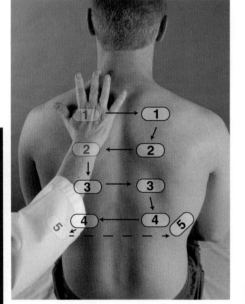

18-15

Symmetry is most important; the vibrations should feel the same in the corresponding area on each side. Avoid palpating over the scapulae because bone damps out sound transmission.

The following factors affect the intensity of tactile fremitus:
- Fremitus is most prominent between the scapulae and around the sternum, sites where the major bronchi are closest to the chest wall. It normally decreases as you progress down because more and more tissue impedes sound transmission.
- Fremitus feels greater over a thin chest wall than over an obese or heavily muscular one where thick tissue damps the vibration.
- A loud, low-pitched voice generates more fremitus than a soft, high-pitched one.

Note any areas of abnormal fremitus. Sound is conducted better through a uniformly dense structure than through a porous one, which changes in shape and solidity (as does the lung tissue during normal respiration). Thus conditions that increase the density of lung tissue make a better conducting medium for sound vibrations and increase tactile fremitus.

Asymmetric findings suggest dysfunction that you can assess further with the stethoscope.

Decreased fremitus occurs with obstructed bronchus, pleural effusion or thickening, pneumothorax, or emphysema. Any barrier that comes between the sound and your palpating hand decreases fremitus.

Increased fremitus occurs with compression or consolidation of lung tissue (e.g., lobar pneumonia). This is present only when the bronchus is patent and the consolidation extends to the lung surface. Note that only gross changes increase fremitus. Small areas of early pneumonia do not significantly affect it.

Rhonchal fremitus is palpable with thick bronchial secretions.

Pleural friction fremitus is palpable with inflammation of the pleura (see Table 18-5, Abnormal Tactile Fremitus, p. 445).

Normal Range of Findings

Using the fingers, gently **palpate the entire chest wall.** This enables you to note any areas of tenderness, to note skin temperature and moisture, to detect any superficial lumps or masses, and to explore any skin lesions noted on inspection.

Percuss the Posterior Chest

Lung Fields

Determine the **predominant note over the lung fields.** Start at the apices and percuss the band of normally resonant tissue across the tops of both shoulders (Fig. 18-16). Then, percussing in the interspaces, make a side-to-side comparison all the way down the lung region. Percuss at 5-cm intervals. Avoid the damping effect of the scapulae and ribs.

18-16 Sequence for percussion.

Resonance is the low-pitched, clear, hollow sound that predominates in healthy lung tissue in the adult (Fig. 18-17). However, resonance is a relative term and has no constant standard. The resonant note may be duller in the athlete with a heavily muscular chest wall and in the heavily obese adult in whom subcutaneous fat produces scattered dullness.

Abnormal Findings

Crepitus is a coarse, crackling sensation palpable over the skin surface. It occurs in subcutaneous emphysema when air escapes from the lung and enters the subcutaneous tissue, as after open thoracic injury or surgery.

Asymmetry is important: one side with prominent dullness or marked hyperresonance indicates underlying disease. **Hyperresonance** is a lower-pitched, booming sound found when too much air is present such as in emphysema or pneumothorax.

A **dull** note (soft, muffled thud) signals abnormal density in the lungs, as with pneumonia, pleural effusion, atelectasis, or tumor.

Objective Data

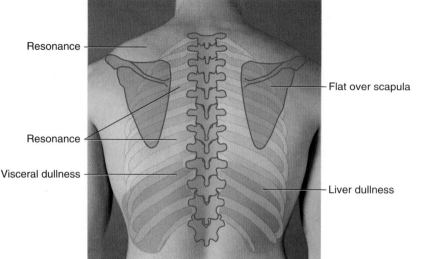

Resonance

Flat over scapula

Resonance

Visceral dullness

Liver dullness

18-17 Expected percussion notes.

The depth of penetration of percussion has limits. Percussion sets into motion only the outer 5 to 7 cm of tissue. It does not penetrate to reveal any change in density deeper than that. In addition, an abnormal finding must be 2 to 3 cm wide to yield an abnormal percussion note. Lesions smaller than that are not detectable by percussion.

Diaphragmatic Excursion

Determine **diaphragmatic excursion** (Fig. 18-18, A). Percuss to map out the lower lung border in both expiration and inspiration. First ask the person to "exhale and hold it" briefly while you percuss down the scapular line until the sound changes from resonant to dull on each side. This estimates the level of the diaphragm separating the lungs from the abdominal viscera. It may be somewhat higher on the right side (about 1 to 2 cm) because of the presence of the liver. Mark the spot.

Now ask the person to "take a deep breath and hold it." Continue percussing down from your first mark and mark the level where the sound changes to dull on this deep inspiration. Measure the vertical difference. This diaphragmatic excursion should be equal bilaterally and measure about 3 to 5 cm in adults, although it may be up to 7 to 8 cm in well-conditioned people (Fig. 18-18, B).

Note an abnormally high level of dullness and absence of excursion. These occur with pleural effusion (fluid in the space between the visceral and parietal pleura) or atelectasis of the lower lobes.

Resonant

Dull

A

B

18-18

Normal Range of Findings	Abnormal Findings

When you are a beginning examiner, you become so involved in the subtle differences of percussion notes that you extend the patient's limits of breath-holding. Always hold your own breath when you ask your patient to do so. When you run out of air, the other person certainly has also, especially if that person has a respiratory problem.

Auscultate the Posterior Chest

The passage of air through the tracheobronchial tree creates a characteristic set of sounds that are audible through the chest wall.

> Breath sounds are changed by obstruction in the passageways or by disease in the lung parenchyma, the pleura, or the chest wall.

Breath Sounds

Evaluate the presence and quality of **normal breath sounds.** The person is sitting, leaning forward slightly, with arms resting comfortably across the lap. Instruct the person to breathe through the mouth, a little bit deeper than usual, but to stop if he or she begins to feel dizzy. Be careful to monitor the breathing throughout the examination, and offer times for the person to rest and breathe normally. The person is usually willing to comply with your instructions in an effort to please you and be a "good patient." Watch that he or she does not hyperventilate to the point of fainting.

Clean the flat diaphragm endpiece of the stethoscope and hold it firmly on the person's chest wall. Listen to at least one full respiration in each location. Side-to-side comparison is most important.

Do not confuse background noise with lung sounds. Become familiar with these extraneous noises that may be confused with lung pathology if not recognized:
1. Examiner's breathing on stethoscope tubing
2. Stethoscope tubing bumping together
3. Patient shivering
4. Patient's hairy chest: movement of hairs under stethoscope sounds like crackles (rales)—minimize this by pressing harder or by wetting the hair with a damp cloth
5. Rustling of paper gown or paper drapes

> Crackles are abnormal lung sounds (see Table 18-6, Adventitious Lung Sounds, p. 446).

While standing behind the person, listen to the following lung areas: posterior from the apices at C7 to the bases (around T10) and laterally from the axilla down to the 7th or 8th rib. Use the sequence illustrated in Fig. 18-19.

18-19

Normal Range of Findings

Continue to visualize approximate locations of the lobes of each lung so you correlate your findings to anatomic areas. As you listen, think (1) what AM I hearing over this spot? and (2) what should I EXPECT to be hearing? You should expect to hear three types of normal breath sounds in the adult and older child: **bronchial** (sometimes called *tracheal* or *tubular*), **bronchovesicular,** and **vesicular.** Study the description of the characteristics of these normal breath sounds in Table 18-1.

Abnormal Findings

TABLE 18-1   Characteristics of Normal Breath Sounds

	PITCH	AMPLITUDE	DURATION	QUALITY	NORMAL LOCATION
BRONCHIAL (TRACHEAL)	High	Loud	Inspiration < expiration	Harsh, hollow tubular	Trachea and larynx
BRONCHOVESICULAR	Moderate	Moderate	Inspiration = expiration	Mixed	Over major bronchi where fewer alveoli are located: posterior, between scapulae especially on right; anterior, around upper sternum in 1st and 2nd intercostal spaces
VESICULAR	Low	Soft	Inspiration > expiration	Rustling, like the sound of the wind in the trees	Over peripheral lung fields where air flows through smaller bronchioles and alveoli

Note the normal location of the three types of breath sounds on the chest wall of the adult and older child (Figs. 18-20 and 18-21).

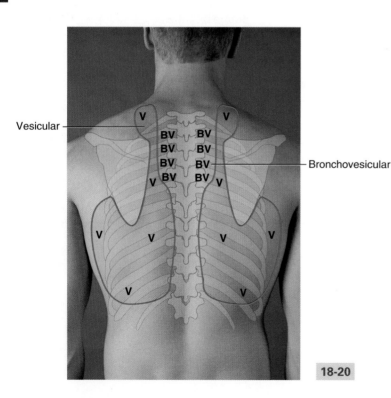

Vesicular

Bronchovesicular

18-20

Decreased or **absent breath sounds** occur:

1. When the bronchial tree is obstructed at some point by secretions, mucus plug, or a foreign body
2. In emphysema as a result of loss of elasticity in the lung fibers and decreased force of inspired air; the lungs also are already hyperinflated, so the inhaled air does not make as much noise
3. When anything obstructs transmission of sound between the lung and your stethoscope such as pleurisy or pleural thickening or air (pneumothorax) or fluid (pleural effusion) in the pleural space

A silent chest means that no air is moving in or out; an ominous sign.

Normal Range of Findings	Abnormal Findings

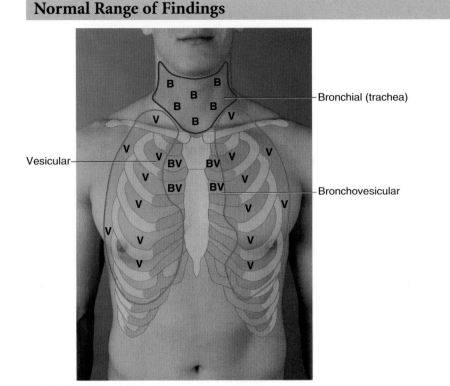

Vesicular —
Bronchial (trachea)
Bronchovesicular

18-21

Adventitious Sounds

Note the presence of any **adventitious sounds.** These are added sounds that are *not* normally heard in the lungs. If present, they are heard as being superimposed on the breath sounds. They are caused by moving air colliding with secretions in the tracheobronchial passageways or by the popping open of previously deflated airways. Sources differ as to the classification and nomenclature of these sounds (see Table 18-6, p. 446), but **crackles** (or rales) and **wheeze** (or rhonchi) are terms commonly used by most examiners. If you hear adventitious sounds, describe them as inspiratory versus expiratory, loudness, pitch, and location on the chest wall.

One type of adventitious sound, **atelectatic crackles,** is not pathologic. They are short, popping, crackling sounds that last only a few breaths. When sections of alveoli are not fully aerated (as in sleepers or in older adults), they deflate slightly and accumulate secretions. Crackles are heard when these sections are expanded by a few deep breaths. Atelectatic crackles are heard only in the periphery, usually in dependent portions of the lungs, and disappear after the first few breaths or after a cough.

Voice Sounds

The spoken voice can be auscultated over the chest wall just as it can be felt in tactile fremitus described earlier. Normal voice transmission is soft, muffled, and indistinct; you can hear sound through the stethoscope but cannot distinguish exactly what is being said. Pathology that increases lung density enhances transmission of voice sounds.

Voice sounds are not elicited routinely. Rather these are supplemental maneuvers performed if you suspect lung pathology on the basis of earlier data. When they are performed, you are testing for the possible presence of **bronchophony, egophony,** and **whispered pectoriloquy** (see Table 18-8, p. 449).

Increased breath sounds mean that sounds are louder than they should be (e.g., bronchial sounds are abnormal when they are heard over an abnormal location, the peripheral lung fields). They have a high-pitched, tubular quality, with a prolonged expiratory phase and a distinct pause between inspiration and expiration. They sound very close to your stethoscope, as if they were right *in* the tubing close to your ear. They occur when consolidation (e.g., pneumonia) or compression (e.g., fluid in the intrapleural space) yields a dense lung area that enhances the transmission of sound from the bronchi. When the inspired air reaches the alveoli, it hits solid lung tissue that conducts sound more efficiently to the surface.

Crackles are discontinuous popping sounds heard over inspiration; **wheezes** are continuous musical sounds heard mainly over expiration. Study Table 18-6 for a complete description of these and other abnormal adventitious breath sounds.

Consolidation or compression of lung tissue will enhance the voice sounds, making the words more distinct.

Objective Data

Normal Range of Findings	Abnormal Findings

Inspect the Anterior Chest

Note the **shape and configuration** of the chest wall. The ribs are sloping downward with symmetric interspaces. The costal angle is within 90 degrees. Development of abdominal muscles is as expected for the person's age, weight, and athletic condition.

Note the person's **facial expression.** The facial expression should be relaxed and benign, indicating an unconscious effort of breathing.

Barrel chest has horizontal ribs and costal angle >90 degrees.

Hypertrophy of abdominal muscles occurs in chronic emphysema.

Tense, strained, tired facies and purse-lipped breathing (the lips in a whistling position) accompany COPD. By exhaling slowly and against a narrow opening, the pressure in the bronchial tree remains positive, and fewer airways collapse.

Assess the **level of consciousness.** The level of consciousness should be alert and cooperative.

Note skin **color and condition.** The lips and nail beds are free of cyanosis or unusual pallor. The nails are of normal configuration. Explore any skin lesions.

Cerebral hypoxia may be reflected by excessive drowsiness or anxiety, restlessness, and irritability.

Clubbing of distal phalanx occurs with COPD because of growth of vascular connective tissue.

Cutaneous angiomas (spider nevi) associated with liver disease or portal hypertension may be evident on the chest.

Assess the quality of **respirations.** Normal relaxed breathing is automatic and effortless, regular and even, and produces no noise. The chest expands symmetrically with each inspiration. Note any localized lag on inspiration.

Noisy breathing occurs with severe asthma or chronic bronchitis.

Unequal chest expansion occurs when part of the lung is obstructed (pneumonia) or collapsed or when guarding to avoid postoperative or pleurisy pain.

No retraction or bulging of the interspaces should occur on inspiration.

Retraction suggests obstruction of respiratory tract or that increased inspiratory effort is needed, as with atelectasis. Bulging indicates trapped air as in the forced expiration associated with emphysema or asthma.

Normally accessory muscles are not used to augment respiratory effort. However, with very heavy exercise the accessory neck muscles (scalene, sternomastoid, trapezius) are used momentarily to enhance inspiration.

Accessory muscles are used in acute airway obstruction and massive atelectasis.

Rectus abdominis and internal intercostal muscles are used to force expiration in COPD.

The respiratory rate is within normal limits for the person's age (see Table 9-2, p. 136), and the pattern of breathing is regular. Occasional sighs normally punctuate breathing.

Tachypnea and hyperventilation, bradypnea and hypoventilation, periodic breathing (see Table 18-4, Respiratory Patterns, p. 444).

Palpate the Anterior Chest

Palpate **symmetric chest expansion.** Place your hands on the anterolateral wall with the thumbs along the costal margins and pointing toward the xiphoid process (Fig. 18-22).

Abnormally wide costal angle with little inspiratory variation occurs with emphysema.

Objective Data

Normal Range of Findings	Abnormal Findings

18-22

Ask the person to take a deep breath. Watch your thumbs move apart symmetrically and note smooth chest expansion with your fingers. Any limitation in thoracic expansion is easier to detect on the anterior chest because greater range of motion exists with breathing here.

A lag in expansion occurs with atelectasis, pneumonia, and postoperative guarding.

A palpable grating sensation with breathing indicates pleural friction fremitus (see Table 18-5, p. 445).

Assess **tactile (vocal) fremitus.** Begin palpating over the lung apices in the supraclavicular areas (Fig. 18-23). Compare vibrations from one side to the other as the person repeats "ninety-nine." Avoid palpating over female breast tissue because breast tissue normally damps the sound.

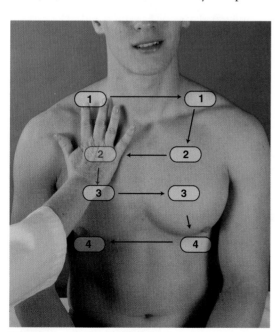

18-23 Assess tactile fremitus.

Normal Range of Findings	Abnormal Findings

Palpate the anterior chest wall to note any tenderness (normally none is present) and detect any superficial lumps or masses (again, normally none are present). Note skin mobility and turgor and skin temperature and moisture.

If any lumps are found in the breast tissue, refer the patient to a specialist.

Percuss the Anterior Chest

Begin percussing the apices in the supraclavicular areas. Then, percussing the interspaces and comparing one side with the other, move down the anterior chest.

Interspaces are easier to palpate on the anterior chest than on the back. Do not percuss directly over female breast tissue because this would produce a dull note. Shift the breast tissue over slightly, using the edge of your stationary hand. In females with large breasts, percussion may yield little useful data. With all people use the sequence illustrated in Fig. 18-24.

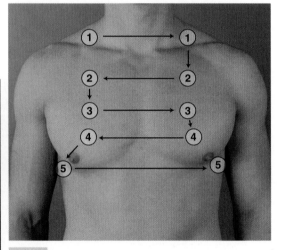

18-24   Sequence for percussion and auscultation.

Note the borders of cardiac dullness normally found on the anterior chest, and do not confuse these with suspected lung pathology (Fig. 18-25). In the right hemithorax, the upper border of liver dullness is located in the 5th intercostal space in the right midclavicular line. On the left, tympany is evident over the gastric space.

Lungs are hyperinflated with chronic emphysema, which results in hyperresonance where you would expect cardiac dullness.

Dullness behind the right breast occurs with right middle lobe pneumonia.

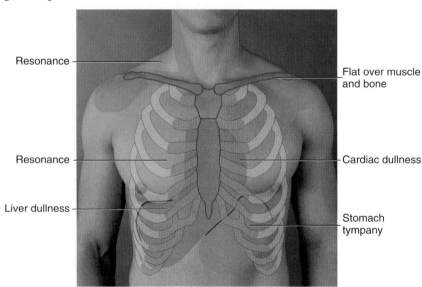

Resonance

Flat over muscle and bone

Resonance

Cardiac dullness

Liver dullness

Stomach tympany

18-25   Expected percussion notes.

Normal Range of Findings	**Abnormal Findings**

Auscultate the Anterior Chest

Breath Sounds

Auscultate the lung fields over the anterior chest from the apices in the supra-clavicular areas down to the 6th rib. Progress from side to side as you move downward and listen to one full respiration in each location. Use the sequence indicated for percussion. Do not place your stethoscope directly over the female breast. Displace the breast and listen directly over the chest wall.

Evaluate normal breath sounds, noting any abnormal breath sounds and adventitious sounds. If the situation warrants, assess the voice sounds on the anterior chest.

> Study Table 18-9, p. 450, for a complete description of abnormal respiratory conditions.

Measurement of Pulmonary Function Status

The **forced expiratory time** is the number of seconds it takes for the person to exhale from total lung capacity to residual volume. It is a screening measure of airflow obstruction. Although the test usually is not performed in the respiratory assessment, it is useful when you wish to screen for pulmonary function.

Ask the person to inhale as deeply as possible and then to blow all out hard, as quickly as possible, with the mouth open. Listen with your stethoscope over the sternum. The normal time for full expiration is 4 seconds or less.

> A forced expiration of 6 seconds or more occurs with obstructive lung disease. Refer this person for more precise pulmonary function studies.

In an ambulatory care setting, a handheld **spirometer** measures lung health in chronic conditions such as asthma. Ask the patient to inhale deeply and then to exhale into the spirometer as fast as possible until the most air possible is exhaled. The *forced vital capacity (FVC)* is the total volume of air exhaled. The *forced expiratory volume in 1 second (FEV1)* is the volume exhaled in the first measured second. A normal outcome is a FEV1/FVC ratio of 75% or greater, meaning that no significant obstruction of airflow is present.

> Mild obstruction of airflow is an FEV1/FCV ratio of 60% to 70%; moderate obstruction is a measure of 50% to 60%; severe obstruction is a ratio of less than 50%.

The **pulse oximeter** is a noninvasive method to assess arterial oxygen saturation (SpO_2) and is described in Chapter 9. A healthy person with no lung disease and no anemia normally has an SpO_2 of 97% to 99%. However, every SpO_2 result must be evaluated in the context of the person's hemoglobin level, acid-base balance, and ventilatory status.

The **6-minute walk test** (6 MWT) is a safer, simple, inexpensive, clinical measure of functional status in aging adults.[20] The 6 MWT is used as an outcome measure for people in pulmonary rehabilitation because it mirrors conditions that are used in everyday life. Locate a flat-surfaced corridor that has little foot traffic, is wide enough to permit comfortable turns, and has a controlled environment. Ensure that the person is wearing comfortable shoes and equip him or her with a pulse oximeter to monitor oxygen saturation. Ask the person to set his or her own pace to cover as much ground as possible in 6 minutes, and assure the person it is all right to slow down or to stop to rest at any time. Use a stopwatch to time the walk. A person who walks >300 meters in 6 minutes is more likely to engage in activities of daily living.

> Ask the person to stop the walk if you measure an SpO_2 below 85% to 88% or if extreme breathlessness occurs.

❖ DEVELOPMENTAL COMPETENCE

Infants and Children

To prepare, let the parent hold an infant supported against the chest or shoulder (Fig. 18-26). Ignore the usual sequence of the physical examination; seize the opportunity with a sleeping infant to inspect and then to listen to lung sounds next. This way you can concentrate on the breath sounds before the baby wakes up and possibly cries. However, infant crying does not have to be a problem for you because it actually enhances palpation of tactile fremitus and auscultation of breath sounds.

Normal Range of Findings	**Abnormal Findings**

18-26

A child may sit upright on the parent's lap. Offer the stethoscope and let the child handle it. This reduces any fear of the equipment. Promote the child's participation; school-age children usually are delighted to hear their own breath sounds when you place the stethoscope properly. While listening to breath sounds, ask the young child to take a deep breath and "blow out" your penlight while you hold the stethoscope with your other hand. Time your letting go of the penlight button so the light goes off after the child blows. Or ask the child to "pant like a dog" while you auscultate.

Inspection. The infant has a rounded thorax with an equal AP–to-transverse chest diameter (Fig. 18-27). By age 6 years the thorax reaches the adult ratio of 1:2 (AP–to-transverse diameter). The newborn's chest circumference is 30 to 36 cm and is 2 cm smaller than the head circumference until 2 years of age. The chest wall is thin with little musculature. The ribs and the xiphoid are prominent; you can both see and feel the sharp tip of the xiphoid process. The thoracic cage is soft and flexible.

Note a barrel shape persisting after age 6 years, which may develop with chronic asthma or cystic fibrosis.

18-27 Round thorax in an infant.

| **Normal Range of Findings** | **Abnormal Findings** |

The newborn's first respiratory assessment is part of the **Apgar scoring system** to measure the successful transition to extrauterine life (Table 18-2). The five standard parameters are scored at 1 minute and 5 minutes after birth. A 1-minute Apgar with a total score of 7 to 10 indicates a newborn in good condition, needing only suctioning of the nose and mouth and otherwise routine care.

In the immediate newborn period, depressed respirations are caused by maternal drugs, interruption of the uterine blood supply, or obstruction of the tracheobronchial tree with mucus or fluid.

A 1-minute Apgar with a total score of 3 to 6 indicates a moderately depressed newborn needing more resuscitation and subsequent close observation. A score of 0 to 2 indicates a severely depressed newborn needing full resuscitation, ventilatory assistance, and subsequent intensive care.

TABLE 18-2 **Apgar Scoring System**			
	2	**1**	**0**
Heart rate	Over 100	Slow (below 100)	Absent
Respiratory effort	Good, sustained cry; regular respirations	Slow, irregular, shallow	Absent
Muscle tone	Active motion, spontaneous flexion	Some flexion of extremities; some resistance to extension	Limp, flaccid
Reflex irritability (response to catheter in nares)	Sneeze, cough, cry	Grimace, frown	No response
Color	Completely pink	Body pink, extremities pale	Cyanotic, pale
			Total score

The infant breathes through the nose rather than the mouth and is an obligate nose breather until 3 months. Slight flaring of the lower costal margins may occur with respirations, but normally no flaring of the nostrils and no sternal retractions or intercostal retractions occur. The diaphragm is the newborn's major respiratory muscle. Intercostal muscles are not well developed. Thus you observe the abdomen bulge with each inspiration but see little thoracic expansion.

Count the respiratory rate for 1 full minute. Normal rates for the newborn are 30 to 40 breaths/min but may spike up to 60 per minute. Obtain the most accurate respiratory rate by counting when the infant is asleep because infants reach rapid rates with very little excitation when awake. The respiratory pattern may be irregular when extremes in room temperature occur or with feeding or sleeping. Brief periods of apnea less than 10 to 15 seconds are common. This periodic breathing is more common in premature infants.

Palpation. Palpate symmetric chest expansion by encircling the infant's thorax with both hands. Further palpation should yield no lumps, masses, or crepitus, although you may feel the costochondral junctions in some normal infants.

Auscultation. Auscultation normally yields bronchovesicular breath sounds in the peripheral lung fields of the infant and young child up to age 5 to 6 years. Their relatively thin chest walls with underdeveloped musculature do not damp off the sound as do the thicker walls of adults; thus breath sounds are louder and harsher.

Marked retractions of sternum and intercostal muscles indicate increased inspiratory effort, as in atelectasis, pneumonia, asthma, and acute airway obstruction.

Rapid respiratory rates accompany pneumonia, fever, pain, heart disease, and anemia.

In an infant tachypnea of 50 to 100 breaths/min during sleep may be an early sign of heart failure.

Asymmetric expansion occurs with diaphragmatic hernia or pneumothorax.

Crepitus is palpable around a fractured clavicle, which may occur with difficult forceps delivery.

Diminished breath sounds occur with pneumonia, atelectasis, pleural effusion, or pneumothorax.

Normal Range of Findings	Abnormal Findings

Fine crackles are the adventitious sounds commonly heard in the immediate newborn period from opening of the airways and clearing of fluid. Because the newborn's chest wall is so thin, transmission of sounds is enhanced; and sound is heard easily all over the chest, making localization of breath sounds a problem. Even bowel sounds are easily heard in the chest. Try using the smaller pediatric diaphragm endpiece or place the bell over the infant's interspaces and not over the ribs. Use the pediatric diaphragm on an older infant or toddler (Fig. 18-28).

Persistent fine crackles that are scattered over the chest occur with pneumonia, bronchiolitis, or atelectasis.

Crackles only in upper lung fields occur with cystic fibrosis; crackles only in lower lung fields occur with heart failure.

Expiratory wheezing occurs with lower airway obstruction (e.g., asthma or bronchiolitis). When unilateral, it may be foreign body aspiration.

Persistent peristaltic sounds with diminished breath sounds on the same side may indicate diaphragmatic hernia.

Stridor is a high-pitched inspiratory crowing sound heard without the stethoscope, occurring with upper airway obstruction (e.g., croup, foreign body aspiration, or acute epiglottitis).

18-28

The Pregnant Woman

The thoracic cage appears wider, and the costal angle widens by about 50%. Respirations are deeper, with a 40% increase in tidal volume.

The Aging Adult

The chest cage commonly shows an increased AP diameter, giving a round barrel shape and **kyphosis** or an outward curvature of the thoracic spine (see Table 18-3, p. 443). The person compensates by holding the head extended and tilted back. You may palpate marked bony prominences because of decreased subcutaneous fat. Chest expansion may be somewhat decreased with the older person, although it still should be symmetric. The costal cartilages become calcified with aging, resulting in a less mobile thorax.

The older person may tire easily, especially during auscultation when deep mouth breathing is required. Take care that this person does not hyperventilate and become dizzy. Allow brief rest periods or quiet breathing. If the person does feel faint, holding the breath for a few seconds restores equilibrium.

The Acutely Ill Person

Ask a second examiner to hold the person's arms and support him or her in the upright position. If no one else is available, you need to roll the person from side to side, examining the uppermost half of the thorax. This obviously prevents you from comparing findings from one side to another. In addition, side flexion of the trunk alters percussion findings because the ribs of the upward side may flex closer together.

Objective Data

Environmental ("Secondhand") Tobacco Smoke (ETS)

According to the National Cancer Institute (NCI), there is no safe level of exposure to environmental tobacco smoke (ETS), commonly referred to as *secondhand* smoke. Research now suggests the risk of secondhand smoke exposure to be an equivalent or stronger risk factor for coronary artery disease than other well-established risks such as high cholesterol, hypertension, and diabetes. According to the Centers for Disease Control (CDC), secondhand smoke, which is a mixture of *side-stream* and *mainstream smoke*, contains more than 7000 chemicals, including hundreds that are toxic and approximately 70 that can cause cancer. *Side-stream* smoke is the smoke given off at the burning end of a tobacco product, whereas *mainstream* smoke is the smoke exhaled from the individual smoking the tobacco product.

Exposure to secondhand smoke, which is involuntary and/or passive, increases an individual's risk for cancer and heart disease in adults. Pregnant women who breathe secondhand smoke have a higher risk of low-weight infants and/or infants who are more likely to die of sudden infant death syndrome (SIDS). It also increases the risk of ear infections, asthma, and lung infections, including pneumonia, in children. To access the CDC Fact Sheet on Secondhand Smoke, go to: http://www.cdc.gov/tobacco/data_statistics/fact_sheets/secondhand_smoke/general_facts/index.htm.

The current problem is that, despite substantial progress in tobacco control policies, people continue to be exposed to secondhand smoke in their homes and workplaces. ETS exposure is higher for people with lower incomes, both overall and in the home; and its effects are seen across the life cycle and environments. Reports estimate that over 50% of children between 3 and 11 years of age have been exposed to secondhand smoke and just under 30% of indoor workers are not protected by smoke-free workplace policies. Occupational disparities in exposure have decreased; but, according to the CDC, African-American, construction, and blue-collar workers continue to experience high levels of ETS exposure relative to others.

When workplaces across the United States first initiated smoke-free policies, workplace productivity was increased, and absenteeism decreased. Conventional air cleaning removes large particles but not the small particles found in secondhand smoke. Further, heating and air-conditioning systems can distribute secondhand smoke throughout a building, increasing exposure of unsuspecting individuals. Although levels of *cotinine*, a biomarker of secondhand smoke exposure, continue to decrease, many nonsmokers, especially African Americans, still have detectable levels in their bloodstream.

For additional information on reducing secondhand smoke exposure, visit the CDC Healthier Worksite Initiative and access its online toolkit for individuals, groups, or communities. Available at http://www.cdc.gov/nccdphp/dnpao/hwi/toolkits/tobacco/index.htm.

Resources

Centers for Disease Control and Prevention (CDC): http://www.cdc.gov/tobacco/basic_information/secondhand_smoke/.

The American Lung Association offers various mechanisms to help individuals stop smoking. One mechanism, the Freedom from Smoking online smoking cessation clinic, can be accessed day or night, 7 days a week, on any schedule a smoker chooses at http://www.ffsonline.org/.

The Environmental Protection Agency (EPA) has developed two valuable resources for families and communities.

Smoke-free Homes Community Action Kit *http://www.epa.gov/smokefree/pdfs/community_action_kit.pdf.*

Secondhand Smoke and the Health of Your Family *(Bilingual-Spanish/English) http://www.epa.gov/smokefree/pdfs/trifold_brochure.pdf.*

DOCUMENTATION AND CRITICAL THINKING

Sample Charting

SUBJECTIVE

No cough, shortness of breath, or chest pain with breathing. No history of respiratory diseases. Has "one or no" colds per year. Has never smoked. Works in well-ventilated office on a smoke-free campus. Last TB skin test 4 years PTA, negative. Never had chest x-ray.

OBJECTIVE

Inspection: AP < transverse diameter. Resp 16/min, relaxed and even.
Palpation: Chest expansion symmetric. Tactile fremitus equal bilaterally. No tenderness to palpation. No lumps or lesions.
Percussion: Resonant to percussion over lung fields. Diaphragmatic excursion 5 cm and = bilaterally.
Auscultation: Vesicular breath sounds clear over lung fields and = bilaterally. No adventitious sounds.

ASSESSMENT

Intact thoracic structures
Lung sounds clear and equal

Clinical Case Study 1

R.B. is a 37-year-old male Caucasian exercise trainer who teaches 10 to 12 clients per day in a small gym and comes to clinic, saying, "I'm really sick." Last visit to care provider was 10 years PTA for ankle sprain. Runs and works out 1 hour most days. Has never smoked. Drinks occasionally on weekends, 1 or 2 beers per occasion. No history of allergies, hospitalizations. No family history of TB, asthma, heart disease, or cancer. No vaccines since childhood.

SUBJECTIVE

2 days PTA—Client in R's gym was coughing productive mucus and dripping on hands and equipment. R cleaned equipment but next day felt sudden-onset overwhelming fatigue and fever. Unable to sleep because of fever of 102° to 104°F (38.9° to 40°C), headache, muscle pain, and stuffy nose that completely obstructs when lying down.

Now—Headache, stuffy nose, sneezing, sore throat, severe cough, chest pain in sternum with coughing, severe muscle aches and pains. No nausea, vomiting, or diarrhea.

OBJECTIVE

Vital signs: Temp 102.8°F (39.3°C). Pulse 88 bpm. Resp 20/min. BP 108/74 mm Hg, L arm sitting.

Ears—TMs clear with landmarks intact.

Nose—Turbinates red and swollen with yellow purulent mucus.

Throat—Tonsils out, throat red, R & L anterior cervical nodes enlarged and tender.

Chest—Respirations not labored, chest expansion symmetric, no tenderness to palpation. Resonant to percussion and = bilaterally. Vesicular breath sounds clear over peripheral lung fields. Loud, low-pitched, gurgling crackles over anterior sternum at 4th and 5th interspace.

Abdomen—Bowel sounds present, soft, no tenderness.

ASSESSMENT

Influenza

Insomnia R/T airway obstruction

Clinical Case Study 2

E.S. is 53-year-old African American line worker at urban automobile plant. Concerned with increasing shortness of breath for past 3 to 4 years. Reports 5 to 6 "colds" per year. Smokes cigarettes starting age 18, 1 PPD × 30 years, 1½ PPD × 5 years. Does not drink alcohol. Takes HCTZ 25 mg for hypertension, no other meds. No allergies. No hospitalizations or injuries. No family history of TB, allergies, heart disease, asthma, cancer.

SUBJECTIVE

Short of breath now after walking 1 flight of stairs or 1 block. Chest tightness. Early morning cough daily, with small amount white sputum × 2-3 years. Fatigue and SOB at work. Has 2-pillow orthopnea at night. Wakes 2-3 times/night to urinate or "catch breath." States thinking of quitting smoking, but previous attempts have not worked.

OBJECTIVE

Vital signs: BP 148/88 mm Hg. Temp 98°F (36.7°C). Pulse 88 bpm. Resp 24/min. Weight 114 lbs.

Inspection: Sitting on side of bed with arms propped on bedside table. Respirations: resting 24/min, regular, shallow with prolonged expiration; resp. ambulating 34/min. Increased use of accessory muscles, AP = transverse diameter with widening of costal angle, tense expression.

Palpation: Minimal but symmetric chest expansion. Tactile fremitus = bilaterally. No lumps, masses, or tenderness to palpation.

Percussion: Diaphragmatic excursion is 1 cm and = bilaterally. Hyperresonance over lung fields.

Auscultation: Breath sounds diminished. Expiratory wheeze throughout posterior chest, R > L. No crackles.

ASSESSMENT

Chronic obstructive pulmonary disease (probable)

Hypertension

Ineffective airway clearance R/T bronchial secretions and obstruction

Activity intolerance R/T imbalance between oxygen supply and demand

Insomnia R/T dyspnea

Anxiety R/T change in health status

A.G. is a 67-year-old Caucasian female retired secretary who is admitted to a surgical unit following uncomplicated cholecystectomy. She has resisted interventions to walk in halls because of incisional pain and obesity (weight is 245 lbs). On 2nd postop day nurse answers call light and finds A.G. sitting bolt upright in bed gasping for breath and clutching bedsheets.

SUBJECTIVE

"I can't breathe, I can't breathe." (Nurse asks when this started.) "Few minutes ago and my chest hurts too, worse when I breathe in."

OBJECTIVE

Vital signs: Temp 99.2°F (37.3°C). Pulse 124 bpm. Resp 32/min, labored. BP 100/70 mm Hg. Pulse oximetry 78% on room air. (Nurse now calls for help, administers O$_2$ 15 L/min via Venturi mask, continues with assessment.)
Mental status: Alert, apprehensive.
Skin: Pale, ashen, cool, diaphoretic, delayed capillary refill.
Chest: Labored breathing, symmetrical expansion, breath sounds labored though present in both lungs, decreased in posterior right base, crackles over posterior right base.

ASSESSMENT

Acute respiratory distress

C.T. is a 9-month-old Caucasian girl who comes to the clinic with her father because of "a bad cold." C.T. attends daycare and lives at home with two school-age siblings, parents, and paternal grandmother who smoke in the home.

SUBJECTIVE

6 days PTA: C.T.'s 4-year-old brother came home from preschool "with a cold that he gave to our whole family."
2 days PTA: C.T. has "cold" with cough, fever (temp unknown because of not having a thermometer at home), and decreased intake of formula.
Now: C.T. "looks and sounds worse. I don't think she's breathing right." Reported last bottle and wet diaper was 6 hours ago.
Birth history: Born at 36 weeks' gestation, spontaneous rupture of membranes (SROM), vaginal birth w/o complications; weight 5 lbs 1 oz (2.3 kg); birth length 19 in (48.2 cm); head circumference 32.5 cm.

OBJECTIVE

Vital signs: Temp 102°F (38.9°C) (axillary). BP 80/56 mm Hg (sitting on exam table). Pulse 192 bpm. Resp 70/min. Weight 13 lbs (5.9 kg). Height 27.5 in. (69.8 cm). Head circumference 41.5 cm.
General appearance: Labored breathing w/ nasal flaring while sitting upright on dad's lap. Attempts to suck from a bottle but gives up, gasping, after latching on for a few seconds.
HEENT: Normocephalic; eyes clear; TM pearly gray bilat; thick, copious amounts of mucus to bilat nares and pharynx.
Cardiovascular: Tachycardic; no abnormal heart sounds.
Respiratory: Tachypneic, crackles at bases, wheezes bilat, and harsh, productive cough; moderate intercostal and subcostal retractions.

ASSESSMENT

Respiratory syncytial virus (RSV) bronchiolitis
Ineffective airway clearance R/T excessive mucus and changes in respiratory rate
Impaired gas exchange R/T infection
Risk for fluid volume deficit R/T deviations affecting intake of fluids
Knowledge deficit R/T dangers of secondhand smoke

ABNORMAL FINDINGS

TABLE 18-3 Configurations of the Thorax

Normal Adult (for Comparison)

The thorax has an elliptical shape with an anteroposterior-to-transverse diameter documented as 1:2 or 0.70.

Barrel Chest

Note equal AP-to-transverse diameter and that ribs are horizontal instead of the normal downward slope. This is associated with normal aging and also with chronic emphysema and asthma as a result of hyperinflation of lungs.

Pectus Excavatum

A markedly sunken sternum and adjacent cartilages (also called *funnel breast*). Depression begins at second intercostal space, becoming depressed most at junction of xiphoid with body of sternum. More noticeable on inspiration. Congenital, usually not symptomatic. When severe, sternal depression may cause embarrassment and a negative self-concept. Surgery may be indicated.

Pectus Carinatum

A forward protrusion of the sternum, with ribs sloping back at either side and vertical depressions along costochondral junctions (pigeon breast). Less common than pectus excavatum, this minor deformity requires no treatment. If severe, surgery may be indicated.

TABLE 18-3   Configurations of the Thorax—cont'd

Scoliosis

A lateral S-shaped curvature of the thoracic and lumbar spine, usually with involved vertebrae rotation. Note unequal shoulder and scapular height and unequal hip levels, rib interspaces flared on convex side. More prevalent in adolescent age-groups, especially girls. Mild deformities are asymptomatic. If severe (>45 degrees) deviation is present, scoliosis may reduce lung volume, and person is at risk for impaired cardiopulmonary function. Primary impairment is cosmetic deformity, negatively affecting self-image. Refer early for treatment, possible surgery.

Kyphosis

An exaggerated posterior curvature of the thoracic spine (humpback) that causes significant back pain and limited mobility. Severe deformities impair cardiopulmonary function. If the neck muscles are strong, compensation occurs by hyperextension of head to maintain level of vision.

Kyphosis has been associated with aging, especially the familiar "dowager's hump" of postmenopausal osteoporotic women. However, it is common well before menopause. It is related to physical fitness; women with adequate exercise habits are less likely to have kyphosis.

TABLE 18-4   Respiratory Patterns*

Inspiration Expiration

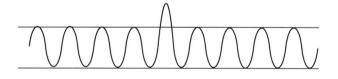

Normal Adult (for Comparison)

Rate—10 to 20 breaths/min
>   Depth—500 to 800 mL
>   Pattern—Even
>   The ratio of pulse to respirations is fairly constant, about 4:1. Both values increase as a normal response to exercise, fear, or fever.
>   Depth—Air moving in and out with each respiration.

Sigh

Occasional sighs punctuate the normal breathing pattern and are purposeful to expand alveoli. Frequent sighs may indicate emotional dysfunction and also may lead to hyperventilation and dizziness.

*Assess the (1) rate, (2) depth (tidal volume), and (3) pattern.

Continued

TABLE 18-4   Respiratory Patterns—cont'd

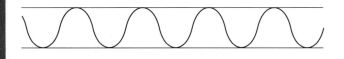

Tachypnea

Rapid, shallow breathing. Increased rate, >24 per minute. This is a normal response to fever, fear, or exercise. Rate also increases with respiratory insufficiency, pneumonia, alkalosis, pleurisy, and lesions in the pons.

Hyperventilation

Increase in both rate and depth. Normally occurs with extreme exertion, fear, or anxiety. Also occurs with diabetic ketoacidosis (Kussmaul respirations), hepatic coma, salicylate overdose (producing a respiratory alkalosis to compensate for the metabolic acidosis), lesions of the midbrain, and alteration in blood gas concentration (either an increase in CO_2 or a decrease in oxygen). Hyperventilation blows off CO_2, causing a decreased level in the blood (alkalosis).

Bradypnea

Slow breathing. A decreased but regular rate (<10 per minute), as in drug-induced depression of the respiratory center in the medulla, increased intracranial pressure, and diabetic coma.

Hypoventilation

An irregular shallow pattern caused by an overdose of narcotics or anesthetics. May also occur with prolonged bed rest or conscious splinting of the chest to avoid respiratory pain.

Cheyne-Stokes Respiration

A cycle in which respirations gradually wax and wane in a regular pattern, increasing in rate and depth and then decreasing. The breathing periods last 30 to 45 seconds, with periods of apnea (20 seconds) alternating the cycle. The most common cause is severe heart failure; other causes are renal failure, meningitis, drug overdose, and increased intracranial pressure. Occurs normally in infants and aging persons during sleep.

Biot Respiration

Similar to Cheyne-Stokes respiration, except that the pattern is irregular. A series of normal respirations (three to four) is followed by a period of apnea. The cycle length is variable, lasting anywhere from 10 seconds to 1 minute. Seen with head trauma, brain abscess, heat stroke, spinal meningitis, and encephalitis.

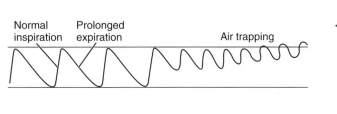

◄ Chronic Obstructive Breathing

Normal inspiration and prolonged expiration to overcome increased airway resistance. In a person with chronic obstructive lung disease, any situation calling for increased heart rate (exercise) may lead to dyspneic episode (air trapping) because the person does not have enough time for full expiration.

TABLE 18-5   Abnormal Tactile Fremitus

Increased Tactile Fremitus

Occurs with conditions that increase the density of lung tissue, thereby making a better conducting medium for vibrations (e.g., compression or consolidation [pneumonia]). There must be a patent bronchus, and consolidation must extend to lung surface for increased fremitus to be apparent.

Decreased Tactile Fremitus

Occurs when anything obstructs transmission of vibrations (e.g., an obstructed bronchus, pleural effusion or thickening, pneumothorax, and emphysema). Any barrier that gets in the way of the sound and your palpating hand decreases fremitus.

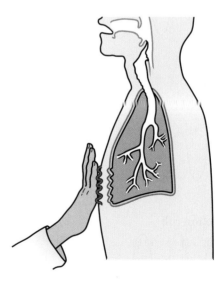

Rhonchal Fremitus

Vibration felt when inhaled air passes through thick secretions in the larger bronchi. This may decrease somewhat by coughing.

Pleural Friction Fremitus

Produced when inflammation of the parietal or visceral pleura causes a decrease in the normal lubricating fluid. The opposing surfaces make a coarse grating sound when rubbed together during breathing. This sound is best detected by auscultation, but it may be palpable and feels like two pieces of leather grating together. It is synchronous with respiratory excursion. Also called a *palpable friction rub*.

TABLE 18-6 Adventitious Lung Sounds

Sound	Description	Mechanism	Clinical Example

Discontinuous Sounds

These are discrete, crackling sounds.

Sound	Description	Mechanism	Clinical Example
Crackles—Fine (formerly called *rales*) *Inspiration* *Expiration*	Discontinuous, high-pitched, short crackling, popping sounds heard during inspiration that are not cleared by coughing; you can simulate this sound by rolling a strand of hair between your fingers near your ear or by moistening your thumb and index finger and separating them near your ear	Inspiratory crackles: inhaled air collides with previously deflated airways; airways suddenly pop open, creating explosive crackling sound Expiratory crackles: sudden airway closing[35]	*Late inspiratory crackles* occur with restrictive disease: pneumonia, heart failure, and interstitial fibrosis *Early inspiratory crackles* occur with obstructive disease: chronic bronchitis, asthma, and emphysema *Posturally induced crackles* (PICs) are fine crackles that appear with a change from sitting to the supine position or with a change from supine to supine with legs elevated
Crackles——Coarse (coarse rales)	Loud, low-pitched bubbling and gurgling sounds that start in early inspiration and may be present in expiration; may decrease somewhat by suctioning or coughing but reappear shortly—sounds like opening a Velcro fastener	Inhaled air collides with secretions in the trachea and large bronchi	Pulmonary edema, pneumonia, pulmonary fibrosis, and the terminally ill who have a depressed cough reflex
Atelectatic crackles (atelectatic rales)	Sound like fine crackles but do not last and are not pathologic; disappear after the first few breaths; heard in axillae and bases (usually dependent) of lungs	When sections of alveoli are not fully aerated, they deflate and accumulate secretions; crackles are heard when these sections reexpand with a few deep breaths	In aging adults, in bedridden persons, or in persons just aroused from sleep
Pleural friction rub	A very superficial sound that is coarse and low pitched; it has a grating quality as if two pieces of leather are being rubbed together; sounds just like crackles, but *close* to the ear; sounds louder if you push the stethoscope harder onto the chest wall; sound is inspiratory and expiratory	Caused when pleurae become inflamed and lose their normal lubricating fluid; their opposing roughened pleural surfaces rub together during respiration; heard best in anterolateral wall where greatest lung mobility exists	Pleuritis, accompanied by pain with breathing (rub disappears after a few days if pleural fluid accumulates and separates pleurae)

TABLE 18-6   Adventitious Lung Sounds—cont'd

Sound	Description	Mechanism	Clinical Example
Continuous Sounds			
These are connected, musical sounds.			
Wheeze—High-pitched (sibilant)	High-pitched, musical squeaking sounds that sound polyphonic (multiple notes as in a musical chord); predominate in expiration but may occur in both expiration and inspiration	Air squeezed or compressed through passageways narrowed almost to closure by collapsing, swelling, secretions, or tumors; the passageway walls oscillate in apposition between the closed and barely open positions; the resulting sound is similar to that of a vibrating reed	Diffuse airway obstruction from acute asthma or chronic emphysema
Wheeze—Low-pitched (sonorous rhonchi)	Low-pitched; monophonic, single note, musical snoring, moaning sounds; they are heard throughout the cycle, although they are more prominent on expiration; may clear somewhat by coughing[7a]	Airflow obstruction as described earlier by the vibrating reed mechanism; the pitch of the wheeze cannot be correlated to the size of the passageway that generates it	Bronchitis, single bronchus obstruction from airway tumor
Stridor	High-pitched, monophonic, inspiratory, crowing sound; louder in neck than over chest wall	Originating in larynx or trachea, upper airway obstruction from swollen, inflamed tissues or lodged foreign body	Croup and acute epiglottitis in children and foreign inhalation; obstructed airway may be life-threatening

ABNORMAL FINDINGS
FOR ADVANCED PRACTICE

TABLE 18-7 Diagnostic Clues to Chronic Dyspnea and Associated Systems

System/Physiology	Example	History	Examination	Diagnostic Study
Pulmonary				
Alveolar	Chronic pneumonia	Fever, productive cough, shortness of breath	Fever, crackles, increased fremitus, bronchophony	Chest radiography, chest CT, bronchoscopy/bronchoalveolar lavage, culture or biopsy
Interstitial	Idiopathic fibrosis	Exertional dyspnea, dry cough, malignancy, prescription or illicit drug use, chemical exposures	Hypoxia, clubbing, persistent inspiratory crackles	Chest radiography (fibrosis, interstitial markings), chest CT, bronchoscopy/biopsy
Obstruction of air flow	Chronic obstructive pulmonary disease	Tobacco use, cough, relief with bronchodilator, increased sputum production, hemoptysis and weight loss with malignancy	Wheezing, barrel chest, decreased breath sounds, accessory muscle use, clubbing, paradoxical pulse	Peak flow, spirometry, chest radiography (hyperinflation), pulmonary function testing (PFT)
Restrictive	Pleural effusion	Pleuritic chest pain, dyspnea not improved with oxygen	Decreased breath sounds, chest morphology, pleural rub, basal dullness	Chest radiography (effusion, anatomic abnormality), spirometry, PFT
Vascular	Chronic pulmonary emboli	Fatigue, pleuritic chest pain, prior emboli/deep venous thrombosis, syncope	Wheezing, lower extremity swelling, pleural rub, prominent P_2, murmur, right ventricular heave, jugular venous distention (JVD)	D-dimer, ventilation/perfusion scan, CT angiography, echocardiography, right heart catheterization
Cardiac				
Arrhythmia	Atrial fibrillation	Palpitations, syncope	Irregular rhythm, pauses	ECG, event recorder, Holter monitor, stress testing
Heart failure	Ischemic cardiomyopathy	Dyspnea on exertion, paroxysmal nocturnal dyspnea, orthopnea, chest pain or tightness, prior coronary artery disease or atrial fibrillation	Edema, JVD, S_3, displaced cardiac apical impulse, hepatojugular reflex, murmur, crackles, wheezing, tachycardia, S_4	ECG, brain natriuretic peptide, echocardiography, stress testing, coronary angiography
Restrictive or constrictive pericardial disease	Metastatic tumor	Viral infection, malignancy, chest radiation, inflammatory diseases	Decreased heart sounds	Echocardiography
Valvular	Aortic stenosis	Dyspnea on exertion	Murmur, JVD	Echocardiography
Gastrointestinal				
Aspiration	Gastroesophageal reflux disease	Postprandial, night cough	Intermittent crackles, wheezes	Chest radiography, esophagography, esophageal pH

TABLE 18-7	**Diagnostic Clues to Chronic Dyspnea and Associated Systems—cont'd**			
System/ Physiology	Example	History	Examination	Diagnostic Study
Neuromuscular				
Respiratory muscle weakness	Phrenic nerve palsy	Known neuromuscular disorders, weakness	Atrophy	Maximal inspiratory and expiratory pressures
Psychological				
—	Anxiety	Anxiety, depression, history of trauma or abuse	Sighing	Normal

From Wahls, S.A. (2012). Causes and evaluation of chronic dyspnea. *Am Fam Phys* 86(2), 173-180.
CT, Computed tomography; *ECG,* electrocardiography; *JVD,* jugular venous distention; *PFT,* pulmonary function testing.

TABLE 18-8	**Voice Sounds**	
Technique	Normal Finding	Abnormal Finding
Bronchophony Ask the person to repeat "ninety-nine" while you listen with the stethoscope over the chest wall; listen especially if you suspect pathology	Normal voice transmission is soft, muffled, and indistinct; you can hear sound through the stethoscope but cannot distinguish exactly what is being said	Pathology that increases lung density enhances transmission of voice sounds; you auscultate a clear "ninety-nine" The words are more distinct than normal and sound close to your ear

Egophony (Greek: "the voice of a goat") Auscultate the chest while the person phonates a long "ee-ee-ee-ee" sound	Normally you should hear "eeeeeee" through your stethoscope	Over area of consolidation or compression the spoken "eeee" sound changes to a bleating long "aaaaa" sound
Whispered Pectoriloquy Ask the person to whisper a phrase such as "one-two-three" as you auscultate	The normal response is faint, muffled, and almost inaudible	With only small amounts of consolidation, the whispered voice is transmitted very clearly and distinctly, although still somewhat faint; it sounds as if the person is whispering right into your stethoscope, "one-two-three"

Abnormal Findings

TABLE 18-9   Assessment of Common Respiratory Conditions

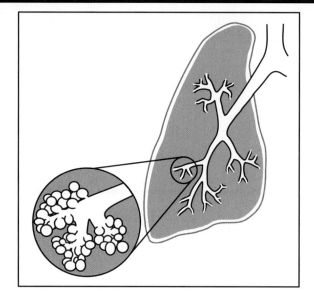

◀ **Normal Lung (for comparison)**

Inspection AP < transverse diameter, relaxed posture, normal musculature; rate 10 to 18 breaths/min, regular; no cyanosis or pallor.

Palpation Symmetric chest expansion. Tactile fremitus present and equal bilaterally, diminishing toward periphery. No lumps, masses, or tenderness.

Percussion Resonant. Diaphragmatic excursion 3 to 5 cm and equal bilaterally.

Auscultation Vesicular over peripheral fields. Bronchovesicular parasternally (anterior) and between scapulae (posterior). Infant and young child—bronchovesicular throughout.

Adventitious Sounds None.

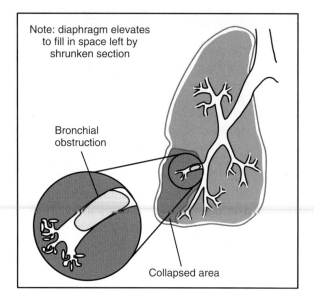

Note: diaphragm elevates to fill in space left by shrunken section

Bronchial obstruction

Collapsed area

◀ **Atelectasis (Collapse)**

Condition Collapsed shrunken section of alveoli or an entire lung as a result of (1) airway obstruction (e.g., the bronchus is completely blocked by thick exudate, aspirated foreign body, or tumor); the alveolar air beyond the obstruction is gradually absorbed by the pulmonary capillaries, and the alveolar walls cave in); (2) compression on the lung; and (3) lack of surfactant (hyaline membrane disease).

Inspection Cough. Lag on expansion on affected side. Increased respiratory rate and pulse. Possible cyanosis.

Palpation Chest expansion decreased on affected side. Tactile fremitus decreased or absent over area. With large collapse, tracheal shift toward affected side.

Percussion Dull over area (remainder of thorax sometimes may have hyperresonant note).

Auscultation Breath sounds decreased vesicular or absent over area. Voice sounds variable, usually decreased or absent over affected area.

Adventitious Sounds None if bronchus is obstructed. Occasional fine crackles if bronchus is patent.

TABLE 18-9   Assessment of Common Respiratory Conditions—cont'd

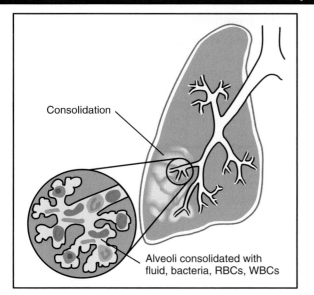

Consolidation

Alveoli consolidated with fluid, bacteria, RBCs, WBCs

◀ Lobar Pneumonia

Condition Infection in lung parenchyma leaves alveolar membrane edematous and porous; thus red blood cells (RBCs) and white blood cells (WBCs) pass from blood to alveoli. Alveoli progressively fill up (become consolidated) with bacteria, solid cellular debris, fluid, and blood cells, which replace alveolar air. This decreases surface area of the respiratory membrane, causing hypoxemia.

History Fever, cough with pleuritic chest pain, blood-tinged sputum, chills, SOB, fatigue.

Inspection Increased respirations >24/min. Guarding and lag on expansion on affected side. Children—Sternal retraction, nasal flaring.

Palpation Chest expansion decreased on affected side. Tactile fremitus increased if bronchus patent, decreased if bronchus obstructed.

Percussion Dull over lobar pneumonia.

Auscultation Tachycardia. Loud bronchial breathing with patent bronchus. Voice sounds have increased clarity; bronchophony, egophony, whispered pectoriloquy present. Children—Diminished breath sounds may occur early.

Adventitious Sounds Crackles, fine to medium.

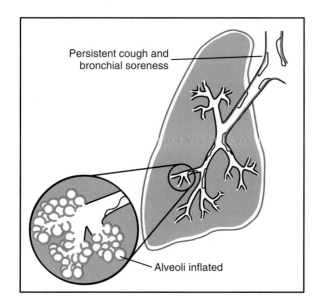

Persistent cough and bronchial soreness

Alveoli inflated

◀ Acute Bronchitis

Condition An acute infection of the trachea and larger bronchi characterized by cough, lasting up to 3 weeks. Most cases are viral and do not require antibiotics. Epithelium of bronchi are inflamed and damaged, releasing proinflammatory mediators. Large airways are narrowed from capillary dilation, increased mucus production, loss of cilia function, and swelling of epithelium. More cases occur with smokers, aging adults, children, and in winter months.

Inspection Cough is productive or nonproductive. Also sore throat, low-grade fever, postnasal drip, fatigue, substernal aching.

Palpation No pain, no increased fremitus.

Percussion Resonance predominates.

Auscultation May be clear and equal bilaterally. No egophony.

Adventitious sounds No crackles (distinguishes the consolidation of pneumonia, no wheeze).

Continued

TABLE 18-9 Assessment of Common Respiratory Conditions—cont'd

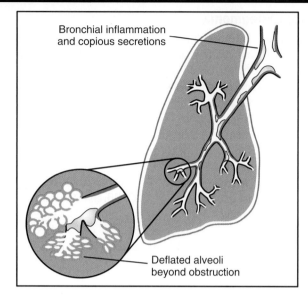

Bronchial inflammation and copious secretions

Deflated alveoli beyond obstruction

◀ Chronic Bronchitis

Condition Proliferation of mucus glands in the passageways, resulting in excessive mucus secretion. Inflammation of bronchi with partial obstruction of bronchi by secretions or constrictions. Sections of lung distal to obstruction may be deflated. Bronchitis may be acute or chronic with recurrent productive cough. Chronic bronchitis is usually caused by cigarette smoking.

Inspection Hacking, rasping cough productive of thick mucoid sputum. Chronic—Dyspnea, fatigue, cyanosis, possible clubbing of fingers.

Palpation Tactile fremitus normal.

Percussion Resonant.

Auscultation Normal vesicular. Voice sounds normal. Chronic—Prolonged expiration.

Adventitious Sounds Crackles over deflated areas. May have wheeze.

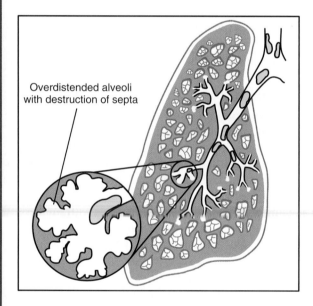

Overdistended alveoli with destruction of septa

◀ Emphysema

Condition Caused by destruction of pulmonary connective tissue (elastin, collagen); characterized by permanent enlargement of air sacs distal to terminal bronchioles and rupture of interalveolar walls. This increases airway resistance, especially on expiration, producing a hyperinflated lung and an increase in lung volume. Cigarette smoking accounts for 80% to 90% of cases of emphysema.

Inspection Increased AP diameter. Barrel chest. Accessory muscles used to aid respiration. Tripod position. SOB, especially on exertion. Respiratory distress. Tachypnea.

Palpation Decreased tactile fremitus and chest expansion.

Percussion Hyperresonant. Decreased diaphragmatic excursion.

Auscultation Decreased breath sounds. May have prolonged expiration. Muffled heart sounds resulting from overdistention of lungs.

Adventitious Sounds Usually none; occasionally, wheeze.

TABLE 18-9   Assessment of Common Respiratory Conditions—cont'd

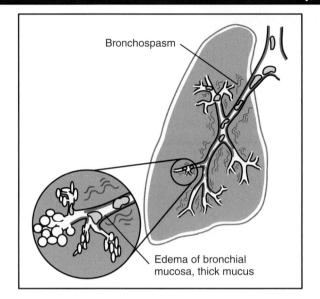

Bronchospasm

Edema of bronchial mucosa, thick mucus

◀ Asthma (Reactive Airway Disease)

Condition An allergic hypersensitivity to certain inhaled allergens (pollen), irritants (tobacco, ozone), microbes, stress, or exercise that produces a complex response characterized by bronchospasm and inflammation, edema in walls of bronchioles, and secretion of highly viscous mucus into airways. These factors greatly increase airway resistance, especially during expiration, and produce the symptoms of wheezing, dyspnea, and chest tightness.

Inspection During severe attack: increased respiratory rate, SOB with audible wheeze, use of accessory neck muscles, cyanosis, apprehension, retraction of intercostal spaces. Expiration labored, prolonged. When chronic, may have barrel chest.

Palpation Tactile fremitus decreased, tachycardia.

Percussion Resonant. May be hyperresonant if chronic.

Auscultation Diminished air movement. Breath sounds decreased, with prolonged expiration. Voice sounds decreased.

Adventitious Sounds Bilateral wheezing on expiration, sometimes inspiratory and expiratory wheezing.

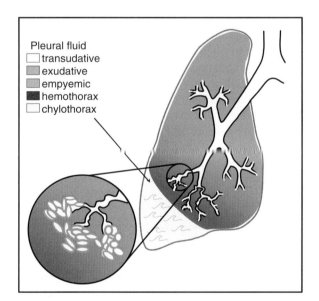

Pleural fluid
☐ transudative
■ exudative
▨ empyemic
■ hemothorax
☐ chylothorax

◀ Pleural Effusion (Fluid) or Thickening

Condition Collection of excess fluid in the intrapleural space, with compression of overlying lung tissue. Effusion may contain watery capillary fluid (transudative), protein (exudative), purulent matter (empyemic), blood (hemothorax), or milky lymphatic fluid (chylothorax). Gravity settles fluid in dependent areas of thorax. Presence of fluid subdues all lung sounds.

Inspection Increased respirations, dyspnea; may have dry cough, tachycardia, cyanosis, asymmetric expansion, abdominal distention.

Palpation Tactile fremitus decreased or absent. Tracheal shift away from affected side. Chest expansion decreased on affected side.

Percussion Dull percussion. No diaphragmatic excursion on affected side.

Auscultation Breath sounds decreased or absent. Voice sounds decreased or absent. When remainder of lung is compressed near the effusion, may have bronchial breath sounds over the compression along with bronchophony, egophony, whispered pectoriloquy.

Adventitious Sounds Crackles, pleural rub.

Continued

TABLE 18-9   Assessment of Common Respiratory Conditions—cont'd

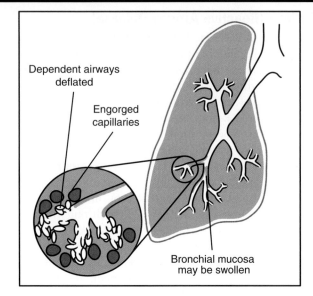

◀ **Heart Failure**

Condition Pump failure with increasing pressure of cardiac overload causes pulmonary congestion or an increased amount of blood present in pulmonary capillaries. Dependent air sacs deflated. Pulmonary capillaries engorged. Bronchial mucosa may be swollen.

Inspection Increased respiratory rate, SOB on exertion, orthopnea, paroxysmal nocturnal dyspnea, nocturia, ankle edema, pallor in light-skinned people.

Palpation Skin moist, clammy. Tactile fremitus normal.

Percussion Resonant.

Auscultation Normal vesicular. Heart sounds include S_3 gallop.

Adventitious Sounds Crackles at lung bases.

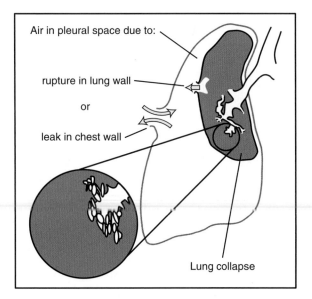

◀ **Pneumothorax**

Condition Free air in pleural space causes partial or complete lung collapse. Air in pleural space neutralizes the usual negative pressure present; thus lung collapses. Usually unilateral. Pneumothorax can be (1) **spontaneous** (air enters pleural space through rupture in lung wall, (2) **traumatic** (air enters through opening or injury in chest wall), or (3) **tension** (trapped air in pleural space increases, compressing lung and shifting mediastinum to the unaffected side).

Inspection Unequal chest expansion. If large, tachypnea, cyanosis, apprehension, bulging in interspaces.

Palpation Tactile fremitus decreased or absent. Tracheal shift to opposite side (unaffected side). Chest expansion decreased on affected side. Tachycardia, decreased BP.

Percussion Hyperresonant. Decreased diaphragmatic excursion.

Auscultation Breath sounds decreased or absent. Voice sounds decreased or absent.

Adventitious Sounds None.

TABLE 18-9 **Assessment of Common Respiratory Conditions—cont'd**

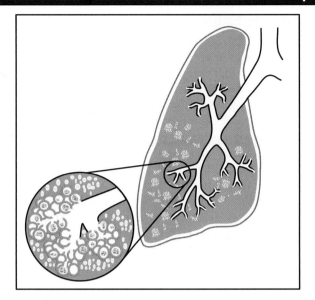

◀ *Pneumocystis jiroveci (P. carinii)* **Pneumonia**

Condition This virulent form of pneumonia is a protozoal infection associated with AIDS. The parasite *P. jiroveci (P. carinii)* is common in the United States and harmless to most people, except to the immunocompromised, in whom a diffuse interstitial pneumonitis ensues. Cysts containing the organism and macrophages form in alveolar spaces, alveolar walls thicken, and the disease spreads to bilateral interstitial infiltrates of foamy, protein-rich fluid.

Inspection Anxiety, SOB, dyspnea on exertion, malaise are common; also tachypnea; fever; a dry, nonproductive cough; intercostal retractions in children; cyanosis.

Palpation Decreased chest expansion.

Percussion Dull over areas of diffuse infiltrate.

Auscultation Breath sounds may be diminished.

Adventitious Sounds Crackles may be present but often are absent.

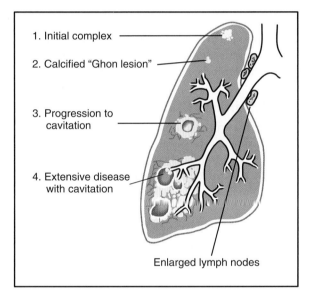

1. Initial complex
2. Calcified "Ghon lesion"
3. Progression to cavitation
4. Extensive disease with cavitation

Enlarged lymph nodes

◀ **Tuberculosis**

Condition Inhalation of tubercle bacilli into the alveolar wall starts: (1) Initial complex is acute inflammatory response—macrophages engulf bacilli but do not kill them. Tubercle forms around bacilli. (2) Scar tissue forms, lesion calcifies and shows on x-ray. (3) Reactivation of previously healed lesion. Dormant bacilli now multiply, producing necrosis, cavitation, and caseous lung tissue (cheeselike). (4) Extensive destruction as lesion erodes into bronchus, forming air-filled cavity. Apex usually has the most damage.

Subjective Initially asymptomatic, showing as positive skin test or on x-ray study. Progressive TB involves weight loss, anorexia, easy fatigability, low-grade afternoon fevers, night sweats. May have pleural effusion, recurrent lower respiratory infections.

Inspection Cough initially nonproductive, later productive of purulent, yellow-green sputum; may be blood tinged. Dyspnea, orthopnea, fatigue, weakness.

Palpation Skin moist at night from night sweats.

Percussion Resonant initially. Dull over any effusion.

Auscultation Normal or decreased vesicular breath sounds.

Adventitious Sounds Crackles over upper lobes common, persist following full expiration and cough.

Continued

TABLE 18-9   Assessment of Common Respiratory Conditions—cont'd

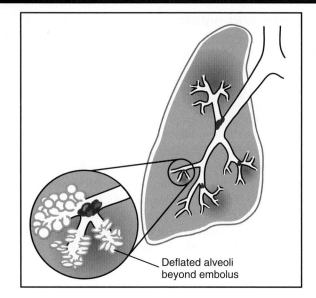

Deflated alveoli beyond embolus

◀ Pulmonary Embolism

Condition Undissolved materials (e.g., thrombus or air bubbles, fat globules) originating in legs or pelvis detach and travel through venous system, returning blood to right heart, and lodge to occlude pulmonary vessels. Over 95% arise from deep vein thrombi in lower legs as a result of stasis of blood, vessel injury, or hypercoagulability. Pulmonary occlusion results in ischemia of downstream lung tissue, increased pulmonary artery pressure, decreased cardiac output, and hypoxia. Rarely, a saddle embolus in bifurcation of pulmonary arteries leads to sudden death from hypoxia. More often small-to-medium pulmonary branches occlude, leading to dyspnea. These may resolve by fibrolytic activity.

Subjective Chest pain, worse on deep inspiration, dyspnea.

Inspection Apprehensive, restless, anxiety, mental status changes, cyanosis, tachypnea, cough, hemoptysis, Pao_2 <80% on pulse oximetry. Arterial blood gases show respiratory alkalosis.

Palpation Diaphoresis, hypotension.

Auscultation Tachycardia, accentuated pulmonic component of S_2 heart sound.

Adventitious Sounds Crackles, wheezes.

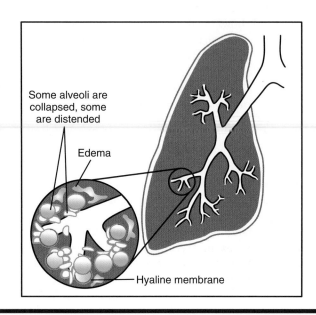

Some alveoli are collapsed, some are distended

Edema

Hyaline membrane

◀ Acute Respiratory Distress Syndrome (ARDS)

Condition An acute pulmonary insult (trauma, gastric acid aspiration, shock, sepsis) damages alveolar capillary membrane, leading to increased permeability of pulmonary capillaries and alveolar epithelium and to pulmonary edema. Gross examination (autopsy) would show dark red, firm, airless tissue, with some alveoli collapsed and hyaline membranes lining the distended alveoli.

Subjective Acute onset of dyspnea, apprehension.

Inspection Restlessness; disorientation; rapid, shallow breathing; productive cough; thin, frothy sputum; retractions of intercostal spaces and sternum. Decreased Pao_2, blood gases show respiratory alkalosis, x-ray films show diffuse pulmonary infiltrates; a late sign is cyanosis.

Palpation Hypotension.

Auscultation Tachycardia.

Adventitious Sounds Crackles, rhonchi.

TABLE 18-9 Assessment of Common Respiratory Conditions—cont'd

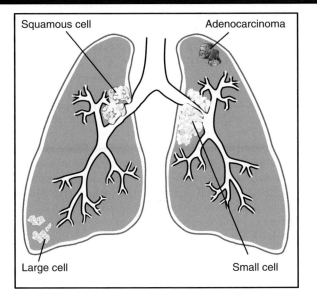

Squamous cell

Adenocarcinoma

Large cell

Small cell

◀ Lung Cancer

Condition This is the most fatal of malignancies, claiming as many lives per year as breast, colorectal, and prostate cancers combined.[15] The major cause is tobacco smoking (85%), followed by exposure to secondhand smoke and asbestos exposure. Four types: squamous cell usually starts in central bronchi near the hilus; adenocarcinoma usually starts in periphery and escapes early detection; large cell also starts in periphery with tumors arranged as clusters; small cell (oat cell) compresses and narrows central bronchi.[15]

Subjective Fatigue, nausea and vomiting, change in taste perception, anorexia. Persistent cough may also be productive; dyspnea; dull poorly localized chest pain. 10%-25% are asymptomatic.

Inspection Weight loss, clubbing, hoarseness, anemia, hemoptysis

Auscultation May have wheezing, atelectasis, pleural effusion, pneumonia distal to obstruction.

Summary Checklist: Thorax and Lung Examination

1. **Inspection**
   Thoracic cage
   Respirations
   Skin color and condition
   Person's position
   Facial expression
   Level of consciousness

2. **Palpation**
   Confirm symmetric expansion
   Tactile fremitus
   Detect any lumps, masses, tenderness

3. **Percussion**
   Percuss over lung fields
   Estimate diaphragmatic excursion

4. **Auscultation**
   Assess normal breath sounds
   Note any abnormal breath sounds
   If abnormal breath sounds present, perform bronchophony, whispered pectoriloquy, egophony
   Note any adventitious sounds

BIBLIOGRAPHY

1. Baker K., Barsamian J., Leone D., et al. (2013). Routine dyspnea assessment on unit admission. *Am J Nurs 112*(11), 42-50.

2. Bel, E. H. (2013). Mild asthma. *New Engl J Med 369*(6), 549-557.

3. Best, D. (2009). Technical report: secondhand and prenatal tobacco smoke exposure. *Pediatrics, 124*(5), e1017-e1044.

4. Blair, K. A., & Evelo, A. J. (2013). COPD: overview and survey of NP knowledge. *Nurse Pract, 38*(6), 18-26.

5. Blood-Siegfried, J., & Rende, E. K. (2010). The long-term effects of prenatal nicotine exposure on neurologic development. *J Midwif Women's Health, 55*(2), 143-152.

6. Blush R. R. (2013). Acute bronchitis evaluation and management. *Nurse Pract, 38*(10), 14-20.

7. Bobrowski, R. A. (2010). Pulmonary physiology in pregnancy. *Clinical Obstetrics and Gynecology, 53*(2), 285.

7a. Bohadana A., Izbicki G., & Kraman S. S. (2014). Fundamentals of lung auscultation. *N Engl J Med, 370*(8), 744-751.

8. Burt, L., & Corbridge, S. (2013). COPD exacerbations. *Am J Nurs, 113*(2), 34-43.

9. Carlsten, C., & Melén, E. (2012). Air pollution, genetics, and allergy. *Curr Opin Allerg Clin Immunol, 12*(5), 455-461.

10. Carlucci, M., Smith, M., & Corbridge, S. J. (2013). Poor sleep, hazardous breathing: an overview of obstructive sleep apnea. *Nurse Pract, 38*(3), 20-28.

11. Centers for Disease Control and Prevention. (2012). National surveillance of asthma: United States, 2001-2010. *Vital Health Stat, 3*(35).

12. Centers for Disease Control and Prevention. (2013). Trends in tuberculosis—United States, 2012. *MMWR, 62*(11), 201-216.

13. Chaney, S. E., & Sheriff, S. (2012). Evidence-based treatments for smoking cessation. *Nurse Pract, 37*(4), 24-31.

14. Chantry, C. J., Howard, C. R., & Auinger, P. (2006). Full breastfeeding duration and associated decrease in respiratory tract infection in U.S. children. *Pediatrics, 117*(2), 425-432.

15. Copstead, L., & Banasik, J. (2013). *Pathophysiology.* (5th ed.) St. Louis: Elsevier.

16. Reference deleted in proofs.

17. Corbridge, S., Wilken, L., Kapella, M. C., et al. (2012). An evidence-based approach to COPD: part 1. *Am J Nurs, 112*(3), 46-57.

18. Crocker, D., Brown, C., Moolenaar, R., et al. (2009). Racial and ethnic disparities in asthma medication usage and health-care utilization. *Chest, 136*(4), 1063-1071.

19. Cunningham, F. G., Leveno, K., Bloom, S., et al. (2010). *Williams obstetrics.* (23rd ed.). New York: McGraw-Hill Professional.

20. Du, H., Newton, P. J., Salamonson, Y., et al. (2009). A review of the six-minute walk test. *Eur J Cardiovasc Nurs, 8*(1), 2-8.

21. Garvey, C. (2011). Best practices in chronic obstructive pulmonary disease. *Nurse Pract, 36*(5):16-22.

22. Goss, L. K. (2011). A close up view of pneumococcal disease. *Nurse Pract, 36*(12), 41-45.

23. Haberg, S. E., Bentdal, Y. E., London, S. J., et al. (2010). Prenatal and postnatal parental smoking and acute otitis media in early childhood. *Acta Paediatrica, 99*(1), 99-105.

24. Hanania, N. A., Mannino, D. M., Yawn, B. P., et al. (2010). Predicting risk of airflow obstruction in primary care: validation of the lung function questionnaire (LFQ). *Resp Med, 104*(8), 1160-1170.

25. Jha, P., Ramasundarahettige, C., Landsman, V., et al. (2013). 21st-century hazards of smoking and benefits of cessation in the United States. *N Engl J Med, 368*(4), 341-350.

25a. Lew, K. B. (2014). Identifying pectus excavatum in the primary care setting. *Nurse Pract, 39*(6), 25-28.

26. McCool, F. D., & Tzelepis, G. E. (2012). Dysfunction of the diaphragm. *N Engl J Med, 366*(10), 932-942.

26a. Musher, D. M., & Thorner, A. R. (2014). Community-acquired pneumonia. *N Engl J Med, 371*(17), 1619-1627.

27. Nicholson, K. N. (2013). Screening for cystic fibrosis. *Nurse Pract, 38*(9), 24-32.

28. O'Laughlen, M. C., & Rance, K. (2012). Update on asthma management in primary care. *Nurse Pract, 37*(11), 32-40.

29. Paksu, S., Paksu, M. S., Kilic, M., et al. (2012). Foreign body aspiration in childhood: evaluation of diagnostic parameters *Pediatr Emerg Care, 28*(3), 259-264.

29a. Quinn, B., Baker, D. L., Cohen, S., et al. (2014). Basic nursing care to prevent nonventilator hospital-acquired pneumonia. *J Nurs Scholar, 46*(1), 11-18.

30. Sleiman, P. M. A., Flory, J., Imielinshi, M., et al. (2010). Variants of DENND1B associated with asthma in children. *N Engl J Med, 362*(1), 36-44.

30a. Tarlo, S. M., Lemiere, C. (2014). Occupational asthma. *N Engl J Med, 370*(7), 640-649.

31. Thun, M. J., Carter, B. D., Feskanich, D., et al. (2013). 50-year trends in smoking-related mortality in the United States. *N Engl J Med, 368*(4), 351-364.

32. U.S. Department of Defense. (2013). *Five A's of counseling patients to quit smoking.* Available at http://www.ucanquit2.org/helpsomeonequit/healthprofessionals/FiveAs.aspx.

33. U.S. Department of Health and Human Services. (2012.) *Preventing tobacco use among youth and young adults.* Atlanta, GA: Centers for Disease Control and Prevention, www.cdc.gov/tobacco.

34. Vazquez, R., Gheorghe, C., Ramos, F., et al. (2010). Gurgling breath sounds may predict hospital-acquired pneumonia. *Chest, 138*(2), 284-288.

35. Vyshedskiy, A., Alhashem, R. M., Paciej, R., et al. (2009). Mechanism of inspiratory and expiratory crackles. *Chest, 135*(1), 156-164.

36. Wahls, S. A. (2012). Causes and evaluation of chronic dyspnea. *Am Fam Phys, 86*(2), 173-180.

37. Wong, C. L., Holroyd-Leduc, J., Straus, S. E. (2009). Does this patient have a pleural effusion? *JAMA, 301*(3), 309-317.

37a. Wunderink R. G., Waterer G. W. (2014). Community-acquired pneumonia. *N Engl J Med, 370*(6), 543-550.

38. Yates, C. (2013). Assessing asthma control: an evidence-based approach. *Nurse Pract, 38*(6), 40-47.

39. Zemek, R., Plint, A., Osmond, M. H., et al. (2012). Triage nurse initiation of corticosteroids in pediatric asthma is associated with improved emergency department efficiency. *Pediatrics, 129*(4), 671-680.

40. Zumla, A., Raviglione, M., Hafner, R., et al. (2013). Tuberculosis. *N Engl J Med, 368*(8), 745-755.

CHAPTER 19

Heart and Neck Vessels

STRUCTURE AND FUNCTION

PRECORDIUM

Base

Apex

1
2
3
4
5
6
7
8

19-1

© Pat Thomas, 2006.

POSITION AND SURFACE LANDMARKS

The cardiovascular (CV) system consists of the **heart** (a muscular pump) and the **blood vessels.** The **precordium** is the area on the anterior chest directly overlying the heart and great vessels (Fig. 19-1). The great vessels are the major arteries and veins connected to the heart. The heart and great vessels are located between the lungs in the middle third of the thoracic cage (**mediastinum).** The heart extends from the 2nd to the 5th intercostal space and from the right border of the sternum to the left midclavicular line.

Inside the body the heart is rotated so its right side is anterior and its left side is mostly posterior. Of the heart's four chambers, the right ventricle is immediately behind the sternum and forms the greatest area of anterior cardiac surface. The left ventricle lies behind the right ventricle and forms the apex and slender area of the left border. The right atrium lies to the right and above the right ventricle and forms the right border. The left atrium is located posteriorly, with only a small portion, the left atrial appendage, showing anteriorly.

459

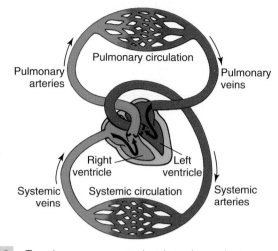

19-2 Two loops—separate but interdependent.

The blood vessels are arranged in two continuous loops, the *pulmonary circulation* and the *systemic circulation* (Fig. 19-2). When the heart contracts, it pumps blood simultaneously into both loops.

Think of the heart as an upside-down triangle in the chest. The "top" of the heart is the broader *base,* and the "bottom" is the *apex,* which points down and to the left (Fig. 19-3). During contraction the apex beats against the chest wall, producing an apical impulse. This is palpable in most people, normally at the fifth intercostal space, 7 to 9 cm from the midsternal line.

The **great vessels** lie bunched above the base of the heart. The **superior** and **inferior vena cava** return unoxygenated venous blood to the right side of the heart. The **pulmonary artery** leaves the right ventricle, bifurcates, and carries the venous blood to the lungs. The **pulmonary veins** return the freshly oxygenated blood to the left side of the heart, and the **aorta** carries it out to the body. The aorta ascends from the left ventricle, arches back at the level of the sternal angle, and descends behind the heart.

HEART WALL, CHAMBERS, AND VALVES

The **heart wall** has numerous layers. The **pericardium** is a tough, fibrous, double-walled sac that surrounds and protects the heart (see its cut edge in Fig. 19-4). It has two layers that contain a few milliliters of serous *pericardial fluid.* This ensures smooth, friction-free movement of the heart muscle. The pericardium is adherent to the great vessels, esophagus, sternum, and pleurae and is anchored to the diaphragm. The **myocardium** is the muscular wall of the heart; it does the pumping. The **endocardium** is the thin layer of endothelial tissue that lines the inner surface of the heart chambers and valves.

The common metaphor is to think of the heart as a pump. But consider that the heart is actually *two* pumps; the right side of the heart pumps blood into the lungs, and the left side simultaneously pumps blood into the body. The two pumps are separated by an impermeable wall, the septum. Each side has an **atrium** and a **ventricle.** The atrium (Latin for "anteroom") is a thin-walled reservoir for holding blood, and the thick-walled ventricle is the muscular pumping chamber. (It is common to use the following abbreviations to refer to the chambers: *RA,* right atrium; *RV,* right ventricle; *LA,* left atrium; and *LV,* left ventricle.)

The four **chambers** are separated by swinging-door–like structures, called *valves,* whose main purpose is to prevent backflow of blood. The valves are unidirectional; they can open only one way. They open and close *passively* in response to pressure gradients in the moving blood.

There are four **valves** in the heart (see Fig. 19-4). The two **atrioventricular** (AV) valves separate the atria and the ventricles. The right AV valve is the **tricuspid,** and the left AV valve is the bicuspid or **mitral** valve (so named because it resembles a bishop's mitered cap). The valves' thin leaflets are anchored by collagenous fibers (**chordae tendineae**) to papillary muscles embedded in the ventricle floor. The AV valves open during the heart's filling phase, or **diastole,** to allow the ventricles to fill with blood. During the pumping phase, or **systole,** the AV valves close to prevent regurgitation

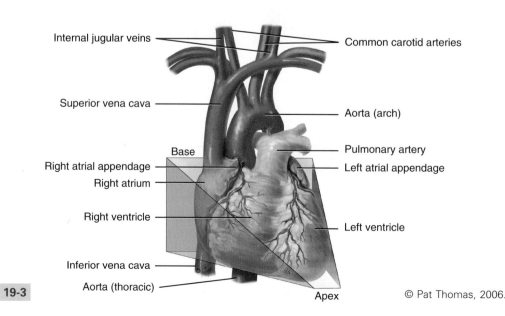

Internal jugular veins

Common carotid arteries

Superior vena cava

Aorta (arch)

Base

Pulmonary artery

Right atrial appendage

Left atrial appendage

Right atrium

Right ventricle

Left ventricle

Inferior vena cava

19-3

Aorta (thoracic)

Apex

© Pat Thomas, 2006.

Aorta (arch)

Cut edge of pericardium

Superior vena cava

Pulmonary artery

Pulmonary veins

Pulmonic valve

Right atrium

Tricuspid (AV) valve

Inferior vena cava

Right ventricle

Pulmonary veins

Left atrium

Aortic valve

Mitral (AV) valve

Chordae tendineae

Left ventricle

Papillary muscle

Endocardium

Myocardium

19-4

© Pat Thomas, 2006.

of blood back up into the atria. The papillary muscles contract at this time so the valve leaflets meet and unite to form a perfect seal without turning themselves inside out.

The **semilunar** (SL) valves are set between the ventricles and the arteries. Each valve has three cusps that look like half moons. The SL valves are the **pulmonic** valve in the right side of the heart and the **aortic** valve in the left side of the heart. They open during pumping, or **systole,** to allow blood to be ejected from the heart.

NOTE: There are no valves between the vena cava and the right atrium or between the pulmonary veins and the left atrium. For this reason abnormally high pressure in the left side of the heart gives a person symptoms of pulmonary congestion, and abnormally high pressure in the right side of the heart shows in the distended neck veins and abdomen.

DIRECTION OF BLOOD FLOW

Think of an unoxygenated red blood cell being drained downstream into the vena cava. It is swept along with the flow of venous blood and follows the route illustrated in Fig. 19-5.

1. From liver to RA through inferior vena cava.

    Superior vena cava drains venous blood from the head and upper extremities.

    From RA venous blood travels through tricuspid valve to RV.

2. From RV venous blood flows through pulmonic valve to pulmonary artery.

    Pulmonary artery delivers unoxygenated blood to lungs.

to head and neck

to arms

to arms

⑤

③

②

①

④

to abdomen and lower extremities

19-5

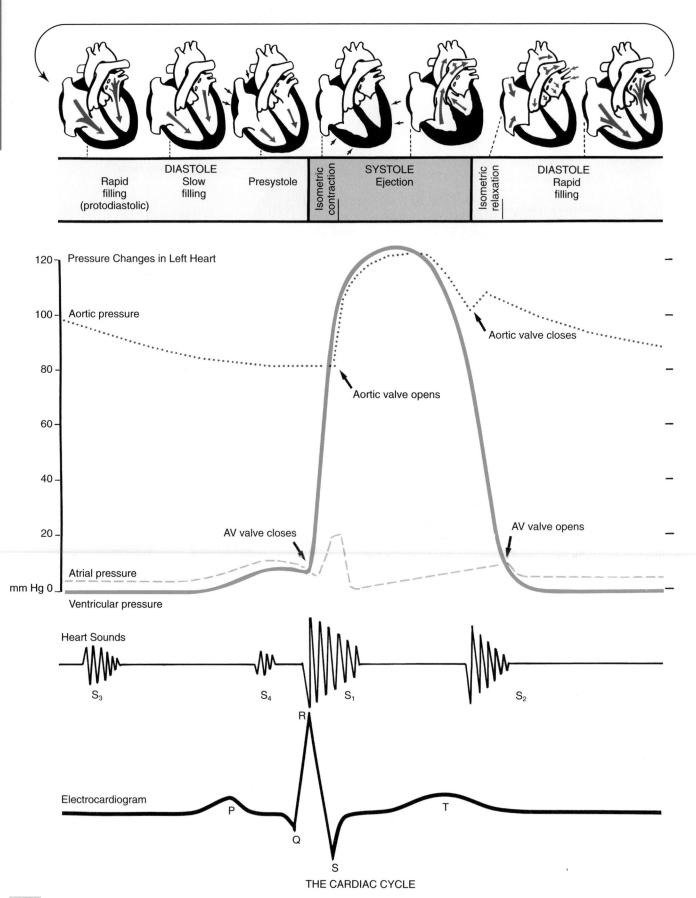

	DIASTOLE			Isometric contraction	SYSTOLE		Isometric relaxation	DIASTOLE
Rapid filling (protodiastolic)	Slow filling	Presystole			Ejection			Rapid filling

Pressure Changes in Left Heart

Aortic pressure

Aortic valve closes

Aortic valve opens

AV valve opens

AV valve closes

Atrial pressure

mm Hg 0

Ventricular pressure

Heart Sounds

S₃   S₄   S₁   S₂

R

P   Q   S   T

THE CARDIAC CYCLE

3. Lungs oxygenate blood.
   Pulmonary veins return fresh blood to LA.
4. From LA arterial blood travels through mitral valve to LV.
   LV ejects blood through aortic valve into aorta.
5. Aorta delivers oxygenated blood to body.

Remember that the circulation is a continuous loop. The blood is kept moving by continually shifting pressure gradients. It flows from an area of higher pressure to one of lower pressure.

CARDIAC CYCLE

The rhythmic movement of blood through the heart is the **cardiac cycle.** It has two phases, **diastole** and **systole.** In **diastole** the ventricles relax and fill with blood. This takes up two thirds of the cardiac cycle. Heart contraction is **systole.** During systole blood is pumped from the ventricles and fills the pulmonary and systemic arteries. This is one third of the cardiac cycle.

Diastole.   In diastole the ventricles are relaxed, and the AV valves (i.e., the tricuspid and mitral) are open (Fig. 19-6). (Opening of the normal valve is acoustically silent.) The pressure in the atria is higher than that in the ventricles; therefore blood pours rapidly into the ventricles. This first passive filling phase is called **early** or **protodiastolic filling.**

Toward the end of diastole the atria contract and push the last amount of blood (about 25% of stroke volume) into the ventricles. This active filling phase is called **presystole,** or **atrial systole,** or sometimes the *atrial kick.* It causes a small rise in left ventricular pressure. (Note that atrial systole occurs during ventricular diastole, a confusing but important point.)

Systole.   Now so much blood has been pumped into the ventricles that ventricular pressure is finally higher than that in the atria; thus the mitral and tricuspid valves swing shut. The closure of the AV valves contributes to the first heart sound (S$_1$) and signals the beginning of systole. The AV valves close to prevent any regurgitation of blood back up into the atria during contraction.

For a very brief moment all four valves are closed. The ventricular walls contract. This contraction against a closed system works to build pressure inside the ventricles to a high level (**isometric contraction**). Consider first the left side of the heart. When the pressure in the ventricle finally exceeds pressure in the aorta, the aortic valve opens, and blood is ejected rapidly.

After the ventricle's contents are ejected, its pressure falls. When pressure falls below pressure in the aorta, some blood flows backward toward the ventricle, causing the aortic valve to swing shut. This closure of the semilunar valves causes the second heart sound (S$_2$) and signals the end of systole.

Diastole Again.   Now all four valves are closed, and the ventricles relax (called **isometric** or **isovolumic relaxation**). Meanwhile the atria have been filling with blood delivered from the lungs. Atrial pressure is now higher than the relaxed ventricular pressure. The mitral valve drifts open, and diastolic filling begins again.

Events in the Right and Left Sides.   The same events are happening at the same time in the right side of the heart, but pressures in the right side of the heart are much lower than those of the left side because less energy is needed to pump blood to its destination, the pulmonary circulation. Also, events occur just slightly later in the right side of the heart because of the route of myocardial depolarization. As a result, two distinct components to each of the heart sounds exist, and sometimes you can hear them separately. In the first heart sound the mitral component (M$_1$) closes just before the tricuspid component (T$_1$). And with S$_2$, aortic closure (A$_2$) occurs slightly before pulmonic closure (P$_2$).

HEART SOUNDS

Events in the cardiac cycle generate sounds that can be heard through a stethoscope over the chest wall. These include normal heart sounds and occasionally extra heart sounds and murmurs (Fig. 19-7).

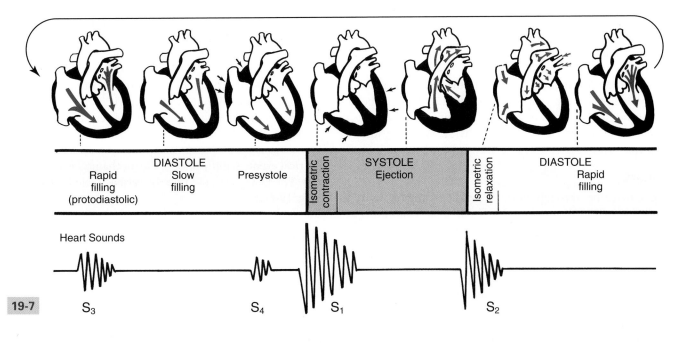

	DIASTOLE			Isometric contraction	SYSTOLE	Isometric relaxation	DIASTOLE
Rapid filling (protodiastolic)	Slow filling	Presystole			Ejection		Rapid filling

Heart Sounds

S$_3$ S$_4$ S$_1$ S$_2$

19-7

Structure and Function

Normal Heart Sounds

The **first heart sound** (S_1) occurs with closure of the AV valves and thus signals the beginning of systole. The mitral component of the first sound (M_1) slightly precedes the tricuspid component (T_1), but you usually hear these two components fused as one sound. You can hear S_1 over all the precordium, but usually it is loudest at the apex.

The **second heart sound** (S_2) occurs with closure of the semilunar valves and signals the end of systole. The aortic component of the second sound (A_2) slightly precedes the pulmonic component (P_2). Although it is heard over all the precordium, S_2 is loudest at the base.

Effect of Respiration. The volume of right and left ventricular systole is just about equal, but this can be affected by respiration. To learn this, consider the phrase:

MoRe to the **R**ight heart,

Less to the **L**eft

That means that during inspiration, intrathoracic pressure is decreased. This pushes more blood into the vena cava, increasing venous return to the right side of the heart, which increases right ventricular stroke volume. The increased volume prolongs right ventricular systole and delays pulmonic valve closure.

Meanwhile on the left side, a greater amount of blood is sequestered in the lungs during inspiration. This momentarily decreases the amount returned to the left side of the heart, decreasing left ventricular stroke volume. The decreased volume shortens left ventricular systole and allows the aortic valve to close a bit earlier. When the aortic valve closes significantly earlier than the pulmonic valve, you can hear the two components separately. This is a *split* S_2.

Extra Heart Sounds

Third Heart Sound (S_3). Normally diastole is a silent event. However, in some conditions ventricular filling creates vibrations that can be heard over the chest. These vibrations are S_3. S_3 occurs when the ventricles are resistant to filling during the early rapid filling phase (protodiastole). This occurs immediately after S_2, when the AV valves open and atrial blood first pours into the ventricles. (See a complete discussion of S_3 in Table 19-8, p. 499.)

Fourth Heart Sound (S_4). S_4 occurs at the end of diastole, at presystole, when the ventricle is resistant to filling. The atria contract and push blood into a noncompliant ventricle. This creates vibrations that are heard as S_4. S_4 occurs just before S_1.

Murmurs

Blood circulating through normal cardiac chambers and valves usually makes no noise. However, some conditions create turbulent blood flow and collision currents. These result in a murmur, much like a pile of stones or a sharp turn in a stream creates a noisy water flow. A murmur is a gentle, blowing, swooshing sound that can be heard on the chest wall. Conditions resulting in a murmur are as follows:

1. Velocity of blood increases (flow murmur) (e.g., in exercise, thyrotoxicosis)
2. Viscosity of blood decreases (e.g., in anemia)
3. Structural defects in the valves (a stenotic or narrowed valve, an incompetent or regurgitant valve) or unusual openings occur in the chambers (dilated chamber, septal defect)

Characteristics of Sound

All heart sounds are described by:

1. Frequency (pitch)—Heart sounds are described as high pitched or low pitched, although these terms are relative because all are low-frequency sounds, and you need a good stethoscope to hear them.
2. Intensity (loudness)—Loud or soft
3. Duration—Very short for heart sounds; silent periods are longer
4. Timing—Systole or diastole

CONDUCTION

Of all organs, the heart has a unique ability—automaticity. The heart can contract by itself, independent of any signals or stimulation from the body. It contracts in response to an electrical current conveyed by a conduction system (Fig. 19-8). Specialized cells in the sinoatrial (SA) node near the superior vena cava initiate an electrical impulse. (Because the SA node has an intrinsic rhythm, it is the "pacemaker.") The current flows in an orderly sequence, first across the atria to the AV node low in the atrial septum. There it is delayed slightly so the atria have time to contract before the ventricles are stimulated. Then the impulse travels to the bundle of His, the right and left bundle branches, and then through the ventricles.

The electrical impulse stimulates the heart to do its work, which is to contract. A small amount of electricity spreads to the body surface, where it can be measured and recorded on the electrocardiograph (ECG). The ECG waves are arbitrarily labeled *PQRST,* which stand for the following elements:

P wave—Depolarization of the atria
PR interval—From the beginning of the P wave to the beginning of the QRS complex (the time necessary for atrial depolarization plus time for the impulse to travel through the AV node to the ventricles)
QRS complex—Depolarization of the ventricles
T wave—Repolarization of the ventricles

Electrical events slightly *precede* the mechanical events in the heart. The ECG juxtaposed on the cardiac cycle is illustrated in Fig. 19-6.

PUMPING ABILITY

In the resting adult, the heart normally pumps between 4 and 6 L of blood per minute throughout the body. This **cardiac output** equals the volume of blood in each systole (called the

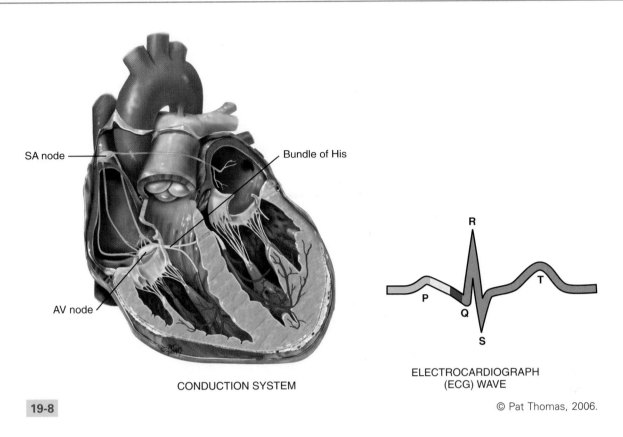

SA node

Bundle of His

AV node

CONDUCTION SYSTEM

19-8

ELECTROCARDIOGRAPH
(ECG) WAVE

© Pat Thomas, 2006.

stroke volume) times the number of beats per minute (rate). This is described as:

$$CO = SV \times R$$

The heart can alter its cardiac output to adapt to the metabolic needs of the body. Preload and afterload affect the heart's ability to increase cardiac output.

Preload is the venous return that builds during diastole. It is the length to which the ventricular muscle is stretched at the end of diastole just before contraction (Fig. 19-9).

When the volume of blood returned to the ventricles is increased (as when exercise stimulates skeletal muscles to contract and force more blood back to the heart), the muscle bundles are stretched beyond their normal resting state to accommodate. The force of this stretch is the preload. According to the Frank-Starling law, the greater the stretch, the stronger is the contraction of the heart. This increased contractility results in an increased volume of blood ejected (increased stroke volume).

Afterload is the opposing pressure the ventricle must generate to open the aortic valve against the higher aortic

PRELOAD

19-9

AFTERLOAD

© Pat Thomas, 2006.

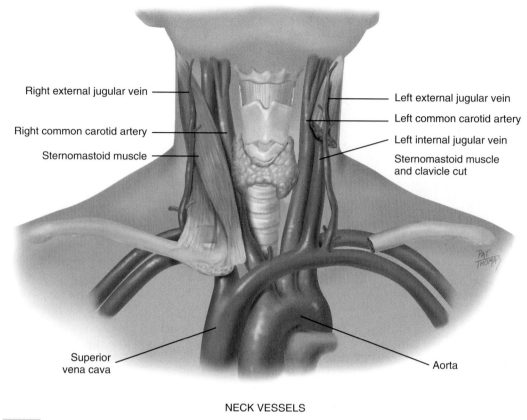

Right external jugular vein

Right common carotid artery

Sternomastoid muscle

Left external jugular vein

Left common carotid artery

Left internal jugular vein

Sternomastoid muscle and clavicle cut

Superior vena cava

Aorta

NECK VESSELS

19-10

pressure. It is the resistance against which the ventricle must pump its blood. Once the ventricle is filled with blood, the ventricular end diastolic pressure is 5 to 10 mm Hg, whereas that in the aorta is 70 to 80 mm Hg. To overcome this difference, the ventricular muscle *tenses* (isovolumic contraction). After the aortic valve opens, rapid ejection occurs.

THE NECK VESSELS

CV assessment includes the survey of vascular structures in the neck—the carotid artery and the jugular veins (Fig. 19-10). These vessels reflect the efficiency of cardiac function.

The Carotid Artery Pulse

Chapter 9 describes the pulse as a pressure wave generated by each systole pumping blood into the aorta. The carotid artery is a central artery (i.e., it is close to the heart). Its timing closely coincides with ventricular systole. (Assessment of the peripheral pulses is found in Chapter 20, and blood pressure [BP] assessment is found in Chapter 9.)

The **carotid artery** is located in the groove between the trachea and the sternomastoid muscle, medial to and alongside that muscle. Note the characteristics of its waveform (Fig. 19-11): a smooth rapid upstroke, a summit that is rounded and smooth, and a downstroke that is more gradual and has a dicrotic notch caused by closure of the aortic valve (marked *D* in the figure).

Jugular Venous Pulse and Pressure

The **jugular veins** empty unoxygenated blood directly into the superior vena cava. Because no cardiac valve exists to separate the superior vena cava from the right atrium, the jugular veins give information about activity on the right side of the heart. Specifically they reflect filling pressure and

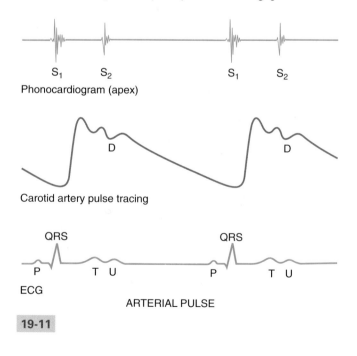

S_1 S_2 S_1 S_2

Phonocardiogram (apex)

D   D

Carotid artery pulse tracing

QRS   QRS

P   T U   P   T U

ECG

ARTERIAL PULSE

19-11

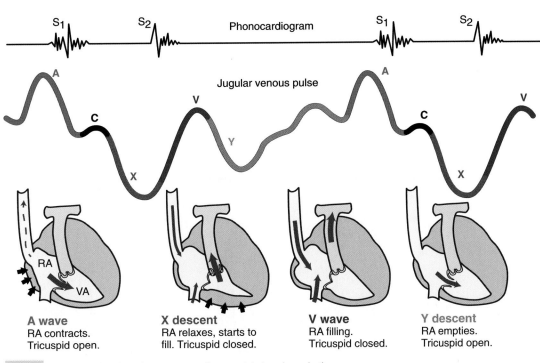

A wave
RA contracts.
Tricuspid open.

X descent
RA relaxes, starts to
fill. Tricuspid closed.

V wave
RA filling.
Tricuspid closed.

Y descent
RA empties.
Tricuspid open.

19-12 **Note:** Match color on waveform with its description.

volume changes. Because volume and pressure increase when the right side of the heart fails to pump efficiently, the jugular veins expose this.

Two jugular veins are present in each side of the neck (see Fig. 19-10). The larger **internal jugular** lies deep and medial to the sternomastoid muscle. It is usually not visible, although its diffuse pulsations may be seen in the sternal notch when the person is supine. The **external jugular** vein is more superficial; it lies lateral to the sternomastoid muscle, above the clavicle.

Although an arterial pulse is caused by a forward propulsion of blood, the jugular venous pulse is different. The jugular pulse results from a backwash, a waveform moving backward caused by events upstream. The jugular pulse has five components, as shown in Fig 19-12.

The five components of the jugular venous pulse occur because of events in the right side of the heart. The A wave reflects atrial contraction because some blood flows backward to the vena cava during right atrial contraction. The C wave, or ventricular contraction, is backflow from the bulging upward of the tricuspid valve when it closes at the beginning of ventricular systole (not from the neighboring carotid artery pulsation). Next the X descent shows atrial relaxation when the right ventricle contracts during systole and pulls the bottom of the atria downward. The V wave occurs with passive atrial filling because of the increasing volume in the right atria and increased pressure. Finally the Y descent reflects passive ventricular filling when the tricuspid valve opens and blood flows from the RA to the RV.

❖ DEVELOPMENTAL COMPETENCE

The Pregnant Woman

The CV system adapts to ensure adequate blood supply to the uterus and placenta, to deliver oxygen and nutrients to the fetus, and to allow the mother to function normally during this altered state.[10] Blood volume increases by 30% to 40% during pregnancy, with the most rapid expansion occurring during the second trimester. This creates an increase in stroke volume and cardiac output and an increased pulse rate of 10 to 15 beats/min. The pulse rate rises in the first trimester, peaks in the third trimester, and returns to baseline within the first 10 postpartum days.[16] Despite the increased cardiac output, arterial BP decreases in pregnancy as a result of peripheral vasodilation. The BP drops to its lowest point during the second trimester and rises after that.

Infants and Children

The fetal heart functions early; it begins to beat at the end of 3 weeks' gestation. The lungs are nonfunctional, but the fetal circulation compensates for this (Fig. 19-13). Oxygenation takes place at the placenta, and the arterial blood is returned to the right side of the fetal heart. There is no point in pumping all this freshly oxygenated blood through the lungs; therefore it is rerouted in two ways. First, about two thirds of it is shunted through an opening in the atrial septum, the **foramen ovale,** into the left side of the heart, where it is pumped out through the aorta. Second, the rest of the oxygenated blood is pumped by the right side of the heart out

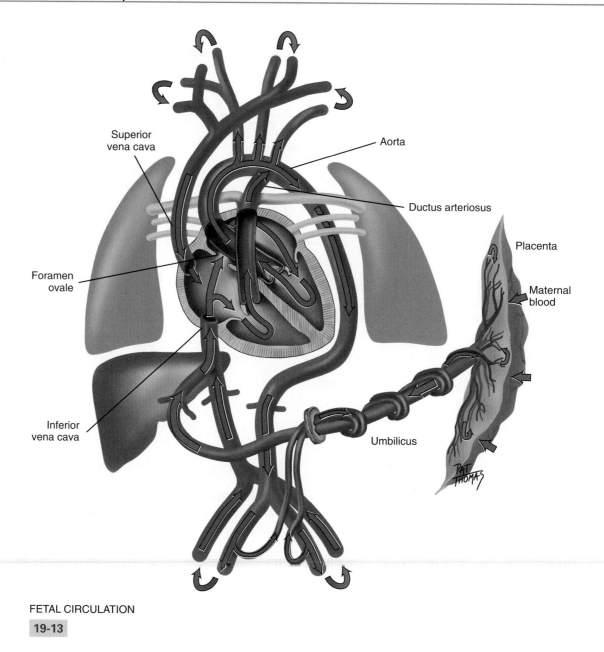

FETAL CIRCULATION

19-13

through the pulmonary artery, but it is detoured through the **ductus arteriosus** to the aorta. Because they are both pumping into the systemic circulation, the right and left ventricles are equal in weight and muscle wall thickness.

Inflation and aeration of the lungs at birth produces circulatory changes. Now the blood is oxygenated through the lungs rather than through the placenta. The foramen ovale closes within the first hour because of the new lower pressure in the right side of the heart than in the left side. The ductus arteriosus closes later, usually within 10 to 15 hours of birth. Now the left ventricle has the greater workload of pumping into the systemic circulation. So by the time the baby has reached 1 year of age, the mass of the left ventricle will have increased to reach the adult ratio of 2 : 1, left ventricle to right ventricle.

The heart's position in the chest is more horizontal in the infant than in the adult; thus the apex is higher, located at the fourth left intercostal space (Fig. 19-14). It reaches the adult position when the child reaches age 7 years.

The Aging Adult

It is difficult to isolate the "aging process" of the CV system *per se* because it is so closely interrelated with lifestyle, habits, and diseases. We know that lifestyle modifies the development of CV disease; smoking, diet, alcohol use, exercise patterns, and stress have an immense influence. Lifestyle also affects the aging process; cardiac changes once thought to be caused by aging are partially the result of the sedentary lifestyle accompanying aging (Fig. 19-15). What is left to be attributed to the aging process alone?

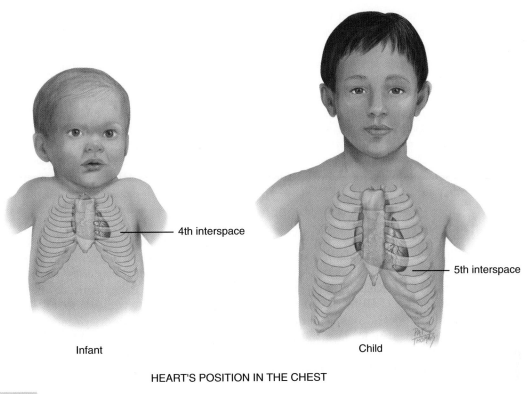

4th interspace

5th interspace

Infant

Child

HEART'S POSITION IN THE CHEST

19-14

Hemodynamic Changes with Aging

With aging there is an increase in systolic BP.[8] This is caused by thickening and stiffening of the large arteries, which in turn are caused by collagen and calcium deposits in vessel walls and loss of elastic fibers. This stiffening (arteriosclerosis) creates an increase in pulse wave velocity because the less compliant arteries cannot store the volume ejected.

The overall size of the heart does not increase with age, but left ventricular wall thickness increases. This is an adaptive mechanism to accommodate the vascular stiffening mentioned earlier that creates an increased workload on the heart.

Diastolic BP may decrease after the sixth decade.[8] Together with a rising systolic pressure, this increases the pulse pressure (the difference between the two).

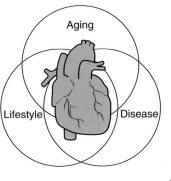

Aging

Lifestyle   Disease

19-15   (Lakatta, 1985.)

No change in resting heart rate occurs with aging.
Cardiac output at rest is not changed with aging.

There is a decreased ability of the heart to augment cardiac output with exercise. This is shown by a decreased maximum heart rate with exercise and diminished sympathetic response. Noncardiac factors also cause a decrease in maximum work performance with aging: decrease in skeletal muscle performance, increase in muscle fatigue, increased sense of dyspnea. However, aerobic exercise conditioning modifies many of the aging changes in CV function.[8]

Dysrhythmias. The presence of supraventricular and ventricular dysrhythmias increases with age. Ectopic beats are common in aging people; although these are usually asymptomatic in healthy older people, they may compromise cardiac output and BP when disease is present.

Tachydysrhythmias may not be tolerated as well in older people. The myocardium is thicker and less compliant, and early diastolic filling is impaired at rest. Thus it may not tolerate a tachycardia as well because of shortened diastole. Also, tachydysrhythmias may further compromise a vital organ whose function has already been affected by aging or disease.

Electrocardiograph. Age-related changes in the ECG occur as a result of histologic changes in the conduction system. These changes include:

- Prolonged P-R interval (first-degree AV block) and prolonged Q-T interval, but the QRS interval is unchanged.
- Left axis deviation from age-related mild LV hypertrophy and fibrosis in left bundle branch.
- Increased incidence of bundle branch block.

Although the hemodynamic changes associated with aging alone do not seem severe or portentous, the fact remains that the incidence of CV disease (CVD) increases with age. CVD is the leading cause of death in those ages 65 years and older. Stage 1 hypertension (systolic >140 mm Hg and/or diastolic >90 mm Hg) and heart failure also increase with age. Certainly, lifestyle habits (smoking, chronic alcohol use, obesity, lack of exercise, diet) play a significant role in the acquisition of heart disease. Also, increasing the physical activity of older adults—even at a moderate level—shows a reduced risk of death from CVDs and respiratory illnesses. Thus health teaching is a crucial treatment parameter.

CULTURE AND GENETICS

Prevalence is an estimate of how many people in a stated geographic location have a disease at a given point in time. In the United States an estimated 83.6 million people (more than 1 in 3) have one or more forms of CVD.[1] The annual rates of first CV event increase with age. For women, comparable rates occur 10 years later in life than for men, but this gap narrows with advancing age.

Causes of CVD include an interaction of genetic, environmental, and lifestyle factors. A peripheral blood test on 23-gene expression may prove useful in diagnosing obstructive coronary artery disease (CAD) in at-risk persons.[22] However, the American Heart Association (AHA) does not recommend genotype testing for CV risk assessment in asymptomatic adults. Further, evidence shows that potentially modifiable risk factors attribute to the overwhelming majority of cardiac risk. For example, myocardial infarction (MI) is an important type of CVD. The INTERHEART study covering 52 countries indicated that 9 potentially modifiable risk factors accounted for 90% of the population attributable risk for MI in men and 94% in women![32] These 9 modifiable factors include abnormal lipids, smoking, hypertension, diabetes, abdominal obesity, psychosocial factors, inadequate consumption of fruits and vegetables, alcohol use, and lack of regular physical activity.

High Blood Pressure. Although all adults have some potential CVD risk, some groups (defined by race, ethnicity, gender, socioeconomic status, educational level) carry an excess burden of CVD. Stage 1 **hypertension** is a systolic BP (SBP) of ≥140 mm Hg or diastolic BP (DBP) of ≥90 mm Hg or currently taking antihypertensive medicine. A higher percentage of men than women have hypertension until age 45 years. From age 45 to 64 years, the percentages are similar; after age 64 years women have a much higher percentage of hypertension than men have.[1] Hypertension also is 2 to 3 times more common among women taking oral contraceptives (especially among obese and older women) than in women who do not take them.

Among racial groups the prevalence of hypertension in Blacks is among the highest in the world, and it is rising. The prevalence of hypertension is 41.4% for African Americans, 25.8% for American Indians or Alaska natives, 28.1% for Whites, 22.2% for Hispanics, and 18.7% for Asians.[1]

Compared with Whites, African Americans develop high BP earlier in life, and their average BPs are much higher. This results in African Americans having a greater rate of stroke, death from heart disease, and end-stage kidney disease.

Smoking. Smoking rates have decreased, but cigarette smoking still is the leading cause of preventable disease, disability, and death in the United States. In the 45 years from 1965 to 2010, U.S. smoking rates declined by 54% among adults 18 years of age and older.[19] The result is that in 2010 21.2% of men and 17.5% of women were smokers. Nicotine increases the risk of MI and stroke by causing the following: increase in oxygen demand with a concomitant decrease in oxygen supply, an activation of platelets and fibrinogen, and an adverse change in the lipid profile.

Serum Cholesterol. High levels of low-density lipoprotein (LDL or "bad" cholesterol) gradually add to the lipid core of thrombus formation in arteries, which results in MI and stroke. The age-adjusted prevalence of LDL cholesterol levels over 130 mg/dL are as follows: 39.9% of Mexican-American men and 30.4% of Mexican-American women; 30.1% of White men and 29.3% of White women; and 33.1% of African-American men and 31.2% of African-American women.[1]

Obesity. The epidemic of obesity in the United States is well known and is referenced in many chapters of this text. Among Americans ages 20 years and older, the prevalence of overweight or obesity (body mass index [BMI] of ≥25 kg/m² for overweight and ≥30.0 for obesity) is as follows: overall 68% are overweight or obese (73% of men and 64% of women); among men, Mexican-Americans (81%), Whites (73%), Blacks (69%); among women, Blacks (80%), Mexican-Americans (78%), Whites (60%). Obesity increases risk of CVD, including hypertension, hyperlipidemia, type 2 diabetes mellitus (DM), sleep-disordered breathing, numerous cancers, nonalcoholic fatty liver disease, gallbladder disease, musculoskeletal disorders, and reproductive problems.[1]

Type 2 Diabetes Mellitus. The risk of CVD is twofold greater among people with DM than without DM. The increased prevalence of DM in the United States is being followed by an increasing prevalence of CVD morbidity and mortality.[1] Diabetes causes damage to the large blood vessels that nourish the brain, heart, and extremities; this results in stroke, CAD, and peripheral vascular disease.

Approximately 12.6% of African Americans 20 years of age and older, 11.8% of Hispanics, 8.4% of Asians, and 7.1% of Whites have DM.[1] The most powerful predictor of type 2 DM is obesity, with abdominal (visceral) fat posing a greater risk than lower-body obesity poses. Evidence from epidemiologic studies shows a strong genetic factor for DM, but no specific antigen type has yet been identified. In the past type 2 DM was diagnosed in adults 40 years of age and older, but now we are finding more children with it. These children are usually overweight or obese; have a family history of DM; and identify with White, American Indian, African-American, Hispanic, or Asian groups.[1]

Sex Differences. Regardless of race or ethnicity, CVD is the leading cause of death in women, claiming more women's lives annually than cancer, COPD, Alzheimer disease, and accidents combined.[17] Within the first year after a heart attack, 26% of women age 45 years and older will die compared to 19% of men.[1] This is partly because women are older than men when they do have heart attacks. However, a lack of awareness of heart attack symptoms and management has been documented widely. A recent survey revealed that only 53% of women said they would call 9-1-1 first thing if they thought they were having a heart attack.[17] Women do not report the same symptom profile for heart attack that men do, and that may affect failure to report and misdiagnosis. Chest pain is a top symptom; but men report it as sharp and crushing, whereas women report it as more like an ache. Other top symptoms that women report are unusual fatigue (67%); difficulty breathing (58%); pain radiating to back, jaw or arm (50%); feeling flushed or cold sweat (40%); dizziness (39%); and nausea (38%).[14]

Recent evidence shows some racial variations regarding heart attack symptom clusters. Older White women were more likely to have a single symptom of "unusual profound fatigue," whereas younger Black women (<50 years) who already had risk factors were more likely to have a cluster of symptoms before heart attack.[15] The largest cluster of acute prodromal symptoms was reported by smoking, younger, obese, diabetic Black women with a history of heart disease.[15]

Because women have been underrepresented in most clinical-trial reporting evidence, the AHA has redefined "ideal CV health" based on effectiveness (i.e., the benefits and risks observed in clinical practice).[17]

SUBJECTIVE DATA

1. Chest pain
2. Dyspnea
3. Orthopnea
4. Cough

5. Fatigue
6. Cyanosis or pallor
7. Edema
8. Nocturia

9. Past cardiac history
10. Family cardiac history
11. Patient-centered care (cardiac risk factors)

Examiner Asks	Rationale
1. **Chest pain.** Any **chest pain** or tightness? • Onset: When did it start? How long have you had it *this* time? Had this type of pain before? How often? • Location: Where did the pain start? Does the pain radiate to any other spot? • Character: How would you describe it? Crushing, stabbing, burning, viselike? Or aching, heaviness? (Allow the person to offer adjectives before you suggest them.) (Note if uses clenched fist to describe pain.)	Angina, an important cardiac symptom, occurs when the heart's own blood supply cannot keep up with metabolic demand. Chest pain also may have pulmonary, musculoskeletal, or gastrointestinal (GI) origin, it is important to differentiate. See Table 19-2, Differential Diagnosis of Chest Pain. A squeezing "clenched fist" sign is characteristic of angina, but the symptoms below may be anginal equivalents in the absence of chest pain.[10,14,33]
• Pain brought on by: activity—what type; rest; emotional upset; after eating; during sexual intercourse; with cold weather? • Any associated symptoms: sweating, ashen gray or pale skin, heart skips beat, shortness of breath, nausea or vomiting, racing of heart?	Diaphoresis, cold sweats, pallor, grayness. Palpitations, dyspnea, nausea, tachycardia, fatigue.
• Pain made worse by moving the arms or neck, breathing, lying flat?	Try to differentiate pain of cardiac versus noncardiac origin.
• Pain relieved by rest or nitroglycerin? How many tablets?	
2. **Dyspnea.** Any shortness of breath? • Which type of activity and how much brings on shortness of breath? How much activity brought it on 6 months ago? • Onset: Does the shortness of breath come on unexpectedly? • Duration: Constant or does it come and go? • Seem to be affected by position? Lying down?	**Dyspnea** on exertion (DOE)—Quantify exactly (e.g., DOE after walking two level blocks). Paroxysmal. Constant or intermittent. Recumbent.

Examiner Asks	Rationale

- Awaken you from sleep at night?

Paroxysmal nocturnal dyspnea (PND) occurs with heart failure. Lying down increases volume of intrathoracic blood, and the weakened heart cannot accommodate the increased load. Typically the person awakens after 2 hours of sleep with the perception of needing fresh air.

- Does the shortness of breath interfere with activities of daily living?

See Table 19-3, Clinical Portrait of Heart Failure, p. 495.

3. **Orthopnea**. How many pillows do you use when sleeping or lying down?

Orthopnea is the need to assume a more upright position to breathe. Note the exact number of pillows used.

4. **Cough**. Do you have a **cough?**
- Duration: How long have you had it?
- Frequency: Is it related to time of day?
- Type: Dry, hacking, barky, hoarse, or congested?
- Do you cough up mucus? Color? Any odor? Blood tinged?

Sputum production, mucoid or purulent. Hemoptysis is often a pulmonary disorder but also occurs with mitral stenosis.

- Associated with: activity, position (lying down), anxiety, talking?
- Does activity make it better or worse (sit, walk, exercise)?
- Relieved by rest or medication?

5. **Fatigue**. Do you seem to tire easily? Able to keep up with your family and co-workers?
- Onset: When did fatigue start? Sudden or gradual? Has any *recent* change occurred in energy level?
- Fatigue related to time of day: all day, morning, evening?

Unusual fatigue is a top prodromal MI symptom for women.[14]

Fatigue from decreased cardiac output is worse in the evening, whereas fatigue from anxiety or depression occurs all day or is worse in the morning.

6. **Cyanosis or pallor**. Ever noted your facial skin turning blue or ashen?

Cyanosis or **pallor** occurs with MI or low cardiac output states as a result of decreased tissue perfusion.

7. **Edema**. Any swelling of your feet and legs?
- Onset: When did you first notice this?
- Any recent change?
- What time of day does the swelling occur? Do your shoes feel tight at the end of day?

Edema is dependent when caused by heart failure.

Cardiac edema is worse at evening and better in morning after elevating legs all night.

- How much swelling would you say there is? Are both legs equally swollen?

Cardiac edema is bilateral; unilateral swelling has a local vein cause.

- Does the swelling go away with: rest, elevation, after a night's sleep?
- Any associated symptoms such as shortness of breath? If so, does the shortness of breath occur before leg swelling or after?

8. **Nocturia**. Do you awaken at night with an urgent need to urinate? How long has this been occurring? Any recent change?

Nocturia—Recumbency at night promotes fluid resorption and excretion; this occurs with heart failure in the person who is ambulatory during the day.

Examiner Asks	Rationale

9. **Past cardiac history.** Any **history** of: hypertension, elevated cholesterol or triglycerides, heart murmur, congenital heart disease, rheumatic fever or unexplained joint pains as child or youth, recurrent tonsillitis, anemia?
   - Ever had heart disease? When was this? Treated by medication or heart surgery?
   - Last ECG, stress ECG, serum cholesterol measurement, other heart tests?

10. **Family cardiac history.** Any **family history** of: hypertension, obesity, diabetes, CAD, sudden death at younger age?

11. **Patient-centered care (cardiac risk factors).**
    - Nutrition: Please describe your usual daily diet. (Note if this diet is representative of the basic food groups, the amount of calories, cholesterol, and any additives such as salt.) What is your usual weight? Has there been any recent change?
    - Smoking: Do you smoke cigarettes or other tobacco? At what age did you start? How many packs per day? For how many years have you smoked this amount? Have you ever tried to quit? If so, how did this go?
    - Alcohol: How much alcohol do you usually drink each week, or each day? When was your last drink? How many drinks during that episode? Have you ever been told you had a drinking problem?
    - Exercise: What is your usual amount of exercise each day or week? What type of exercise (state type or sport)? If a sport, what is your usual amount (light, moderate, heavy)?
    - Drugs: Do you take any antihypertensives, beta-blockers, calcium channel blockers, digoxin, diuretics, aspirin/anticoagulants, over-the-counter or street drugs?

Risk factors for CAD—Collect data regarding elevated cholesterol, elevated BP, blood sugar levels above 100 mg/dL or known DM, obesity, cigarette smoking, low activity level, and length of any hormone replacement therapy for postmenopausal women.

Encourage men ages 45 to 79 years and women age 55 to 79 years to use aspirin if the potential benefit of preventing MI outweighs the potential risk of GI bleeding.[26,30] Vitamin D replacement may be considered; vitamin D deficiency may increase risk of CVD and is associated with hypertension, diabetes, metabolic syndrome, left ventricular hypertrophy, and chronic vascular inflammation.[23]

Additional History for Infants

1. How was the mother's health during pregnancy? Any unexplained fever, rubella first trimester, other infection, hypertension, drugs taken?

2. Have you noted any cyanosis while nursing, crying? Is the baby able to eat, nurse, or finish bottle without tiring?

To screen for heart disease in infant, note fatigue during feeding. Infant with heart failure takes fewer ounces each feeding; becomes dyspneic with sucking; may be diaphoretic, then falls into exhausted sleep; awakens after a short time hungry again.

3. **Growth:** Has this baby grown as expected by growth charts and about the same as siblings or peers?

Poor weight gain.

4. **Activity:** Were this baby's motor milestones achieved as expected? Is the baby able to play without tiring? How many naps does the baby take each day? How long does a nap last?

Subjective Data

Additional History for Children

1. **Growth:** Has this child grown as expected by growth charts?

   Poor weight gain.

2. **Activity:** Is this child able to keep up with siblings or age mates? Is the child willing or reluctant to go out to play? Is the child able to climb stairs, ride a bike, walk a few blocks? Does the child squat to rest during play or to watch television or assume a knee-chest position while sleeping? Have you noted "blue spells" during exercise?

   Fatigue. Record specific limitations.

   Cyanosis occurs in some congenital defects: tetralogy of Fallot or transposition of the great arteries.

3. Has the child had any chest pain?

   Serious causes of chest pain are not common. Most frequent causes are musculoskeletal pain, including costochondritis, and respiratory causes, including asthma. GI and psychogenic causes are less common, and cardiac causes occur <5% of occasions.[25] However, families are worried about cardiac cause; a careful history and physical examination always is important.

4. Does the child have frequent respiratory infections? How many per year? How are they treated? Have any of these proved to be streptococcal infections?

5. **Family history:** Does the child have a sibling with heart defect? Is anyone in the child's family known to have chromosomal abnormalities such as Down syndrome?

Additional History for the Pregnant Woman

1. Have you had any high BP during this or earlier pregnancies?
   - What was your usual BP level before pregnancy? How has your BP been monitored during the pregnancy?
   - If high BP, what treatment has been started?
   - Any associated symptoms: weight gain; protein in urine; swelling in feet, legs, or face?

2. Have you had any faintness or dizziness with this pregnancy?

Additional History for the Aging Adult

1. Do you have any known heart or lung disease: hypertension, CAD, chronic emphysema, or bronchitis?
   - What efforts to treat this have been started?
   - Usual symptoms changed recently? Does your illness interfere with activities of daily living?

   Risk of CVD increases with advancing age.

2. Do you take any medications for your illness such as digitalis? Aware of side effects? Have you recently stopped taking your medication? Why?

   Noncompliance may be related to side effects or lack of finances.

3. **Environment:** Does your home have any stairs? How often do you need to climb them? Does this have any effect on activities of daily living?

OBJECTIVE DATA

PREPARATION

To evaluate the carotid arteries, the person can be sitting up. To assess the jugular veins and the precordium, the person should be supine with the head and chest elevated between 30 and 45 degrees.

Stand on the person's right side; this facilitates your hand placement, viewing of the neck veins, and auscultation of the precordium.

The room must be warm—Chilling makes the person uncomfortable, and shivering interferes with heart sounds. Take scrupulous care to ensure *quiet*; heart sounds are very soft, and any ambient room noise masks them.

Ensure the female's privacy by keeping her breasts draped. The female's left breast overrides part of the area you will need to examine. Gently displace the breast upward, or ask the woman to hold it out of the way.

When performing a regional CV assessment, use this order:

1. Pulse and BP (see Chapter 9)
2. Extremities (see Chapter 20)
3. Neck vessels
4. Precordium

The logic of this order is that you begin observations peripherally and move in toward the heart. For choreography of these steps in the complete physical examination, see Chapter 27.

EQUIPMENT NEEDED

Marking pen
Small centimeter ruler
Stethoscope with diaphragm and bell
  endpieces
Alcohol wipe (to clean endpiece)

Normal Range of Findings	Abnormal Findings

The Neck Vessels

Palpate the Carotid Artery

Located central to the heart, the carotid artery yields important information on cardiac function.

Palpate each carotid artery medial to the sternomastoid muscle in the neck (Fig. 19-16). Avoid excessive pressure on the carotid sinus area higher in the neck; excessive vagal stimulation here could slow down the heart rate, especially in older adults. Take care to palpate gently. Palpate only one carotid artery at a time to avoid compromising arterial blood to the brain.

Carotid sinus hypersensitivity is the condition in which pressure over the carotid sinus leads to a decreased heart rate, decreased BP, and cerebral ischemia with syncope. This may occur in older adults with hypertension or occlusion of the carotid artery.

19-16

Normal Range of Findings

Feel the contour and amplitude of the pulse. Normally the contour is smooth with a brisk upstroke and slower downstroke, and the normal strength is moderate. Your findings should be the same bilaterally.

Auscultate the Carotid Artery

For people middle-age or older or who show symptoms or signs of CVD, auscultate each carotid artery for the presence of a **bruit** (pronounced brú-ee) (Fig. 19-17). This is a blowing, swishing sound indicating blood flow turbulence; normally none is present.

19-17

Keep the neck in a neutral position. Lightly apply the bell of the stethoscope over the carotid artery at three levels: (1) the angle of the jaw, (2) the midcervical area, and (3) the base of the neck (see Fig. 19-17). Avoid compressing the artery because this could create an artificial bruit, and it could compromise circulation if the carotid artery is already narrowed by atherosclerosis. Ask the person to take a breath, exhale, and hold it briefly while you listen so tracheal breath sounds do not mask or mimic a carotid artery bruit. (Holding the breath on inhalation also tenses the levator scapulae muscles, which makes it hard to hear the carotids.) Sometimes you can hear normal heart sounds transmitted to the neck; do not confuse these with a bruit.

Inspect the Jugular Venous Pulse

From the jugular veins you can assess the **central venous pressure (CVP)** and thus judge the heart's efficiency as a pump and the intravascular volume status. Stand on the person's right side because the veins there have a direct route to the heart. You may use either the external or the internal jugular veins because

Abnormal Findings

Diminished pulse feels small and weak (decreased stroke volume as in cardiogenic shock).

Increased pulse feels full and strong in hyperkinetic states (see Table 20-1, Variations in Pulse Contour, p. 530).

A bruit indicates turbulence from a local vascular cause and is a marker for atherosclerotic disease. This increases the risk of transient ischemic attack (TIA) and ischemic stroke.[20] However, a bruit also occurs in 5% of those age 45 to 80 years who have no significant carotid disease.[8a]

A carotid bruit is audible when the lumen is occluded by ½ to ⅔. Bruit loudness increases as the atherosclerosis worsens until the lumen is occluded by ⅔. After that, bruit loudness decreases. When the lumen is completely occluded, the bruit disappears. Thus absence of a bruit does not ensure absence of a carotid lesion.

A murmur sounds much the same but is caused by a cardiac disorder. Some aortic valve murmurs (aortic stenosis) radiate to the neck and must be distinguished from a local bruit.

Normal Range of Findings	Abnormal Findings

measurements in both are similar.[13] You can see the top of the external jugular vein distention overlying the sternomastoid muscle or the pulsation of the internal jugular vein in the sternal notch. The latter is harder to see because of its deep position.

Position the person supine anywhere from a 30- to a 45-degree angle, wherever you can best see the top of the vein or pulsations. In general the higher the venous pressure is, the higher the position you need. Remove the pillow to avoid flexing the neck; the head should be in the same plane as the trunk. Turn the person's head slightly away from the examined side and direct a strong light tangentially onto the neck to highlight pulsations and shadows.

Note the external jugular veins overlying the sternomastoid muscle. In some people the veins are not visible at all, whereas in others they are full in the supine position. As the person is raised to a sitting position, these external jugulars flatten and disappear, usually at 45 degrees.

Unilateral distention of external jugular veins is caused by local cause (kinking or aneurysm).

Full distended external jugular veins above 45 degrees signify increased CVP as with heart failure.

Now look for pulsations of the internal jugular veins in the area of the suprasternal notch or around the origin of the sternomastoid muscle around the clavicle. You must be able to distinguish internal jugular vein pulsation from that of the carotid artery. It is easy to confuse them because they lie close together. Use the guidelines shown in Table 19-1.

TABLE 19-1	**Characteristics of Jugular versus Carotid Pulsations**	
	Internal Jugular Pulse	**Carotid Pulse**
1. Location	Lower, more lateral, under or behind the sternomastoid muscle	Higher and medial to this muscle
2. Quality	Undulant and diffuse; two visible waves per cycle	Brisk and localized; one wave per cycle
3. Respiration	Varies with respiration, its level descends during inspiration when intrathoracic pressure is decreased	Does not vary
4. Palpable	No	Yes
5. Pressure	Light pressure at the base of the neck easily obliterates	No change
6. Position of person	Level of pulse drops and disappears as the person is brought to a sitting position	Unaffected

Estimate the Jugular Venous Pressure

Think of the jugular veins as a CVP manometer attached directly to the right atrium. You can "read" the CVP at the highest level of pulsations. Use the angle of Louis (sternal angle) as an arbitrary reference point, and compare it with the highest level of the distended vein or venous pulsation.

Hold a vertical ruler on the sternal angle. Align a straightedge on the ruler like a T-square and adjust the level of the horizontal straightedge to the level of pulsation (Fig. 19-18, *A*). Read the level of intersection on the vertical ruler; normal jugular venous pulsation is 2 cm or less above the sternal angle. Also state the person's position (e.g., "internal jugular vein pulsations 3 cm above sternal angle when elevated 30 degrees").

Normal Range of Findings	Abnormal Findings

A

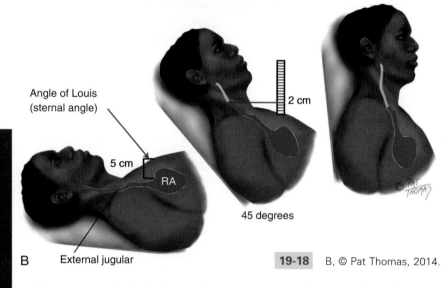

Angle of Louis
(sternal angle)

5 cm

RA

2 cm

45 degrees

B   External jugular

19-18   B, © Pat Thomas, 2014.

If you cannot find the internal jugular veins, use the external jugular veins and note the point where they look collapsed. Be aware that the technique of estimating venous pressure is difficult and is not always a reliable predictor of CVP. Consistency in grading among examiners is difficult to achieve.

If venous pressure is elevated or if you suspect heart failure, perform the **abdominojugular test** (formerly **hepatojugular reflux**) (Fig. 19-19). Position the person comfortably supine, and instruct him or her to breathe quietly through an open mouth. Hold your right hand over the midabdomen and watch the level of jugular pulsation as you push in with your hand. Exert firm sustained pressure for 30 seconds. This displaces venous blood out of the splanchnic vessels and adds its volume to the venous system. If the heart is able to pump this additional volume (i.e., if no elevated CVP is present), the jugular veins will rise for a few seconds and then recede back to the previous level.

Elevated pressure is a level of pulsation that is >3 cm above the sternal angle while at 45 degrees (Fig. 19-18, *B*). This occurs with heart failure, cardiac tamponade, and constrictive pericarditis.

If heart failure is present, the jugular veins will elevate more than 4 cm and stay elevated as long as you push.

19-19   Abdominojugular test.

Normal Range of Findings	Abnormal Findings

The Precordium

Inspect the Anterior Chest

Arrange tangential lighting to accentuate any flicker of movement.

Pulsations. You may or may not see the **apical impulse,** the pulsation created as the left ventricle rotates against the chest wall during systole. When visible, it occupies the 4th or 5th intercostal space, at or inside the midclavicular line. It is easier to see in children and in those with thinner chest walls.

A **heave** or **lift** is a sustained forceful thrusting of the ventricle during systole. It occurs with ventricular hypertrophy as a result of increased workload. A right ventricular heave is seen at the sternal border; a left ventricular heave is seen at the apex (see Table 19-9, Abnormal Pulsations on the Precordium, p. 501).

Palpate the Apical Impulse

Localize the **apical impulse** precisely by using one finger pad (Fig. 19-20, *A*). Asking the person to "exhale and then hold it" helps the examiner locate the pulsation. You may need to roll the person midway to the left to find it; note that this also displaces the apical impulse farther to the left (Fig. 19-20, *B*). You feel it best at the end of expiration when the heart is closest to the chest wall; then it moves quickly away from your finger.

19-20   The apical impulse.

NOTE:
- *Location*—The apical impulse should occupy only one interspace, the 4th or 5th, and be at or medial to the midclavicular line
- *Size*—Normally 1 × 2 cm
- *Amplitude*—Normally a short, gentle tap
- *Duration*—Short; normally occupies only first half of systole

Cardiac enlargement:
Left ventricular dilation (volume overload) displaces impulse down and to left and increases size more than one space. A diameter of ≥4 cm is likely a dilated heart.[13] This occurs with heart failure and cardiomyopathy.

A **sustained** impulse with increased force and duration but no change in location occurs with left ventricular hypertrophy and no dilation (pressure overload) (see Table 19-9).

The apical impulse is palpable in the supine position in 25% to 40% of adults and in the left lateral position in 50% to 73% of adults.[13] It is not palpable in obese persons or in people with thick chest walls. With high cardiac output states (anxiety, fever, hyperthyroidism, anemia) the apical impulse increases in amplitude and duration.

Not palpable with pulmonary emphysema because of overriding lungs.

Objective Data

Normal Range of Findings	Abnormal Findings

Palpate Across the Precordium

Using the palmar aspects of your four fingers, gently palpate the apex, the left sternal border, and the base, searching for any other pulsations (Fig. 19-21). Normally none occur. If any are present, note the timing. Use the carotid artery pulsation as a guide, or auscultate as you palpate.

A **thrill** is a palpable vibration. It feels like the throat of a purring cat. The thrill signifies turbulent blood flow and directs you to locate the origin of loud murmurs. However, absence of a thrill does not rule out the presence of a murmur.

Accentuated first and second heart sounds and extra heart sounds also may cause abnormal pulsations.

19-21

Percussion*

Auscultation

Identify the auscultatory areas where you will listen. These include the four traditional valve "areas" (Fig. 19-22). The valve areas are not over the actual anatomic locations of the valves but are the sites on the chest wall where sounds produced by the valves are best heard. The sound radiates with the direction of blood flow.

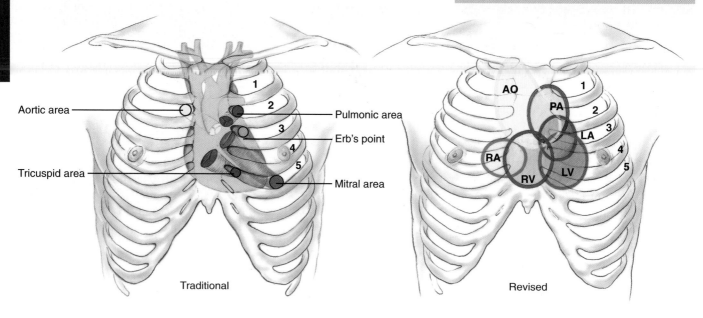

Aortic area — Pulmonic area — Erb's point — Tricuspid area — Mitral area

Traditional

AO — PA — LA — RA — RV — LV

Revised

AUSCULTATORY AREAS

19-22

*Percussion to outline the borders of the heart has been replaced by the chest x-ray image or echocardiogram. Evidence shows that these are more accurate in detecting heart enlargement. When the right ventricle enlarges, it does so in the anteroposterior diameter, which is better seen on x-ray image. Evidence from numerous comparison studies shows that the percussed cardiac border correlates "only moderately" with the true cardiac border.[13] In addition, percussion is of limited usefulness with the female breast tissue or in an obese person or a person with a muscular chest wall.

Normal Range of Findings	**Abnormal Findings**

The valve areas are:
- Second right interspace—Aortic valve area
- Second left interspace—Pulmonic valve area
- Left lower sternal border—Tricuspid valve area
- Fifth interspace at around left midclavicular line—Mitral valve area

Do not limit your auscultation to only four locations. Sounds produced by the valves may be heard all over the precordium. (For this reason many experts even discourage the naming of the valve areas.) Thus learn to inch your stethoscope in a rough **Z** pattern, from the base of the heart across and down and over to the apex. Or start at the apex and work your way up. Include the sites shown in Fig. 19-22.

Recall the characteristics of a good stethoscope (see Chapter 8). Clean the endpieces with an alcohol wipe; you will use both endpieces. Although all heart sounds are low frequency, the diaphragm detects relatively higher-pitched sounds, and the bell detects relatively lower-pitched ones. Make sure that your earpieces fit snugly and are aimed forward, toward your nose, to avoid air leak. These heart sounds are soft; enhance your success with a completely quiet room—no television, no radio, no talking, please.

Before you begin, alert the person: "I always listen to the heart in a number of places on the chest. Just because I'm listening for a long time, it does not necessarily mean that something is wrong."

After you place the stethoscope, try closing your eyes briefly to tune out any distractions. Concentrate and listen selectively to *one sound at a time.* Consider that at least 2, and perhaps 3 or 4, sounds may be happening in less than 1 second. You cannot process everything at once. Begin with the diaphragm endpiece and use the following routine: (1) note the rate and rhythm, (2) identify S_1 and S_2, (3) assess S_1 and S_2 separately, (4) listen for extra heart sounds, and (5) listen for murmurs.

Note the Rate and Rhythm. The rate ranges normally from 50 to 95 beats/ min. (Review the full discussion of the pulse in Chapter 9 and the normal rates across age-groups.) The rhythm should be regular, although **sinus arrhythmia** occurs normally in young adults and children. With sinus arrhythmia, the rhythm varies with the person's breathing, increasing at the peak of inspiration and slowing with expiration. Note any other irregular rhythm. If one occurs, check if it has any pattern or if it is totally irregular.

When you notice any irregularity, check for a **pulse deficit** by auscultating the apical beat while simultaneously palpating the radial pulse. Count a serial measurement (one after the other) of apical beat and radial pulse. Normally every beat you hear at the apex should perfuse to the periphery and be palpable. The two counts should be identical. When different, subtract the radial rate from the apical, and record the remainder as the pulse deficit.

Identify S_1 and S_2. This is important because S_1 is the start of systole and thus serves as the reference point for the timing of all other cardiac sounds. You must learn to distinguish systole from diastole before you can attach meaning to all other sounds. Usually you can identify S_1 instantly because you hear a pair of sounds close together (lub-dup) and S_1 is the first of the pair. This guideline works, except in the cases of the tachydysrhythmias (rates >100 beats/min). Then the diastolic filling time is shortened, and the beats are too close together to distinguish.

Premature beat—An isolated beat is early, or a pattern occurs in which every third or fourth beat sounds early.

Irregularly irregular—No pattern to the sounds; beats come rapidly and at random intervals as in atrial fibrillation.

A **pulse deficit** signals a weak contraction of the ventricles; it occurs with atrial fibrillation, premature beats, and heart failure.

Objective Data

Normal Range of Findings

Abnormal Findings

Timing. It is crucial to define the murmur by its occurrence in systole or diastole. You must be able to identify S_1 and S_2 accurately to do this. Try to further describe the murmur as being in early, mid, or late systole or diastole; throughout the cardiac event (termed *pansystolic, holosystolic/pandiastolic,* or *holodiastolic);* and whether it obscures or muffles the heart sounds.

A systolic murmur may occur with a healthy heart or with heart disease; a diastolic murmur always indicates heart disease.

Normal heart tones[13]	**Lub** S_1	**Dup** S_2	**Lub** S_1	**Dup** S_2
Early systolic murmur	**LSHSHSH** S_1	**Dup** S_2	**LSHSHSH** S_1	**Dup** S_2
Midsystolic murmur	**LubSHSHDup** S_1 S_2		**LubSHSHDup** S_1 S_2	
Late systolic murmur	**Lub** S_1	**SHSHP** S_2	**Lub** S_1	**SHSHP** S_2
Late systolic murmur and click (C) of mitral valve prolapse	**Lub** S_1	**KSHSHP** C S_2	**Lub** S_1	**KSHSHP** C S_2
Holosystolic murmur	**SHSHSHSHSH** S_1 S_2		**SHSHSHSHSH** S_1 S_2	

Loudness. Describe the intensity in terms of six "grades." For example, record a grade 2 murmur as "2/6."
Grade 1—Barely audible; heard only in a quiet room and then with difficulty
Grade 2—Clearly audible but faint
Grade 3—Moderately loud; easy to hear
Grade 4—Loud; associated with a thrill palpable on the chest wall
Grade 5—Very loud; heard with one corner of the stethoscope lifted off the chest wall; associated thrill
Grade 6—Loudest; still heard with entire stethoscope lifted just off the chest wall; associated thrill

Pitch. Describe the pitch as high, medium, or low. The pitch depends on the pressure and rate of blood flow producing the murmur.

Pattern. The intensity may follow a pattern during the cardiac phase, growing louder (crescendo), tapering off (decrescendo) or increasing to a peak, and then decreasing (crescendo-decrescendo or diamond shaped). Because the whole murmur is just milliseconds long, it takes practice to diagnose any pattern.

Quality. Describe the quality as musical, blowing, harsh, or rumbling.

The murmur of mitral stenosis is low-pitched and rumbling, whereas that of aortic stenosis is harsh (see Table 19-11).

Location. Describe the area of maximum intensity of the murmur (where it is best heard) by noting the valve area or intercostal spaces.
Radiation. The murmur may be transmitted downstream in the direction of blood flow and may be heard in another place on the precordium, the neck, the back, or the axilla.
Posture. Some murmurs disappear or are enhanced by a change in position.
Some murmurs are common in healthy children or adolescents and are termed *innocent* or *functional.* **Innocent** indicates having no valvular or other

Objective Data

Normal Range of Findings	**Abnormal Findings**

pathologic cause; **functional** is caused by increased blood flow in the heart (e.g., in anemia, fever, pregnancy, hyperthyroidism). The contractile force of the heart is greater in children. This increases blood flow velocity. The increased velocity plus a smaller chest measurement makes an audible murmur.

The innocent murmur is generally soft (grade 2), midsystolic, short, crescendo-decrescendo, and with a vibratory or musical quality ("vooot" sound like fiddle strings). It is heard at the 2nd or 3rd left intercostal space and disappears with sitting, and the young person has no associated signs of cardiac dysfunction. It is important to distinguish innocent murmurs from pathologic ones. Diagnostic tests such as ECG and echocardiogram will establish an accurate diagnosis.

Change Position. After auscultating in the supine position, roll the person toward his or her left side. Listen with the bell at the apex for the presence of any diastolic filling sounds (i.e., the S_3 or S_4) (Fig. 19-28).

S_3 and S_4 and the murmur of mitral stenosis sometimes may be heard only when on the left side.

19-28

Ask the person to sit up, lean forward slightly, and exhale. Listen with the diaphragm firmly pressed at the base, right, and left sides. Check for the soft, high-pitched, early diastolic murmur of aortic or pulmonic regurgitation (Fig. 19-29).

The soft diastolic murmur of aortic regurgitation may be heard only when the person is leaning forward in the sitting position.

19-29

Objective Data

Normal Range of Findings	Abnormal Findings

❖ DEVELOPMENTAL COMPETENCE

Infants

The transition from fetal to pulmonic circulation occurs in the immediate newborn period. Fetal shunts normally close within 10 to 15 hours but may take up to 48 hours. Thus you should assess the CV system during the first 24 hours and again in 2 to 3 days.

Note any extracardiac signs that may reflect heart status (particularly in the skin), liver size, and respiratory status. The skin color should be pink to pinkish brown, depending on the infant's genetic heritage. If cyanosis occurs, determine its first appearance—at or shortly after birth versus after the neonatal period. Normally the liver is not enlarged, and the respirations are not labored. In addition, note the expected parameters of weight gain throughout infancy.

Palpate the apical impulse to determine the size and position of the heart. Because the infant's heart has a more horizontal placement, expect to palpate the apical impulse at the 4th intercostal space just lateral to the midclavicular line. It may or may not be visible.

The heart rate is best auscultated because radial pulses are hard to count accurately. Use the small (pediatric size) diaphragm and bell (Fig. 19-30). The heart rate may range from 100 to 180 beats/min immediately after birth and stabilize to an average of 120 to 140 beats/min. Infants normally have wide fluctuations with activity, from 170 beats/min or more with crying or being active to 70 to 90 beats/min with sleeping. Variations are greatest at birth and are even more so with premature babies.

Abnormal Findings:

Failure of shunts to close (e.g., patent ductus arteriosus [PDA], atrial septal defect [ASD]); see Table 19-10, Congenital Heart Defects.

Cyanosis at or just after birth signals oxygen desaturation of congenital heart disease (see Table 19-10).

The most important signs of heart failure in an infant are persistent tachycardia, tachypnea, and liver enlargement. Engorged veins, gallop rhythm, and pulsus alternans also are signs. Respiratory crackles (rales) are an important sign in adults but not in infants.

Failure to thrive occurs with cardiac disease.

The apex is displaced with:
- Cardiac enlargement, shifts to the left.
- Pneumothorax, shifts away from the affected side.
- Diaphragmatic hernia, shifts usually to right because this hernia occurs more often on the left.
- Dextrocardia, a rare anomaly in which the heart is located on right side of chest.

Persistent tachycardia is >200 beats/min in newborns or >160 beats/min in infants.

Bradycardia is <90 beats/min in newborns or <60 beats/min in older infants or children. This causes a serious drop in cardiac output because the small muscle mass of their hearts cannot increase stroke volume significantly.

19-30

Normal Range of Findings

Expect the heart rhythm to have sinus arrhythmia, the phasic speeding up or slowing down with the respiratory cycle.

Rapid rates make it more challenging to evaluate heart sounds. Expect heart sounds to be louder in infants than in adults because of the infant's thinner chest wall. Also, S_2 has a higher pitch and is sharper than S_1. Splitting of S_2 just after the height of inspiration is common, not at birth but beginning a few hours after birth.

Murmurs in the immediate newborn period do not necessarily indicate congenital heart disease. They are relatively common in the first 2 to 3 days because of fetal shunt closure. These murmurs are usually grade 1 or 2, are systolic, accompany no other signs of cardiac disease, and disappear in 2 to 3 days. The murmur of PDA is a continuous machinery murmur, which disappears by 2 to 3 days. On the other hand, absence of a murmur in the immediate newborn period does not ensure a healthy heart; congenital defects can be present that are not signaled by an early murmur. It is best to listen frequently and to note and describe any murmur according to the characteristics listed on p. 484.

Children

Note any extracardiac or cardiac signs that may indicate heart disease: poor weight gain, developmental delay, persistent tachycardia, tachypnea, DOE, cyanosis, and clubbing. Note that clubbing of fingers and toes usually does not appear until late in the first year, even with severe cyanotic defects.

The apical impulse is sometimes visible in children with thin chest walls. Note any obvious bulge or any heave—these are not normal.

Palpate the apical impulse in the fourth intercostal space to the left of the midclavicular line until age 4 years; at the fourth interspace at the midclavicular line from ages 4 to 6 years, and in the fifth interspace to the right of the midclavicular line at age 7 years (Fig. 19-31).

19-31

Abnormal Findings

Investigate any irregularity except sinus arrhythmia.

Fixed split S_2 indicates atrial septal defect (see Table 19-10).

Congenital defects are associated with: harsh murmur quality, location (right upper sternal border, left lower sternal border, apex), and timing (pansystolic, diastolic, or continuous).[12]

A precordial bulge to the left of the sternum with a hyperdynamic precordium signals cardiac enlargement. The bulge occurs because the cartilaginous rib cage is more compliant.

A substernal heave occurs with right ventricular enlargement; an apical heave occurs with left ventricular hypertrophy.

The apical impulse moves laterally with cardiac enlargement.

Thrill (palpable vibration).

Objective Data

Normal Range of Findings

The average heart rate slows as the child grows older, although it is still variable with rest or activity.

The heart rhythm remains characterized by sinus arrhythmia. Physiologic S_3 is common in children (see Table 19-8). It occurs in early diastole, just after S_2, and is a dull soft sound that is best heard at the apex.

A **venous hum**—caused by turbulence of blood flow in the jugular venous system—is common in healthy children and has no pathologic significance. It is a continuous, low-pitched, soft hum that is heard throughout the cycle, although it is loudest in diastole. Listen with the bell over the supraclavicular fossa at the medial third of the clavicle, especially on the right, or over the upper anterior chest.

The venous hum is usually not affected by respiration, may sound louder when the child stands, and is easily obliterated by occluding the jugular veins in the neck with your fingers.

A **carotid bruit** is a benign murmur heard just above the clavicles. It is slightly harsh, early or midsystolic, often louder on the left, and will disappear completely by carotid artery compression.

Heart murmurs that are innocent (or functional) in origin are very common through childhood (often termed *Still's murmur*). They may have a 30% occurrence, although some authors say that nearly all children may demonstrate a murmur at some time. Most innocent murmurs have these characteristics: soft, relatively short, early or midsystolic ejection murmur; medium pitch; vibratory; best heard at the left lower sternal or midsternal border, with no radiation to the apex, base, or back.

For the child whose murmur has been shown to be innocent, it is very important that the parents understand this completely. They need to believe that this murmur is just a "noise" and has no pathologic significance. Otherwise the parents may become overprotective and limit activity for the child, which may result in the child developing a negative self-concept.

The Pregnant Woman

The vital signs usually yield an increase in resting pulse rate of 10 to 15 beats/min and a drop in BP from the normal prepregnancy level. The BP decreases to its lowest point during the second trimester and then slowly rises during the third trimester. It varies with position. It is usually lowest in the left lateral recumbent position, a bit higher when supine, and highest when sitting.[6]

Inspection of the skin often shows a mild hyperemia in light-skinned women because the increased cutaneous blood flow tries to eliminate the excess heat generated by the increased metabolism. Palpation of the apical impulse is higher and lateral compared with the normal position because the enlarging uterus elevates the diaphragm and displaces the heart up and to the left and rotates it on its long axis.

Auscultation of the heart sounds shows changes caused by the increased blood volume and workload. An exaggerated splitting of S_1 and increased loudness of S_1 are common, as is a loud, easily heard S_3. An ejection systolic murmur is common; heard at left sternal border; grade 1, 2 or 3 in intensity.[27]

A continuous murmur from breast vasculature is termed a **mammary souffle** (pronounced soof' f'l), which occurs near term or when the mother is lactating; it is caused by increased blood flow through the internal mammary artery. The murmur is heard in the 2nd, 3rd, or 4th intercostal space; it is continuous, although it is accented in systole. You can obliterate it by pressure with the stethoscope or one finger lateral to the murmur.

Abnormal Findings

This latter maneuver helps differentiate the venous hum from other cardiac murmurs (e.g., PDA).

Distinguish innocent murmurs from pathologic ones. This may involve referral to another examiner or performing diagnostic tests (e.g., ECG or echocardiography).

Gestational hypertension is BP $\geq$140/90 mm Hg on two separate measures without proteinuria, starting after 20th week of pregnancy. This returns to baseline by 12 weeks after delivery.[27]

Murmurs of aortic valve disease cannot be obliterated.

Objective Data

Normal Range of Findings	Abnormal Findings

The ECG has no changes except for a slight left axis deviation caused by the change in the heart's position.

The Aging Adult

A gradual rise in SBP is common with aging; the DBP stays fairly constant with a resulting widening of pulse pressure. Some older adults experience **orthostatic hypotension,** a sudden drop in BP when rising to sit or stand.

Use caution in palpating and auscultating the carotid artery. Avoid pressure in the carotid sinus area, which could cause a reflex slowing of the heart rate. Also, pressure on the carotid artery could compromise circulation if the artery is already narrowed by atherosclerosis.

The chest often increases in anteroposterior diameter with aging. This makes it more difficult to palpate the apical impulse and hear the splitting of S_2. The S_4 often occurs in older people with no known cardiac disease. Systolic murmurs are common, occurring in over 50% of aging people.

The S_3 is associated with heart failure and is always abnormal over age 35 years (see Table 19-8).

Occasional premature ectopic beats are common and do not necessarily indicate underlying heart disease. When in doubt, obtain an ECG. However, consider that the ECG records for only one isolated minute in time and may need to be supplemented by a test of 24-hour ambulatory heart monitoring.

Objective Data

PROMOTING A HEALTHY LIFESTYLE
The Heart Truth: Women and Heart Attacks

When someone complains of chest pain or pain radiating down the left arm, think that it could be a heart attack or MI. After all, these are the symptoms that typically occur, aren't they? Yes and no. These are the most "typical" symptoms for men having an MI but not for women. Women's symptoms can be quite different. Their "atypical" symptoms may be one of the reasons that more women than men are dying from heart disease these days. According to the Women's Heart Foundation, almost a third of women experience no chest pain at all when having a heart attack. Instead they report extreme fatigue and flulike symptoms up to a month before the attack. Other signs for women include:

- Uncomfortable pressure, squeezing, sense of fullness in the chest that either lasts a few minutes or goes away, but then comes back.
- Pain or discomfort in one or both arms, back, neck, jaw, lower chest, and/or upper abdomen.
- Shortness of breath, with or without chest discomfort.
- Breaking out in a cold sweat, nausea, and light-headedness.

The problem is that women tend to minimize their symptoms or more often attribute them to something else such as the flu, menopause, or normal aging. This is because of a lack of awareness. One of the most effective outreach efforts aimed directly at women is a simple video, called *Just a Little Heart Attack,* starring and directed by Emmy-nominated actress Elizabeth Banks. It can be accessed through the AHA *Go Red For Women*™ campaign website or directly at: http://www.youtube.com/watch?v=t7wmPWTnDbE.

The AHA and the National Heart, Lung, and Blood Institute (NHLBI) have joined forces to raise awareness of women and heart disease. The NHLBI introduced the red dress as a national symbol for women and heart disease awareness, and the AHA adopted this symbol, hoping that by working together the two organizations could have a greater impact.

The Heart Truth® is another effective national awareness and prevention campaign about heart disease in women, sponsored by the NHLBI. *The Red Dress*® is the centerpiece of this campaign, the primary message of which is *Heart Disease Doesn't Care What You Wear—It's the #1 Killer of Women*®. The idea behind using a red dress as the symbol was to draw attention to the idea that heart disease is not only a man's issue. National *Wear Red Day*® is the first Friday in February. Plan to wear red and raise awareness. You may save a life!

References
American Heart Association: www.heart.org.
Be sure to take their Women's Heart Disease Risk Quiz: *http://www.womensheart.org/content/HeartDisease/heart_disease_risk_quiz.asp.*
Go Red For Women™: http://www.goredforwomen.org/.
National Institutes of Health National Heart, Lung, and Blood Institute: www.nhlbi.nih.gov.
The Heart Truth®: *Awareness and Prevention: http://www.nhlbi.nih.gov/educational/hearttruth/, where you can also sign up to receive bimonthly e-newsletters about The Heart Truth® campaign and women's heart health.*
The Women's Heart Foundation at http://www.womensheart.org/.

DOCUMENTATION AND CRITICAL THINKING

Sample Charting

SUBJECTIVE

No chest pain, dyspnea, orthopnea, cough, fatigue, or edema. No history of hypertension, abnormal blood tests, heart murmur, or rheumatic fever in self. Last ECG 2 yrs. PTA, result normal. No stress ECG or other heart tests.

Family history: Father with obesity, smoking, and hypertension, treated $\bar{c}$ diuretic medication. No other family history significant for CV disease.

Personal habits: Diet balanced in 4 food groups, 2 to 3 c. regular coffee/day; no smoking; alcohol, 1 to 2 beers occasionally on weekend; exercise, runs 2 miles, 3 to 4 ×/week; no prescription or OTC medications or street drugs.

OBJECTIVE

Neck: Carotids' upstrokes are brisk and = bilaterally. No bruit. Internal jugular vein pulsations present when supine and disappear when elevated to a 45-degree position.

Precordium: Inspection. No visible pulsations; no heave or lift.

Palpation: Apical impulse in 5th ICS at left midclavicular line; no thrill.

Auscultation: Rate 68 bpm, rhythm regular, S_1-S_2 are crisp, not diminished or accentuated, no S_3, no S_4 or other extra sounds, no murmurs.

ASSESSMENT

Neck vessels healthy by inspection and auscultation
Heart sounds normal, no murmurs

Clinical Case Study 1

H.J. is a 56-year-old obese Latino male with a past medical history of MI 6 months PTA, hypertension × 30 years, 50–pack/year history of smoking, type 2 diabetes × 1 year. Current medications include a beta-blocker, ACE-inhibitor, aspirin, oral antidiabetic medication, and a platelet inhibitor. H.J. is at the clinic for a 6-month follow-up with his cardiologist. Reports taking all medication except that he ran out of the beta-blocker last week.

SUBJECTIVE

H.J. reports increased breathlessness, nocturia, and fatigue 2 weeks PTA. For the past week, "my ankles look like melons after a day at work," and reports dizziness and palpitations ×2 days.

Family history includes father with MI resulting in death at age 50. Mother died in childbirth at age 21. Brother with hypertension and "some type of heart thing."

Personal habits: Smokes 2 ppd, drinks 1 to 2 beers at least 2 days per week. Caffeine intake of 1 to 2 cups of coffee each morning. "I try to eat healthy." Unable to provide 24-hour diet recall, but reports "salting everything, even my watermelon."

OBJECTIVE

Vital signs: Temperature 98.6° F (37° C). Pulse 130 bpm. Resp 22/min. BP 96/60 mm Hg, right arm, sitting.

Extremities: Skin cool, tan, no cyanosis. Bilateral upper extremities—no clubbing, no edema, capillary refill <3 seconds. Bilateral lower extremities—2+ pitting edema, no hair growth 10 cm below knees.

Cardiovascular, pulses: Carotid 2+, brachial 2+, radial 2+, femoral 2+, popliteal 0, PT 1+, DP 1+ (all pulses equal bilaterally).

Neck: Internal jugular vein pulsations 5 cm above sternal angle when elevated 30 degrees.

Heart Inspection: Apical impulse not visible. No heave. Palpation: Apical impulse not palpable. No thrill. Auscultation: Apical rate 120 bpm, irregularly irregular. S_1S_2 present. S_1 varying intensity. S_3 gallop at apex and left lower sternal border. No murmur.

ASSESSMENT

Systolic heart failure
Atrial fibrillation
Decreased cardiac output R/T reduction in stroke volume
Ineffective tissue perfusion R/T decreased cardiac output
Knowledge deficit R/T effects of smoking, extra salt, alcohol on heart, recommended dosing of beta blocker

Clinical Case Study 2

M.B. is a 35-year-old immigrant from Northern India. Past medical history of rheumatic fever at age 10 years. No medications. All immunizations up to date.

SUBJECTIVE

M.B. reports worsening fatigue and dyspnea on exertion. "I've never had the same endurance as my friends, but my doctors in India told me that was normal." Substernal chest pain rated at 4/10 with exertion or stress. Relieved by rest. No family history of heart disease. No stress ECG or other heart tests. Nonsmoker. Reports no alcohol use. Denies use of illicit drugs. Eats a "balanced" diet in all food groups. 1 to 2 caffeinated beverages per day.

OBJECTIVE

Vital signs: Temperature 98.6° F (37° C). Pulse 74 bpm. Resp 14/min. BP 102/70 mm Hg, right arm, sitting.
Neck: Carotids 2+, equal bilaterally. Internal jugular vein pulsation present when supine, disappears when elevated 45 degrees.
Heart: Inspection: Lift at apex. Apical impulse visible 5th intercostal space, 4 cm left of midclavicular line. Palpation: Apical impulse 5th intercostal space, 4 cm left of midclavicular line, 2 cm × 2 cm. No thrills. Auscultation: S_1S_2 present. S_1 accentuated. No S_3 or S_4. Low-pitched diastolic murmur grade 2/6 heard best at apex.

ASSESSMENT

Mitral stenosis secondary to childhood rheumatic fever
Fatigue R/T decreased cardiac output
Risk for decreased cardiac output R/T mitral stenosis

Clinical Case Study 3

N.V. is a 53-year-old Caucasian male crane operator admitted to the CCU at University Medical Center (UMC) with chest pain.

SUBJECTIVE

1 year PTA—N.V. admitted to UMC with crushing substernal chest pain radiating to L shoulder, accompanied by nausea, vomiting, diaphoresis. Diagnosed as MI, hospitalized 7 days, discharged with nitroglycerin prn for anginal pain. Did not return to work. Activity included walking 1 mile/day, hunting. Had occasional episodes of chest pain with exercise, relieved by rest.
1 day PTA—Had increasing frequency of chest pain, about every 2 hours, lasting few minutes. Saw pain as warning to go to MD.
Day of admission—Severe substernal chest pain ("like someone sitting on my chest") unrelieved by rest. Saw personal MD; while in office had episode of chest pain similar to last year's, accompanied by diaphoresis; no N&V or SOB, relieved by 1 nitroglycerin. Transferred to UMC by paramedics. No further pain since admission 2 hours ago.
Family hx—Mother died of MI at age 57.
Personal habits—Smokes 1½ pack cigarettes daily × 34 years; no alcohol; diet—trying to limit fat and fried food, still high in added salt.

OBJECTIVE

Extremities: Skin tan pink, no cyanosis. Upper extrem.—capillary refill sluggish, no clubbing. Lower extrem.—no edema, no hair growth 10 cm below knee bilaterally.

Pulses:

Carotid	Brachial	Radial	Femoral	Popliteal	P.T.	D.P.	
2+	2+	2+	2+	0	0	1+	All = Bilaterally

BP R arm 104/66 mm Hg

Neck: External jugulars flat. Internal jugular pulsations present when supine and absent when elevated to 45 degrees.

Precordium: Inspection. Apical impulse visible 5th ICS, 7 cm left of midsternal line; no heave.

Palpation: Apical impulse palpable in 5th and 6th ICS; no thrill.

Auscultation: Apical rate 92 bpm, regular; S_1-S_2 are normal, not diminished or accentuated; no S_3 or S_4; grade 3/6 systolic murmur present at left lower sternal border.

ASSESSMENT

Substernal chest pain

Systolic murmur

Ineffective tissue perfusion R/T interruption in flow

Decreased cardiac output R/T reduction in stroke volume

Knowledge deficit R/T effects of smoking

Clinical Case Study 4

L.B. is a 7-week-old Asian-American female who is being admitted to the hospital for observation due to failure to thrive (FTT). The C-R monitor alarms, so you enter the room to find mom holding a sleeping baby. The monitor indicates a narrow QRS tachycardia.

SUBJECTIVE

Mom reports, "L.B. has always been a poor eater," vomits often with feeds, and is "overall less active and alert than my other kids were as babies." **Birth history:** Born at 40 weeks' gestation, SROM, vaginal birth w/o complications; weight 9 lbs (4.08 kg); birth length 21.5 in (56.6 cm); head circumference 34.5 cm.

OBJECTIVE

Vital signs: Temp 97.4°F (36.3°C, axillary). BP (unable to obtain). Pulse 236 bpm (sleeping). Resp 48/min. Weight 9 lbs 7 oz (4.3 kg). Head circumference 38 cm.

General appearance: Sleeping and pale w/labored breathing.

HEENT: Anterior and posterior fontanels flat; eyes clear; TM pearly gray bilat; nares patent bilat.

Cardiovascular: Tachycardic.

Respiratory: Tachypneic w/sternal and intercostal retractions; crackles to bilat lung bases.

Extremities: Mottled and cool to touch; 1+ pulses bilat.

ASSESSMENT

Supraventricular tachycardia (SVT)

Decreased cardiac output R/T altered electrical conduction

Imbalanced nutrition: less than body requirements R/T biological factors

Ineffective tissue perfusion: cerebral R/T interruption of cerebral arterial flow secondary to decreased cardiac output

Documentation and Critical Thinking

TABLE 19-2   Differential Diagnosis of Chest Pain

	Common Pain Description	Location/Radiation	Possible Associated Symptoms
Cardiovascular (Ischemic)			
Angina pectoris: stable (no change in pain pattern within last 60 days)	Pressurelike discomfort (e.g., tightness, squeezing, burning, heaviness that lasts 3-5 minutes precipitated by activity and often resolves with rest)	Generalized substernal or retrosternal: can radiate to teeth, jaw, neck, one or both arms or shoulders; or there may be no pain and only associated symptoms	Diaphoresis, nausea, vomiting, dyspnea
Prinzmetal or variant angina	Pressurelike discomfort often occurring at rest and early morning hours	Retrosternal: can radiate to jaw, neck, left arm, or shoulder	Palpitations, syncope, or feelings of syncope
Acute coronary syndrome (unstable angina, myocardial infarction)	Heaviness; viselike, squeezing, crushing, tightness; vague, burning, constricting, or pressure; poorly localized pain lasting 20-30 minutes to hours and does not resolve with rest	Generalized substernal or retrosternal: can radiate to teeth, jaw, neck, one or both arms or shoulders; or there may be no pain and only associated symptoms	Indigestion-like feeling, nausea, vomiting, dizziness, flushing, perspiration, palpitations, dyspnea
Cardiovascular (Nonischemic)			
Pericarditis	Sudden sharp and stabbing pain relieved often by sitting or leaning forward and worsens by lying down or with inspiration	Substernal, which can radiate to trapezius muscle region	Dry cough, muscle and joint aches, fever
Mitral valve prolapse	Sharp pain not associated with activity	Chest pain without radiation	Fatigue, light-headedness, dyspnea, irregular heartbeat, palpitations, exercise intolerance
Aortic dissection	Sudden severe pain with change in location and/or tearing sensation lasting for hours	Anterior chest pain with radiation to the neck, jaw, or intrascapular region of the back	Mental status changes, limb pain and weakness, dyspnea
Pulmonary hypertension (secondary)	Cardiac-like chest pain with exertion	Chest region	Dyspnea, lower-extremity edema, fatigue
Pulmonary			
Pulmonary embolism	Sharp, stabbing pain worsening with deep breaths	Pain can be experienced in chest, back, shoulder, or upper abdomen	Dyspnea, hemoptysis, cough
Pneumonia	Sharp or stabbing pain associated with cough	Mostly generalized to one side of chest but can have upper abdominal pain	Cough, fever, dyspnea, chills, sputum, myalgia, malaise
Pneumothorax	Acute/sudden and sharp	Lateral region of the chest but can have referred pain to shoulder	Acute dyspnea, cough

Continued

TABLE 19-2 Differential Diagnosis of Chest Pain—cont'd

	Common Pain Description	Location/Radiation	Possible Associated Symptoms
Gastrointestinal			
Gastroesophageal reflux	May be angina-like; however, usually burning sensation with eating large meals reproduced by lying down and relieved by sitting up	Retrosternal region	Cough, regurgitation of food, abdominal pain
Esophageal spasm	Crushing chest pain	Substernal	Dysphagia, sensation of object in throat or esophagus
Cholecystitis	Sudden onset of pain that crescendos and can last for up to 20 minutes, usually after eating a fatty meal	Epigastrium or right upper abdomen that can radiate to right intrascapular region, shoulder, or back	Nausea, vomiting, anorexia, fever
Pancreatitis	Sudden dull, boring, steady pain unrelieved by lying supine; leaning forward or the fetal position may ease pain	Epigastrium or periumbilical pain radiating to back	Nausea, vomiting, anorexia, and sometimes diarrhea
Dermatologic			
Herpes zoster	Unilateral, burning, borelike pain	Chest region in dermatome distribution	Tingling, itching, burning
Musculoskeletal/Neurologic			
Costochondritis	Sharp, pleuritic-type pain worsens with deep breathing, palpation, or movement	Area from 2nd through 5th intercostal spaces; can radiate to arm, depending on where initial inflammation occurs	Chest tightness, warmth at area of pain
Chest wall muscle strain	Sharp pain with moving, stretching, or pushing movements of the arms; palpation of area reproduces the pain	Area around the strained muscle, sternum, or ribs	Muscle spasm, crepitation, swelling, loss of strength
Psychogenic			
Depression	Heaviness	Chest region	Fatigue, restlessness, withdrawal, weight gain or loss, depressed mood
Anxiety	Sharp pain	Chest region	Palpitations, dizziness, sweating, shaking, restlessness, fatigue, irritability

From Zitkus, B. S. (2010). Take chest pain to heart. *Nurse Pract, 35*(9), 41-47.

TABLE 19-3   Clinical Portrait of Heart Failure

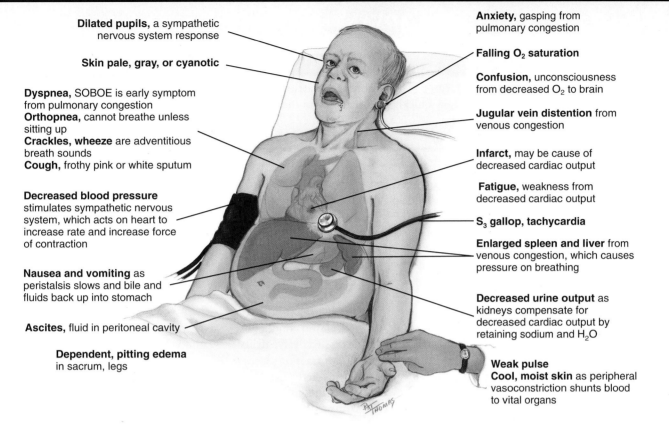

Dilated pupils, a sympathetic nervous system response

Skin pale, gray, or cyanotic

Dyspnea, SOBOE is early symptom from pulmonary congestion
Orthopnea, cannot breathe unless sitting up
Crackles, wheeze are adventitious breath sounds
Cough, frothy pink or white sputum

Decreased blood pressure stimulates sympathetic nervous system, which acts on heart to increase rate and increase force of contraction

Nausea and vomiting as peristalsis slows and bile and fluids back up into stomach

Ascites, fluid in peritoneal cavity

Dependent, pitting edema in sacrum, legs

Anxiety, gasping from pulmonary congestion

Falling O$_2$ saturation

Confusion, unconsciousness from decreased O$_2$ to brain

Jugular vein distention from venous congestion

Infarct, may be cause of decreased cardiac output

Fatigue, weakness from decreased cardiac output

S$_3$ gallop, tachycardia

Enlarged spleen and liver from venous congestion, which causes pressure on breathing

Decreased urine output as kidneys compensate for decreased cardiac output by retaining sodium and H$_2$O

Weak pulse
Cool, moist skin as peripheral vasoconstriction shunts blood to vital organs

Decreased cardiac output occurs when the heart fails as a pump and the circulation becomes backed up and congested.
Signs and symptoms of heart failure come from two basic mechanisms: (1) the heart's inability to pump enough blood to meet the metabolic demands of the body; and (2) the kidney's compensatory mechanisms of abnormal retention of sodium and water to compensate for the decreased cardiac output. This increases blood volume and venous return, which causes further congestion.
Onset of heart failure may be: (1) *acute,* as following a myocardial infarction when direct damage to the heart's contracting ability has occurred; or (2) *chronic,* as with hypertension, when the ventricles must pump against chronically increased pressure.

SOBOE, Shortness of breath on exertion.

ABNORMAL FINDINGS
FOR ADVANCED PRACTICE

TABLE 19-4 Variations in S_1

The intensity of S_1 depends on three factors: (1) position of the atrioventricular valve (AV) valve at the start of systole, (2) structure of the valve leaflets, and (3) how quickly pressure rises in the ventricle.

	Factor	Examples
Loud (Accentuated) S_1		
S_1 S_2	1. Position of AV valve at start of systole—Wide open and no time to drift together	Hyperkinetic states in which blood velocity is increased: exercise, fever, anemia, hyperthyroidism
	2. Change in valve structure—Calcification of valve; needs increasing ventricular pressure to close the valve against increased atrial pressure	Mitral stenosis with leaflets still mobile
Faint (Diminished) S_1		
S_1 S_2	1. Position of AV valve—Delayed conduction from atria to ventricles. Mitral valve drifts shut before ventricular contraction closes it	First-degree heart block (prolonged PR interval)
	2. Change in valve structure—Extreme calcification, which limits mobility	Mitral insufficiency
	3. More forceful atrial contraction into noncompliant ventricle; delays or diminishes ventricular contraction	Severe hypertension—Systemic or pulmonary
Varying Intensity of S_1		
S_1 S_2 S_1 S_2	1. Position of AV valve varies before closing from beat to beat	Atrial fibrillation—Irregularly irregular rhythm
	2. Atria and ventricles beat independently	Complete heart block with changing PR interval
Split S_1		
S_1 S_2 T M	Mitral and tricuspid components are heard separately	Normal but uncommon

TABLE 19-5 Variations in S_2

		Condition	Example
Accentuated S_2			
S_1	S_2	1. Higher closing pressure	Systemic hypertension, ringing or booming S_2
		2. Exercise and excitement increase pressure in aorta	
		3. Pulmonary hypertension	Mitral stenosis, heart failure
		4. Semilunar valves calcified but still mobile	Aortic or pulmonic stenosis
Diminished S_2			
S_1	S_2	1. A fall in systemic blood pressure causes a decrease in valve strength	Shock
		2. Semilunar valves thickened and calcified, with decreased mobility	Aortic or pulmonic stenosis

TABLE 19-6 Variations in Split S_2

Normal Splitting

		Condition	Example
Fixed Split		A fixed split is unaffected by respiration; the split is always there.	Atrial septal defect
			Right ventricular failure
Paradoxical Split		Conditions that delay aortic valve closure cause the opposite of a normal split. In inspiration, P_2 is normally delayed; thus with a paradoxical split the sounds fuse. In expiration you hear the split in the order of P_2A_2.	Aortic stenosis
			Left bundle branch block
			Patent ductus arteriosus
Wide Split		When the right ventricle has delayed electrical activation, the split is very wide on inspiration and is still there on expiration.	Right bundle branch block (which delays P_2)

TABLE 19-7 Systolic Extra Sounds

Early systolic:
  Ejection click
  Aortic prosthetic valve sounds

Mid/late systolic:
  Midsystolic (mitral) click

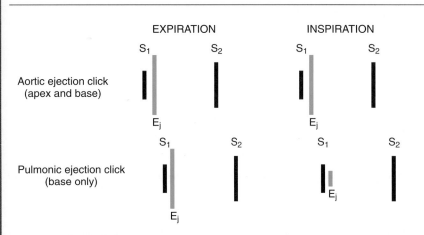

Ejection Click

The ejection click occurs early in systole at the start of ejection because it results from opening of the semilunar (SL) valves. Normally the SL valves open silently, but in the presence of stenosis (e.g., aortic stenosis, pulmonic stenosis) their opening makes a sound. It is short and high pitched, with a click quality and is heard better with the diaphragm.

   The aortic ejection click is heard at the 2nd right interspace and apex and may be loudest at the apex. Its intensity does not change with respiration. The pulmonic ejection click is best heard in the 2nd left interspace and often grows softer with inspiration.

"Ball-in-cage"
AO = aortic opens
AC = aortic closes

Aortic Prosthetic Valve Sounds

As a sequela of modern technologic intervention for heart problems, some people now have *iatrogenically* induced heart sounds. The opening of a mechanical aortic ball-in-cage prosthesis produces an early systolic sound. This sound is less intense with a tilting disk prosthesis and is absent with a biologic tissue prosthesis (e.g., porcine).

Apex
C = click

Midsystolic Click

Although it is systolic, this is not an ejection click. It is associated with **mitral valve prolapse,** in which the mitral valve leaflets not only close with contraction but balloon back up into the left atrium. During ballooning the sudden tensing of the valve leaflets and the chordae tendineae creates the click.

   The sound occurs in mid-to-late systole and is short and high pitched with a click quality. It is best heard with the diaphragm, at the apex, but also may be heard at the left lower sternal border. The click usually is followed by a systolic murmur. The click and murmur move with postural change; when the person assumes a squatting position, the click may move closer to S_2, and the murmur may sound louder and delayed. The Valsalva maneuver also moves the click closer to S_2.

TABLE 19-8   Diastolic Extra Sounds

Early diastole:
  Opening snap
  Mitral prosthetic valve sound

Mid-diastole:
  Third heart sound
  Summation sound (S_3 + S_4)

Late diastole:
  Fourth heart sound
  Pacemaker-induced sound

Opening Snap

Normally the opening of the AV valves is silent. In the presence of stenosis, increasingly higher atrial pressure is required to open the valve. The deformed valve opens with a noise: the opening snap. It is sharp and high pitched with a snapping quality. It sounds after S_2 and is best heard with the diaphragm at the 3rd or 4th left interspace at the sternal border, less well at the apex.

The opening snap usually is not an isolated sound. As a sign of mitral stenosis, the opening snap usually ushers in the low-pitched diastolic rumbling murmur of that condition.

Mitral Prosthetic Valve Sound

An iatrogenic sound, the opening of a ball-in-cage mitral prosthesis gives an early diastolic sound: an opening click just after S_2. It is loud, heard over the whole precordium, and loudest at the apex and left lower sternal border.

Third Heart Sound

The S_3 is a ventricular filling sound. It occurs in early diastole during the rapid filling phase. Your hearing quickly accommodates to the S_3; thus it is best heard when you listen initially. It sounds after S_2 but later than an opening snap would be. It is a dull, soft sound; and it is low pitched, like "distant thunder." It is heard best in a quiet room, at the apex, with the bell held lightly (just enough to form a seal), and with the person in the left lateral position.

The S_3 can be confused with a split S_2. Use these guidelines to distinguish the S_3:
- *Location*—The S_3 is heard at the apex or left lower sternal border; the split S_2 at the base.
- *Respiratory variation*—The S_3 does not vary in timing with respirations; the split S_2 does.
- *Pitch*—The S_3 is lower pitched; the pitch of the split S_2 stays the same.

The S_3 may be normal (physiologic) or abnormal (pathologic). The **physiologic** S_3 is heard frequently in children and young adults; it occasionally may persist after 40 years, especially in women. The normal S_3 usually disappears when the person sits up.

In adults the S_3 is usually abnormal. The **pathologic** S_3 is also called a **ventricular gallop** or an S_3 gallop, and it persists when sitting up. The S_3 indicates decreased compliance of the ventricles, as in heart failure. It may be the earliest sign of heart failure. The S_3 may originate from either the left or the right ventricle; a left-sided S_3 is heard at the apex in the left lateral position, and a right-sided S_3 is heard at the left lower sternal border with the person supine and is louder in inspiration.

The S_3 also occurs with conditions of volume overload such as mitral regurgitation and aortic or tricuspid regurgitation. The S_3 is also found in high cardiac output states in the absence of heart disease such as hyperthyroidism, anemia, and pregnancy. When the primary condition is corrected, the gallop disappears.

Continued

TABLE 19-8   Diastolic Extra Sounds—cont'd

Fourth Heart Sound

The S_4 is a ventricular filling sound. It occurs when the atria contract late in diastole. It is heard immediately before S_1. This is a very soft sound, of very low pitch. You need a good bell, and you must be listening for it. It is heard best at the apex, with the person in left lateral position.

A **physiologic** S_4 may occur in adults older than 40 or 50 years with no evidence of cardiovascular disease, especially after exercise.

A **pathologic** S_4 is termed an **atrial gallop** or an S_4 **gallop**. It occurs with decreased compliance of the ventricle (e.g., coronary artery disease, cardiomyopathy) and systolic overload (afterload), including outflow obstruction to the ventricle (aortic stenosis) and systemic hypertension. A left-sided S_4 occurs with these conditions. It is heard best at the apex, in the left lateral position.

A right-sided S_4 is less common. It is heard at the left lower sternal border and may increase with inspiration. It occurs with pulmonary stenosis or pulmonary hypertension.

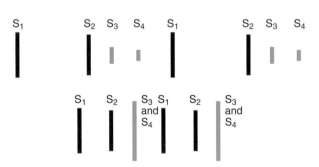

Summation Sound

When both the pathologic S_3 and S_4 are present, a quadruple rhythm is heard. Often in cases of cardiac stress, one response is tachycardia. During rapid rates the diastolic filling time shortens, and the S_3 and S_4 move closer together. They sound superimposed in mid-diastole, and you hear one loud, prolonged, summated sound, often louder than either S_1 or S_2.

Extracardiac Sounds

Pericardial Friction Rub

Inflammation of the pericardium gives rise to a friction rub. The sound is high pitched and scratchy, like sandpaper being rubbed. It is best heard with the diaphragm, with the person sitting up and leaning forward and the breath held in expiration.

A friction rub can be heard any place on the precordium but usually is best heard at the apex and left lower sternal border, places where the pericardium comes in close contact with the chest wall. Timing may be systolic and diastolic. The friction rub of pericarditis is common during the 1st week after a myocardial infarction and may last only a few hours.

TABLE 19-9   Abnormal Pulsations on the Precordium

Base

A **thrill** in the 2nd and 3rd right interspaces occurs with severe aortic stenosis and systemic hypertension.
A **thrill** in the 2nd and 3rd left interspaces occurs with pulmonic stenosis and pulmonic hypertension.

Left Sternal Border

A **lift (heave)** occurs with right ventricular hypertrophy, as found in pulmonic valve disease, pulmonic hypertension, and chronic lung disease. You feel a diffuse lifting impulse during systole at the left lower sternal border. It may be associated with retraction at the apex because the left ventricle is rotated posteriorly by the enlarged right ventricle.

Apex

Cardiac enlargement displaces the apical impulse laterally and over a wider area when left ventricular hypertrophy and dilation are present. This is **volume overload,** as in heart failure, mitral regurgitation, aortic regurgitation, and left-to-right shunts.

Apex

The apical impulse is increased in force and duration but is not necessarily displaced to the left when left ventricular hypertrophy occurs alone without dilation. This is **pressure overload,** as found in aortic stenosis or systemic hypertension.

TABLE 19-10	Congenital Heart Defects	
	Description	Clinical Data

Patent Ductus Arteriosus (PDA)

Persistence of the channel joining left pulmonary artery to aorta. This is normal in the fetus and usually closes spontaneously within hours of birth.

S: Usually no symptoms in early childhood; growth and development are normal.

O: Blood pressure has wide pulse pressure and bounding peripheral pulses from rapid runoff of blood into low-resistance pulmonary bed during diastole. Thrill is often palpable at left upper sternal border. The continuous murmur heard in systole and diastole is called a *machinery murmur.*

Atrial Septal Defect (ASD)

Abnormal opening in the atrial septum, resulting usually in left-to-right shunt and causing large increase in pulmonary blood flow.

S: Defect is remarkably well tolerated. Symptoms in infants are rare; growth and development normal. Children and young adults have mild fatigue and DOE.

O: Sternal lift is often present. S_2 has fixed split, with P_2 often louder than A_2. Murmur is systolic, ejection, medium pitch, best heard at base in 2nd left interspace. Murmur is caused not by shunt itself but by increased blood flow through pulmonic valve.

Ventricular Septal Defect (VSD)

Abnormal opening in septum between the ventricles, usually subaortic area. The size and exact position vary considerably.

S: Small defects are asymptomatic. Infants with large defects have poor growth, slow weight gain; later they look pale, thin, delicate. May have feeding problems; DOE; frequent respiratory infections; and, when the condition is severe, heart failure.

O: Loud, harsh holosystolic murmur, best heard at left lower sternal border, may be accompanied by thrill. Large defects also have soft diastolic murmur at apex (mitral flow murmur) caused by increased blood flow through mitral valve.

TABLE 19-10   Congenital Heart Defects—cont'd

	Description	Clinical Data

Tetralogy of Fallot

Four components: (1) right ventricular outflow stenosis, (2) VSD, (3) right ventricular hypertrophy, and (4) overriding aorta. *Result:* shunts a lot of venous blood directly into aorta away from pulmonary system; thus blood never gets oxygenated.

S: Severe cyanosis, not in first months of life but develops as infant grows and right ventricular outflow (i.e., pulmonic) stenosis gets worse. Cyanosis with crying and exertion at first, then at rest. Uses squatting posture after starts walking. DOE is common. Development is slowed.

O: Thrill palpable at left lower sternal border. S_1 normal; S_2 has A_2 loud and P_2 diminished or absent. Murmur is systolic, loud, crescendo-decrescendo.

Coarctation of the Aorta

Severe narrowing of descending aorta, usually at the junction of the ductus arteriosus and the aortic arch, just distal to the origin of the left subclavian artery. Results in increased workload on left ventricle.

Associated with defects of aortic valve in most cases, associated patent ductus arteriosus, and associated VSD.

S: In infants with associated lesions or symptoms, diagnosis occurs in the early months as heart failure develops. For asymptomatic children, growth and development are normal. Diagnosis follows abnormal BP findings. Adolescents may complain of vague lower-extremity cramping, worse with exercise.

O: Arm hypertension over 20 mm Hg higher than leg measures is a hallmark of coarctation. Another important sign is absent or greatly diminished femoral pulses. A systolic murmur is heard best at the left sternal border, radiating to the back.

S, Subjective data; *O,* objective data.

Images © Pat Thomas, 2006.

TABLE 19-11   Murmurs Caused by Valvular Defects

Midsystolic Ejection Murmurs

Caused by forward flow through semilunar valves. Examples below have the murmur pictured here:

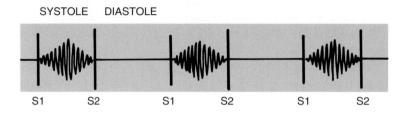

	Description	Clinical Data
Aortic Stenosis	Calcification of aortic valve cusps restricts forward flow of blood during systole; LV hypertrophy develops.	S: Fatigue, DOE, palpitation, dizziness, fainting, anginal pain. O: Pallor, slow diminished radial pulse, low BP, and auscultatory gap are common. Apical impulse sustained and displaced to left. Thrill in systole over 2nd and 3rd right interspaces and right side of neck. S_1 normal, often ejection click present, often paradoxical split S_2, S_4 present with LV hypertrophy. Murmur: Loud, harsh, midsystolic, crescendo-decrescendo, loudest at second right interspace, radiates widely to side of neck, down left sternal border, or apex.
Pulmonic Stenosis	Calcification of pulmonic valve restricts forward flow of blood	O: Thrill in systole at 2nd and 3rd left interspace, ejection click often present after S_1, diminished S_2 and usually with wide split, S_4 common with RV hypertrophy. Murmur: Systolic, medium pitch, coarse, crescendo-decrescendo (diamond shape), best heard at 2nd left interspace, radiates to the left and neck.

TABLE 19-11   Murmurs Caused by Valvular Defects—cont'd

Pansystolic Regurgitant Murmurs

Caused by backward flow of blood from area of higher pressure to one of lower pressure. Examples below have the murmur pictured here:

Description	Clinical Data

Mitral Regurgitation

Stream of blood regurgitates back into LA during systole through incompetent mitral valve. In diastole, blood passes back into LV again along with new flow; results in LV dilation and hypertrophy.

S: Fatigue, palpitation, orthopnea, PND.
O: Thrill in systole at apex. Lift at apex. Apical impulse displaced down and to left. S_1 diminished, S_2 accentuated, S_3 at apex often present.
Murmur: Pansystolic, often loud, blowing; best heard at apex; radiates well to left axilla.

Tricuspid Regurgitation

Backflow of blood through incompetent tricuspid valve into RA.

O: Engorged pulsating neck veins, liver enlarged. Lift at sternum if RV hypertrophy present; often thrill at left lower sternal border.
Murmur: Soft, blowing, pansystolic; best heard at left lower sternal border; increases with inspiration.

Continued

TABLE 19-11   Murmurs Caused by Valvular Defects—cont'd

Diastolic Rumbles of AV Valves

Filling murmurs at low pressures, best heard with bell lightly touching skin. Examples below have the murmur pictured here:

	Description	Clinical Data

Mitral Stenosis

Calcified mitral valve does not open properly, impedes forward flow of blood into LV during diastole. Results in LA enlarged and LA pressure increased.

S: Fatigue, palpitations, DOE, orthopnea, occasional PND or pulmonary edema.

O: Diminished, often irregular arterial pulse. Lift at apex, diastolic thrill common at apex. S_1 accentuated; opening snap after S_2 heard over wide area of precordium, followed by murmur.

Murmur: Low-pitched diastolic rumble, best heard at apex, with person in left lateral position; does not radiate.

Tricuspid Stenosis

Calcification of tricuspid valve impedes forward flow into RV during diastole.

O: Diminished arterial pulse, jugular venous pulse prominent.

Murmur: Diastolic rumble; best heard at left lower sternal border; louder in inspiration.

TABLE 19-11   Murmurs Caused by Valvular Defects—cont'd

Early Diastolic Murmurs

Caused by Semilunar valve incompetence. Examples below have the murmur pictured here:

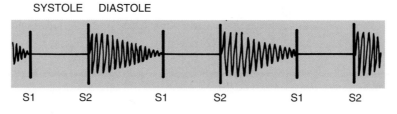

	Description	Clinical Data
Aortic Regurgitation	Stream of blood regurgitates back through incompetent aortic valve into LV during diastole. LV dilation and hypertrophy caused by increased LV stroke volume. Rapid ejection of large stroke volume into poorly filled aorta, then rapid runoff in diastole as part of blood pushed back into LV.	S: Only minor symptoms for many years, then rapid deterioration: DOE, PND, angina, dizziness. O: Bounding "water-hammer" pulse in carotid, brachial, and femoral arteries. Blood pressure has wide pulse pressure. Pulsations in cervical and suprasternal area, apical impulse displaced to left and down, apical impulse feels brief. Murmur starts almost simultaneously with S_2: soft, high pitched, blowing diastolic, decrescendo, best heard at 3rd left interspace at base as person sits up and leans forward, radiates down.
Pulmonic Regurgitation	Backflow of blood through incompetent pulmonic valve from pulmonary artery to RV.	Murmur has same timing and characteristics as that of aortic regurgitation, and is hard to distinguish on physical examination

O, Objective data; *S,* subjective data.

Images © Pat Thomas, 2006.

Summary Checklist: Heart and Neck Vessels Examination

Neck
1. Carotid pulse—Observe and palpate
2. Observe jugular venous pulse
3. Estimate jugular venous pressure

Precordium

Inspection and palpation
1. Describe location of apical impulse.
2. Note any heave (lift) or thrill.

Auscultation
1. Identify anatomic areas where you listen.
2. Note rate and rhythm of heartbeat.
3. Identify S_1 and S_2 and note any variation.
4. Listen in systole and diastole for any extra heart sounds.
5. Listen in systole and diastole for any murmurs.
6. Repeat sequence with bell.
7. Listen at the apex with person in left lateral position
8. Listen at the base with person in sitting position.

BIBLIOGRAPHY

1. American Heart Association. (2013). Heart disease and stroke statistics—2013 update. *Circulation, 127*(1), e6-e245.
2. American Heart Association. *Women and cardiovascular diseases*. (2013). Available at http://www.heart.org/idc/groups/heart-public/@wcm/@sop/@smd/documents/downloadable/ucm_319576.pdf.
3. Berry, J. D., Dyer, A., Cai, X., et al. (2012). Lifetime risks of cardiovascular disease. *N Engl J Med, 366*(4), 321-329.
4. Caboral, M. F. (2013). Update on cardiovascular disease prevention in women. *Am J Nurs, 113*(3):26-34.
4a. Caboral-Stevens, M. F. (2014). A snapshot of the latest heart failure guidelines. *Nurse Pract, 39*(7), 49-54.
5. Conn, R. D., & O'Keefe, J. H. (2009). Cardiac physical diagnosis in the digital age: an important but increasingly neglected skill (from stethoscopes to microchips). *Am J Cardiol, 104*(4), 590-595.
6. Cunningham, F. G., Leveno, K. J., Bloom, S. L., et al. (2014). *Williams obstetrics* (24th ed.). New York: McGraw-Hill.
7. Fang, J. C., & O'Gara, P. T. (2012). The history and physical examination: an evidence-based approach. In R. O. Bonow, D. L. Mann, D. P. Zipes, et al. (Eds.). *Braunwald's heart disease* (9th ed.). Philadelphia: Elsevier. pp. 107-125.
8. Fleg, J. L., & Strait, J. (2012). Age-associated changes in cardiovascular structure and function: a fertile milieu for future disease. *Heart Failure Rev, 17*(4-5), 545-554.
8a. Grotta, J. C. (2013). Carotid stenosis. *N Engl J Med, 369*(12), 1143-1149.
9. Hickey, K. T., & Rezzadeh, K. (2013). Hypertrophic cardiomyopathy: a clinical and genetic update. *Nurse Pract, 38*(5), 22-31.
10. Jones, I. D., & Slovis, C. M. (2010). Pitfalls in evaluating the low-risk chest pain patient. *Emerg Med Clin North Am, 28*(1), 183-201.
11. Luttenberger, K., & DiNapoli, M. (2011). Subacute bacterial endocarditis: making the diagnosis. *Nurse Pract, 36*(3), 31-38.
12. Mackie, A. S., Jutras, L. C., Dancea, A. B., et al. (2009). Can cardiologists distinguish innocent from pathologic murmurs in neonates? *J Pediatr, 154*(1), 50-54.
13. McGee, S. (2012). *Evidence-based physical diagnosis* (3rd ed.). Philadelphia: Elsevier.
14. McSweeney, J. C., Cody, M., O'Sullivan, P., et al. (2003). Women's early warning symptoms of acute myocardial infarction. *Circulation, 108*(21), 2619-2623.
15. McSweeney, J. C., Cleves, M. A., Zhao, W., et al. (2010). Cluster analysis of women's prodromal and acute myocardial infarction symptoms by race and other characteristics. *J Cardiovasc Nurs, 25*(4), 311.
16. Melchiorre, K., Sharma, R., & Thilaganathan, B. (2012). Cardiac structure and function in normal pregnancy. *Curr Opin Obstetr Gynecol, 24*(6), 413-421.
17. Mosca, L., Benjamin, E. J., Berra, K., et al. (2011). Effectiveness-based guidelines for the prevention of cardiovascular disease in women—2011 update. *Circulation 123*(11):1243-1262.
18. Reference deleted in proofs.
19. National Center for Health Statistics. (2011). *Health, United States, 2011*. Hyattsville, MD: Author. Available at www.cdc.gov/nchs/hus/hus/contents2011.pdf.
20. Pickett, C. A., Jackson, J. L., Hemann, B. A., et al. (2010). Carotid bruits and cerebrovascular disease risk: a meta-analysis. *Stroke, 41*(10), 2295-2302.
21. Ramani, G. V., Uber, P. A., & Mehra, M. R. (2010). *Chronic heart failure*. Mayo Clinic Proceedings, 85(2), 180-195.
22. Rosenberg, S., Elashoff, M. R., Beineke, P., et al. (2010). Multicenter validation of the diagnostic accuracy of a blood-based gene expression test. *Ann Intern Med, 153*(7):425-434.
23. Sarkinen, B. E. (2011). Vitamin D deficiency and heart disease. *Nurse Pract, 36*(3), 46-53.
24. Spencer, A., Jablonski, R., & Loeb, S. J. (2012). Hypertensive African American women and the DASH diet. *Nurse Pract, 37*(2), 41-46.
25. Thull-Freedman, J. (2010). Evaluation of chest pain in the pediatric patient. *Med Clin North Am, 94*(2), 327-347.
26. U.S. Preventive Services Task Force. (2009). Aspirin for the prevention of cardiovascular disease. *Ann Intern Med, 150*(6), 396-404.
27. Warnes, C. A. Pregnancy and heart disease. In Bonow, R. O., Mann, D. L., Zipes, D. P., et al. (2012). *Braunwald's heart disease* (9th ed.). Philadelphia: Elsevier.
28. Wells, M., & Kalman, M. (2011). Women & heart disease: symptoms and treatment guidelines. *Nurse Pract, 36*(9), 22-27.
29. Wierwille, L. (2011). Pediatric heart murmurs: evaluation and management in primary care. *Nurse Pract, 36*(3), 22-29.
30. Wolf, T., Miller, T., & Ko, S. (2009). Aspirin for the primary prevention of cardiovascular events. *Ann Intern Med, 150*(6), 405-410.
31. Wood, J., & Gordon, P. (2012). Preventing CVD in women: the NP's role. *Nurse Pract, 37*(2), 26-33.
32. Yusuf, S., Hawken, S., Ôunpuu, S., et al. (2004). Effect of potentially modifiable risk factors associated with myocardial infarction in 52 countries (the INTERHEART study). *Lancet, 364*(9438), 937-952.
33. Zitkus, B. S. (2010). Take chest pain to heart. *Nurse Pract, 35*(9), 41-47.

CHAPTER 20

Peripheral Vascular System and Lymphatic System

STRUCTURE AND FUNCTION

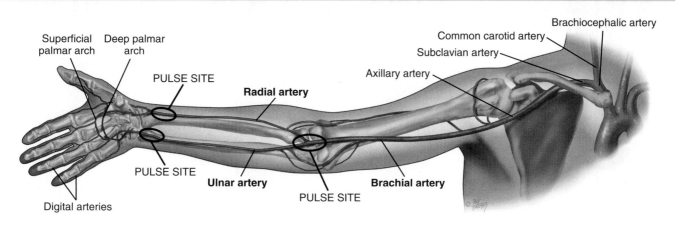

Superficial palmar arch
Deep palmar arch
PULSE SITE
Radial artery
Brachiocephalic artery
Common carotid artery
Subclavian artery
Axillary artery
PULSE SITE
Ulnar artery
PULSE SITE
Digital arteries
Brachial artery

20-1

© Pat Thomas, 2010.

The vascular system consists of the vessels for transporting fluid such as the blood or lymph. Any disease in the vascular system impairs the delivery of oxygen and nutrients to the tissues and retards the elimination of carbon dioxide and waste products from cellular metabolism.

ARTERIES

The heart pumps freshly oxygenated blood through the arteries to all body tissues (Fig. 20-1). The pumping heart makes this a high-pressure system. The artery walls are strong, tough, and tense to withstand pressure demands. Arteries contain elastic fibers, which allow their walls to stretch with systole and recoil with diastole. They also contain muscle fibers (vascular smooth muscle [VSM]), which control the amount of blood delivered to the tissues. The VSM contracts or dilates, which changes the diameter of the arteries to control the rate of blood flow.

Each heartbeat creates a pressure wave, which makes the arteries expand and then recoil. It is the recoil that propels blood through like a wave. All arteries have this pressure wave, or **pulse,** throughout their length, but you can feel it only at body sites where the artery lies close to the skin and over a bone. The following arteries are accessible to examination.

Temporal Artery. The temporal artery is palpated in front of the ear, as discussed in Chapter 13.

Carotid Artery. The carotid artery is palpated in the groove between the sternomastoid muscle and the trachea, as discussed in Chapter 19.

Arteries in the Arm. The major artery supplying the arm is the **brachial** artery, which runs in the biceps-triceps furrow of the upper arm and surfaces at the antecubital fossa in the elbow medial to the biceps tendon (see Fig. 20-1). Immediately below the elbow the brachial artery bifurcates into the ulnar and radial arteries. These run distally and form two arches supplying the hand; these are called the *superficial and deep palmar arches.* The radial pulse lies just medial to the radius at the wrist; the ulnar artery is in the same relation to the ulna, but it is deeper and often difficult to feel.

Arteries in the Leg. The major artery to the leg is the **femoral** artery, which passes under the inguinal ligament (Fig. 20-2). The femoral artery travels down the thigh. At the lower thigh it courses posteriorly; then it is termed the **popliteal** artery. Below the knee the popliteal artery divides. The anterior tibial artery travels down the front of the leg on to the dorsum of the foot, where it becomes the **dorsalis pedis.** In back of the leg the **posterior tibial** artery travels down behind the medial malleolus and forms the plantar arteries in the foot.

The function of the arteries is to supply oxygen and essential nutrients to the tissues. **Ischemia** is a deficient supply of oxygenated arterial blood to a tissue caused by obstruction of

509

20-2 Arteries in the leg.

20-3 Veins in the leg.   © Pat Thomas, 2010.

a blood vessel. A complete blockage leads to death of the distal tissue. A partial blockage creates an insufficient supply, and the ischemia may be apparent only at exercise when oxygen needs increase. **Peripheral artery disease (PAD)** affects noncoronary arteries and usually refers to arteries supplying the limbs. It usually is caused by atherosclerosis, and less commonly by embolism, hypercoagulable states, or arterial dissection.

VEINS

The course of the veins is parallel to the arteries, but the direction of flow is opposite; the veins absorb CO_2 and waste products from the periphery and carry them back to the heart. The body has more veins, and they lie closer to the skin surface. The following veins are accessible to examination.

Jugular Veins. Assessment of the jugular veins is presented in Chapter 19.

Veins in the Arm. Each arm has two sets of veins: superficial and deep. The superficial veins are in the subcutaneous tissue and are responsible for most of the venous return.

Veins in the Leg. The legs have three types of veins (Fig. 20-3):
1. The **deep veins** run alongside the deep arteries and conduct most of the venous return from the legs. These are the **femoral** and **popliteal** veins. As long as these veins remain intact, the superficial veins can be excised without harming the circulation.
2. The **superficial veins** are the **great** and **small saphenous** veins. The great saphenous vein, inside the leg, starts at the medial side of the dorsum of the foot. You can see it ascend in front of the medial malleolus; then it crosses the tibia obliquely and ascends along the medial side of the thigh. The small saphenous vein, outside the leg, starts on the lateral side of the dorsum of the foot and ascends behind the lateral malleolus, up the back of the leg, where it joins

the popliteal vein. Blood flows from the superficial veins into the deep leg veins.

3. **Perforators** (not illustrated) are connecting veins that join the two sets. They also have one-way valves that route blood from the superficial into the deep veins and prevent reflux to the superficial veins.

VENOUS FLOW

Veins drain the deoxygenated blood with its waste products from the tissues and return it to the heart. Unlike the arteries, veins are a low-pressure system. Because they do not have a pump to generate their blood flow, they need a mechanism to keep blood moving (Fig. 20-4). This is accomplished by (1) the contracting skeletal muscles that milk the blood proximally, back toward the heart; (2) the pressure gradient caused by breathing, in which inspiration makes the thoracic pressure decrease and the abdominal pressure increase; and (3) the intraluminal valves, which ensure unidirectional flow. Each valve is a paired semilunar pocket that opens toward the heart and closes tightly when filled to prevent backflow of blood.

In the legs this mechanism is called the *calf pump* or *peripheral heart*. When walking, the calf muscles alternately contract (systole) and relax (diastole). In the contraction phase the gastrocnemius and soleus muscles squeeze the veins and direct the blood flow proximally. Because of the valves, venous blood flows just one way—toward the heart.

Besides the presence of intraluminal valves, venous structure differs from arterial structure. Because venous pressure is lower, walls of the veins are thinner than those of the arteries. Veins have a larger diameter and are more distensible;

② Inspiration: ⬇Thoracic pressure ⬆Abdominal pressure

① Skeletal muscle pressure

③ Intraluminal valves

Open   Closed

MECHANISMS OF VENOUS FLOW

20-4

Structure and Function

they can expand and hold more blood when blood volume increases. This is a compensatory mechanism to reduce stress on the heart. Because of this ability to stretch, veins are called **capacitance vessels.**

Efficient venous return depends on contracting skeletal muscles, competent valves in the veins, and a patent lumen. Problems with any of these three elements lead to venous stasis. At risk for venous disease are people who undergo prolonged standing, sitting, or bed rest because they do not benefit from the milking action that walking accomplishes. Hypercoagulable states and vein wall trauma are other factors that increase risk for venous disease. Also, dilated and tortuous (varicose) veins create **incompetent valves,** wherein the lumen is so wide that the valve cusps cannot approximate. This condition increases venous pressure, which further dilates the vein. Some people have a genetic predisposition to varicose veins, but venous pooling also occurs in obese people and women following multiple pregnancies.

20-5 Microcirculation. © Pat Thomas, 2014.

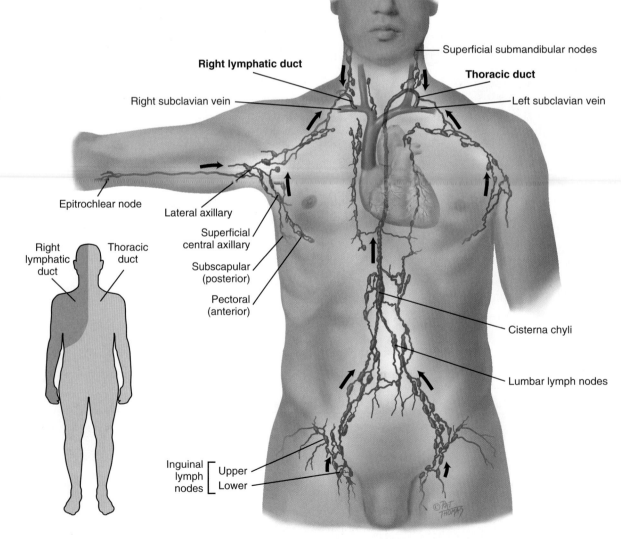

LYMPHATIC DUCTS AND DRAINAGE PATTERNS

20-6 © Pat Thomas, 2010.

LYMPHATICS

The lymphatics form a completely separate vessel system that retrieves excess fluid and plasma proteins from the interstitial spaces and returns it to the bloodstream (Fig. 20-5). Fluid moves according to a pressure gradient (filtration). At the arterial end the *hydrostatic pressure* is caused by the pumping action of the heart and pushes somewhat more fluid out of the capillaries than the venules can absorb. This fluid is vacuumed out of the interstitial spaces by the lymph vessels. Without lymphatic drainage, fluid would build up in the interstitial spaces and produce edema.

Substances pass around the microcirculation by a concentration gradient (diffusion). Most plasma proteins are too big to be pushed out of the arterioles; they remain and create the force for *colloid osmotic pressure* that pulls interstitial fluid back into the venules. A few smaller plasma proteins do escape the arterioles; they are captured by the lymph vessels and eventually returned to the bloodstream.

The vessels converge and drain into two main trunks, which empty into the venous system at the subclavian veins (Fig. 20-6):

1. The **right lymphatic duct** empties into the right subclavian vein. It drains the right side of the head and neck, right arm, right side of the thorax, right lung and pleura, right side of the heart, and right upper section of the liver.
2. The **thoracic duct** drains the rest of the body. It empties into the left subclavian vein.

The functions of the lymphatic system are to (1) conserve fluid and plasma proteins that leak out of the capillaries, (2) form a major part of the immune system that defends the body against disease, and (3) absorb lipids from the small intestine.

The immune system is a complicated network of organs and cells that work together to protect the body. It detects and eliminates foreign pathogens, both those that come in from the environment and those arising from inside (abnormal or mutant cells). It accomplishes this by phagocytosis (digestion) of the substances by neutrophils and monocytes/macrophages and by production of specific antibodies or specific immune responses by the lymphocytes.

The lymphatic vessels have a unique structure. Lymphatic capillaries start as microscopic open-ended tubes, which siphon interstitial fluid. The capillaries converge to form vessels and drain into larger ones. The vessels have valves; therefore flow is one way from the tissue spaces into the bloodstream. The many valves make the vessels look beaded. The flow of lymph is slow compared with that of the blood. Lymph flow is propelled by contraction of the skeletal muscles, by pressure changes secondary to breathing, and by contraction of the vessel walls themselves.

Lymph nodes are small, oval clumps of lymphatic tissue located at intervals along the vessels. Most nodes are arranged in groups, both deep and superficial, in the body. Nodes filter the fluid before it is returned to the bloodstream and filter out microorganisms that could be harmful to the body. The pathogens are exposed to B and T lymphocytes in the lymph nodes, and these mount an antigen-specific response to eliminate the pathogens. With local inflammation the nodes in that area become swollen and tender.

The superficial groups of nodes are accessible to inspection and palpation and give clues to the status of the lymphatic system:

- **Cervical nodes** drain the head and neck and are described in Chapter 13.
- **Axillary nodes** drain the breast and upper arm. They are described in Chapter 17.
- The **epitrochlear node** is in the antecubital fossa and drains the hand and lower arm.
- The **inguinal nodes** in the groin drain most of the lymph of the lower extremity, the external genitalia, and the anterior abdominal wall.

Related Organs

The spleen, tonsils, and thymus aid the lymphatic system (Fig. 20-7). The **spleen** is located in the left upper quadrant of the abdomen. It has four functions: (1) to destroy old red blood cells; (2) to produce antibodies; (3) to store red blood cells; and (4) to filter microorganisms from the blood.

The **tonsils** (palatine, pharyngeal, and lingual) are located at the entrance to the respiratory and gastrointestinal tracts and respond to local inflammation.

The **thymus** is the flat, pink-gray gland located in the superior mediastinum behind the sternum and in front of the aorta. It is relatively large in the fetus and young child and atrophies after puberty. It is important in developing the T lymphocytes of the immune system in children. The B lymphocytes originate in the bone marrow and mature in the lymphoid tissue.

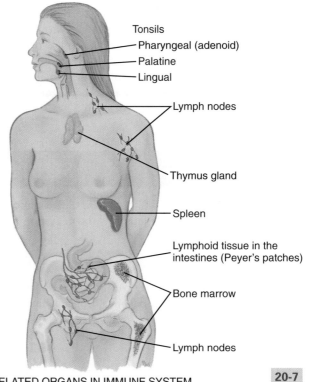

Tonsils
Pharyngeal (adenoid)
Palatine
Lingual
Lymph nodes
Thymus gland
Spleen
Lymphoid tissue in the intestines (Peyer's patches)
Bone marrow
Lymph nodes

RELATED ORGANS IN IMMUNE SYSTEM   **20-7**

❖ DEVELOPMENTAL COMPETENCE

Infants and Children

The lymphatic system has the same function in children as in adults. Lymphoid tissue is well developed at birth and grows rapidly until age 10 or 11 years. By 6 years of age the lymphoid tissue reaches adult size; it surpasses adult size by puberty, and then it slowly atrophies. It is possible that the excessive antigen stimulation in children causes the early rapid growth.

Lymph nodes are relatively large in children, and the superficial ones often are palpable even when the child is healthy. With infection, excessive swelling and hyperplasia occur. Enlarged tonsils are familiar signs in respiratory infections. The excessive lymphoid response also may account for the common childhood symptom of abdominal pain with seemingly unrelated problems such as upper respiratory infection (URI). Possibly the inflammation of mesenteric lymph nodes produces the abdominal pain.

The Pregnant Woman

Hormonal changes cause vasodilation and the resulting drop in blood pressure described in Chapter 19. The growing uterus obstructs drainage of the iliac veins and the inferior vena cava. This condition causes low blood flow and increases venous pressure. This in turn causes dependent edema, varicosities in the legs and vulva, and hemorrhoids.

The Aging Adult

Peripheral blood vessels grow more rigid with age, termed **arteriosclerosis.** This condition produces the rise in systolic blood pressure discussed in Chapter 9. Do not confuse this process with **atherosclerosis,** or the deposition of fatty plaques on the intima of the arteries. Both processes are present with PAD in aging adults. PAD is underdiagnosed and undertreated, yet it is a large cause of morbidity (painful walking, poor wound healing) and mortality in the United States. It increases dramatically with age and is present in 29% of those over 70 years and in those between 50 to 69 years with a history of cigarette smoking or diabetes.[19]

During the middle-aged years, more men have PAD than women. In people over 85 years, the prevalence in women is 39% compared to 27% of men. It is not clear why women develop PAD a decade later than men do. When women do develop PAD, they also may have arthritis or peripheral neuropathy that masks their symptoms and delays diagnosis.[14] (If you are old, are disabled, and cannot walk, you will not show leg pain.) Despite its prevalence and the risk for coronary artery disease (CAD), only 70% to 80% of those diagnosed with PAD are treated with antiplatelet or lipid-lowering drugs[1]; the rest are untreated. Many more are undiagnosed.

Aging produces a progressive enlargement of the intramuscular calf veins. Prolonged bed rest, prolonged immobilization, and heart failure increase the risk for deep vein thrombosis (DVT) and subsequent pulmonary embolism. These conditions are common in aging and also with malignancy and myocardial infarction (MI). Low-dose anticoagulant medication reduces the risk for venous thromboembolism.

Loss of lymphatic tissue leads to fewer numbers of lymph nodes in older people and to a decrease in the size of remaining nodes.

🌐 CULTURE AND GENETICS

The American Heart Association considers PAD a CAD risk equivalent; thus screening and treatment are important. Some diseases have a defined genetic component, but PAD seems to result from changes in "dozens or hundreds of genes" that interact with one another and the environment.[9] Current smoking is the strongest risk factor; together with diabetes mellitus, dyslipidemia, and hypertension, these factors account for >50% of the cause of PAD.[9] The ethnic group with PAD who also has the highest risk of these PAD risk factors is non-Hispanic Black.[2] The ankle-brachial index (ABI) test (see p. 525) is a relatively simple noninvasive screening for PAD. The AHA recommends this screening for all people over 70 years and for people ages 50 to 69 years who have a history of smoking or diabetes. However this office-based technique is underused.

SUBJECTIVE DATA

1. Leg pain or cramps
2. Skin changes on arms or legs
3. Swelling in arms or legs
4. Lymph node enlargement
5. Medications
6. Smoking history

Examiner Asks	Rationale
1. **Leg pain or cramps.** Any leg pain (cramps)? Where? • Describe the type of pain. Is it burning, aching, cramping, stabbing? Did this come on gradually or suddenly?	Peripheral vascular disease (PVD) includes PAD and venous disease—see pain profiles in Table 20-3, p. 532.

Examiner Asks	Rationale
• Is it aggravated by activity, walking?	With PAD, blood flow cannot match muscle demand during exercise; therefore people feel muscle fatigue or pain when walking (claudication). But only 10% of those with PAD have this classic symptom; 40% do not have leg pain, and 50% have varying leg symptoms.[1]
• How many blocks (stairs) does it take to produce this pain?	**Claudication distance** is the number of blocks walked or stairs climbed to produce pain.
• Has this amount changed recently? • Is the pain worse with elevation? Worse with cool temperatures? • Does the pain wake you up at night?	Note sudden decrease in claudication distance or pain not relieved by rest. Night leg pain is common in aging adults. It may indicate the ischemic rest pain of PVD, severe night muscle cramping (usually the calf), or restless leg syndrome.
• Any recent change in exercise, a new exercise, or an increase in exercise?	Pain of musculoskeletal origin rather than vascular.
• What relieves this pain: dangling, walking, rubbing? Is the leg pain associated with any skin changes? • Is it associated with any change in sexual function (males)?	Aortoiliac occlusion is associated with erectile dysfunction (Leriche syndrome).
• Any history of vascular problems, heart problems, diabetes, obesity, pregnancy, hypertension, trauma, prolonged standing, or bed rest?	Risk factors for PVD. Diabetes and smoking are stronger risk factors for PVD than they are even for heart disease.
2. Skin changes on arms or legs. Any **skin changes** on arms or legs? What color: redness, pallor, blueness, brown discolorations?	
• Any change in temperature—excess warmth or coolness? • Do your leg veins look bulging and crooked? How have you treated these? • Do you use support hose?	Coolness occurs with PAD. Varicose veins. Avoid compression stockings with PAD since they further impede blood flow. They are indicated to prevent leg swelling in standing workers or thrombus formation.
• Any leg sores or ulcers? Where on the leg? Any pain with the leg ulcer?	Leg ulcers occur with chronic arterial and venous disease (see Table 20-4, p. 533).
3. Swelling in arms or legs. Swelling in one or both legs? When did this swelling start?	**Edema** is bilateral when the cause is generalized (heart failure) or unilateral when it is the result of a local obstruction or inflammation.
• What time of day is the swelling at its worst: morning or after being up most of the day? • Does the swelling come and go, or is it constant? • What seems to bring it on: trauma, standing all day, sitting? • What relieves swelling: elevation, support hose? • Is swelling associated with pain, heat, redness, ulceration, hardened skin?	
4. Lymph node enlargement. Any "swollen glands" (lumps, kernels)? Where in body? How long have you had them?	Enlarged lymph nodes occur with infection, malignancies, and immunologic diseases.
• Any recent change? • How do they feel to you: hard, soft? • Are the swollen glands associated with pain, local infection?	

Examiner Asks	Rationale
5. **Medications.** Which medications are you taking (e.g., oral contraceptives, hormone replacement)?	These may cause a hypercoagulable state. Also note that low-dose aspirin or clopidogrel are used to prevent blood clots in selected people.
6. **Smoking history.** Do you smoke cigarettes? How many packs per day, would you say? At what age did you start? How many years have you smoked? Have you tried to quit? What helped for you? What did not help?	Tobacco constricts arteries, increases coagulability, injures endothelium, and promotes inflammation. Smoking is the strongest risk factor for PAD; starting smoking at ≤16 years more than doubles future PAD risk.[19]

OBJECTIVE DATA

PREPARATION

During a complete physical examination, examine the arms at the very beginning when you are checking the vital signs and the person is sitting. Examine the legs directly after the abdominal examination while the person is still supine. Then have the person stand to evaluate the leg veins.

Examination of the arms and legs includes peripheral vascular characteristics (following here), the skin (see Chapter 12), musculoskeletal findings (see Chapter 22), and neurologic findings (see Chapter 23). A method of integrating these steps is discussed in Chapter 27.

Room temperature should be about 22°C (72°F) and draftless to prevent vasodilation or vasoconstriction. Use inspection and palpation. Compare your findings with the opposite extremity.

EQUIPMENT NEEDED

Occasionally need:
Paper tape measure
Tourniquet or blood pressure cuff
Stethoscope
Doppler ultrasonic probe

Normal Range of Findings	Abnormal Findings
Inspect and Palpate the Arms	
Lift both the person's hands in your hands. Inspect and then turn the person's hands over, noting color of skin and nail beds; temperature, texture, and turgor of skin; and the presence of any lesions, edema, or clubbing. Use the **profile sign** (viewing the finger from the side) to detect early clubbing. The normal nail-bed angle is 160 degrees. (See Chapter 12 for a full discussion of skin color, lesions, and clubbing.)	Flattening of angle and clubbing (diffuse enlargement of terminal phalanges) occur with congenital cyanotic heart disease and cor pulmonale.
With the person's hands near the level of his or her heart, check **capillary refill.** This is an index of peripheral perfusion and cardiac output. Depress and blanch the nail beds; release and note the time for color return. Usually the vessels refill within a fraction of a second. Consider it normal if the color returns in less than 1 or 2 seconds. Note conditions that can skew your findings: a cool room, decreased body temperature, cigarette smoking, peripheral edema, and anemia.	Refill lasting more than 1 or 2 seconds signifies vasoconstriction or decreased cardiac output (hypovolemia, heart failure, shock). The hands are cold, clammy, and pale.
The two arms should be symmetric in size.	Edema of upper extremities occurs when lymphatic drainage is obstructed after breast surgery or radiation (see Table 20-2, p. 531).

Objective Data

Normal Range of Findings

Note the presence of any scars on hands and arms. Many occur normally with usual childhood abrasions or occupations involving hand tools.

Palpate both radial pulses, noting rate, rhythm, elasticity of vessel wall, and equal force (Fig. 20-8). Grade the force (amplitude) on a 3-point scale:
3+, Increased, full, bounding
2+, **Normal**
1+, Weak
0, Absent

20-8

It usually is not necessary to palpate the ulnar pulses. If indicated, reach your hand under the person's arm and palpate along the medial side of the inner forearm (Fig. 20-9), although the ulnar pulses often are not palpable in the healthy person.

20-9   Palpate ulnar pulse.

Abnormal Findings

Needle tracks in hands, arms, antecubital fossae occur with intravenous drug use; linear scars in wrists may signify past self-inflicted injury.

Full, bounding pulse (3+) occurs with hyperkinetic states (exercise, anxiety, fever), anemia, and hyperthyroidism.

Weak, "thready" pulse (1+) occurs with shock and PAD. See Table 20-1, p. 530, for illustrations of these and irregular pulse rhythms.

Objective Data

Normal Range of Findings	Abnormal Findings

Palpate the brachial pulses if you suspect arterial insufficiency—their force should be equal bilaterally (Fig. 20-10).

20-10

Check the epitrochlear lymph nodes in the depression above and behind the medial condyle of the humerus. Do this by "shaking hands" with the person and reaching your other hand under the person's elbow to the groove between the biceps and triceps muscles, above the medial epicondyle (Fig. 20-11). These nodes normally are not palpable.

An enlarged epitrochlear node occurs with infection of the hand or forearm.

Epitrochlear nodes occur in conditions of generalized lymphadenopathy: palpable in 25%-30% of lymphoma, chronic lymphocytic leukemia, sarcoidosis, and up to 55% in mononucleosis conditions.[11]

20-11 Search epitrochlear area.

The **modified Allen test** is used to evaluate the adequacy of collateral circulation before cannulating the radial artery (Fig. 20-12). **A,** Firmly occlude both the ulnar and radial arteries of one hand while the person makes a fist several times. This causes the hand to blanch. **B,** Ask the person to open the hand without hyperextending it; then release pressure on the ulnar artery while maintaining pressure on the radial artery. Adequate circulation is suggested by a palmar blush, a return to the normal color of the hand in approximately 2 to 5 seconds. Although this test is simple and useful, it is relatively crude and subject to error (i.e., you must occlude both arteries uniformly with 11 pounds of pressure for the test to be accurate).

C, Pallor persists, or a sluggish return to color suggests occlusion of the collateral arterial flow. Avoid radial artery cannulation until adequate circulation is shown.

| **Normal Range of Findings** | **Abnormal Findings** |

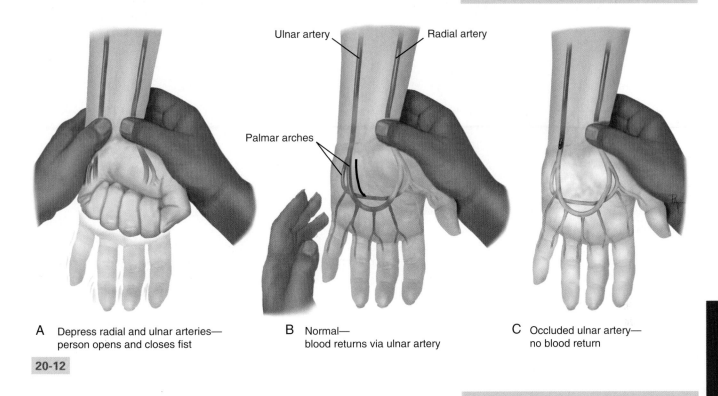

A   Depress radial and ulnar arteries— person opens and closes fist

B   Normal— blood returns via ulnar artery

C   Occluded ulnar artery— no blood return

20-12

Limitations of the modified Allen test are that it is subjective and requires patient cooperation that may not occur in emergency or critical care situations— just the times you need to cannulate the radial artery. The laser Doppler gives a quantifiable measurement of blood flow that is recordable and reproducible. A small, flat probe is taped to the palm at the end of the patient's index finger. A baseline value for blood flow is recorded and then compared for change when the two arteries are occluded.

Inspect and Palpate the Legs

Uncover the legs while keeping the genitalia draped. Inspect both legs together, noting skin color, hair distribution, venous pattern, size (swelling or atrophy), and any skin lesions or ulcers.

Normally hair covers the legs. Even if leg hair is shaved, you will still note hair on the dorsa of the toes.

The venous pattern normally is flat and barely visible. Note obvious varicosities, although these are best assessed while standing.

Both legs should be symmetric in size without any swelling or atrophy. If the lower legs look asymmetric or if DVT is suspected, measure the calf circumference with a nonstretchable tape measure (Fig. 20-13). Measure at the widest point, taking care to measure the other leg in exactly the same place (i.e., the same number of centimeters down from the patella or other landmark). If lymphedema is suspected, measure also at the ankle, distal calf, knee, and thigh. Record your findings in centimeters.

Pallor with vasoconstriction; erythema with vasodilation; cyanosis.

Malnutrition: thin, shiny, atrophic skin; thick-ridged nails; loss of hair; ulcers; gangrene. Malnutrition, pallor, and coolness occur with arterial insufficiency.

Diffuse bilateral edema occurs with systemic illnesses.

Acute, unilateral, painful swelling and asymmetry of calves of 1 cm or more is abnormal; refer the person to determine whether DVT is present.

Objective Data

Normal Range of Findings	Abnormal Findings

Normal Range of Findings

20-13 Measure calf circumference.

In the presence of skin discoloration, skin ulcers, or gangrene, note the size and the exact location.

Palpate for temperature along the legs down to the feet, comparing symmetric spots (Fig. 20-14). The skin should be warm and equal bilaterally. Bilateral cool feet may be caused by environmental factors such as cool room temperature, apprehension, and cigarette smoking. If any increase in temperature is present higher up the leg, note if it is gradual or abrupt.

20-14

Flex the person's knee and then gently compress the gastrocnemius (calf) muscle anteriorly against the tibia; no tenderness should be present.

Palpate the inguinal lymph nodes. It is not unusual to find palpable nodes that are small (1 cm or less), movable, and nontender.

Abnormal Findings

Asymmetry of 1 to 3 cm occurs with mild lymphedema; 3 to 5 cm with moderate lymphedema; and more than 5 cm with severe lymphedema (see Table 20-2).

Brown discoloration occurs with chronic venous stasis caused by hemosiderin deposits from red blood cell degradation.

Venous ulcers occur usually at medial malleolus because of bacterial invasion of poorly drained tissues (see Table 20-4).

With arterial deficit, ulcers occur on tips of toes, metatarsal heads, and lateral malleoli.

A unilateral cool foot or leg or a sudden temperature drop as you move down the leg occurs with arterial deficit.

Calf pain occurs in 35% of cases of DVT. It is not specific for this because it occurs also with superficial phlebitis, Achilles tendinitis, gastrocnemius and plantar muscle injury, and lumbosacral disorders.

Nodes that are enlarged, tender, or fixed in area.

Normal Range of Findings

Palpate these peripheral arteries in both legs: femoral, popliteal, dorsalis pedis, and posterior tibial. Grade the force on the three-point scale. Locate the **femoral arteries** just below the inguinal ligament halfway between the pubis and anterior superior iliac spines (Fig. 20-15). To help expose the femoral area, particularly in obese people, ask the person to bend his or her knees to the side in a froglike position. Press firmly and then slowly release, noting the pulse tap under your fingertips. If this pulse is weak or diminished, auscultate the site for a bruit.

20-15 Femoral pulse.

The **popliteal pulse** is a more diffuse pulse and can be difficult to localize. With the leg extended but relaxed, anchor your thumbs on the knee and curl your fingers around into the popliteal fossa (Fig. 20-16). Press your fingers forward hard to compress the artery against the bone (the lower edge of the femur or the upper edge of the tibia). Often it is just lateral to the medial tendon.

20-16 Popliteal pulse.

If you have difficulty, turn the person prone and lift up the lower leg (Fig. 20-17). Let the leg relax against your arm and press in deeply with your two thumbs. Often a normal popliteal pulse is impossible to palpate.

Abnormal Findings

A bruit occurs with turbulent blood flow, indicating partial occlusion (see Table 20-6, p. 535).

Normal Range of Findings	**Abnormal Findings**

20-17 Popliteal pulse while prone.

For the **posterior tibial** pulse, curve your fingers around the medial malleolus (Fig. 20-18). Press softly. You will feel the tapping right behind it in the groove between the malleolus and the Achilles tendon. If you cannot, try passive dorsiflexion of the foot to make the pulse more accessible.

20-18 Posterior tibial pulse.

The **dorsalis pedis** pulse requires a very light touch. Normally it is just lateral to and parallel with the extensor tendon of the big toe (Fig. 20-19). Do not mistake the pulse in your own fingertips for that of the person.

20-19 Dorsalis pedis pulse.

Normal Range of Findings	**Abnormal Findings**

In adults older than 45 years, occasionally either the dorsalis pedis or the posterior tibial pulse may be hard to find, but not both on the same foot.

Check for pretibial edema. Firmly depress the skin over the tibia or the medial malleolus for 5 seconds and release (Fig. 20-20, *A*). Normally your finger should leave no indentation, although a pit commonly is seen if the person has been standing all day or during pregnancy.

Bilateral, dependent pitting edema occurs with heart failure, diabetic neuropathy, and hepatic cirrhosis (Fig. 20-20, *B*).

A

B

20-20 **A,** Check pretibial edema.

B, Pitting edema. (Bloom, Watkins, & Ireland, 1992.)

If pitting edema is present, grade it on the following scale:
1+, Mild pitting, slight indentation, no perceptible swelling of the leg
2+, Moderate pitting, indentation subsides rapidly
3+, Deep pitting, indentation remains for a short time, leg looks swollen
4+, Very deep pitting, indentation lasts a long time, leg is grossly swollen and distorted

This classic method of capturing pit depth and recovery time is commonly used. But it has not been proven to be an objective, reliable, or sensitive measurement for edema. The amount of pressure used is arbitrary, as is the judgment of the depth and rate of pitting. Ankle circumference is more reliable using a nonstretchable tape at a point 7 cm proximal to the midpoint of the medial malleolus. Because peripheral edema is a common clinical sign in a great number of conditions, it is important to detect true changes in the most accurate way available. Check with your own institution to conform to a consistently used scale.

Unilateral edema occurs with occlusion of a deep vein. Unilateral or bilateral edema occurs with lymphatic obstruction. With these factors it is "brawny" or nonpitting and feels hard to the touch.

Bilateral pitting edema calls for an examination of the neck veins (see Chapter 19). If the neck veins are abnormally distended, the peripheral edema may be related to heart disease or pulmonary hypertension).[11] If neck veins are normal, something else may cause the edema (e.g., liver disease, nephrosis, chronic venous insufficiency, antihypertensive or hormonal medications).

Ask the person to stand up so you can assess the venous system. Note any visible, dilated, and tortuous veins. If varicose veins are present, ask if they cause pain, swelling, fatigue, cramping.

Varicosities occur in the saphenous veins (see Table 20-5). Examination techniques to assess valve incompetency within varicose veins are not reliable because varicosities occur below or between even competent valves).[12] Imaging by Doppler ultrasound is an objective, noninvasive measure of valvular incompetency.

Normal Range of Findings	Abnormal Findings

Color Changes

If you suspect an arterial deficit, raise the legs about 30 cm (12 inches) off the table and ask the person to wag the feet for about 30 seconds to drain off venous blood (Fig. 20-21). The skin color now reflects only the contribution of arterial blood. A light-skinned person's feet normally look a little pale but still should be pink. A dark-skinned person's feet are more difficult to evaluate, but the soles should reveal extreme color change.

Elevational pallor (marked) indicates arterial insufficiency.

20-21

Now have the person sit up with the legs over the side of the table (Fig. 20-22, *A*). Compare the color of both feet. Note the time it takes for color to return to the feet—the normal time is 10 seconds or less. Note also the time it takes for the superficial veins around the feet to fill—the normal time is about 15 seconds. This test is unreliable if the person has concomitant venous disease with incompetent valves.

Dependent rubor (deep blue-red color) occurs with severe arterial insufficiency (Fig. 20-22, *B*). Chronic hypoxia produces loss of vasomotor tone and pooling of blood in the veins.

Delayed venous filling occurs with arterial insufficiency.

A

20-22

B

(**B,** Lemmi & Lemmi, 2011.)

Test the lower legs for strength (see Chapter 22) and sensation (see Chapter 23).

Motor loss occurs with severe arterial deficit.

Sensory loss occurs with arterial deficit, especially diabetes.

Normal Range of Findings	**Abnormal Findings**

The Doppler Ultrasonic Probe

Use this device to detect a weak peripheral pulse, to monitor blood pressure in infants or children, or to measure a low blood pressure or blood pressure in a lower extremity (Fig. 20-23). The Doppler probe magnifies pulsatile sounds from the heart and blood vessels. Position the person supine, with the legs externally rotated so you can reach the medial ankles easily. Place a drop of coupling gel on the end of the handheld transducer. Place the transducer over a pulse site at a 90-degree angle. Apply very light pressure; locate the pulse site by the swishing, whooshing sound.

20-23

The Ankle-Brachial Index

Use of the Doppler stethoscope is a highly specific, noninvasive, and readily available way to determine the extent of peripheral arterial disease (PAD).

The patient is lying flat with the head and heels fully supported.[1] Confirm no smoking within 2 hours of the measurement and allow a 5- to 10-minute rest period supine before measurement. Choose the correct cuff width for the arm and the ankle; width should be 40% of limb circumference. Position the ankle cuff just above the malleoli with straight wrapping.

Use the Doppler probe for both brachial and ankle measurements. In all sites locate the pulse by Doppler and inflate the cuff 20 mm Hg above disappearance of flow signal; then deflate slowly to detect reappearance of flow signal.[1] Moving counterclockwise, measure: right arm, right posterior tibial (PT), right dorsalis pedis (DP), left PT, left DP, left arm. Calculate both ABI using this formula:

$$\text{Right ABI} = \frac{\text{Highest right ankle pressure (DP or PT)}}{\text{Highest arm pressure (right or left)}}$$

$$\text{Example:} \quad \frac{132 \text{ ankle systolic}}{124 \text{ arm systolic}} = \frac{1.06 \text{ or } 106\%, \text{ indicating}}{\text{no flow reduction}}$$

$$\text{Left ABI} = \frac{\text{Highest left ankle pressure (DP or PT)}}{\text{Highest arm pressure (right or left)}}$$

See Jarvis, *Lab Manual for Physical Examination and Health Assessment* (7th ed, Ch. 20), for a grid format to record your findings and for a link to an online calculator.

People with diabetes mellitus or renal failure may have calcified arteries that occasionally are noncompressible and give a falsely high ankle pressure. Thus the presence or severity of PAD may be underestimated.[3]

An ABI between 0.91 and 1 is borderline cardiovascular risk.[1]

An ABI of 0.90 or less indicates PAD:
- 0.90 to 0.71—Mild PAD
- 0.70 to 0.41—Moderate PAD
- 0.40 to 0.30—Severe PAD, usually with rest pain except in the presence of diabetic neuropathy
- <0.30—Ischemia, with impending loss of tissue

Normal Range of Findings	Abnormal Findings

The Wells Score for Leg Deep Vein Thrombosis[17]

Many of the assessment findings for DVT are unreliable and also occur with other conditions. Wells and others have combined findings into a simple scoring system. These criteria separate patients into groups of low, moderate, or high probability of DVT.[11]

Clinical Model for Predicting Pretest Probability of Deep-Vein Thrombosis*

Clinical Characteristic	Score
Active cancer (treatment ongoing, administered within previous 6 mo or palliative)	1
Paralysis, paresis, or recent plaster immobilization of the lower extremities	1
Recently bedridden >3 d or major surgery within previous 12 wk requiring general or regional anesthesia	1
Localized tenderness along the distribution of the deep venous system	1
Swelling of entire leg	1
Calf swelling >3 cm larger than asymptomatic side (measured 10 cm below tibial tuberosity)	1
Pitting edema confined to the symptomatic leg	1
Collateral superficial veins (nonvaricose)	1
Previously documented DVT	1
Alternative diagnosis at least as likely as DVT	-2

From Scarvelis, D., & Wells, P. S. (2006). Diagnosis and treatment of deep-vein thrombosis. *Can Med Assoc J, 175*(9), 1087-1092.
*A score of 0 or less = Low probability of DVT.

Abnormal Findings: Score of 1 or 2 = moderate probability; score of 3 points or more = high probability of DVT.

❖ DEVELOPMENTAL COMPETENCE

Infants and Children

Transient acrocyanosis and skin mottling at birth are discussed in Chapter 12. Pulse force should be normal and symmetric. It also should be the same in the upper and lower extremities.

Abnormal Findings: Weak pulses occur with vasoconstriction of diminished cardiac output.

Full, bounding pulses occur with patent ductus arteriosus from the large left-to-right shunt.

Diminished or absent femoral pulses while upper-extremity pulses are normal suggest coarctation of aorta.

Palpable lymph nodes occur often in healthy infants and children. They are small, firm (shotty), mobile, and nontender. They may be the sequelae of past infection such as inguinal nodes from a diaper rash or cervical nodes from a respiratory infection. Vaccinations also can produce local lymphadenopathy. Note characteristics of any palpable nodes and whether they are local or generalized.

Abnormal Findings: Enlarged, warm, tender nodes indicate current infection. Look for source of infection.

The Pregnant Woman

Expect diffuse bilateral pitting edema in the lower extremities, especially at the end of the day and into the third trimester. Nearly 80% of pregnant women have some peripheral edema.[8] Varicose veins in the legs also are common in the third trimester.

Abnormal Findings: Remain alert for generalized edema plus hypertension, which suggests preeclampsia, a dangerous obstetric condition.

The Aging Adult

The DP and PT pulses may become more difficult to find. Trophic changes associated with arterial insufficiency (thin, shiny skin; thick-ridged nails; loss of hair on lower legs) also occur normally with aging.

PROMOTING A HEALTHY LIFESTYLE

Foot Care

According to the National Institute on Aging (NIA), foot problems are often the first sign of more serious health conditions such as arthritis, diabetes, and nerve or circulatory disorders. Although health care providers advise patients to take care of their feet, they often do not take the time to explain what "good" foot care entails. "Good" foot care includes:

- Checking your feet every day.
  - If you are unable to see the bottoms of your feet, use a mirror or ask someone to help you.
  - Dry feet carefully after a shower or bath. Examine each foot for red spots or sensitive areas, discoloration of skin or nails, ingrown nails, pain, cuts, swelling, or blisters.
  - Keep toenails trimmed, straight across, and filed at the edges with an emery board or nail file.
  - Nail polish … do's and don'ts.
    - Chipped nail polish may support the growth of larger numbers of organisms on nails. This is especially important for those already at risk for infection.
    - Do not use nail polish to cover up discolored nails. Nail polish locks out moisture and keeps the nail bed from being able to "breathe."
- Keeping blood flowing to your feet.
  - Walking is a great way to exercise your feet, or try foot exercises such as:
    - Sitting down and rotating your ankles in one direction, then the other, or try writing the alphabet from A to Z!
    - In bare feet curl your toes and spread them out.
    - When an individual is not able to walk, putting the feet up when sitting or lying down, stretching, wiggling toes,

or having a gentle foot massage or warm foot bath is a great alternative.

- Wearing shoes that fit and are comfortable.
  - The best time to measure feet is toward the end of the day, when feet tend to be the largest.
  - Individuals often have one foot that is larger than the other. They should fit their shoes to the larger foot.
  - Select shoes that are shaped like one's feet. The ball of the foot should fit comfortably into the widest part of the shoe. Toes should not be crowded.
  - For women, low-heeled shoes are safer and less damaging than high-heeled shoes.
- Keeping skin soft and smooth.
  - Use mild soap.
  - Be careful about adding oils to bath water. They can make your feet and the bathtub both very slippery.
  - A thin coat of skin lotion over the tops and bottoms of one's feet helps to keep skin soft and smooth.

Resources

National Institute on Aging. http://www.nia.nih.gov/.

National Institute on Aging. Foot care pamphlet. http://www.nia.nih.gov/sites/default/files/foot_care.pdf.

National Diabetes Education Program. Take care of your feet for a lifetime. http://www.ndep.nih.gov/publications/PublicationDetail.aspx?PubId=67&redirect=true.

Sign up for foot health updates from the U.S. National Library of Medicine/NIH at http://www.nlm.nih.gov/medlineplus/foothealth.html.

DOCUMENTATION AND CRITICAL THINKING

Sample Charting

SUBJECTIVE

No leg pain, no skin changes, no swelling or lymph node enlargement. No history of heart or vascular problems, diabetes, or obesity. Does not smoke. On no medications.

OBJECTIVE

Inspection: Extremities have pink-tan color without redness, cyanosis, or any skin lesions. Extremity size is symmetric without swelling or atrophy.

Palpation: Temperature is warm and = bilaterally. All pulses present, 2+ and = bilaterally. No lymphadenopathy.

ASSESSMENT

Healthy tissue integrity
Effective tissue perfusion

Case Study 1

S.E. is a 30-year-old Caucasian male with no significant past medical history. Family history unremarkable. Recent basketball injury resulting in torn Achilles tendon.

SUBJECTIVE

3 weeks PTA—R ankle surgery to repair torn Achilles tendon. S.E. placed in non–weight-bearing cast.
1 week PTA—Intermittent right calf pain. "Felt like cramping."
Present—Constant right calf pain. Rated at 7/10. Described as cramping, burning muscle pain. S.E. reports that "the cast feels tight."
Cast removed for assessment.

OBJECTIVE

Extremities inspection: Right calf red, toes pale. No cyanosis. Right calf 40 cm, left calf 36 cm in diameter. No varicosities. Left leg pink-tan. Right leg pink-tan with red area over posterior calf. Leg hair present.
Palpation: Right calf warm, toes cool. 2+ nonpitting edema. Tender to palpation.
Pulses: Femoral 2+, popliteal 0, DP 2+, PT 2+. All pulses equal bilaterally.

ASSESSMENT

Deep vein thrombosis R/T postoperative immobilization
Ineffective tissue perfusion R/T decreased venous circulation
Activity intolerance R/T recent surgery and DVT formation
Acute pain R/T inflammatory process

Clinical Case Study 2

J.K. is a 43-year-old, married, Caucasian male city sanitation worker, admitted to University Medical Center today for "bypass surgery tomorrow to fix my aorta and these black toes."

SUBJECTIVE

6 years PTA—Motorcycle accident with handlebars jammed into groin. Treated and released at local hospital. No apparent injury, although MD now thinks accident may have precipitated present stenosis of aorta.
1 year PTA—Radiating pain in right calf on walking 1 mile. Pain relieved by stopping walking.
3 months PTA—Problems with sex; unable to maintain erection during intercourse.
1 month PTA—Leg pain present after walking two blocks. Numbness and tingling in right foot and calf. Tips of three toes on right foot look black. Saw MD. Diagnostic studies showed stenosis of aorta "below vessels that go to my kidneys."
Present—Leg pain at rest, constant and severe, worse at night, partially relieved by dangling leg over side of bed.
Past History—No history of heart or vessel disease, hypertension, diabetes, obesity.
Personal habits—Smokes cigarettes, 3 packs per day (PPD) × 23 years. Now cut down to 1 PPD.
Walking is part of occupation, although has been driving city truck past 3 months because of leg pain. On no medications.

OBJECTIVE

Inspection: Lower extremity size = bilaterally with no swelling or atrophy. No varicosities. Color L leg pink-tan, R leg pink-tan when supine, but marked pallor to R foot on elevation. Black gangrene at tips of R 2nd, 3rd, 4th toes. Leg hair present but absent on involved toes.
Palpation: R foot cool and temperature gradually warms as proceed palpating up R leg.
Pulses: Femorals—both 1+; popliteals—both 0; PT—both 0 but present with Doppler; DP—0, but left DP is present with Doppler, and right is not present with Doppler.

ASSESSMENT

Ischemic rest pain R leg
Ineffective tissue perfusion R/T interruption of flow
Impaired tissue integrity R/T altered circulation
Activity intolerance R/T leg pain
Sexual dysfunction R/T effects of disease

Case Study 3

A.P. is a 17-year-old African-American male who presents to the ED with pain and discoloration of his fingers. He is accompanied by his grandmother.

SUBJECTIVE

4 hours PTA—A.P. was waiting outside for the school bus "that took longer than usual 'cause of all the snow and ice." A.P. reports, "The tips of all my fingers are hard and feel like they're on fire. My grandma told me to run them under water to warm them up, but that made it hurt real bad."

OBJECTIVE

Vital signs: Temp 97.4° F (36.3° C) (oral). BP 118/78 mm Hg (sitting). Pulse 80 bpm (at rest). Resp 16/min.
General appearance: Grimacing with hands resting on thighs, palmar side up; not dressed appropriate for weather conditions (i.e., no gloves, hat, or winter coat).
Extremities: Skin brown with erythema, edema, waxy appearance, hard white plaques, and sensory deficit to phalanges (#1-5) bilat., distal portions of phalanges (#1-5) are cool to touch.

ASSESSMENT

Frostbite (stage I)
Acute pain R/T decreased circulation from prolonged exposure to cold
Impaired tissue integrity R/T freezing of the skin and tissues
Ineffective peripheral tissue perfusion R/T damage to extremities from prolonged exposure to cold

Summary Checklist: Peripheral Vascular Examination

1. Inspect arms for color, size, any lesions.
2. Palpate pulses: radial, brachial.
3. Check epitrochlear node.
4. Inspect legs for color, size, any lesions, trophic skin changes.
5. Palpate temperature of feet and legs.
6. Palpate inguinal nodes.
7. Palpate pulses: femoral, popliteal, posterior tibial, dorsalis pedis.

BIBLIOGRAPHY

1. American Heart Association. (2012). Measurement and interpretation of the ankle-brachial index. *Circulation, 126*(24), 2890-2909.
1a. Anastasi, J. K., Capili, B., & Chang, M. (2013). HIV peripheral neuropathy and foot care management. *Am J Nurs, 113*(12), 34-41.
2. Aponte, J. (2012). The prevalence of peripheral arterial disease (PAD) and PAD risk factors among different ethnic groups in the U.S. population. *J Vasc Nurs, 30*(2), 37-43.
3. Aronow, W. S. (2012). Peripheral arterial disease of the lower extremities. *Arch Med Sci, 8*(2), 375-388.
4. Brazziel, T., Cox, L., Drury, C., et al. (2011). Stopping the wave of PAD. *Nurse Pract, 36*(11), 28-33.
5. Collins, L., & Seraj, S. (2010). Diagnosis and treatment of venous ulcers. *Am Fam Physician, 81*(8), 989.
6. Gay, S. E. (2010). An inside view of venous thromboembolism. *Nurse Pract, 35*(9), 32-39.
7. Kessenich, C. R., & Cronin, K. (2012). Venous ultrasound of the lower extremities. *Nurse Pract, 37*(5), 20-21.
8. Koo, L. W., Reedy, S., & Smith, J. K. (2010). Patient history key to diagnosing peripheral edema. *Nurse Pract, 35*(3), 44-52.
8a. Lancaster, S. L., Owens, A., Bryant, A. S., et al. (2010). Upper-extremity deep vein thrombosis. *Am J Nurs, 110*(5), 48-52.
9. Leeper, N. J., Kullo, I. J., & Cooke, J. P. (2012). Genetics of peripheral artery disease. *Circulation, 125*(25), 3220-3228.
10. Lyons, R. (2012). Treating venous thromboembolic events in the pediatric population. *Nurse Pract, 37*(3), 47-52.
11. McGee, S. (2012). *Evidence-based physical diagnosis.* (3rd ed.). Philadelphia: Saunders.
12. Oklu, R., Habito, R., & Mayr, M., et al. (2012). Pathogenesis of varicose veins. *J Vasc Interv Radiol, 23*(1), 33-39.
13. Paskett, E. D., Dean, J. A., Oliveri, J. M., et al. (2012). Cancer-related lymphedema risk factors, diagnosis, treatment, and impact: a review. *J Clin Oncol, 30*(30), 3726-3733.
14. Peripheral arterial disease. (2012). *Harvard Women's Health Watch,* April, 4-6.
15. Ridner, S. H. (2013). Pathophysiology of lymphedema. *Semin Oncol Nurs, 29*(1), 4-11).
16. Roger, V. L., Go, A. S., Lloyd-Jones, D. M., et al. (2012). Heart disease and stroke statistics—2012 update. *Circulation, 125*(1), e2-e220.
17. Scarvelis, D., & Wells, P. S. (2006). Diagnosis and treatment of deep-vein thrombosis. *Can Med Assoc J, 175*(9), 1087-1092.
18. Simanovsky, N., & Hiller, N. (2007). Importance of sonographic detection of enlarged abdominal lymph nodes in children. *J Ultrasound Med, 26*(5), 581-584.
19. Simmons, A., & Steffen, K. (2011). Peripheral arterial disease in women. *Rev Cardiovasc Med, 12*(3), 123-131.
20. Thomas, D. R. (2013). Managing peripheral arterial disease and vascular ulcers. *Clin Geriatr Med, 29*(2), 425-431.
21. Werchek, S. (2010). Diagnosis and treatment of venous leg ulcers. *Nurse Pract, 35*(12), 46-53.
22. Wiley, M., & Kumar, A. (2012). Peripheral arterial disease: diagnosis and treatment. *Consultant, 52*, 601-610.

CHAPTER 21

Abdomen

http://evolve.elsevier.com/Jarvis/

STRUCTURE AND FUNCTION

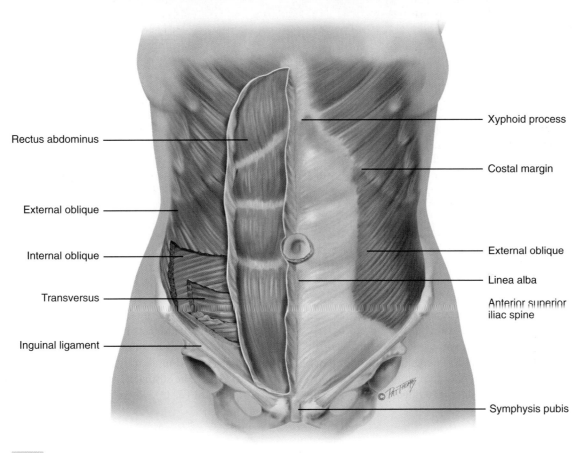

Rectus abdominus

External oblique

Internal oblique

Transversus

Inguinal ligament

Xyphoid process

Costal margin

External oblique

Linea alba

Anterior superior iliac spine

Symphysis pubis

21-1

© Pat Thomas, 2006.

SURFACE LANDMARKS

The **abdomen** is a large, oval cavity extending from the diaphragm down to the brim of the pelvis. It is bordered in back by the vertebral column and paravertebral muscles, and at the sides and front by the lower rib cage and abdominal muscles (Fig. 21-1). Four layers of large, flat muscles form the ventral abdominal wall. These are joined at the midline by a tendinous seam, the **linea alba.** One set, the **rectus abdominis,** forms a strip extending the length of the midline, and its edge is often palpable. The muscles protect and hold the organs in place, and they flex the vertebral column.

INTERNAL ANATOMY

Inside the abdominal cavity all the internal organs are called the **viscera.** It is important that you know the location of these organs so well that you could draw a map of them on the skin. You must be able to visualize each organ that you listen to or palpate through the abdominal wall.

The **solid viscera** are those that maintain a characteristic shape (liver, pancreas, spleen, adrenal glands, kidneys, ovaries, and uterus) (Fig. 21-2). The liver fills most of the right upper quadrant (RUQ) and extends over to the left midclavicular line (MCL). The lower edge of the liver and the right kidney

537

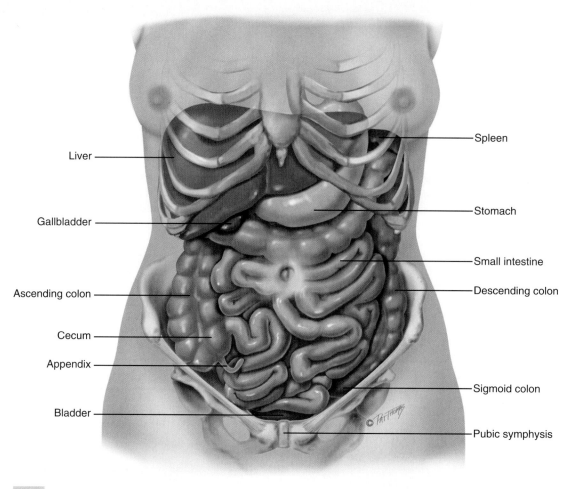

21-2

© Pat Thomas, 2006.

normally may be palpable. The ovaries normally are palpable only on bimanual examination during the pelvic examination.

The shape of the **hollow viscera** (stomach, gallbladder, small intestine, colon, and bladder) depends on the contents. They usually are not palpable, although you may feel a colon distended with feces or a bladder distended with urine. The stomach is just below the diaphragm, between the liver and spleen. The gallbladder rests under the posterior surface of the liver, just lateral to the right MCL. Note that the small intestine is located in all four quadrants. It extends from the pyloric valve of the stomach to the ileocecal valve in the right lower quadrant (RLQ), where it joins the colon.

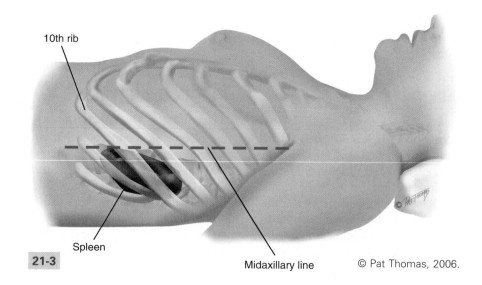

21-3

© Pat Thomas, 2006.

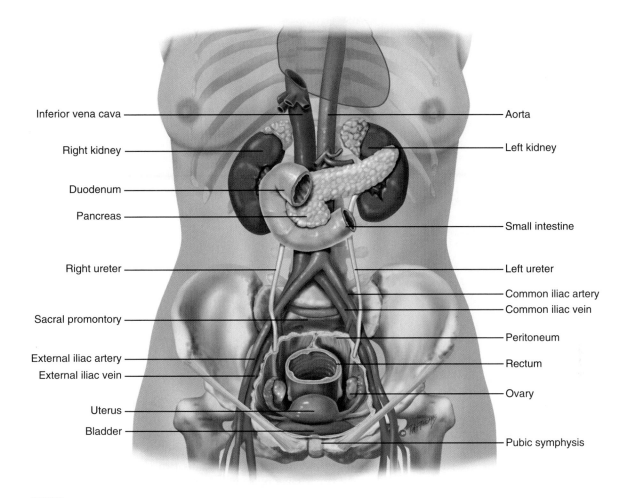

Inferior vena cava

Right kidney

Duodenum

Pancreas

Right ureter

Sacral promontory

External iliac artery

External iliac vein

Uterus

Bladder

Aorta

Left kidney

Small intestine

Left ureter

Common iliac artery

Common iliac vein

Peritoneum

Rectum

Ovary

Pubic symphysis

21-4

© Pat Thomas, 2006.

The **spleen** is a soft mass of lymphatic tissue on the posterolateral wall of the abdominal cavity, immediately under the diaphragm (Fig. 21-3). It lies obliquely with its long axis behind and parallel to the 10th rib, lateral to the midaxillary line. Its width extends from the 9th to the 11th rib, about 7 cm. It is not palpable normally. If it becomes enlarged, its lower pole moves downward and toward the midline.

The **aorta** is just to the left of midline in the upper part of the abdomen (Fig. 21-4). It descends behind the peritoneum, and at 2 cm below the umbilicus it bifurcates into the right and left common iliac arteries opposite the 4th lumbar vertebra. You can palpate the aortic pulsations easily in the upper anterior abdominal wall. The right and left iliac arteries become the femoral arteries in the groin area. Their pulsations are easily palpated at a point halfway between the anterior superior iliac spine and the symphysis pubis.

The **pancreas** is a soft, lobulated gland located behind the stomach. It stretches obliquely across the posterior abdominal wall to the left upper quadrant.

The bean-shaped **kidneys** are retroperitoneal, or posterior to the abdominal contents (Fig. 21-5). They are well protected by the posterior ribs and musculature. The 12th rib forms an angle with the vertebral column, the **costovertebral angle.** The left kidney lies here at the 11th and 12th ribs. Because of

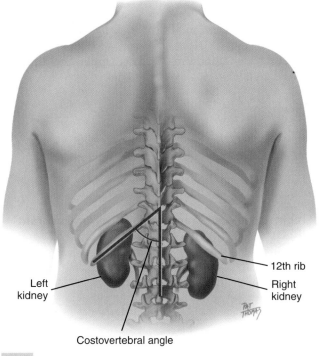

Left kidney

12th rib

Right kidney

Costovertebral angle

21-5

21-6   Four quadrants

the placement of the liver, the right kidney rests 1 to 2 cm lower than the left kidney and sometimes may be palpable.

For convenience in description, the abdominal wall is divided into **four quadrants** by a vertical and a horizontal line bisecting the umbilicus (Fig. 21-6). (An older, more complicated scheme divided the abdomen into nine regions; and some regional names persist such as **epigastric** for the area between the costal margins, **umbilical** for the area around the umbilicus, and **hypogastric** or **suprapubic** for the area above the pubic bone.)

The anatomic location of the organs by quadrants is:

Right Upper Quadrant (RUQ)

Liver
Gallbladder
Duodenum
Head of pancreas
Right kidney and adrenal
Hepatic flexure of colon
Part of ascending and
   transverse colon

Right Lower Quadrant (RLQ)

Cecum
Appendix
Right ovary and tube
Right ureter
Right spermatic cord

Left Upper Quadrant (LUQ)

Stomach
Spleen
Left lobe of liver
Body of pancreas
Left kidney and adrenal
Splenic flexure of colon
Part of transverse and
   descending colon

Left Lower Quadrant (LLQ)

Part of descending colon
Sigmoid colon
Left ovary and tube
Left ureter
Left spermatic cord

Midline

Aorta
Uterus (if enlarged)
Bladder (if distended)

❖ DEVELOPMENTAL COMPETENCE

Infants and Children

In the newborn the umbilical cord shows prominently on the abdomen. It contains two arteries and one vein. The liver takes up proportionately more space in the abdomen at birth than in later life. In a healthy term neonate the lower edge may be palpated 0.5 to 2.5 cm below the right costal margin. Age-related values of expected liver span are listed in the Objective Data section. The urinary bladder is located higher in the abdomen than in the adult. It lies between the symphysis and the umbilicus. In addition, during early childhood the abdominal wall is less muscular; therefore the organs may be easier to palpate.

The Pregnant Woman

Nausea and vomiting, or "morning sickness," is an early sign of pregnancy for most pregnant women, starting between the 1st and 2nd missed periods. The cause may be the result of hormonal changes such as the production of human chorionic gonadotropin (hCG). Another symptom is "acid indigestion" or heartburn (pyrosis) caused by esophageal reflux. Gastrointestinal (GI) motility decreases, which prolongs gastric emptying time. The decreased motility causes more water to be resorbed from the colon, which leads to constipation. The constipation, in addition to increased venous pressure in the lower pelvis, may lead to hemorrhoids.

The enlarging uterus displaces the intestines upward and posteriorly. Bowel sounds are diminished. The appendix may be displaced upward and to the right, but any appendicitis-related pain during pregnancy would still be felt in the RLQ.[28] Finally skin changes on the abdomen such as striae and linea nigra are discussed later in this chapter on p. 547 and in Chapter 12.

The Aging Adult

Aging alters the appearance of the abdominal wall. After middle age, some fat accumulates in the suprapubic area in females as a result of decreased estrogen levels. Males also show some fat deposits in the abdominal area, which accentuates with a more sedentary lifestyle. With further aging adipose tissue is redistributed away from the face and extremities and to the abdomen and hips. The abdominal musculature relaxes.

Age-related changes occur in the GI system but do not significantly affect function as long as no disease is present.

- Salivation decreases, causing a dry mouth and a decreased sense of taste (discussed in Chapter 16).
- Esophageal emptying is delayed. If an aging person is fed in the supine position, it increases risk for aspiration.
- Gastric acid secretion decreases with aging. This may cause pernicious anemia (because it interferes with vitamin B_{12} absorption), iron deficiency anemia, and malabsorption of calcium.
- The incidence of gallstones increases with age, occurring in 10% to 20% of middle-age and older adults, being more common in females.
- Liver size decreases by 25% between the ages of 20 and 70 years, although most liver function remains normal. Drug metabolism by the liver is impaired, in part because blood flow through the liver and liver size are decreased.[26] Therefore the liver metabolism that is responsible for the enzymatic oxidation, reduction, and hydrolysis of drugs is substantially decreased with age. Prolonged liver metabolism causes increased side effects (e.g., older people taking benzodiazepines have an increased risk of falling and thus of hip fracture).
- Aging people frequently report constipation. Those reporting constipation included 26% of women and 16% of men in younger adults, whereas 34% of women and 28% of men ages ≥84 years reported constipation.[3] Because many adults are confused as to what defines constipation, the Rome III standardizes symptom criteria for functional constipation. These symptoms include reduced stool frequency (less than 3 bowel movements per week) and other common and troubling associated symptoms (i.e., straining, lumpy or hard stool, feeling of incomplete evacuation, feeling of anorectal blockage, use of manual maneuvers).

Constipation is not a physiologic consequence of aging. Common causes of constipation include decreased physical activity, inadequate intake of water, a low-fiber diet, side effects of medications (opioids, tricyclic antidepressants), irritable bowel syndrome, bowel obstruction, hypothyroidism, and inadequate toilet facilities (i.e., difficulty ambulating to the toilet may cause the person to deliberately retain the stool until it becomes hard and difficult to pass).

🌐 CULTURE AND GENETICS

Lactase is the digestive enzyme necessary for absorption of the carbohydrate *lactose* (milk sugar). In some racial groups lactase activity is high at birth but declines to low levels by adulthood. These people are **lactose intolerant** and have abdominal pain, bloating, and flatulence when milk products are consumed. Millions of American adults have the potential for lactose-intolerance symptoms; traditional estimated rates were that 15% of Whites, 50% of Mexican Americans, and 80% of African Americans had the condition. Yet a recent study found that the prevalence rates in practical life settings are significantly lower than previously estimated rates.[27] When subjects were screened for symptoms following a typical serving of dairy food in the home setting, lactose-intolerance prevalence estimates were 7.72% for Whites, 19.5% for African Americans, and 10% for Hispanics.[27] This is clinically significant because dairy foods meet crucial nutritional requirements, including calcium, magnesium, potassium, proteins, and vitamins A, D, B_{12}, and riboflavin. If people perceive themselves to be lactose intolerant based on racial heritage, the lowered calcium intake may affect bone health. Health care providers should encourage low-fat or fat-free dairy foods and monitor any symptoms.[7]

Obesity is the accumulation of excess body fat. It is caused by a complex interaction of genetic predisposition, dietary intake, physical inactivity, and what is now called an *obesogenic* environment[19] (i.e., one that encourages large portions of high-fat, energy-dense food). The prevalence of obesity has increased in the United States and globally. Currently 35.7% of U.S. adults are obese (BMI ≥30 kg/m^2).[10]

Data from the National Health and Nutrition Examination Survey (NHANES) show significant differences among racial groups.[10] Among men the obesity rates are similar across groups: 36.2% of Whites, 38.8% of Blacks, and 36.6% of Mexican Americans are obese. However among women 32.2% of White women are obese, whereas 58.5% of Black women and 44.9% of Mexican-American women are obese.

Obesity in adults results in comorbidities of type 2 diabetes and cardiovascular disease (CVD). Obese children have an increased risk for asthma, diabetes, liver disease, CVD, sleep apnea, and joint problems; and they risk becoming obese adults.[22] Controlling the obesity epidemic will be important in containing health care costs. Do Americans view obesity as a threat in the same way they now view the dangers of smoking? A change in public awareness and public thinking to regard obesity as a "common enemy" has been proposed to garner public support.[22] The areas for needed change are vast and include personal, community, and government strategies. Recommendations include the following[22]:

Making healthful food and beverages more widely available; providing access to healthier food by locating stores in underserved areas; and decreasing the availability of less healthful food and beverages....discourage consumption of sugar-sweetened beverages; increased support for breastfeeding; linkages between local farms and institutions to increase fruit and vegetable consumption; shifts in agricultural policy; and improved community infrastructure to promote biking, walking, and use of public transit.

SUBJECTIVE DATA

1. Appetite	4. Abdominal pain	7. Past abdominal history
2. Dysphagia	5. Nausea/vomiting	8. Medications
3. Food intolerance	6. Bowel habits	9. Nutritional assessment

Examiner Asks	Rationale
1. Appetite • Any change in **appetite?** Is it a loss of appetite? • Any change in weight? How much weight gained or lost? Over what time period? Is the weight loss caused by diet?	**Anorexia** is a loss of appetite from GI disease as a side effect to some medications, with pregnancy, or with mental health disorders.
2. Dysphagia • Any difficulty swallowing? When did you first notice it?	**Dysphagia** occurs with disorders of the throat or esophagus.
3. Food intolerance • Are there any foods you cannot eat? What happens if you do eat them: allergic reaction, heartburn, belching, bloating, indigestion? • Do you use antacids? How often?	**Food intolerance** (e.g., lactase deficiency resulting in bloating or excessive gas after taking milk products). **Pyrosis** (heartburn), a burning sensation in esophagus and stomach, from reflux of gastric acid. Eructation (belching).
4. Abdominal pain • Any **abdominal pain?** Please point to it. • Is the pain in one spot, or does it move around? • How did it start? How long have you had it? • Constant, or does it come and go? Occur before or after meals? Does it peak? When? • How would you describe the character: cramping (colic type), burning in pit of stomach, dull, stabbing, aching? • Is the pain relieved by food or worse after eating? • Is the pain associated with menstrual period or irregularities, stress, dietary indiscretion, fatigue, nausea and vomiting, gas, fever, rectal bleeding, frequent urination, vaginal or penile discharge? • What makes the pain worse: food, position, stress, medication, activity? • What have you tried to relieve pain: rest, heating pad, change in position, medication?	Abdominal pain may be *visceral* from an internal organ (dull, general, poorly localized); *parietal* from inflammation of overlying peritoneum (sharp, precisely localized, aggravated by movement); or *referred* from a disorder in another site (see Table 21-3, p. 570). Acute pain requiring urgent diagnosis occurs with appendicitis, cholecystitis, bowel obstruction, or a perforated organ. Chronic pain of gastric ulcers occurs usually on an empty stomach; pain of duodenal ulcers occurs 2 to 3 hours after a meal and is relieved by more food.
5. Nausea/vomiting • Any **nausea** or **vomiting?** How often? How much comes up? What is the color? Is there an odor? • Is it bloody? • Is the nausea or vomiting associated with colicky pain, diarrhea, fever, chills? • What foods did you eat in the past 24 hours? Where? At home, school, restaurant? Is there anyone else in the family with same symptoms in past 24 hours?	Nausea/vomiting is common with GI disease, many medications, and early pregnancy. **Hematemesis** occurs with stomach or duodenal ulcers and esophageal varices. Consider food poisoning.

Examiner Asks	Rationale
• Any recent travel? Where to? Drink the local water or eat fruit? Swimming in public beaches or pools?	GI upset and diarrhea occur when exposed to new local pathogens in developing countries. Water supply may be contaminated.

6. Bowel habits
- How often do you have a **bowel movement?**
- What is the color? Consistency?
- Any diarrhea or constipation? How long?
- Any recent change in bowel habits?
- Use laxatives? Which ones? How often do you use them?

Assess usual **bowel habits.**

Black stools may be tarry due to occult blood (melena) from GI bleeding or nontarry from iron medications. Gray stools occur with hepatitis.

Red blood in stools occurs with GI bleeding or localized bleeding around the anus.

7. Past abdominal history
- Any **history** of GI problems: ulcer, gallbladder disease, hepatitis/jaundice, appendicitis, colitis, hernia?
- Ever had any abdominal operations? Please describe.
- Any problems after surgery?
- Any abdominal x-ray studies? How were the results?

8. Medications
- Which **medications** are you taking currently?
- How about alcohol—how much would you say you drink each day? Each week? When was your last alcoholic drink?
- How about cigarettes—do you smoke? How many packs per day? For how long?

Peptic ulcer disease occurs with frequent use of nonsteroidal antiinflammatory drugs (NSAIDs), alcohol, smoking, and *Helicobacter pylori* infection.

9. Nutritional assessment
- Now I would like to ask you about your diet. Please tell me all the food you ate yesterday, starting with breakfast.
- Which fresh food markets are located in your neighborhood?

Nutritional assessment via 24-hour recall (see Chapter 11 for full discussion). Many inner-city neighborhoods are fresh food "deserts," lacking produce markets but full of fast-food restaurants.

Additional History for Infants and Children

1. Are you breastfeeding or bottle-feeding the baby? If bottle-feeding, how does baby tolerate the formula?

2. Which table foods have you introduced? How does the infant tolerate the food?

Consider a new food as a possible allergen. Adding only one new food at a time to the infant's diet helps identify allergies.

3. How often does your toddler/child eat? Does he or she eat regular meals? How do you feel about your child's eating problems?
- Please describe all that your child had to eat yesterday, starting with breakfast. Which foods does the child eat for snacks?

- Does toddler/child ever eat nonfoods: grass, dirt, paint chips?

Irregular eating patterns are common and a source of parental anxiety. As long as the child shows normal growth and development and only nutritious foods are offered, parents may be reassured.

Pica: Although a toddler may attempt nonfoods at some time, he or she should recognize edibles by age 2 years.

4. Does your child have constipation? How long?
- What is the number of stools/day? Stools/week?
- How much water, juice is in the diet?

Examiner Asks	Rationale

Subjective Data

- Does the constipation seem to be associated with toilet training?
- What have you tried to treat the constipation?

5. Does the child have abdominal pain? Please describe what you have noticed and when it started.

Pain is hard to assess with children. Many conditions of unrelated organ systems have vague abdominal pain (e.g., otitis media). They cannot articulate specific symptoms and often focus on "the tummy." Abdominal pain accompanies inflammation of the bowel, constipation, urinary tract infection, and anxiety.

6. For the overweight child: How long has weight been a problem?
- At what age did the child first seem overweight? Did any change in diet pattern occur then?
- Describe the diet pattern now.
- Do any others in family have a similar problem?
- How does child feel about his or her own weight?

Reduced physical activity and food marketing practices contribute to current obesity epidemic.

Family history of obesity.

Assess body image and social adjustment.

Additional History for Adolescents

1. What do you eat at regular meals? Do you eat breakfast? What do you eat for snacks?

- How many calories do you figure you consume?

Adolescent takes control of eating and may reject family values (e.g., skipping breakfast, consuming junk foods and soda pop). The only control parents have is what food is in the house.

You probably cannot change adolescent eating pattern, but you can supply nutritional facts.

2. What is your exercise pattern?

Boys need an average 4000 cal/day to maintain weight; more calories if exercise is pursued. Girls need 20% fewer calories and the same nutrients as boys. Fast food is high in fat, calories, and salt and has no fiber.

3. If weight is less than body requirements: How much have you lost? By diet, exercise, or how?

Screen any extremely thin teenager for **anorexia nervosa,** a serious psychosocial disorder that includes loss of appetite, voluntary starvation, and grave weight loss. This person may augment weight loss by purging (self-induced vomiting) and use of laxatives.

- How do you feel? Tired, hungry? How do you think your body looks?

Denial of these feelings is common. Although thin, teen insists that she looks fat, "disgusting." Distorted body image.

- What is your activity pattern?

The anorectic adolescent may have healthy activity and exercise but often is hyperactive.

- Is the weight loss associated with any other body change such as menstrual irregularity?
- What do your parents say about your eating? What do your friends say?

Amenorrhea is common with anorexia nervosa.

This is a family problem involving control issues. Anyone at risk warrants immediate referral to a physician and mental health professional.

Examiner Asks	Rationale

Additional History for the Aging Adult

1. How do you acquire your groceries and prepare your meals?

Assess risk for nutritional deficit: limited access to grocery store, income, or cooking facilities; physical disability (impaired vision, decreased mobility, decreased strength, neurologic deficit).

2. Do you eat alone or share meals with others?

Assess risk for nutritional deficit if living alone; may not bother to prepare all meals; social isolation; depression.

3. Please tell me all that you had to eat yesterday, starting with breakfast.

NOTE: 24-hour recall may not be sufficient because daily pattern may vary. Attempt week-long diary of intake. Food pattern may differ during the month if monthly income (e.g., Social Security check) runs out.

- Do you have any trouble swallowing these foods?
- What do you do right after eating: walk, take a nap?

4. How often do your bowels move?
- If the person reports constipation: What do you mean by constipation? How much liquid is in your diet? How much bulk or fiber?
- Do you take anything for constipation such as laxatives? Which ones? How often?

- Which medications do you take?

Consider GI side effects (e.g., nausea, upset stomach, anorexia, dry mouth).

OBJECTIVE DATA

PREPARATION

The lighting should include a strong overhead light and a secondary stand light. Expose the abdomen so it is fully visible. Drape the genitalia and female breasts.
The following measures enhance abdominal wall relaxation:
- The person should have emptied the bladder, saving a urine specimen if needed.
- Keep the room warm to avoid chilling and tensing of muscles.
- Position the person supine, with the head on a pillow, the knees bent or on pillow, and the arms at the sides or across the chest. (NOTE: Discourage the person from placing his or her arms over the head because this tenses abdominal musculature.)
- To avoid abdominal tensing, the stethoscope endpiece must be warm, your hands must be warm, and your fingernails must be very short.
- Inquire about any painful areas. Examine such an area last to avoid any muscle guarding.
- Finally learn to use distraction: Enhance muscle relaxation through breathing exercises; emotive imagery; your low, soothing voice; engaging in conversation; or having the person relate his or her abdominal history while you palpate.

EQUIPMENT NEEDED

Stethoscope
Small centimeter ruler
Skin-marking pen
Alcohol wipe (to clean endpiece)

Objective Data

Normal Range of Findings	Abnormal Findings

Inspect the Abdomen

Contour

Stand on the person's right side and look down on the abdomen. Then stoop or sit to gaze across the abdomen. Your head should be slightly higher than the abdomen. Determine the profile from the rib margin to the pubic bone. The contour describes the nutritional state and normally ranges from flat to rounded (Fig. 21-7).

Scaphoid abdomen caves in. Protuberant abdomen, abdominal distention (see Table 21-1, p. 567-568).

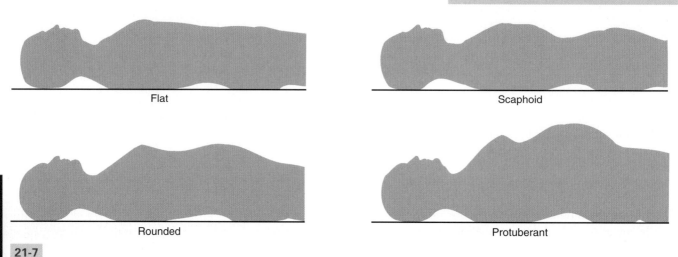

Flat   Scaphoid

Rounded   Protuberant

21-7

Symmetry

Shine a light across the abdomen toward you or lengthwise across the person. The abdomen should be symmetric bilaterally (Fig. 21-8). Note any localized bulging, visible mass, or asymmetric shape. Even small bulges are highlighted by shadow. Step to the foot of the examination table to recheck symmetry.

Bulges, masses.
Hernia—Protrusion of abdominal viscera through abnormal opening in muscle wall (see Table 21-4, Abnormalities on Inspection, p. 571).
Sister Mary Joseph nodule is a hard nodule in umbilicus that occurs with metastatic cancer of stomach, large intestine, ovary. or pancreas.[25]

21-8

Ask the person to take a deep breath to further highlight any change. The abdomen should stay smooth and symmetric. Or ask the person to perform a sit-up without pushing up with his or her hands.

Note any localized bulging.
Hernia or enlarged liver or spleen may show.

Umbilicus

Normally it is midline and inverted, with no sign of discoloration, inflammation, or hernia. It becomes everted and pushed upward with pregnancy.

The umbilicus is a common site for piercings in young women. The site should not be red or crusted.

Everted with ascites or underlying mass (see Table 21-1).
Deeply sunken with obesity.
Enlarged, everted with umbilical hernia.
Bluish periumbilical color occurs (though rarely) with intraperitoneal bleeding (Cullen sign).

Normal Range of Findings	Abnormal Findings

Skin

The surface is smooth and even, with homogeneous color. This is a good area to judge pigment because it is often protected from sun.

Redness with localized inflammation. Jaundice (shows best in natural daylight).
Skin glistening and taut with ascites. Striae also occur with ascites.

One common pigment change is **striae** (lineae albicantes)—silvery white, linear, jagged marks about 1 to 6 cm long (Fig. 21-9). They occur when elastic fibers in the reticular layer of the skin are broken after rapid or prolonged stretching as in pregnancy or excessive weight gain. Recent striae are pink or blue; then they turn silvery white.

Striae look purple-blue with Cushing syndrome (excess adrenocortical hormone causes the skin to be fragile and easily broken from normal stretching).

21-9   Striae.

Pigmented nevi (moles)—circumscribed brown macular or papular areas—are common on the abdomen.

Unusual color or change in shape of mole (see Chapter 12).
Petechiae.
Cutaneous angiomas (spider nevi) occur with portal hypertension or liver disease.
Lesions, rashes (see Chapter 12).
Underlying adhesions are inflammatory bands that connect opposite sides of serous surfaces after trauma or surgery.

Normally no lesions are present, although you may note well-healed surgical scars. If a scar is present, draw its location in the person's record, indicating the length in centimeters (Fig. 21-10). (NOTE: Infrequently a person may forget a past operation when providing the history. If you note a scar now, ask about it.) A surgical scar alerts you to the possible presence of underlying adhesions and excess fibrous tissue.

6 cm

11 cm

21-10

Normal Range of Findings	Abnormal Findings

Veins usually are not seen, but a fine venous network may be visible in thin persons.

Prominent, dilated veins occur with portal hypertension, cirrhosis, ascites, or vena caval obstruction. Veins are more visible with malnutrition as a result of thinned adipose tissue.

Good skin turgor reflects healthy nutrition. Gently pinch up a fold of skin; then release to note the immediate return of the skin to original position.

Poor turgor occurs with dehydration, which often accompanies GI disease.

Pulsation or Movement

Normally you may see the pulsations from the aorta beneath the skin in the epigastric area, particularly in thin people with good muscle wall relaxation. Respiratory movement also shows in the abdomen, particularly in males. Finally, waves of peristalsis sometimes are visible in very thin people. They ripple slowly and obliquely across the abdomen.

Marked pulsation of aorta occurs with widened pulse pressure (e.g., hypertension, aortic insufficiency, thyrotoxicosis) and aortic aneurysm.

Marked visible peristalsis, together with a distended abdomen, indicates intestinal obstruction.

Hair Distribution

The pattern of pubic hair growth normally has a diamond shape in adult males and an inverted triangle shape in adult females (see Chapters 24 and 26).

Patterns alter with endocrine or hormone abnormalities, chronic liver disease.

Demeanor

A comfortable person is relaxed quietly on the examining table and has a benign facial expression and slow, even respirations.

Restlessness and constant turning to find comfort occur with the colicky pain of gastroenteritis or bowel obstruction (see Table 21-2, p. 569, and Table 21-3, p. 570).

Absolute stillness, resisting any movement, occurs with the pain of peritonitis.

Knees flexed up, facial grimacing, and rapid, uneven respirations also indicate pain.

Auscultate Bowel Sounds and Vascular Sounds

Depart from the usual examination sequence and auscultate the abdomen next. This is done because percussion and palpation can increase peristalsis, which would give a false interpretation of bowel sounds. Use the diaphragm endpiece because bowel sounds are relatively high-pitched. Hold the stethoscope lightly against the skin; pushing too hard may stimulate more bowel sounds (Fig. 21-11). Begin in the RLQ at the ileocecal valve area because bowel sounds normally are always present here.

21-11

Normal Range of Findings

Bowel Sounds

Note the character and frequency of bowel sounds. They originate from the movement of air and fluid through the stomach and large and small intestine. Depending on the time elapsed since eating, a wide range of normal sounds can occur. Bowel sounds are high-pitched, gurgling, cascading sounds, occurring irregularly anywhere from 5 to 30 times per minute. Do not bother to count them. In addition, because the sounds radiate widely over the abdomen, the gurgle you hear in the RLQ may originate in the stomach. Therefore listening in all four quadrants usually is not necessary.[25] Just judge if they are present or are hypoactive or hyperactive.

One type of hyperactive bowel sounds is fairly common: hyperperistalsis, when you feel your "stomach growling," termed **borborygmus.** A perfectly "silent abdomen" is uncommon; you must listen for 5 minutes by your watch before deciding if bowel sounds are completely absent.

Vascular Sounds

As you listen to the abdomen, note the presence of any vascular sounds or **bruits.** Using firmer pressure, check over the aorta, renal arteries, iliac, and femoral arteries, especially in people with hypertension (Fig. 21-12). Usually no such sound is present. However, about 4% to 20% of healthy people (usually younger than 40 years) may have a normal bruit originating from the celiac artery.[25] It is systolic, medium to low in pitch, and heard between the xiphoid process and the umbilicus.

21-12

For safe practice, one assessment for which you should *NOT* use auscultation of the abdomen is for the correct placement of nasogastric feeding tubes. Despite evidence showing that auscultation of an air bolus is not adequate to determine placement in stomach or lung, you may see some nurses still practicing this method. Current evidence mandates confirming initial placement by chest x-ray and continuing assessment by measuring the external portion of the tube, testing the pH of stomach aspirates (stomach pH is 1.0 to 3.0, whereas intestinal pH is 6.0 to 9.0).[29] Visualizing gastric aspirates can be helpful in distinguishing gastric (grassy green or colorless) versus intestinal (yellow, bile stained, clear or cloudy) placement but is not helpful in determining respiratory placement.[29]

Abnormal Findings

Two distinct patterns of abnormal bowel sounds may occur:
1. **Hyperactive sounds** are loud, high-pitched, rushing, tinkling sounds that signal increased motility.
2. **Hypoactive or absent sounds** follow abdominal surgery or with inflammation of the peritoneum (see Table 21-5, Abnormal Bowel Sounds, p. 572, and Table 21-2 Clinical Portrait of Intestinal Obstruction, p. 569).

Note location, pitch, and timing of a vascular sound.

A systolic bruit is a pulsatile blowing sound and occurs with stenosis or occlusion of an artery.

Venous hum and peritoneal friction rub are rare (see Table 21-6, Friction Rubs and Vascular Sounds, p. 573).

The auscultation method can wrongly suggest that the feeding tube is correctly placed in the stomach; serious harm or even fatality can result from administering tube-feeding material into the lung.

Objective Data

Normal Range of Findings	Abnormal Findings

Percuss General Tympany, Liver Span, and Splenic Dullness

Percuss to assess the relative density of abdominal contents, to locate organs, and to screen for abnormal fluid or masses.

General Tympany

First percuss lightly in all four quadrants to determine the prevailing amount of tympany and dullness (Fig. 21-13). Move clockwise. Tympany should predominate because air in the intestines rises to the surface when the person is supine.

Dullness occurs over a distended bladder, adipose tissue, fluid, or a mass. Hyperresonance is present with gaseous distention.

21-13

Liver Span

Next percuss to map out the boundaries of certain organs. Measure the height of the liver in the right MCL. (For a consistent placement of the MCL line landmark, remember to palpate the acromioclavicular and sternoclavicular joints and judge the line at a point midway between the two.)

Begin in the area of lung resonance and percuss down the interspaces until the sound changes to a dull quality (Fig. 21-14). Mark the spot, usually in the 5th intercostal space. Then find abdominal tympany and percuss up in the MCL. Mark where the sound changes from tympany to a dull sound, normally at the right costal margin.

21-14

Normal Range of Findings

Measure the distance between the two marks; the normal liver span in the adult ranges from 6 to 12 cm (Fig. 21-15). The height of the liver span correlates with the height of the person; taller people have longer livers. Males also have a larger liver span than females of the same height. Overall the mean liver span is 10.5 cm for males and 7 cm for females.

21-15

One variation occurs in people with chronic emphysema, in which the liver is displaced downward by the hyperinflated lungs. Although you hear a dull percussion note well below the right costal margin, the overall span is still within normal limits.

Clinical estimation of liver span screens for hepatomegaly and monitors changes in liver size. However, this measurement is a gross estimate; the liver span usually is underestimated because clinicians place the upper border too low and/or the lower border too high.[25]

Scratch Test. This traditional technique uses auscultation to detect the lower border of the liver. Place the stethoscope over the xiphoid while lightly stroking the skin with one finger up the MCL from the RLQ and parallel to the liver border. When you reach the liver edge, the sound is magnified in the stethoscope. However, there are many variations in the technique, and evidence is mixed as to its value.[25] One recent study found moderate agreement between the results by scratch test and ultrasound.[16] They recommend the scratch test if the abdomen is distended, obese, or too tender for palpation or if muscles are rigid or guarded.[16]

Splenic Dullness

Often the spleen is obscured by stomach contents, but you may locate it by percussing for a dull note from the 9th to 11th intercostal space just behind the left midaxillary line (Fig. 21-16). The area of splenic dullness normally is not wider than 7 cm in the adult and should not encroach on the normal tympany over the gastric air bubble.

Abnormal Findings

An enlarged liver span indicates liver enlargement or **hepatomegaly.**

Accurate detection of liver borders is confused by dullness above the 5th intercostal space, which occurs with lung disease (e.g., pleural effusion or consolidation). Accurate detection at the lower border is confused when dullness is pushed up with ascites or pregnancy or with gas distention in the colon, which obscures the lower border.

Objective Data

Normal Range of Findings	Abnormal Findings

21-16

Now percuss in the lowest interspace in the left *anterior* axillary line. Tympany should result. Ask the person to take a deep breath. Normally tympany remains through full inspiration.

Costovertebral Angle Tenderness

Indirect fist percussion causes the tissues to vibrate instead of producing a sound. To assess the kidney place one hand over the 12th rib at the costovertebral angle on the back (Fig. 21-17). Thump that hand with the ulnar edge of your other fist. The person normally feels a thud but no pain. (Although this step is explained here with percussion techniques, its usual sequence in a complete examination is with thoracic assessment, when the person is sitting up and you are standing behind.)

21-17

Abnormal Findings

A dull note forward of the midaxillary line indicates enlargement of the spleen, as occurs with mononucleosis, trauma, and infection.

In this site, the *anterior* axillary line, a change in percussion from tympany to a dull sound with full inspiration is a **positive spleen percussion sign,** indicating splenomegaly. This method detects mild-to-moderate splenomegaly before the spleen becomes palpable, as in mononucleosis, malaria, or hepatic cirrhosis.

Sharp pain occurs with inflammation of the kidney or paranephric area.

Normal Range of Findings	Abnormal Findings

Special Procedures

At times you may suspect that a person has ascites (free fluid in the peritoneal cavity) because of a distended abdomen, bulging flanks, and an umbilicus that is protruding and displaced downward. You can differentiate ascites from gaseous distention by performing two percussion tests.

Ascites occurs with heart failure, portal hypertension, cirrhosis, hepatitis, pancreatitis, and cancer.

Fluid Wave. First test for a **fluid wave** by standing on the person's right side. Place the ulnar edge of another examiner's hand or the patient's own hand firmly on the abdomen in the midline (Fig. 21-18). (This stops transmission across the skin of the upcoming tap.) Place your left hand on the person's right flank. With your right hand reach across the abdomen and give the left flank a firm strike.

21-18   Fluid wave.

If ascites is present, the blow will generate a fluid wave through the abdomen, and you will feel a distinct tap on your left hand. If the abdomen is distended from gas or adipose tissue, you will feel no change.

A positive fluid wave test occurs with large amounts of ascitic fluid. Also note edema in the legs.

Shifting Dullness. The second test for ascites is percussing for **shifting dullness.** In a supine person ascitic fluid settles by gravity into the flanks, displacing the air-filled bowel to the periumbilical space. You will hear a tympanitic note as you percuss over the top of the abdomen because gas-filled intestines float over the fluid (Fig. 21-19). Then percuss down the side of the abdomen. If fluid is present, the note will change from tympany to dull as you reach its level. Mark this spot.

Tympany
Dullness

21-19

Normal Range of Findings	Abnormal Findings

Now turn the person onto the right side (roll him or her toward you) (Fig. 21-20). The fluid will gravitate to the dependent (in this case, right) side, displacing the lighter bowel upward. Begin percussing the upper side of the abdomen and move downward. The sound changes from tympany to a dull sound as you reach the fluid level; but this time the level of dullness is higher, upward toward the umbilicus. This **shifting level of dullness** indicates the presence of fluid.

This test has less diagnostic value than the fluid wave test. Shifting dullness is positive with a large volume of ascitic fluid; it will not detect less than 500 to 1100 mL of fluid.[25]

Tympany

Shifting level of dullness

21-20

Both tests, fluid wave and shifting dullness, are not completely reliable. Ultrasound study is the definitive tool.

Palpate Surface and Deep Areas

Perform palpation to judge the size, location, and consistency of certain organs and to screen for an abnormal mass or tenderness. Review comfort measures on p. 545. Because most people are naturally inclined to protect the abdomen, you need to use additional measures to enhance complete muscle relaxation.

1. Bend the person's knees.
2. Keep your palpating hand low and parallel to the abdomen. Holding the hand high and pointing down would make anyone tense up.
3. Teach the person to breathe slowly (in through the nose and out through the mouth).
4. Keep your own voice low and soothing. Conversation may relax the person.
5. Try "emotive imagery." For example, you might say, "Now I want you to imagine that you are dozing on the beach, with the sun warming your muscles and the sound of the waves lulling you to sleep. Let yourself relax."
6. With a very ticklish person, keep the person's hand under your own with your fingers curled over his or her fingers. Move both hands around as you palpate; people are not ticklish to themselves.
7. Alternatively perform palpation just after auscultation. Keep the stethoscope in place and curl your fingers around it, palpating as you pretend to auscultate. People do not perceive a stethoscope as a ticklish object. You can slide the stethoscope out when the person is used to being touched.

Normal Range of Findings	Abnormal Findings

Light and Deep Palpation

Begin with **light palpation.** With the first four fingers close together, depress the skin about 1 cm (Fig. 21-21). Make a gentle rotary motion, sliding the fingers and skin together. Then lift the fingers (do not drag them) and move clockwise to the next location around the abdomen. The objective here is not to search for organs but to form an overall impression of the skin surface and superficial musculature. Save the examination of any identified tender areas until last. This method avoids pain and the resulting muscle rigidity that would obscure deep palpation later in the examination.

Muscle guarding.
Rigidity.
Large masses.
Tenderness.

21-21

As you circle the abdomen, discriminate between voluntary muscle guarding and involuntary rigidity. **Voluntary guarding** occurs when the person is cold, tense, or ticklish. It is bilateral, and you will feel the muscles relax slightly during exhalation. Use the relaxation measures to try to eliminate this type of guarding, or it will interfere with deep palpation. If the rigidity persists, it is probably involuntary.

Involuntary rigidity is a constant, boardlike hardness of the muscles. It is a protective mechanism accompanying acute inflammation of the peritoneum. It may be unilateral, and the same area usually becomes painful when the person increases intra-abdominal pressure by attempting a sit-up.

Now perform **deep palpation** using the technique described earlier but push down about 5 to 8 cm (2 to 3 inches) (Fig. 21-22). Moving clockwise, explore the entire abdomen.

21-22

Normal Range of Findings

To overcome the resistance of a very large or obese abdomen, use a bimanual technique. Place your two hands on top of one another (Fig. 21-23). The top hand does the pushing; the bottom hand is relaxed and can concentrate on the sense of palpation. With either technique note the location, size, consistency, and mobility of any palpable organs and the presence of any abnormal enlargement, tenderness, or masses.

21-23

Making sense of what you are feeling is more difficult than it looks. Inexperienced examiners complain that the abdomen "all feels the same," as if they are pushing their hand into a soft sofa cushion. It helps to memorize the anatomy and visualize what is under each quadrant as you palpate. Also remember that some structures are normally palpable, as illustrated in Fig. 21-24.

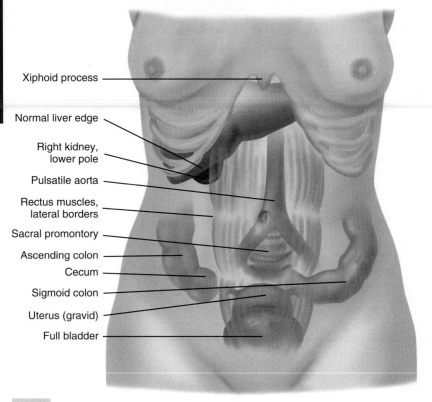

Xiphoid process

Normal liver edge

Right kidney, lower pole

Pulsatile aorta

Rectus muscles, lateral borders

Sacral promontory

Ascending colon

Cecum

Sigmoid colon

Uterus (gravid)

Full bladder

21-24   NORMALLY PALPABLE STRUCTURES

Mild tenderness normally is present when palpating the sigmoid colon. Any other tenderness should be investigated.

Abnormal Findings

Tenderness occurs with local inflammation, inflammation of the peritoneum or underlying organ, and with an enlarged organ whose capsule is stretched.

Normal Range of Findings	Abnormal Findings

Normal Range of Findings

If you identify a mass, first distinguish it from a normally palpable structure or an enlarged organ. Then note the following:
1. Location
2. Size
3. Shape
4. Consistency (soft, firm, hard)
5. Surface (smooth, nodular)
6. Mobility (including movement with respirations)
7. Pulsatility
8. Tenderness

Liver

Next palpate for specific organs, beginning with the liver in the RUQ (Fig. 21-25). Place your left hand under the person's back parallel to the 11th and 12th ribs and lift up to support the abdominal contents. Place your right hand on the RUQ, with fingers parallel to the midline. Push deeply down and under the right costal margin. Ask the person to breathe slowly. With every exhalation, move your palpating hand up 1 or 2 cm. It is normal to feel the edge of the liver bump your fingertips as the diaphragm pushes it down during inhalation. It feels like a firm, regular ridge. Often the liver is not palpable and you feel nothing firm.

Abnormal Findings

Except with a depressed diaphragm, a liver palpated more than 1 to 2 cm below the right costal margin is enlarged. Record the number of centimeters it descends and note its consistency (hard, nodular) and tenderness (see Table 21-7, Palpation of Enlarged Organs, p. 573).

21-25

Hooking Technique. An alternative method of palpating the liver is to stand up at the person's shoulder and swivel your body to the right so you face the person's feet (Fig. 21-26). Hook your fingers over the costal margin from above. Ask the person to take a deep breath. Try to feel the liver edge bump your fingertips.

21-26

Objective Data

Normal Range of Findings	Abnormal Findings

Spleen

Normally the spleen is not palpable and must be enlarged 3 times its normal size to be felt. To search for it, reach your left hand over the abdomen and behind the left side at the 11th and 12th ribs (Fig. 21-27, *A*). Lift up for support. Place your right hand obliquely on the LUQ with the fingers pointing toward the left axilla and just inferior to the rib margin. Push your hand deeply down and under the left costal margin and ask the person to take a deep breath. You should feel nothing firm.

The spleen enlarges with mononucleosis, trauma, leukemias and lymphomas, portal hypertension, and HIV infection (see Table 21-7). If you feel an enlarged spleen, refer the person but do not continue to palpate it. An enlarged spleen is friable and can rupture easily with overpalpation.

Describe the number of centimeters that it extends below the left costal margin.

21-27

When enlarged, the spleen slides out and bumps your fingertips. It can grow so large that it extends into the lower quadrants. When this condition is suspected, start low so you will not miss it. An alternative position is to roll the person onto his or her right side to displace the spleen more forward and downward (Fig. 21-27, *B*). Then palpate as described earlier.

Normal Range of Findings	Abnormal Findings

Kidneys

Search for the right kidney by placing your hands together in a "duck-bill" position at the person's right flank (Fig. 21-28, *A*). Press your two hands together firmly (you need deeper palpation than that used with the liver or spleen) and ask the person to take a deep breath. In most people you will feel no change. Occasionally you may feel the lower pole of the right kidney as a round, smooth mass that slides between your fingers. Either condition is normal.

Enlarged kidney.
Kidney mass.

21-28

The left kidney sits 1 cm higher than the right kidney and is not palpable normally. Search for it by reaching your left hand across the abdomen and behind the left flank for support (Fig. 21-28, *B*). Push your right hand deep into the abdomen and ask the person to breathe deeply. You should feel no change with the inhalation.

Aorta

Using your opposing thumb and fingers, palpate the aortic pulsation in the upper abdomen slightly to the left of midline (Fig. 21-29). Normally it is 2.5 to 4 cm wide in the adult and pulsates in an anterior direction.

Widened with aneurysm (see Table 21-6, p. 573, and Table 21-7, p. 573).
Prominent lateral pulsation with aortic aneurysm pushes the examiner's two fingers apart.

21-29

Objective Data

Normal Range of Findings	Abnormal Findings

Normal Range of Findings

Special Procedures for Advanced Practice

Rebound Tenderness (Blumberg Sign). Assess rebound tenderness when the person reports abdominal pain or when you elicit tenderness during palpation. Choose a site away from the painful area. Hold your hand 90 degrees, or perpendicular, to the abdomen. Push down slowly and deeply (Fig. 21-30, *A*); then lift up *quickly* (Fig. 21-30, *B*). This makes structures that are indented by palpation rebound suddenly. A normal, or negative, response is no pain on release of pressure. Perform this test at the end of the examination because it can cause severe pain and muscle rigidity.

21-30   Rebound tenderness.

Inspiratory Arrest (Murphy Sign). Normally palpating the liver causes no pain. In a person with inflammation of the gallbladder (cholecystitis), pain occurs. Hold your fingers under the liver border. Ask the person to take a deep breath. A normal response is to complete the deep breath without pain. (NOTE: This sign is less accurate in patients older than 60 years; evidence shows that 25% of them do not have any abdominal tenderness.[25])

Iliopsoas Muscle Test. Perform the iliopsoas muscle test when the acute abdominal pain of appendicitis is suspected. With the person supine, lift the right leg straight up, flexing at the hip (Fig. 21-31); then push down over the lower part of the right thigh as the person tries to hold the leg up. When the test is negative, the person feels no change.

21-31   Iliopsoas muscle test.

For the obturator test, lift the person's right leg, flexing at the hip, and 90 degrees at the knee. Hold his or her ankle and rotate the leg internally and externally. There should be no pain. This test is less specific.[25]

Abnormal Findings

Pain on release of pressure confirms rebound tenderness, which is a reliable sign of peritoneal inflammation. Peritoneal inflammation accompanies appendicitis.

Cough tenderness that is localized to a specific spot also signals peritoneal irritation. Refer the person with suspected appendicitis for computed tomography (CT) scanning.

When the test is positive, as the descending liver pushes the inflamed gallbladder onto the examining hand, the person feels sharp pain and abruptly stops inspiration midway.

When the iliopsoas muscle is inflamed (which occurs with an inflamed or perforated appendix), pain is felt in the RLQ.

An inflamed appendix irritates the obturator muscle, and this leg movement produces pain.

Normal Range of Findings

The Alvarado Score. This scoring system combines findings to assist evaluation in patients with RLQ pain. Also called the **MANTRELS score**, from the mnemonic in the following list, a score of 4 or less significantly decreases the probability of appendicitis.[25]

Finding	Points
Symptoms	
Migration to right iliac fossa	1
Anorexia*	1
Nausea and vomiting	1
Signs	
Tenderness, RLQ	2
Rebound tenderness	1
Elevation of temperature (oral ≥37.3° C)	1
Laboratory Findings	
Leukocytosis (white blood cell count >10,000/µL)	2
Shift to the left (>75% neutrophils)	1
Total Possible Points	10

*For *anorexia,* may substitute acetone in urine.[25]

❖ DEVELOPMENTAL COMPETENCE

The Infant

Inspection. The contour of the abdomen is protuberant because of the immature abdominal musculature. The skin contains a fine, superficial venous pattern. This may be visible in lightly pigmented children up to the age of puberty.

Inspect the umbilical cord throughout the neonatal period. At birth it is white and contains two umbilical arteries and one vein surrounded by mucoid connective tissue, called *Wharton's jelly.* The umbilical stump dries within a week, hardens, and falls off by 10 to 14 days. Skin covers the area by 3 to 4 weeks.

The abdomen should be symmetric, although two bulges are common. You may note an **umbilical hernia.** It appears at 2 to 3 weeks and is especially prominent when the infant cries. The hernia reaches maximum size at 1 month (up to 2.5 cm or 1 inch) and usually disappears by 1 year. Another common variation is **diastasis recti,** a separation of the rectus muscles with a visible bulge along the midline (see Table 21-4). The condition is more common with Black infants, and it usually disappears by early childhood.

The abdomen shows respiratory movement. The only other abdominal movement you should note is occasional peristalsis, which may be visible because of the thin musculature.

Auscultation. Auscultation yields only bowel sounds, the metallic tinkling of peristalsis. No vascular sounds should be heard.

Percussion. Percussion finds tympany over the stomach (the infant swallows some air with feeding) and dullness over the liver. The spleen is not percussed. The abdomen sounds tympanitic, although it is normal to percuss dullness over the bladder. This dullness may extend up to the umbilicus.

Palpation. Aid palpation by flexing the baby's knees with one hand while palpating with the other (Fig. 21-32). Alternatively you may hold the upper back and flex the neck slightly with one hand. Offer a pacifier to a crying baby.

Abnormal Findings

An Alvarado score of ≥7 increases the probability of appendicitis.

Scaphoid shape occurs with dehydration.
Dilated veins.

The presence of only one artery signals the risk for congenital defects.
Inflammation.
Drainage after cord falls off.
Refer any umbilical hernia larger than 2.5 cm (see Table 21-4); continuing to grow after 1 month; or lasting for more than 2 years in a White child or for more than 7 years in a Black child.
Refer diastasis recti lasting more than 6 years.
Marked peristalsis with pyloric stenosis (see Table 21-5, p. 572).

Bruit.
Venous hum.

Normal Range of Findings	Abnormal Findings

21-32

The liver fills the RUQ. It is normal to feel the liver edge at the right costal margin or 1 to 2 cm below. Normally you may palpate the spleen tip and both kidneys and the bladder. Also easily palpated are the cecum in the RLQ and the sigmoid colon, which feels like a sausage in the left inguinal area.

Make note of the newborn's first stool, a sticky, greenish-black meconium stool within 24 hours of birth. By the 4th day, stools of breastfed babies are golden yellow, pasty, and smell like sour milk, whereas those of formula-fed babies are brown-yellow, firmer, and more fecal smelling.

The Child

Younger than 4 years, the abdomen looks protuberant when the child is both supine and standing. After age 4 years the potbelly remains when standing because of lumbar lordosis, but the abdomen looks flat when supine. Normal movement on the abdomen includes respirations, which remain abdominal until 7 years of age.

To palpate the abdomen, position the young child on the parent's lap as you sit knee-to-knee with the parent. Flex the knees up and elevate the head slightly. The child can "pant like a dog" to further relax abdominal muscles. Hold your entire palm flat on the abdominal surface for a moment before starting palpation. This accustoms the child to being touched (Fig. 21-33). If the child is very ticklish, hold his or her hand under your own as you palpate or apply the stethoscope and palpate around it.

A scaphoid abdomen is associated with dehydration or malnutrition.

Younger than 7 years, the absence of abdominal respirations occurs with inflammation of the peritoneum.

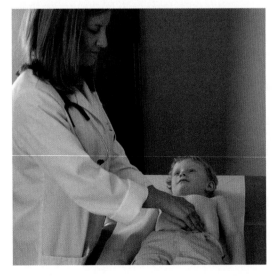

21-33

Normal Range of Findings	**Abnormal Findings**

The liver remains easily palpable 1 to 2 cm below the right costal margin. The edge is soft and sharp and moves easily. On the left the spleen also is easily palpable with a soft, sharp, movable edge. Usually you can feel 1 to 2 cm of the right kidney and the tip of the left kidney. Percussion of the liver span measures about 3.5 cm at age 2 years, 5 cm at age 6 years, and 6 to 7 cm during adolescence.

In assessing abdominal tenderness, remember that the young child often answers this question affirmatively no matter how the abdomen actually feels. Use objective signs to aid assessment such as a cry changing in pitch as you palpate, facial grimacing, moving away from you, and guarding.

The school-age child has a slim abdominal shape as he or she loses the potbelly. This slimming trend continues into adolescence. Variation in body image means that some adolescents are comfortable with exposure to the abdomen and others may be embarrassed. Be sensitive to this and use adequate draping or keep her or him in personal clothing (Fig. 21-34). The physical findings are the same as those listed for the adult.

21-34

The Aging Adult

On inspection you may note increased deposits of subcutaneous fat on the abdomen and hips because it is redistributed away from the extremities. The abdominal musculature is thinner and has less tone than that of the younger adult; thus in the absence of obesity, you may note peristalsis.

Because of the thinner, softer abdominal wall, the organs may be easier to palpate (in the absence of obesity). The liver is easier to palpate. Normally you will feel the liver edge at or just below the costal margin. With distended lungs and a depressed diaphragm, the liver is palpated lower, descending 1 to 2 cm below the costal margin with inhalation. The kidneys are easier to palpate.

Abdominal rigidity with acute abdominal conditions is less common in aging.

With an acute abdomen the aging person often complains of less pain than a younger person would.

PROMOTING A HEALTHY LIFESTYLE

Probiotics

The National Center for Complementary and Alternative Medicine (NCCAM) provides information and research findings about complementary health products and practices. One topic that draws public attention and the attention of clinicians and researchers is probiotics. Probiotics, referred to as *good bacteria,* are bacteria or other live microorganisms similar to the microorganisms normally found in the human digestive tract. Currently they are available in oral products such as dietary supplements and yogurts and in suppositories and creams. The two most common organisms in probiotics include *Lactobacillus* and *Bifidobacterium;* however, there are many specific types of bacteria within each of these two broad groups, and health benefits associated with one type may not hold true for others. Also important is that the effects may vary from person to person.

What is important to know is that our current understanding of probiotics is still a work in progress because scientific evidence supporting specific uses is limited and the Food and Drug Administration (FDA) has not approved any of the health claims for probiotics. To this end the National Institutes of Health has established the *Probiotic and Prebiotic Working Group* (PPWG) as a trans-NIH effort to identify gaps and challenges in research. Clinicians can join the listserv and stay up to date on their progress at http://sigs.nih.gov/PPWG/Pages/JointheSIG.aspx. Preliminary evidence already exists for several uses of probiotics, from shortening duration of diarrhea and reducing stool frequency in acute infectious diarrhea to reducing side effects associated with treatment for *Helicobacter pylori* infection, the cause of most stomach ulcers. There is also strong evidence that probiotics may reduce the risk of necrotizing enterocolitis, a severe intestinal condition of premature newborns. Other potential future applications include use in reducing cholesterol levels, treating obesity, and managing irritable bowel syndrome.

Resources

An overview of probiotics, including current use and research, is available through NCCAM at http://nccam.nih.gov/health/probiotics/introduction.htm.

The NCCAM site also includes a reproducible handout for patients and families: http://nccam.nih.gov/sites/nccam.nih.gov/files/Get_The_Facts_Probiotics_01-08-2013.pdf?nav=gsa.

DOCUMENTATION AND CRITICAL THINKING

Sample Charting

SUBJECTIVE

States appetite is good with no recent change, no dysphagia, no food intolerance, no pain, no nausea/vomiting. Has one formed BM/day. Takes OTC multivitamins, no other prescribed or over-the-counter medication. No history of abdominal disease, injury, or surgery. Diet recall of past 24 hours listed at end of history.

OBJECTIVE

Inspection: Abdomen flat, symmetric, with no apparent masses. Skin smooth with no striae, scars, or lesions.
Auscultation: Bowel sounds present, no bruits.
Percussion: Tympany predominates in all 4 quadrants, liver span is 8 cm in right MCL. Splenic dullness located at 10th intercostal space in left midaxillary line.
Palpation: Abdomen soft, no organomegaly, no masses, no tenderness.

ASSESSMENT

Healthy abdomen; bowel sounds present

Clinical Case Study 1

O.W. is a 33-year-old Caucasian male who underwent gastric bypass surgery 1 week PTA. Preoperative BMI 62.8 (height 180 cm; weight 204 kg). Past medical history of type 2 diabetes mellitus, morbid obesity, hypertension, obstructive sleep apnea, and venous stasis ulcers on bilateral lower extremities.

Documentation and Critical Thinking

SUBJECTIVE

1 week PTA—Endoscopic gastric bypass surgery performed without complication.
5 days PTA—Patient discharged home in stable condition on a pureed diet. No postoperative complications.
1 day PTA—O.W. noticed increased nausea and nonspecific shoulder pain.
Present—"I feel terrible." Reports fever with chills, nausea, constant pain in back and shoulders, abdominal pain, and palpitations. O.W. denies changes in diet or deviation from prescribed diet.

OBJECTIVE

Vital signs: Temp 102° F (39° C). Pulse 130 bpm. Resp 20/min. BP 90/56 mm Hg, right arm, supine.
Inspection: Lying on side with knees tucked. Abdomen uniformly round. Grimacing with movement.
Auscultation: Hypoactive bowel sounds. No vascular sounds.
Percussion: Tympany predominates. Scattered dullness caused by adipose tissue. Percussion elicits tenderness.
Palpation: Extreme tenderness. Rebound tenderness present RLQ and LLQ. Unable to palpate organs because of tenderness and obesity.

ASSESSMENT

Acute abdomen
Possible anastomotic leaking at gastric bypass site
Acute pain R/T peritoneal inflammation
Risk for infection R/T anastomotic leak of stomach contents into abdominal cavity

Clinical Case Study 2

E.J. is a 63-year-old retired homemaker with a history of lung cancer with metastasis to the liver.

SUBJECTIVE

Feeling "puffy and bloated" for the past week. States unable to get comfortable. Also short of breath "all the time now." Difficulty sleeping. "I feel like crying all the time now."

OBJECTIVE

Inspection: Weight increase of 8 lbs in 1 week. Abdomen is distended with everted umbilicus and bulging flanks. Girth at umbilicus is 85 cm. Prominent dilated venous pattern present over abdomen.
Auscultation: Bowel sounds present. No vascular sounds.
Percussion: When supine, tympany present at dome of abdomen, dullness over flanks. Shifting dullness present. Positive fluid wave present. Liver span is 12 cm in right MCL.
Palpation: Abdominal wall firm, able to feel liver with deep palpation at 6 cm below right costal margin. Liver feels firm, nodular, nontender. 4+ pitting edema in both ankles.

ASSESSMENT

Ascites
Grieving
Ineffective breathing pattern R/T increased intra-abdominal pressure
Pain R/T distended abdomen
Risk for impaired skin integrity R/T ascites, edema, and faulty metabolism
Insomnia

Clinical Case Study 3

D.G. is a 17-year-old African-American male high school student who enters the emergency department with abdominal pain for 2 days.

SUBJECTIVE

2 days PTA, D.G. noted general abdominal pain in umbilical region. Now pain is sharp and severe, and he points to location in RLQ. No BM for 2 days. No appetite. Nausea and vomiting off and on 1 day; no blood in vomitus.

OBJECTIVE

Inspection: Temp 100.4° F (38° C). Pulse 116 bpm. Resp 18/min. BP 112/70 mm Hg.
Lying on side with knees drawn up under chin. Resists any movement. Face tight and occasionally grimacing. Cries out with any sudden movement.
Auscultation: No bowel sounds present. No vascular sounds.
Percussion: Tympany. Percussion over RLQ leads to tenderness.
Palpation: Abdominal wall is rigid and boardlike. Extreme tenderness to palpation in RLQ. Rebound tenderness is present in RLQ. Positive iliopsoas muscle test. Alvarado score 7 with no laboratory results available yet.

ASSESSMENT

Acute abdomen, possible appendicitis
Acute abdominal pain in RLQ
Nausea

Clinical Case Study 4

G.C. is a 5-week-old Latino male who was brought to the clinic today by his parents for vomiting.

SUBJECTIVE

Since birth G.C. has been a "great eater who nursed all the time without problems."
10 days PTA—G.C. continues to want to nurse all the time but now "projectile vomits" soon after feeds and "never appears comfortable."
4 days PTA—Vomiting continued post-feeds; last reported stool at that time; 7 wet diapers/day.
1 day PTA—Vomiting continued; "only had 3 wet diapers today."
Birth weight—9 lbs 9 oz (4.3 kg)

OBJECTIVE

Vital signs: Temp 98.6°F (37°C) (axillary). Pulse 128 bpm. Resp 42/min. Weight 11 lbs 3oz (5.1 kg). BP 76/40 mm Hg (sleeping).
General appearance: Infant resting comfortably in mom's arms.
HEENT: Anterior and posterior fontanels slightly sunken; eyes clear and moist; TM pearly gray bilat; nares patent bilat; oral mucosa slightly moist
Cardiovascular: Sinus arrhythmia; no abnormal heart sounds.
Respiratory: Breath sounds clear and equal bilat; unlabored.
Abdomen: Visible gastric peristalsis and olive-shaped mass palpated in the epigastrium just right of umbilicus.

ASSESSMENT

Pyloric stenosis
Imbalanced nutrition: less than body requirements R/T vomiting secondary to pyloric sphincter obstruction
Acute pain R/T abdominal fullness
Risk for imbalanced fluid volume R/T vomiting, dehydration

ABNORMAL FINDINGS

TABLE 21-1 Abdominal Distention

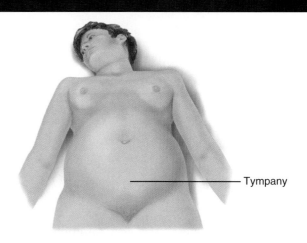

Obesity

Inspection. Uniformly rounded. Umbilicus sunken (it adheres to peritoneum, layers of fat are superficial to it).
Auscultation. Normal bowel sounds.
Percussion. Tympany. Scattered dullness over adipose tissue.
Palpation. Normal. May be hard to feel through thick abdominal wall.

Air or Gas

Inspection. Single round curve.
Auscultation. Depends on cause of gas (e.g., decreased or absent bowel sounds with ileus); hyperactive with early intestinal obstruction.
Percussion. Tympany over large area.
Palpation. May have muscle spasm of abdominal wall.

Ascites

Inspection. Single curve. Everted umbilicus. Bulging flanks when supine. Taut, glistening skin; recent weight gain; increase in abdominal girth.
Auscultation. Normal bowel sounds over intestines. Diminished over ascitic fluid.
Percussion. Tympany at top where intestines float. Dull over fluid. Produces fluid wave and shifting dullness.
Palpation. Taut skin and increased intra-abdominal pressure limit palpation.

Ovarian Cyst (Large)

Inspection. Curve in lower half of abdomen, midline. Everted umbilicus.
Auscultation. Normal bowel sounds over upper abdomen where intestines pushed superiorly.
Percussion. Top dull over fluid. Intestines pushed superiorly. Large cyst produces fluid wave and shifting dullness.
Palpation. Transmits aortic pulsation, whereas ascites does not.

Continued

TABLE 21-1 Abdominal Distention—cont'd

Fetal
heart tones

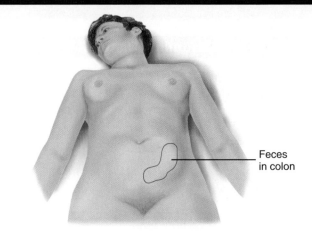

Feces
in colon

Pregnancy*

Inspection. Single curve. Umbilicus protruding. Breasts engorged.
Auscultation. Fetal heart tones. Bowel sounds diminished.
Percussion. Tympany over intestines. Dull over enlarging uterus.
Palpation. Fetal parts. Fetal movements.

Feces

Inspection. Localized distention.
Auscultation. Normal bowel sounds.
Percussion. Tympany predominates. Scattered dullness over fecal mass.
Palpation. Plastic-like or ropelike mass with feces in intestines.

◀ **Tumor**

Inspection. Localized distention.
Auscultation. Normal bowel sounds.
Percussion. Dull over mass if reaches up to skin surface.
Palpation. Define borders. Distinguish from enlarged organ or normally palpable structure.

*Obviously a normal finding, pregnancy is included for comparison of conditions causing abdominal distention.

TABLE 21-2   Clinical Portrait of Intestinal Obstruction

- History of previous abdominal surgery with adhesions

- Vomiting

- Absence of stool or gas passage

- Distended abdomen (after 2nd day)

- X-ray shows dilated air-filled loops of small bowel with multiple air-fluid levels

- Hyperactive bowel sounds in early obstruction; hypoactive or silent in late obstruction

- Dehydration and loss of electrolytes

- Accumulation of fluid and gas in bowel proximal (above) to obstruction

- Colicky pain from strong peristalsis above the obstruction

- Fever

- Pressure from excess fluid and gas may ➡leaking fluid into peritoneum

- Hypovolemic shock
  (⬇BP, ⬆pulse, cool skin if left untreated)

© Pat Thomas, 2014.

TABLE 21-3   Common Sites of Referred Abdominal Pain

When a person gives a history of abdominal pain, the pain's location may not necessarily be directly over the involved organ because the human brain has no felt image for internal organs. Rather pain is referred to a site where the organ was located in fetal development. Although the organ migrates during fetal development, its nerves persist in referring sensations from the former location. The following are examples, not a complete list.

Liver. Hepatitis may have mild-to-moderate dull pain in right upper quadrant (RUQ) or epigastrium, along with anorexia, nausea, malaise, low-grade fever.

Esophagus. Gastroesophageal reflux disease (GERD) is a complex of symptoms of esophagitis, including burning pain in midepigastrium or behind lower sternum that radiates upward or "heartburn." Occurs 30 to 60 minutes after eating; aggravated by lying down or bending over.

Gallbladder. Cholecystitis is biliary colic, sudden pain in RUQ that may radiate to right or left scapula and that builds over time, lasting 2 to 4 hours, after ingestion of fatty foods, alcohol, or caffeine. Associated with nausea and vomiting and with positive Murphy sign or sudden stop in inspiration with RUQ palpation.

Pancreas. Pancreatitis has acute, boring midepigastric pain radiating to the back and sometimes to the left scapula or flank, severe nausea, and vomiting.

Duodenum. Duodenal ulcer typically has dull, aching, gnawing pain; does not radiate; may be relieved by food; and may awaken the person from sleep.

Stomach. Gastric ulcer pain is dull, aching, gnawing epigastric pain, usually brought on by food and radiates to back or substernal area. Pain of perforated ulcer is burning epigastric pain of sudden onset that refers to one or both shoulders.

Appendix. Appendicitis typically starts as dull, diffuse pain in periumbilical region that later shifts to severe, sharp, persistent pain and tenderness localized in RLQ (McBurney point). Pain is aggravated by movement, coughing, deep breathing; associated with anorexia, then nausea and vomiting, fever.

Kidney. Kidney stones prompt a sudden onset of severe, colicky flank or lower abdominal pain.

Small intestine. Gastroenteritis has diffuse, generalized abdominal pain with nausea, diarrhea.

Colon. Large bowel obstruction has moderate, colicky pain of gradual onset in lower abdomen and bloating. Irritable bowel syndrome (IBS) has sharp or burning cramping pain over a wide area; does not radiate. Brought on by meals; relieved by bowel movement.

Image © Pat Thomas, 2006.

TABLE 21-4   Abnormalities on Inspection

Umbilical Hernia

This is a soft, skin-covered mass, the protrusion of the omentum or intestine through a weakness or incomplete closure in the umbilical ring. It is accentuated by increased intra-abdominal pressure as with crying, coughing, vomiting, or straining; but the bowel rarely incarcerates or strangulates. More common in premature infants. Most resolve spontaneously by 1 year; parents should avoid affixing a belt or coin at the hernia because this will not help closure and may cause contact dermatitis. In an adult it occurs with pregnancy, chronic ascites, or chronic intrathoracic pressure (e.g., asthma, chronic bronchitis).

Incisional Hernia

A bulge near an old operative scar that may not show when person is supine but is apparent when the person increases intra-abdominal pressure by a sit-up, by standing, or by the Valsalva maneuver.

Epigastric Hernia

Protrusion of abdominal structures presents as a small, fatty nodule at epigastrium in midline, through the linea alba. Usually one can feel it rather than observe it. May be palpable only when standing.

Diastasis Recti

A midline longitudinal ridge that is a separation of the abdominal rectus muscles. Ridge is revealed when intra-abdominal pressure is increased by raising head while supine. Occurs congenitally (here), and as a result of pregnancy or marked obesity in which prolonged distention or a decrease in muscle tone has occurred. It is not clinically significant.

See Illustration Credits for source information.

TABLE 21-5   Abnormal Bowel Sounds

◄ Succussion Splash

Unrelated to peristalsis, this is a very loud splash auscultated over the upper abdomen when the infant is rocked side to side. It indicates increased air and fluid in the stomach, as seen with pyloric obstruction or large hiatus hernia.

Marked peristalsis together with projectile vomiting in the newborn suggests pyloric stenosis, an obstruction of the pyloric valve of the stomach. Pyloric stenosis is a congenital defect and appears in the 2nd or 3rd week. After feeding, pronounced peristaltic waves cross from left to right, leading to projectile vomiting. Then one can palpate an olive-size mass in the RUQ midway between the right costal margin and umbilicus. Refer promptly because of risk for weight loss.

Hypoactive Bowel Sounds

Diminished or absent bowel sounds signal decreased motility as a result of inflammation as seen with peritonitis; from paralytic ileus as following abdominal surgery; or from late bowel obstruction. Occurs also with pneumonia.

Hyperactive Bowel Sounds

Loud, gurgling sounds, **"borborygmi,"** signal increased motility. They occur with early mechanical bowel obstruction (high-pitched), gastroenteritis, brisk diarrhea, laxative use, and subsiding paralytic ileus.

TABLE 21-6 Friction Rubs and Vascular Sounds

◄ **Peritoneal Friction Rub**

A rough, grating sound, like two pieces of leather rubbed together, indicates peritoneal inflammation. Occurs rarely. Usually occurs over organs with a large surface area in contact with the peritoneum.

Liver—Friction rub over lower right rib cage from abscess or metastatic tumor.

Spleen—Friction rub over lower left rib cage in left anterior axillary line from abscess, infection, or tumor.

◄ **Vascular Sounds**

Arterial—A **bruit** indicates turbulent blood flow, as found in constricted, abnormally dilated, or tortuous vessels. Listen with the bell. Occurs with the following:

- *Aortic aneurysm*—Murmur is harsh, systolic, or continuous and accentuated with systole. Note in person with hypertension.
- *Renal artery stenosis*—Murmur is midline or toward flank, soft, low-to-medium pitch.
- *Partial occlusion of femoral arteries.*

Venous hum—Occurs rarely. Heard in periumbilical region. Originates from inferior vena cava. Medium pitch, continuous sound, pressure on bell may obliterate it. May have palpable thrill. Occurs with portal hypertension and cirrhotic liver.

Peritoneal friction rub

Vascular sounds

TABLE 21-7 Palpation of Enlarged Organs

Enlarged Liver

An enlarged, smooth, nontender liver occurs with fatty infiltration, portal obstruction or cirrhosis, high obstruction of inferior vena cava, and lymphocytic leukemia.

The liver feels enlarged and smooth but is tender to palpation with early heart failure, acute hepatitis, or hepatic abscess.

Enlarged Nodular Liver

An enlarged and nodular liver occurs with late portal cirrhosis, metastatic cancer, or tertiary syphilis. Often with cirrhosis the liver is smaller, but the edge is firmer than normal, and the edge is easily palpable.

Abnormal Findings

TABLE 21-7 Palpation of Enlarged Organs—cont'd

Enlarged Gallbladder

An enlarged, tender gallbladder suggests acute cholecystitis. Feel it behind the liver border as a smooth and firm mass like a sausage, although it may be difficult to palpate because of involuntary rigidity of abdominal muscles. The area is exquisitely painful to fist percussion, and inspiratory arrest (Murphy sign) is present.

An enlarged, nontender gallbladder also feels like a smooth, sausagelike mass. It occurs when the gallbladder is filled with stones, as with common bile duct obstruction.

Enlarged Spleen

Because any enlargement superiorly is stopped by the diaphragm, the spleen enlarges down and to the midline. When extreme, it can extend down to the left pelvis. It retains the splenic notch on the medial edge. When splenomegaly occurs with acute infections (mononucleosis), it is moderately enlarged and soft, with rounded edges. When the result of a chronic cause, the enlargement is firm or hard, with sharp edges. An enlarged spleen is usually not tender to palpation; it is tender only if the peritoneum is also inflamed.

Enlarged Kidney

Enlarged with hydronephrosis, cyst, or neoplasm. May be difficult to distinguish an enlarged kidney from an enlarged spleen because they have a similar shape. Both extend forward and down. However, the spleen may have a sharp edge, whereas the kidney never does. The spleen retains the splenic notch, whereas the kidney has no palpable notch. Percussion over the spleen is dull, whereas over the kidney it is tympanitic because of the overriding bowel.

Aortic Aneurysm

Most aortic aneurysms (>95%) are located below the renal arteries and extend to the umbilicus. A focal bulging >5 cm is palpable in about 80% of cases during routine physical examination and feels like a pulsating mass in the upper abdomen just to the left of midline. You will hear a bruit. Femoral pulses are present but decreased. Additional information on abdominal aneurysm is illustrated in Table 21-6.

Summary Checklist: Abdomen Examination

1. **Inspection**
   Contour
   Symmetry
   Umbilicus
   Skin
   Pulsation or movement
   Hair distribution
   Demeanor

2. **Auscultation**
   Bowel sounds
   Note any vascular sounds
3. **Percussion**
   Percuss all four quadrants
   Percuss borders of liver, spleen

4. **Palpation**
   Light palpation in all four
      quadrants
   Deeper palpation in all four
      quadrants
   Palpate for liver, spleen, kidneys

BIBLIOGRAPHY

1. Ambinder, M. (2010, May). Beating obesity. *The Atlantic*, 72-83.
2. Anastasi, J. K., Capili, B., & Chang, M. (2013). Managing irritable bowel syndrome. *Am J Nurs, 113*(7), 42-52.
3. Bailes, B. K. & Reeve, K. (2013). Constipation in older adults. *Nurse Pract, 38*(8), 21-25.
4. Budd, G. M., & Falkenstein, K. (2009). Bariatric surgery: putting the squeeze on obesity. *Nurse Pract, 34*(7), 39-46.
5. Camilleri, M. (2012). Peripheral mechanisms in irritable bowel syndrome. *N Engl J Med, 367*(17), 1626-1635.
6. Campbell, B. H., & Mendelson, M. H. (2010). Acute abdomen: the basics. *Emerg Med, 42*(7), 8-12.
7. Carter, S. L., & Attel, S. (2013). The diagnosis and management of patients with lactose-intolerance. *Nurse Pract, 38*(7), 23-28.
8. Cross, S. (2011). Barrett esophagus: a practical challenge for primary care. *Nurse Pract, 36*(11), 18-21.
9. Ferrara, L. R., & Saccomano, S. J. (2012). Crohn disease: recognition is key. *Nurse Pract, 37*(12), 22-28.
10. Flegal, K. M., Carroll, M. D., Kit, B. K., et al. (2012). Prevalence of obesity and trends in the distribution of body mass index among U.S. adults, 1999-2010. *JAMA, 307*(5), 491-497.
11. Fournier, M., & Zanoff, J. (2012). Understanding aortic aneurysms. *OR Nurse 2012, 6*(4), 26-34.
12. Fowler, C. (2013). Management of patients with complications of cirrhosis. *Nurse Pract, 38*(4), 14-22.
13. Gainer, C. L. (2011). Celiac disease: helping patients live gluten-free. *Nurse Pract, 36*(9), 14-19.
14. Gallagher, P., & O'Mahony, D. (2009). Constipation in old age. *Best Pract Res Clin Gastroenterol, 23*(6), 875-887.
15. Gujral, H., & Collantes, R. S. (2009). Understanding viral hepatitis: a guide for primary care. *Nurse Pract, 34*(12), 23-32.
16. Gupta, K., Dhawan, A., Abel, C., et al. (2013). A re-evaluation of the scratch test for locating the liver edge. *BMC Gastroenterol, 13*(1), 35.
17. Halpert, A. D. (2010). Importance of early diagnosis in patients with irritable bowel syndrome. *Postgrad Med, 122*(2), 102-111.
18. Hart, A. M. (2013). Evidence-based recommendations for GERD treatment. *Nurse Pract, 38*(8), 26-34.
19. Heber, D. (2010). An integrative view of obesity. *Am J Clin Nutr, 91*(1), 280S-283S.
20. Keith, J. N., Nicholls, J., Reed, A., et al. (2011). The prevalence of self-reported lactose intolerance and the consumption of dairy foods among African American adults are less than expected. *J Natl Med Assoc, 103*(1), 36.
21. King, J. (2009). Infectious mononucleosis: update and considerations. *Nurse Pract, 34*(11), 42-45.
22. Klein, J. D., & Dietz, W. (2010). Childhood obesity: the new tobacco. *Health affairs, 29*(3), 388-392.
23. Madsen, D., Sebolt, T., Cullen, L., et al. (2005). Listening to bowel sounds: an evidence-based practice project. *Am J Nurs, 105*(12), 40-50.
24. McCabe, M. A., Toughill, E. H., Parkhill, A. M., et al. (2012). Celiac disease: a medical puzzle. *Am J Nurs, 112*(10), 34-44.
25. McGee, S. (2012). *Evidence-based physical diagnosis* (3rd ed.). Philadelphia: Saunders.
26. McLachlan, A. J., & Pont, L. C. (2012). Drug metabolism in older people—a key consideration in achieving optimal outcomes with medicines. *J Gerontol Series, 67*(2), 175-180.
27. Nicklas, T. A., Qu, H., Hughes, S. O., et al. (2009). Prevalence of self-reported lactose intolerance in a multiethnic sample of adults. *Nutr Today, 44*(5), 222-229.
28. Pates, J. A., Avendiano, T. C., Zaretsky, M. V., et al. (2009). The appendix in pregnancy: confirming historical observations with a contemporary modality. *Obstet Gynecol, 114*(4), 805-808.
28a. Saccomano, S. J., & Ferrara, L. R. (2013). Evaluation of acute abdominal pain. *Nurse Pract 38*(11):46-53.
29. Simons, S. R., & Abdallah, L. M. (2012). Bedside assessment of enteral tube placement: aligning practice with evidence. *Am J Nurs, 112*(2), 40-46.
30. Tyson, R. L. (2010). Diagnosis and treatment of abdominal angina. *Nurse Pract, 35*(11), 16-22.
31. Wadlund, D. L. (2012). Meeting the challenge of IBS. *Nurse Pract, 37*(5), 22-30.

CHAPTER 22

Musculoskeletal System

STRUCTURE AND FUNCTION

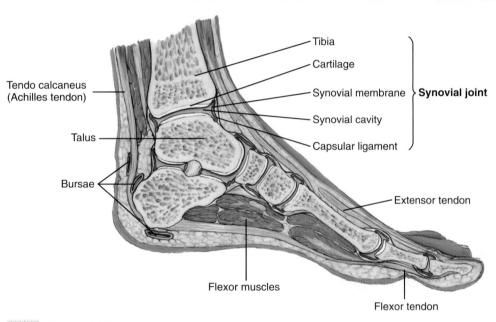

22-1 Synovial joints.

The musculoskeletal system consists of the body's **bones, joints,** and **muscles**. Humans need this system (1) for *support* to stand erect, and (2) for *movement*. The musculoskeletal system also functions (3) to encase and *protect* the inner vital organs (e.g., brain, spinal cord, heart); (4) to *produce* the red blood cells, white blood cells, and platelets in the bone marrow (hematopoiesis); and (5) as a *reservoir* for *storage* of essential minerals such as calcium and phosphorus in the bones.

MUSCULOSKELETAL COMPONENTS

The skeleton is the bony framework of the body. It has 206 bones, which support the body like the posts and beams of a building. **Bone** and cartilage are specialized forms of connective tissue. Bone is hard, rigid, and very dense. Its cells are continually turning over and remodeling. The **joint** (or articulation) is the place of union of two or more bones. Joints are the functional units of the musculoskeletal system because they permit the mobility needed for activities of daily living (ADLs).

Nonsynovial or Synovial Joints

In **nonsynovial** joints, the bones are united by fibrous tissue or cartilage and are immovable (e.g., the sutures in the skull) or only slightly movable (e.g., the vertebrae). **Synovial** joints are freely movable because they have bones that are separated from one another and enclosed in a joint cavity (Fig. 22-1). This cavity is filled with a lubricant, or synovial fluid. Just like grease on gears, synovial fluid allows sliding of opposing surfaces, and this sliding permits movement.

In synovial joints a layer of resilient **cartilage** covers the surface of opposing bones. Cartilage is avascular; it receives nourishment from synovial fluid that circulates during joint movement. It is a very stable connective tissue with a slow cell turnover. It has a tough, firm consistency yet is flexible. This cartilage cushions the bones and gives a smooth surface to facilitate movement.

The joint is surrounded by a fibrous capsule and supported by ligaments. **Ligaments** are fibrous bands running directly from one bone to another bone that strengthen the joint and help prevent movement in undesirable directions. A **bursa** is an enclosed sac filled with viscous synovial fluid,

577

much like a joint. Bursae are located in areas of potential friction (e.g., subacromial bursa of the shoulder, prepatellar bursa of the knee) and help muscles and tendons glide smoothly over bone.

Muscles

Muscles account for 40% to 50% of body weight. When they contract they produce movement. Muscles are of three types: skeletal, smooth, and cardiac. This chapter is concerned with **skeletal,** or voluntary, muscles—those under conscious control.

Each **skeletal muscle** is composed of bundles of muscle fibers or **fasciculi.** The skeletal muscle is attached to bone by a **tendon**—a strong fibrous cord. Skeletal muscles produce the following movements (Fig. 22-2):

1. Flexion—Bending a limb at a joint
2. Extension—Straightening a limb at a joint
3. Abduction—Moving a limb away from the midline of the body
4. Adduction—Moving a limb toward the midline of the body
5. Pronation—Turning the forearm so the palm is down
6. Supination—Turning the forearm so the palm is up

7. Circumduction—Moving the arm in a circle around the shoulder
8. Inversion—Moving the sole of the foot inward at the ankle
9. Eversion—Moving the sole of the foot outward at the ankle
10. Rotation—Moving the head around a central axis
11. Protraction—Moving a body part forward and parallel to the ground
12. Retraction—Moving a body part backward and parallel to the ground
13. Elevation—Raising a body part
14. Depression—Lowering a body part

Temporomandibular Joint

The temporomandibular joint (TMJ) is the articulation of the mandible and the temporal bone (Fig. 22-3). You can feel it in the depression anterior to the tragus of the ear. The TMJ permits jaw function for speaking and chewing. The joint allows three motions: (1) hinge action to open and close the jaws; (2) gliding action for protrusion and retraction; and (3) gliding for side-to-side movement of the lower jaw.

SKELETAL MUSCLE MOVEMENTS

22-2

© Pat Thomas, 2006.

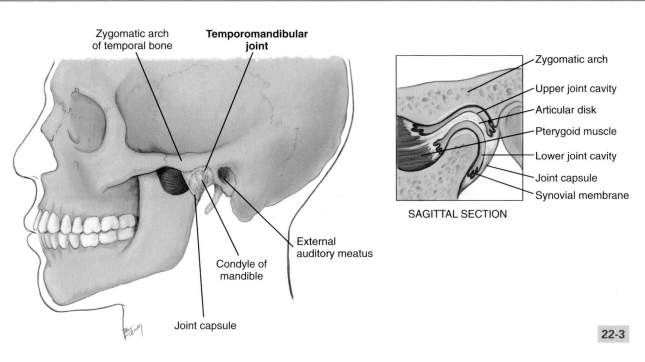

Zygomatic arch
of temporal bone

**Temporomandibular
joint**

Condyle of
mandible

External
auditory meatus

Joint capsule

Zygomatic arch

Upper joint cavity

Articular disk

Pterygoid muscle

Lower joint cavity

Joint capsule

Synovial membrane

SAGITTAL SECTION

22-3

Spine

The **vertebrae** are 33 connecting bones stacked in a vertical column (Fig. 22-4). You can feel their spinous processes in a furrow down the midline of the back. The furrow has paravertebral muscles mounded on either side down to the sacrum, where it flattens. Humans have 7 cervical, 12 thoracic, 5 lumbar, 5 sacral, and 3 or 4 coccygeal vertebrae. The following surface landmarks will orient you to their levels:

- The spinous processes of C7 and T1 are prominent at the base of the neck (see Fig. 22-4).
- The inferior angle of the scapula normally is at the level of the interspace between T7 and T8.
- An imaginary line connecting the highest point on each iliac crest crosses L4.
- An imaginary line joining the two symmetric dimples that overlie the posterior superior iliac spines crosses the sacrum.

A lateral view shows that the vertebral column has four curves (a double-S–shape) (Fig. 22-5). The cervical and lumbar curves are concave (inward or anterior), and the thoracic and

T1

T7

T8

L1

Iliac crest

Posterior
superior
iliac spine

C7

Scapula

T12

L4

S2

Coccyx

22-4   LANDMARKS OF THE SPINE

22-5

22-6   The vertebrae.

sacrococcygeal curves are convex. The balanced or compensatory nature of these curves, together with the resilient intervertebral disks, allows the spine to absorb a great deal of shock.

The **intervertebral disks** are elastic fibrocartilaginous plates that constitute one fourth of the length of the column

(Fig. 22-6). Each disk center has a **nucleus pulposus** made of soft, semifluid, mucoid material that has the consistency of toothpaste in the young adult. The disks cushion the spine like a shock absorber and help it move. As the spine moves, the elasticity of the disks allows compression on one side, with compensatory expansion on the other. Sometimes

22-7

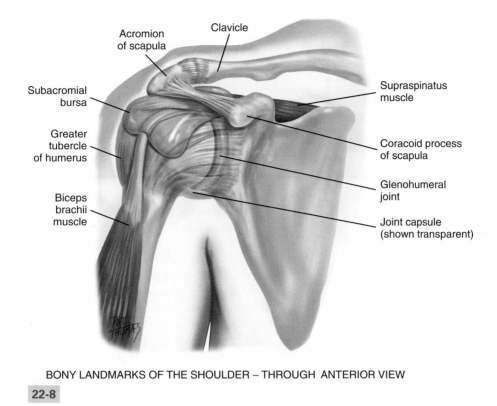

BONY LANDMARKS OF THE SHOULDER – THROUGH ANTERIOR VIEW

22-8

compression can be too great. The disk then can rupture; and the nucleus pulposus can herniate out of the vertebral column, compressing on the spinal nerves and causing pain.

The unique structure of the spine enables both upright posture and flexibility for motion. The motions of the vertebral column are flexion (bending forward), extension (bending back), abduction (to either side), and rotation.

Shoulder

The **glenohumeral joint** is the articulation of the humerus with the glenoid fossa of the scapula (Fig. 22-7). Its ball-and-socket action allows great mobility of the arm on many axes. The joint is enclosed by a group of four powerful muscles and tendons that support and stabilize it. Together these are called the **rotator cuff** of the shoulder. The large **subacromial bursa** helps during abduction of the arm, so the greater tubercle of the humerus moves easily under the acromion process of the scapula.

The bones of the shoulder have palpable landmarks to guide your examination (Fig. 22-8). The scapula and the clavicle connect to form the shoulder girdle. You can feel the bump of the scapula's **acromion process** at the very top of the shoulder. Move your fingers in a small circle outward, down, and around. The next bump is the **greater tubercle** of the humerus a few centimeters down and laterally, and from that the **coracoid process** of the scapula is a few centimeters medially. These surround the deeply situated joint.

Elbow

The elbow joint contains the three bony articulations of the humerus, radius, and ulna of the forearm (Fig. 22-9). Its

hinge action moves the forearm (radius and ulna) on one plane, allowing flexion and extension. The olecranon bursa lies between the olecranon process and the skin.

Palpable landmarks are the **medial** and **lateral epicondyles** of the humerus and the large **olecranon process** of the ulna between them. The sensitive ulnar nerve runs between the olecranon process and the medial epicondyle.

The radius and ulna articulate with one another at two radioulnar joints, one at the elbow and one at the wrist. These move together to permit pronation and supination of the hand and forearm.

22-9   RIGHT ELBOW – POSTERIOR VIEW

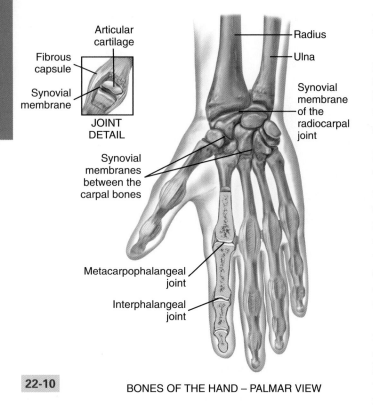

22-10   BONES OF THE HAND – PALMAR VIEW

Wrist and Carpals

Of the body's 206 bones, over half are in the hands and feet. The wrist, or **radiocarpal joint,** is the articulation of the radius (on the thumb side) and a row of carpal bones (Fig. 22-10). Its condyloid action permits movement in two planes at right angles: flexion and extension, and side-to-side devia-

tion. You can feel the groove of this joint on the dorsum of the wrist.

The **midcarpal** joint is the articulation between the two parallel rows of carpal bones. It allows flexion, extension, and some rotation. The **metacarpophalangeal** and the **interphalangeal** joints permit finger flexion and extension. The flexor tendons of the wrist and hand are enclosed in synovial sheaths.

Hip

The hip joint is the articulation between the acetabulum and the head of the femur (Fig. 22-11). As in the shoulder, ball-and-socket action permits a wide range of motion (ROM) on many axes. The hip has somewhat less ROM than the shoulder, but it has more stability as befits its weight-bearing function. Hip stability is the result of powerful muscles that spread over the joint, a strong fibrous articular capsule, and the very deep insertion of the head of the femur. Three bursae facilitate movement.

Palpation of these bony landmarks will guide your examination. You can feel the entire iliac crest, from the **anterior superior iliac spine** to the posterior. The **ischial tuberosity** lies under the gluteus maximus muscle and is palpable when the hip is flexed. The **greater trochanter** of the femur is normally the width of the person's palm below the iliac crest and halfway between the anterior superior iliac spine and the ischial tuberosity. Feel it when the person is standing, in a flat depression on the upper lateral side of the thigh.

Knee

The knee joint is the articulation of three bones—the femur, the tibia, and the patella (kneecap)—in one common articular cavity (Fig. 22-12). It is the largest joint in the body and

HIP JOINT

22-11

LEFT KNEE – MEDIAL VIEW

SAGITTAL SECTION

22-12

is complex. It is a hinge joint, permitting flexion and extension of the lower leg on a single plane.

The knee's synovial membrane is the largest in the body. It forms a sac at the superior border of the patella, called the **suprapatellar pouch** (or bursa), which extends up as much as 6 cm behind the quadriceps muscle. Two wedge-shaped cartilages, called the **medial** and **lateral menisci,** cushion the tibia and femur. The joint is stabilized by two sets of ligaments. The **cruciate ligaments** (not shown) crisscross within

the knee; they give anterior and posterior stability and help control rotation. The **collateral ligaments** connect the joint at both sides; they give medial and lateral stability and prevent dislocation. Numerous bursae prevent friction. One, the **prepatellar bursa,** lies between the patella and the skin. The **infrapatellar fat pad** is a small, triangular fat pad below the patella behind the patellar ligament.

Landmarks of the knee joint start with the large **quadriceps** muscle, which you can feel on your anterior and lateral thigh (Fig. 22-13). The muscle's four heads merge into a common tendon that continues down to enclose the round bony patella. Then the tendon inserts down on the **tibial tuberosity,** which you can feel as a bony prominence in the midline. Move to the sides and a bit superiorly and note the lateral and medial condyles of the tibia. Superior to these on either side of the patella are the medial and lateral epicondyles of the femur.

Ankle and Foot

The ankle, or **tibiotalar joint,** is the articulation of the tibia, fibula, and talus (Fig. 22-14). It is a hinge joint, limited to flexion (dorsiflexion) and extension (plantar flexion) on one plane. Landmarks are two bony prominences on either side: the **medial malleolus** and the **lateral malleolus.** Strong, tight medial and lateral ligaments extend from each malleolus onto the foot. These help the lateral stability of the ankle joint, although they may be torn in eversion or inversion sprains of the ankle.

Joints distal to the ankle give additional mobility to the foot. The subtalar joint permits inversion and eversion of the foot. The foot has a longitudinal arch, with weight-bearing distributed between the parts that touch the ground—the heads of the metatarsals and the calcaneus (heel).

LANDMARKS OF THE RIGHT KNEE JOINT

22-13

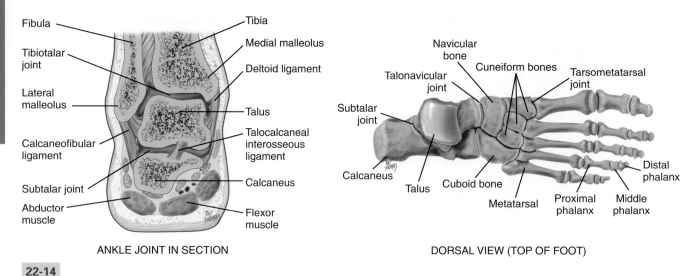

ANKLE JOINT IN SECTION

DORSAL VIEW (TOP OF FOOT)

22-14

⟡ DEVELOPMENTAL COMPETENCE

Infants and Children

By 3 months' gestation, the fetus has formed a "scale model" of the skeleton that is made up of cartilage. During succeeding months in utero, the cartilage ossifies into true bone and starts to grow. Bone growth continues after birth—rapidly during infancy and then steadily during childhood—until adolescence, when both boys and girls undergo a rapid growth spurt.

Long bones grow in two dimensions. They increase in width or diameter by deposition of new bony tissue around the shafts. Lengthening occurs at the **epiphyses,** or growth plates. These specialized growth centers are transverse disks located at the ends of long bone. Any trauma or infection at this location puts the growing child at risk for bone deformity. This longitudinal growth continues until closure of the epiphyses; the last closure occurs at about age 20 years.

Skeletal contour changes are apparent at the vertebral column. At birth the spine has a single C-shaped curve. At 3 to 4 months, raising the baby's head from prone position develops the anterior curve in the cervical neck region. From 1 year to 18 months, standing erect develops the anterior curve in the lumbar region.

Although the skeleton contributes to linear growth, muscles and fat are significant for weight increase. Individual muscle fibers grow throughout childhood, but growth is marked during the adolescent growth spurt. Then muscles respond to increased secretion of growth hormone to adrenal androgens and in boys to further stimulation by testosterone. Muscles vary in size and strength in different people. This is because of genetic programming, nutrition, and exercise. All through life muscles increase with use and atrophy with disuse.

Obesity and osteoporosis have their beginnings in young childhood. Evidence from a study of children ages 3.8 to 7.8 years showed that diets rich in dark green and deep yellow vegetables (spinach, romaine lettuce, broccoli, carrots, sweet potatoes) and low in fried foods help prevent obesity and promote bone mass accrual.[31]

The Pregnant Woman

Increased levels of circulating hormones (estrogen, relaxin from the corpus luteum, and corticosteroids) cause increased mobility in the joints. Increased mobility in the sacroiliac, sacrococcygeal, and symphysis pubis joints in the pelvis contributes to the noticeable changes in maternal posture. The most characteristic change is progressive **lordosis,** which compensates for the enlarging fetus; otherwise the center of balance would shift forward. Lordosis compensates by shifting the weight farther back on the lower extremities. This shift in balance in turn creates strain on the low back muscles, which in some women is felt as low back pain during late pregnancy.

Anterior flexion of the neck and slumping of the shoulder girdle are other postural changes that compensate for the lordosis. These upper-back changes may put pressure on the ulnar and median nerves during the third trimester. Nerve pressure creates aching, numbness, and weakness in the upper extremities in some women.

The Aging Adult

Bone **remodeling** is a cyclic process of bone resorption and deposition. The balance favors deposition until skeletal maturity at 25 to 35 years, when bone mass reaches its peak.[20] After age 40 loss of bone matrix (resorption) occurs more rapidly than new bone formation. The net effect is a gradual loss of bone density, or **osteoporosis.** Although some degree of osteoporosis is nearly universal, women have more than men because, for 5 years after menopause, the lack of estrogen leads to accelerated bone loss.

Postural changes are evident with aging, especially decreased height. Long bones do not shorten with age. Decreased height is caused by shortening of the vertebral column, which is caused by loss of water content and thinning of the intervertebral disks and by a decrease in the height of individual vertebrae from osteoporosis.

Both men and women can expect a progressive decrease in height beginning in the 40s, although this is not significant until 60 years. A greater decrease occurs in the 70s and 80s as a result of osteoporotic collapse of the vertebrae. Other postural changes are kyphosis, a backward head tilt to compensate for the kyphosis, and a slight flexion of hips and knees.

The distribution of subcutaneous fat changes through life. Usually men and women gain weight in their 40s and 50s. They begin to lose fat in the face and deposit it in the abdomen and hips. In the 80s and 90s, fat further decreases in the periphery, which is especially noticeable in the forearms and increasingly apparent over the abdomen and hips.

Loss of subcutaneous fat leaves bony prominences more marked (e.g., tips of vertebrae, ribs, iliac crests) and body hollows deeper (e.g., cheeks, axillae). An absolute loss in muscle mass occurs; some muscles decrease in size, and some atrophy, producing weakness. The contour of muscles becomes more prominent, and muscle bundles and tendons feel more distinct.

Lifestyle affects musculoskeletal changes; a sedentary lifestyle hastens musculoskeletal changes of aging. However, physical exercise increases skeletal mass and helps prevent or delay osteoporosis. Physical activity delays or prevents bone loss in postmenopausal women in a dose-dependent manner.[25] Fast walking is the best prevention for osteoporosis; the faster the pace, the higher the preventive effect on the risk for hip fracture. Physical activity also improves muscle strength to prevent falls and increase balance and posture control, decreases back pain, and increases quality of life.[25] Additional evidence shows that older adults who had a physical activity–training program with resistance, balance, and functional

training showed significant increases in strength, flexibility, heart rate after exercise, and balance.[27] Flexibility and balance remained improved at the end of 3 months of detraining.

CULTURE AND GENETICS

Substantial racial/ethnic differences exist in bone mineral density (BMD) among women in the United States and globally. A higher BMD value means a denser bone; a low BMD value is a strong and consistent predictor of hip and vertebral fracture among postmenopausal women. Evidence comparing BMD in older women in four countries showed in comparison with U.S. Caucasian women that the BMD hip site measurements were 21% to 31% higher in Afro-Caribbean women and 13% to 23% higher in African-American women, similar in Hong Kong Chinese women, and higher in South Korean women.[17] The higher BMD values confer a lower fracture risk among women of African heritage. Why such high hip BMD values for Afro-Caribbean women? Perhaps it was that they reported all their parents and grandparents to be of African ancestry with little European mixture, higher weight-bearing activity, and more sun exposure in Caribbean countries.[17]

Women have been studied regarding age at attaining peak BMD. In the spine, women of all races gained BMD up to 30 to 33 years of age.[2] But at the femoral neck in the hip joint, BMD peaked earlier among White women (≤16 years) than among African Americans (21 years) and Hispanics (20 years). An earlier peak BMD and a more rapid decline following is a trend that may explain the increased fracture risk for White women later in life. These data plus physical activity data discussed earlier suggest that weight-bearing physical activity (e.g., fast walking) is imperative during the reproductive and middle adult years to slow the process of decline in BMD.

SUBJECTIVE DATA

1. Joints
   Pain
   Stiffness
   Swelling, heat, redness
   Limitation of movement
2. Knee joint (if injured)

3. Muscles
   Pain (cramps)
   Weakness
4. Bones
   Pain
   Deformity
   Trauma (fractures, sprains, dislocations)

5. Functional assessment (ADLs)
6. Patient-centered care

Examiner Asks	Rationale
1. Joints • Any problems with your joints? Any **pain?**	**Joint pain** and loss of function are the most common musculoskeletal concerns that prompt a person to seek care.

Examiner Asks	Rationale
• Location: Which joints? On one side or both sides?	Rheumatoid arthritis (RA) involves symmetric joints; other musculoskeletal illnesses involve isolated or unilateral joints. Exquisitely tender with acute inflammation.
• Quality: What does the pain feel like: aching, stiff, sharp or dull, shooting? Severity: How strong is it? • Onset: When did it start? • Timing: What time of day does the pain occur? How long does it last? How often does it occur?	RA pain is worse in the morning when arising; osteoarthritis is worse later in the day; tendinitis is worse in the morning, improves during the day.
• Is the pain aggravated by movement, rest, position, weather? Is it relieved by rest, medications, application of heat or ice?	Movement increases most joint pain except in RA, in which movement decreases pain.
• Is the pain associated with chills, fever, recent sore throat, trauma, repetitive activity?	Joint pain 10 to 14 days after an untreated strep throat suggests rheumatic fever. Joint injury occurs from trauma or repetitive motion.
• Any **stiffness** in your joints?	RA stiffness occurs in the morning and after rest periods.
• Any **swelling, heat, redness** in the joints? • Any tick bite? • Any **limitation of movement** in any joint? Which joint? • Which activities give you problems? (See Functional Assessment on p. 587 and on p. 616.)	Suggests acute inflammation. Assess risk of Lyme disease. Decreased ROM may be caused by joint injury to cartilage or capsule or to muscle contracture.

2. Knee joint (if injury reported)

Examiner Asks	Rationale
• How did you injure your knee? Hit inside of knee? Outside? Twisting or pivoting? Overuse such as jumping or kneeling?	Inside knee injury can strain or rupture medial ligament; outside injury can strain or rupture lateral ligament; abrupt twisting can injure anterior cruciate ligament.[26]
• Hear a "pop" at injury? Can you stand on that leg? Can you flex the knee? Point to where it hurts the most.	Pop may mean tear in ligament or fracture. With direct knee trauma, obtain x-ray if the patient is unable to flex knee to 90 degrees or unable to bear weight, if pain is experienced at fibula head or patella, or if patient is over age 55 years (Ottawa knee rules).[26]

3. Muscles

Examiner Asks	Rationale
• Any problems in the muscles such as any **pain** or **cramping?** Which muscles? • If in calf muscles: Is the pain with walking? Does it go away with rest?	**Myalgia** is usually felt as cramping or aching. Suggests intermittent claudication (see Chapter 20).
• Are your muscle aches associated with fever, chills, the "flu"? • Any **weakness** in muscles? • Location: Where is the weakness? How long have you noticed it? • Do the muscles look smaller there?	Viral illness often includes myalgia. Weakness may involve musculoskeletal or neurologic systems (see Chapter 23). Atrophy.

4. Bones

Examiner Asks	Rationale
• Any **bone pain?** Is the pain affected by movement? • Any **deformity** of any bone or joint? Is the deformity caused by injury or trauma? Does it affect ROM? • Any **accidents** or **trauma** ever affected the bones or joints: fractures; joint strain, sprain, dislocation? Which ones? • When did this occur? What treatment was given? Any problems or limitations now as a result?	Fracture causes sharp pain that increases with movement. Other bone pain usually feels "dull" and "deep" and is unrelated to movement.

Examiner Asks	Rationale
• Any back pain? In which part of your back? Is pain felt anywhere else, such as shooting down leg? • Any numbness and tingling? Any limping?	
5. Functional assessment (ADLs). Do your joint (muscle, bone) problems create any limits on your usual ADLs? Which ones? (NOTE: Ask about each category; if the person answers "yes," ask specifically about each activity in category.) • Bathing—Getting in and out of the tub, turning faucets? • Toileting—Urinating, moving bowels, able to get self on/off toilet, wipe self? • Dressing—Doing buttons or zipper, fastening opening behind neck, pulling dress or sweater over head, pulling up pants, tying shoes, getting shoes that fit? • Grooming—Shaving, brushing teeth, brushing or fixing hair, applying makeup? • Eating—Preparing meals, pouring liquids, cutting up foods, bringing food to mouth, drinking? • Mobility—Walking, walking up or down stairs, getting in/out of bed, getting out of house? • Communicating—Talking, using phone, writing?	**Functional assessment** screens the safety of independent living, the need for home health services, and quality of life (see Chapter 31). Assess any self-care deficit. Impaired physical mobility. Impaired verbal communication.
6. Patient-centered care. Any occupational hazards that could affect the muscles and joints? Does your work involve heavy lifting? Or any repetitive motion or chronic stress to joints? Any efforts to alleviate these? • Tell me about your exercise program. Describe the type of exercise, frequency, the warm-up program. • Any pain during exercise? How do you treat it? • Have you had any recent weight gain? Please describe your usual daily diet. (Note the person's usual caloric intake, all four food groups, daily amount of protein, calcium.) • Are you taking any medications for musculoskeletal system: aspirin, anti-inflammatory, muscle relaxant, pain reliever? Hormone therapy? • How about supplemental medications, calcium, or vitamin D? How many dairy products eaten per day? How many over-the-counter (OTC) medications taken daily? • If person has chronic disability or crippling illness: How has your illness affected: Your interaction with family? Your interaction with friends? The way you view yourself? • How about cigarettes—How much do you smoke per day? And alcohol use—How many drinks per day? Per week?	Assess risk for back pain or carpal tunnel syndrome. A strict program of regular high-dose exercises increases bone strength and reduces fracture risk.[23] Review daily aspirin and NSAID schedule; screen for adverse effects such as GI pain. Menopausal hormone therapy (estrogen) increases BMD and reduces fracture rates, although benefits disappear in a few years once hormones are discontinued.[23] Dietary calcium is better absorbed than supplements. Serum levels of vitamin D can be checked, and supplements recommended. Assess for: • Self-esteem disturbance. • Loss of independence. • Body image disturbance. • Role performance disturbance. • Social isolation. Smoking increases bone loss and risk of fracture in older women; moderate-to-heavy alcohol drinking increases falls risk.

Subjective Data

Objective Data

Examiner Asks	Rationale

Additional History for Infants and Children

1. Were you told about any trauma to infant during labor and delivery? Did the baby's come head first? Was there a need for forceps? Did the baby need resuscitation?

   Traumatic delivery increases risk for fractures, (e.g., humerus, clavicle).
   Period of anoxia may result in hypotonia of muscles.

2. Were the baby's motor milestones achieved at about the same time as siblings or age-mates?

3. Has your child ever broken any bones? Any dislocations? How were these treated?

4. Have you ever noticed any bone deformity? Spinal curvature? Unusual shape of toes or feet? At what age? Have you ever sought treatment for any of these?

Additional History for Adolescents

1. Involved in any sports at school or after school? How frequently (times per week)? How does your sport fit in with other school demands and other activities?

   Assess safety of sport for child. Note if child's height and weight are adequate for the particular sport (e.g., football).

2. Do you use any special equipment? Does any training program exist for your sport?

   Use of safety equipment and presence of adult supervision decrease risk for sports injuries.

3. What do you do if you get hurt?

   Students may not report injury or pain for fear of limiting participation in sport.

Additional History for the Aging Adult

Use functional assessment history questions to elicit any loss of function, self-care deficit, or safety risk that may occur as a process of aging or musculoskeletal illness. (Review the complete functional assessment in Chapter 31.)

1. Any change in weakness over the past months or years? Any increase in falls or stumbling over the past months or years?

   Encourage exercise to the best of person's ability and safety.
   A history of falls increases risk of future falling.

   • Do you use any mobility aids to help you get around: cane, walker?

   The U.S. government recommends screening women ages 65 years or older for osteoporosis with a low dose x-ray called DXA. Have you had that image? Know the results? Do you have access to that test?

   Screening interval of 2 years is suggested to measure any change in BMD.[4] Recent evidence shows if baseline BMD is normal or osteopenia is mild, rescreening intervals of 15 years may suffice, and intervals of 5 years for women with moderate osteopenia.[10]

OBJECTIVE DATA

PREPARATION

The purposes of the musculoskeletal examination are to assess function for ADLs and to screen for any abnormalities. You already will have considerable data regarding ADLs through the history. Note additional ADL data as the person

EQUIPMENT NEEDED

Tape measure
Skin marking pen

goes through the motions necessary for an examination: gait; posture; how the person sits in a chair, rises from chair, takes off jacket, manipulates small object such as a pen, raises from supine.

A **screening** musculoskeletal examination suffices for most people:

- Inspection and palpation of joints integrated with each body region
- Observation of ROM as person proceeds through motions described earlier
- Age-specific screening measures such as Ortolani sign for infants or scoliosis screening for adolescents

A **complete** musculoskeletal examination as described in this chapter is appropriate for people with articular disease, a history of musculoskeletal symptoms, or any problems with ADLs.

Make the person comfortable before and throughout the examination. Drape for full visualization of the body part you are examining without needlessly exposing the person. Take an orderly approach—head to toe, proximal to distal (from the midline outward).

Support each joint at rest. Muscles must be soft and relaxed to assess the joints under them accurately. Take care when examining any inflamed area where rough manipulation could cause pain and muscle spasm. To avoid this, use firm support, gentle movement, and gentle return to a relaxed state.

Compare corresponding paired joints. Expect symmetry of structure and function and normal parameters for that joint.

Normal Range of Findings	Abnormal Findings

Order of the Examination

Inspection

Note the **size** and **contour** of every joint. Inspect the skin and tissues over the joints for **color, swelling,** and any **masses** or **deformity.** Presence of swelling is significant and signals joint irritation.

Swelling may be excess joint fluid (effusion), thickening of the synovial lining, inflammation of surrounding soft tissue (bursae, tendons), or bony enlargement.

Deformities include **dislocation** (complete loss of contact between the two bones in a joint), **subluxation** (two bones in a joint stay in contact, but their alignment is off), **contracture** (shortening of a muscle leading to limited ROM of joint), or **ankylosis** (stiffness or fixation of a joint).

Palpation

Palpate each joint, including its skin for temperature, its muscles, bony articulations, and area of joint capsule. Notice any heat, tenderness, swelling, or masses. Joints normally are not tender to palpation. If any tenderness does occur, try to localize it to specific anatomic structures (e.g., skin, muscles, bursae, ligaments, tendons, fat pads, or joint capsule).

The synovial membrane normally is not palpable. When thickened, it feels "doughy" or "boggy." A small amount of fluid is present in the normal joint, but it is not palpable.

Warmth and tenderness signal inflammation.

Palpable fluid is abnormal. Because fluid is contained in an enclosed sac, if you push on one side of the sac, the fluid will shift and cause a visible bulging on another side.

| **Normal Range of Findings** | **Abnormal Findings** |

Range of Motion

Ask for **active (voluntary) ROM** while modeling the movements yourself as appropriate; thus you can use your own movements as a control. You may stabilize the body area proximal to that being moved. Familiarize yourself with the type of each joint and its normal ROM so you can recognize limitations. If you see a limitation, gently attempt **passive motion** with the person's muscles relaxed while you move the body part. Anchor the joint with one hand while your other hand slowly moves it to its limit. The normal ranges of active and passive motion should be the same.

Joint motion normally causes no tenderness, pain, or crepitation. Do not confuse crepitation with the normal discrete "crack" heard as a tendon or ligament slips over bone during motion, such as when you do a knee bend.

Limitation in ROM is the most sensitive sign of joint disease.[14] The amount of limitation may alert you to the cause of disease. **Articular** disease (inside the joint capsule [e.g., arthritis]) produces swelling and tenderness around the whole joint, and it limits all planes of ROM in both active and passive motion. **Extra-articular** disease (injury to a specific tendon, ligament, nerve) produces swelling and tenderness to that one spot in the joint and affects only certain planes of ROM, especially during active (voluntary) motion.

Crepitation is an audible and palpable crunching or grating that accompanies movement. It occurs when the articular surfaces in the joints are roughened, as with RA (see Table 22-1, Abnormalities Affecting Multiple Joints, p. 620).

Muscle Testing

Test the strength of the prime-mover muscle groups for each joint. Repeat the motions that you elicited for active ROM. Now ask the person to flex and hold as you apply opposing force. Muscle strength should be equal bilaterally and fully resist your opposing force. (NOTE: Muscle status and joint status are interdependent and should be interpreted together. Chapter 23 discusses the examination of muscles for size and development, tone, and presence of tenderness.)

A wide variability of strength exists among people. You may wish to use a grading system from no voluntary movement to full strength, as shown.

Grade	Description	% Normal	Assessment
5	Full ROM against gravity, full resistance	100	Normal
4	Full ROM against gravity, some resistance	75	Good
3	Full ROM with gravity	50	Fair
2	Full ROM with gravity eliminated (passive motion)	25	Poor
1	Slight contraction	10	Trace
0	No contraction	0	Zero

Temporomandibular Joint

With the person seated, **inspect** the area just anterior to the ear. Place the tips of your first two fingers in front of each ear and ask the person to open and close the mouth. Drop your fingers into the depressed area over the joint and note smooth motion of the mandible. An audible and palpable snap or click occurs in many healthy people as the mouth opens (Fig. 22-15). Then ask the person to:

Swelling looks like a round bulge over the joint, although it must be moderate or marked to be visible.

Crepitus and pain occur with TMJ dysfunction.

Normal Range of Findings	**Abnormal Findings**

22-15

Instructions to Person

- Open mouth maximally.

- Partially open mouth, protrude lower jaw, and move it side to side.
- Stick out lower jaw.

Motion and Expected Range

Vertical motion. You can measure the space between the upper and lower incisors. Normal is 3 to 6 cm or three fingers inserted sideways.

Lateral motion. Normal extent is 1 to 2 cm (Fig. 22-16).

Protrude without deviation.

Lateral motion may be lost earlier and more significantly than vertical.

22-16

Palpate the contracted temporalis and masseter muscles as the person clenches the teeth. Compare right and left sides for size, firmness, and strength. Ask the person to move the jaw forward and laterally against your resistance and open mouth against resistance. This also tests the integrity of cranial nerve V (trigeminal).

Normal Range of Findings	**Abnormal Findings**

Cervical Spine

Inspect the alignment of head and neck. The spine should be straight, and the head erect. **Palpate** the spinous processes and the sternomastoid, trapezius, and paravertebral muscles. They should feel firm, with no muscle spasm or tenderness.

Ask the person to follow these motions (Fig. 22-17)*:

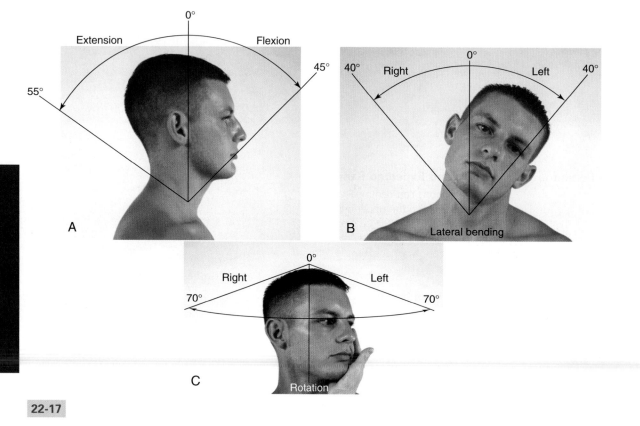

22-17

Instructions to Person	**Motion and Expected Range**
• Touch chin to chest.	Flexion of 45 degrees (Fig. 22-17, *A*).
• Lift the chin toward the ceiling.	Hyperextension of 55 degrees.
• Touch each ear toward the corresponding shoulder. Do not lift the shoulder.	Lateral bending of 40 degrees (Fig. 22-17, *B*).
• Turn the chin toward each shoulder.	Rotation of 70 degrees (Fig. 22-17, *C*).

Repeat the motions while applying opposing force. The person normally can maintain flexion against your full resistance. This also tests the integrity of cranial nerve XI (spinal).

*Do not attempt if you suspect neck trauma.

Abnormal Findings (right column):

Head tilted to one side.
Asymmetry of muscles.
Tenderness and hard muscles with muscle spasm.

Limited ROM.

Pain with movement.

The person cannot hold flexion.

Objective Data

Normal Range of Findings	Abnormal Findings

Upper Extremity

Shoulder

Inspect and compare both shoulders posteriorly and anteriorly. Check the size and contour of the joint and compare shoulders for equality of bony landmarks. Normally no redness, muscular atrophy, deformity, or swelling is present. Check the anterior aspect of the joint capsule and the subacromial bursa for abnormal swelling.

Redness.
Inequality of bony landmarks.
Atrophy, shows as lack of fullness.
Dislocated shoulder loses normal rounded shape and looks flattened laterally.
Swelling from excess fluid is best seen anteriorly. Considerable fluid must be present to cause a visible distention because the capsule normally is so loose (see Table 22-2, Shoulder Abnormalities, p. 621).
Swelling of subacromial bursa is localized under deltoid muscle and may be accentuated when the person tries to abduct the arm.

If the person reports any shoulder pain, ask that he or she point to the spot with the hand of the unaffected side. Be aware that shoulder pain may be from local causes or it may be referred pain from a hiatal hernia or a cardiac or pleural condition, which could be potentially serious. Pain from a local cause is reproducible during the examination by palpation or motion.

While standing in front of the person, **palpate** both shoulders, noting any muscular spasm or atrophy, swelling, heat, or tenderness. Start at the clavicle and methodically explore the acromioclavicular joint, scapula, greater tubercle of the humerus, area of the subacromial bursa, the biceps groove, and anterior aspect of the glenohumeral joint. Palpate the pyramid-shaped axilla; no adenopathy or masses should be present.

Swelling.
Hard muscles with muscle spasm.
Tenderness or pain.

Test ROM by asking the person to perform four motions (Fig. 22-18). Cup one hand over the shoulder during ROM to note any crepitation; normally none is present.

Objective Data

Forward flexion   180°   Up to 50°   Hyperextension   0°

Internal rotation   90°

A   B

22-18

Normal Range of Findings	**Abnormal Findings**

C

D

22-18 Continued

Instructions to Person

- With arms at sides and elbows extended, move both arms forward and up in wide vertical arcs and then move them back.
- Rotate arms internally behind back; place back of hands as high as possible toward scapulae.
- With arms at sides and elbows extended, raise both arms in wide arcs in the coronal plane. Touch palms together above head.
- Touch both hands behind the head with elbows flexed and rotated posteriorly.

Motion and Expected Range

Forward flexion of 180 degrees. Hyperextension up to 50 degrees (Fig. 22-18, *A*).

Internal rotation of 90 degrees (Fig. 22-18, *B*).

Abduction of 180 degrees. Adduction of 50 degrees (Fig. 22-18, *C*).

External rotation of 90 degrees (Fig. 22-18, *D*).

Limited ROM.
Asymmetry.
Pain with motion.

Crepitus with motion.
Rotator cuff lesions may cause limited ROM, pain, and muscle spasm during abduction; whereas forward flexion stays fairly normal.

Test the strength of the shoulder muscles by asking the person to shrug the shoulders, flex forward and up, and abduct against your resistance. The shoulder shrug also tests the integrity of cranial nerve XI, the spinal accessory.

Elbow

Inspect the size and contour of the elbow in both flexed and extended positions. Look for any deformity, redness, or swelling. Check the olecranon bursa and the normally present hollows on either side of the olecranon process for abnormal swelling.

Subluxation of the elbow shows the forearm dislocated posteriorly.
Swelling and redness of olecranon bursa are localized and easy to observe because of the close proximity of the bursa to skin.
Effusion or synovial thickening shows first as a bulge or fullness in groove on either side of the olecranon process, and it occurs with gouty arthritis.

Normal Range of Findings	Abnormal Findings

Normal Range of Findings

Palpate with the elbow flexed about 70 degrees and as relaxed as possible (Fig. 22-19). Use your left hand to support the person's left forearm and palpate the extensor surface of the elbow—the olecranon process and the medial and lateral epicondyles of the humerus—with your right thumb and fingers.

With your thumb in the lateral groove and your index and middle fingers in the medial groove, palpate either side of the olecranon process using varying pressure. Normally present tissues and fat pads feel fairly solid. Check for any synovial thickening, swelling, nodules, or tenderness.

22-19

Palpate the area of the olecranon bursa for heat, swelling, tenderness, consistency, or nodules.

Test ROM by asking the person to:

Instructions to Person

- Bend and straighten the elbow (Fig. 22-20)

- Movement of 90 degrees in pronation and supination (Fig. 22-21).

Motion and Expected Range

Flexion of 150 to 160 degrees; extension at 0. Some healthy people lack 5 to 10 degrees of full extension, and others have 5 to 10 degrees of hyperextension.

Hold the hand midway; then touch front and back sides of hand to table.

Flexion
160°
0°
Extension

22-20

0°
Pronation 90°   90° Supination

22-21

Abnormal Findings

Epicondyles, head of radius, and tendons are common sites of inflammation and local tenderness, or "tennis elbow."

Soft, boggy, or fluctuant swelling in both grooves occurs with synovial thickening or effusion.

Local heat or redness (signs of inflammation) can extend beyond synovial membrane.

Subcutaneous nodules are raised, firm, and nontender, and overlying skin moves freely. Common sites are in the olecranon bursa and along the extensor surface of the ulna. These nodules occur with RA (see Table 22-3, Elbow Abnormalities, p. 623).

Objective Data

TABLE 22-2 Shoulder Abnormalities—cont'd

Frozen Shoulder—Adhesive Capsulitis

Fibrous tissues form in the joint capsule, causing stiffness, progressive limitation of motion, and pain. Motion limited in abduction and external rotation; unable to reach overhead. It may lead to atrophy of shoulder girdle muscles. Gradual onset; unknown cause. It is associated with prolonged bed rest or shoulder immobility. May resolve spontaneously.

Subacromial Bursitis

Inflammation and swelling of subacromial bursa over the shoulder cause limited ROM and pain with motion. Localized swelling under deltoid muscle may increase by partial passive abduction of the arm. Caused by direct trauma, strain during sports, local or systemic inflammatory process, or repetitive motion with injury.

See Illustration Credits for source information.

TABLE 22-3 Elbow Abnormalities

Olecranon Bursitis

Large, soft knob, or "goose egg," and redness from inflammation of olecranon bursa. Localized and easy to see because bursa lies just under skin.

Gouty Arthritis

Joint effusion or synovial thickening, seen first as bulge or fullness in grooves on either side of olecranon process. Redness and heat can extend beyond area of synovial membrane. Soft, boggy, or fluctuant fullness to palpation. Limited extension of elbow.

TABLE 22-3   Elbow Abnormalities—cont'd

Subcutaneous Nodules

Raised, firm, nontender nodules that occur with rheumatoid arthritis. Common sites are in the olecranon bursa and along extensor surface of arm. The skin slides freely over the nodules.

Epicondylitis—Tennis Elbow

Chronic disabling pain at lateral epicondyle (LE) of humerus; radiates down extensor surface of forearm. Pain can be located with one finger. Resisting extension of the hand increases the pain. Occurs with activities combining excessive pronation and supination of forearm with an extended wrist (e.g., racquet sports or using a screwdriver).

See Illustration Credits for source information.

TABLE 22-4   Wrist and Hand Abnormalities

Ganglion Cyst

Round, cystic, nontender nodule overlying a tendon sheath or joint capsule, usually on dorsum of wrist. Flexion makes it more prominent. The fluid-filled mass is more common in women ages 30 to 60 years. Nonpainful ganglion cysts are a cosmetic concern; painful ones may compress the median or ulnar nerve, causing numbness and tingling or weakness.

Colles Fracture (not illustrated)

Nonarticular fracture of distal radius, with or without fracture of ulna at styloid process. Usually from a fall on an outstretched hand; occurs more often in older women. Wrist looks puffy with "silver fork" deformity, a characteristic hump when viewed from the side.

Carpal Tunnel Syndrome With Atrophy of Thenar Eminence

Atrophy occurs from interference with motor function from compression of the median nerve inside the carpal tunnel. Caused by chronic repetitive motion; occurs between 40 and 60 years and is more common in women. Symptoms of carpal tunnel syndrome include pain, burning and numbness, positive findings on Phalen test, positive Tinel sign, and often atrophy of thenar muscles.

Continued

Abnormal Findings

TABLE 22-4 Wrist and Hand Abnormalities—cont'd

Ankylosis

Wrist in extreme flexion with ruptures of wrist and finger extensors, caused by severe rheumatoid arthritis (RA). This is a functionally compromised hand because, when the wrist is palmar flexed, a good deal of power is lost from the fingers, and often the thumb cannot oppose the fingers.

Dupuytren Contracture

Chronic hyperplasia of the palmar fascia causes flexion contractures of the digits, first in the 4th digit, then the 5th digit, and then the 3rd digit. Note the bands that extend from the midpalm to the digits and the puckering of palmar skin. The condition occurs commonly in men older than 40 years and is usually bilateral. It occurs with diabetes, epilepsy, and alcoholic liver disease and as an inherited trait. The contracture is painless but impairs hand function.

Conditions Caused by Chronic Rheumatoid Arthritis

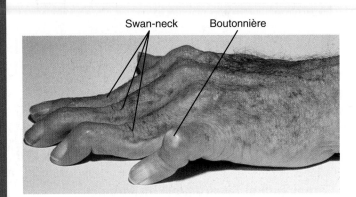

Swan-neck   Boutonnière

Swan-Neck and Boutonnière Deformity

Flexion contracture resembles curve of a **swan's neck**, as in metacarpophalangeal joint. Then hyperextension of the proximal interphalangeal joint, and flexion of the distal interphalangeal joint. It occurs with chronic RA and is often accompanied by ulnar drift of the fingers. In **boutonnière deformity** the knuckle looks as if it is being pushed through a buttonhole. It is a common deformity and includes flexion of the proximal interphalangeal joint with compensatory hyperextension of distal interphalangeal joint.

Ulnar Deviation or Drift

Fingers drift to the ulnar side because of stretching of the articular capsule and muscle imbalance. Also note subluxation and swelling in the joints and muscle atrophy on the dorsa of the hands. This is caused by chronic RA.

TABLE 22-4   Wrist and Hand Abnormalities—cont'd

Osteoarthritis (OA)

Different from RA, OA is characterized by hard, nontender, noninflammatory nodules, 2 to 3 mm or more. These osteophytes (bony overgrowths) of the distal interphalangeal joints are called *Heberden nodes*. Those of the proximal interphalangeal joints are called *Bouchard nodes* and are less common.

Acute Rheumatoid Arthritis

Painful swelling and stiffness of joints, with fusiform or spindle-shaped swelling of the soft tissue of proximal interphalangeal joints. Fusiform swelling is usually symmetric, the hands are warm, and the veins are engorged. The inflamed joints have a limited range of motion.

Polydactyly

Extra digits are a congenital deformity, usually occurring at the 5th finger or the thumb. Surgical removal is considered for cosmetic appearance. The 6th finger shown here was not removed because it had full ROM and sensation and a normal appearance.

Syndactyly

Webbed fingers are a congenital deformity, usually requiring surgical separation. The metacarpals and phalanges of the webbed fingers are different lengths, and the joints do not line up. To leave the fingers fused would thus limit their flexion and extension.

◀ Gout in Thumb

See explanation in Table 22-6.

See Illustration Credits for source information.

TABLE 22-5   **Knee Abnormalities**

Osgood-Schlatter Disease

Painful swelling of the tibial tubercle just below the knee, probably from repeated stress on the patellar tendon. Occurs most in puberty during rapid growth and most often in males. Pain increases with kicking, running, bike riding, stair climbing, or kneeling. The condition is usually self-limited, and symptoms resolve with rest.

Post-Polio Muscle Atrophy

Right leg and foot muscle atrophy as a result of childhood polio. Poliomyelitis epidemics peaked in the United States in the 1940s and 1950s. The development of the oral polio vaccine (1962) has almost eradicated the disease. However, thousands of polio survivors have this muscle atrophy.

Mild Synovitis

Loss of normal hollows on either side of the patella, which are replaced by mild distention. Occurs with synovial thickening or effusion (excess fluid). Also note mild distention of the suprapatellar pouch.

Prepatellar Bursitis

Localized swelling on anterior knee between patella and skin. A tender, fluctuant mass indicates swelling; infection may spread to surrounding soft tissue. The condition is limited to the bursa, and the knee joint itself is not involved. Overlying skin may be red, shiny, atrophic, or coarse and thickened.

TABLE 22-5   Knee Abnormalities—cont'd

◀ Swelling of Menisci

Localized soft swelling from cyst in lateral meniscus shows at the midpoint of the anterolateral joint line. Semiflexion of the knee makes swelling more prominent.

See Illustration Credits for source information.

TABLE 22-6   Ankle and Foot Abnormalities

Achilles Tenosynovitis

Inflammation of a tendon sheath near the ankle (here the Achilles tendon) produces a superficial linear swelling and a localized tenderness along the route of the sheath. Movement of the involved tendon usually causes pain.

Tophi with Chronic Gout

Hard, painless nodule (tophi) over metatarsophalangeal joint of first toe. Tophi are collections of sodium urate crystals caused by chronic gout in and around the joint that cause extreme swelling and joint deformity. They sometimes burst with a chalky discharge.

◀ Acute Gout

Gout is a common chronic arthritis characterized by excess uric acid in the blood and deposits of urate crystals in the joint space. Acute episodes involve history of unusual walking with joint injury, alcohol intake, and dehydration; episodes are characterized by redness, swelling, heat, and extreme pain such as a continuous throbbing. Increased prevalence is caused by increases in obesity, metabolic syndrome, and diuretic use.[13]

Continued

TABLE 22-6 Ankle and Foot Abnormalities—cont'd

Hallux Valgus with Bunion and Hammertoes

Hallux valgus, a common deformity from RA, is a lateral or outward deviation of the great toe with medial prominence of the head of the 1st metatarsal. The **bunion** is the inflamed bursa that forms at the pressure point. The great toe loses power to push off while walking; this stresses the 2nd and 3rd metatarsal heads, and they develop calluses and pain. Chronic sequelae include corns, calluses, hammertoes, and joint subluxation.

Note the **hammertoe** deformities in the 2nd, 3rd, 4th, and 5th toes that include hyperextension of the metatarsophalangeal joint and flexion of the proximal interphalangeal joint. **Corns** (thickening of soft tissue) develop on the dorsum over the bony prominence from prolonged pressure from shoes.

Callus

Hypertrophy of the epithelium develops because of prolonged pressure, commonly on the plantar surface of the 1st metatarsal head in the hallux valgus deformity or as shown here, dorsally over the bony prominences of the joints in hammertoes. The condition is not painful.

Ingrown Toenail

A misnomer; the nail does not grow in, but the soft tissue grows over the nail and obliterates the groove. It occurs almost always on the great toe on the medial or lateral side. It is caused by trimming the nail too short or toe crowding in tight shoes. The area becomes infected when the nail grows and its corner penetrates the soft tissue.

Plantar Wart

Vascular papillomatous growth is probably caused by a virus and occurs on the sole of the foot, commonly at the ball. The condition is extremely painful.

See Illustration Credits for source information.

TABLE 22-7   Spine Abnormalities

◄ Scoliosis

Lateral curvature of thoracic and lumbar segments of the spine, usually with some rotation of involved vertebral bodies.

Functional scoliosis is flexible; it is apparent with standing and disappears with forward bending. It may be compensatory for other abnormalities such as leg length discrepancy.

Structural scoliosis is fixed; the curvature shows both on standing and on bending forward. Note rib hump with forward flexion. When the person is standing, note unequal shoulder elevation, unequal scapulae, obvious curvature, and unequal hip level. More common in females 10 years of age through adolescence during the peak of the growth spurt.

Herniated Nucleus Pulposus   ▶

The nucleus pulposus (at the center of the intervertebral disk) ruptures into the spinal canal and puts pressure on the local spinal nerve root. Usually occurs from stress such as lifting, twisting, continuous flexion with lifting, or fall on buttocks. Occurs mostly in men 20 to 45 years of age. Lumbar herniations occur mainly in interspaces L4 to L5 and L5 to S1. NOTE: Sciatic pain, numbness, and paresthesia of involved dermatome; listing away from affected side; decreased mobility; low back tenderness; and decreased motor and sensory function in leg. Straight leg raising tests reproduce sciatic pain.

See Illustration Credits for source information.

TABLE 22-8   Congenital or Pediatric Abnormalities

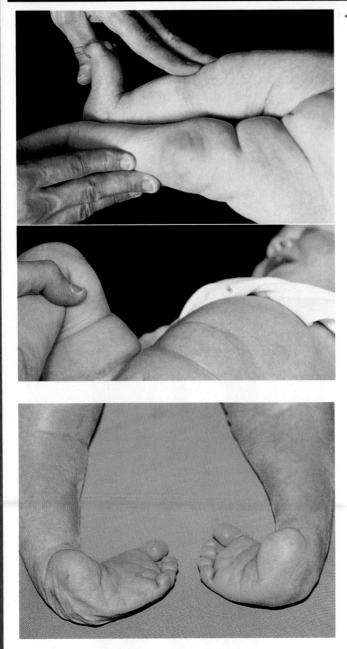

◀ **Congenital Dislocated Hip**

Head of the femur is displaced out of the cup-shaped acetabulum. The degree of the condition varies; subluxation may occur as stretched ligaments allow partial displacement of femoral head, and acetabular dysplasia may develop because of excessive laxity of hip joint capsule.

Occurrence is 1:500 to 1:1000 births; common in girls by 7:1 ratio. Signs include limited abduction of flexed thigh, positive indications of Ortolani and Barlow signs, asymmetric skin creases or gluteal folds, limb length discrepancy, and positive indication of Trendelenburg sign in older children.

Talipes Equinovarus (Clubfoot)

Congenital, rigid, and fixed malposition of foot, including (1) inversion, (2) forefoot adduction, and (3) foot pointing downward (equinus). A common birth defect, with an incidence of 1:1000 to 3:1000 live births. Males are affected twice as frequently as females.

Spina Bifida

Incomplete closure of posterior part of vertebrae results in a neural tube defect. Seriousness varies from skin defect along the spine to protrusion of the sac containing meninges, spinal fluid, or malformed spinal cord. The most serious type is myelomeningocele (shown here), in which the meninges and neural tissue protrude. In these cases the child is usually paralyzed below the level of the lesion.

Coxa Plana (Legg-Calvé-Perthes Syndrome) (not illustrated)

Avascular necrosis of the femoral head, occurring primarily in males between 3 and 12 years of age, with peak at age 6 years. In initial inflammatory stage interruption of blood supply to femoral epiphysis occurs, halting growth. Revascularization and healing occur later, but significant residual deformity and dysfunction may be present.

See Illustration Credits for source information.

TABLE 22-9   Fibromyalgia Syndrome

1990 Criteria

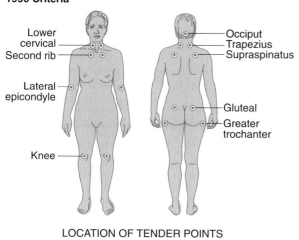

LOCATION OF TENDER POINTS

◀ Chronic disorder of unknown cause with widespread musculoskeletal pain lasting >3 months, associated with fatigue, insomnia, and psychosocial distress. Most (90%) are adult women. The 1990 diagnostic criteria included: (1) pain on both sides of the body, above and below the waist, and axial skeletal pain (cervical, thoracic, lumbar spine, or anterior chest); and (2) point tenderness on digital palpation in 11 of 18 specified sites shown here, included with a force of 4 kg (same as needed to blanch or whiten the nail bed). These criteria have since been criticized because it was not possible to measure 4 kg of force from the examiner's thumb; thus the physical examination was unreliable.

The 2010 revised criteria stopped the tender point count and substituted interview criteria.[30] These include a widespread pain index or a 0-19 count of the person's report of the number of painful body regions. The 2010 criteria also assess characteristic symptoms (fatigue, nonrefreshed sleep, cognitive problems, somatic symptoms) on a 0-3 severity scale.

© Pat Thomas, 2010.

Abnormal Findings

Summary Checklist: Musculoskeletal Examination

For each joint to be examined:
1. **Inspection**
   Size and contour of joint
   Skin color and characteristics
2. **Palpation of joint area**
   Skin
   Muscles

Bony articulations
Joint capsule
3. **ROM**
   Active
   Passive (if limitation in active ROM is present)

Measure with goniometer (if abnormality in ROM is present)
4. **Muscle testing**

BIBLIOGRAPHY

1. Antonelli, M. C., & Starz, T. W. (2012). Assessing for risk and progression of osteoarthritis. *Am J Nurs, 112*(3), S26-S31.
2. Berenson, A. B., Rahman, M., & Wilkinson, G. (2009). Racial difference in the correlates of bone mineral content/density and age at peak among reproductive-aged women. *Osteopor Int, 20*(8), 1439-1449.
3. Bolland, M. J., Grey, A., Avenell, A., et al. (2011). Calcium supplements with or without vitamin D and risk of cardiovascular events. *Br Med J, 342*, 1-9.
4. Calonge, N., et al. Screening for osteoporosis. (2011). *Ann Intern Med, 154*(5), 356-364.
5. Copstead L., & Banasik J. (2013). *Pathophysiology.* (5th ed.) St. Louis: Elsevier.
6. Corrarino, J. E. (2012). Stress fractures in runners. *Nurse Pract, 37*(6), 18-28.
7. Dadabhoy, D., McCarberg, B., & Hassett, A. L. (2010). Managing fibromyalgia in primary care. *Prim Psychiatry, 17*(2), 2-16.
8. Dewing, K., Belza, B., Zierler, B., et al. (2013). Health maintenance module improves BMD testing. *Nurse Pract, 38*(4), 37-41.
9. Firestone, K. A., Holton, K., Mist, S. D., et al. (2012). Optimizing fibromyalgia management. *Nurse Pract, 37*(4), 13-21.
10. Gourlay, M. L., Fine, J. P., Preisser, J. S., et al. (2012). Bone-density testing interval and transition to osteoporosis in older women. *N Engl J Med, 366*(3), 225-233.
11. Hardy, E. (2011). Gout diagnosis and management: what NPs need to know. *Nurse Pract, 36*(6), 14-19.
12. Hresko, M. T. (2013). Idiopathic scoliosis in adolescents. *N Engl J Med, 368*(9), 834-841.
13. Kessenich, C. R. (2011). Uric acid and gout. *Nurse Pract, 36*(3), 11-12.
14. McGee, S. (2012). *Evidence-based physical diagnosis.* (3rd ed.). St. Louis: Saunders.
15. McInnes, I. B., & Schett, G. (2011). The pathogenesis of rheumatoid arthritis. *N Eng J Med, 365*(23), 2205-2219.

16. Moyer, V. A. (2012). Prevention of falls in community-dwelling older adults. *Ann Intern Med, 157*(3), 197-204.

17. Nam, H. S., Kweon, S. S., Choi, J. S. et al. (2013). Racial/ethnic differences in bone mineral density among older women. *J Bone Mineral Metabol, 31*(2), 190-198.

18. Palumbo, A., & Anderson, K. (2011). Multiple myeloma. *N Engl J Med, 364,* 1046-1060.

19. Peltola, H., & Paakkonen, M. (2014). Acute osteomyelitis in children. *N Engl J Med, 370*(4), 352-360.

20. Pigozzi, E., Rizzo, M., Giombini, A., et al. (2009). Bone mineral density and sport: effect of physical activity. *J Sports Med Phys Fitness, 49*(2), 177-183.

21. Ralston, S. H. (2013). Paget's disease of bone. *N Engl J Med, 368*(7), 644-650.

22. Rosen, C. J. (2011). Vitamin D insufficiency. *N Engl J Med, 364*(3), 248-254.

23. Roush K. (2011). Prevention and treatment of osteoporosis in postmenopausal women: review. *Am J Nurs 111*(8), 26-37.

24. Salt, E., & Crofford, L. (2012). Rheumatoid arthritis: new treatments, better outcomes. *Nurse Pract, 37*(11), 16-22.

25. Schmitt, N. M., Schmitt, J., & Doren, M. (2009). The role of physical activity in the prevention of osteoporosis in postmenopausal women. *Maturitas, 63*(1), 34-38.

26. Schraeder, T. L., Terek, R. M., & Smith, C. C. (2010). Clinical evaluation of the knee. *N Engl J Med, 363*(4).

27. Seco, J., Abecia, L. C., & Echevarría, E., et al. (2013). A long-term physical activity training program increases strength and flexibility, and improves balance in older adults. *Rehabil Nurs, 38*(1), 37-47.

28. Shelton, L. R. (2013). A closer look at osteoarthritis. *Nurse Pract, 38*(7), 30-36.

29. U.S. Preventive Services Task Force. (2005). Screening for idiopathic scoliosis for adolescents. *Am Fam Physician, 71,* 1975-1976.

30. Wolfe, F., & Hauser, W. (2011). Fibromyalgia diagnosis and diagnostic criteria. *Ann Med, 4*(7), 495-502.

31. Wosje, K. S., Khoury, P. R., & Claytor, R. P., et al. (2010). Dietary patterns associated with fat and bone mass in young children. *Am J Clin Nutr, 92*(2), 294-303.

32. Zychowicz, M. E. (2013). A closer look at hand and wrist complaints. *Nurse Pract, 38*(3), 46-53.

CHAPTER 23

Neurologic System

STRUCTURE AND FUNCTION

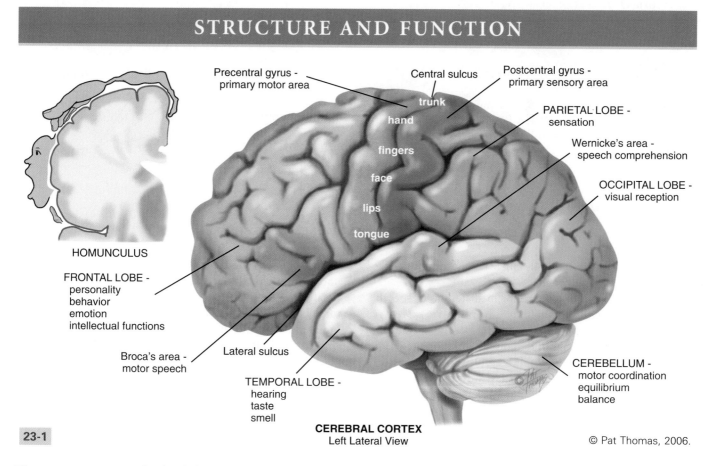

Precentral gyrus -
primary motor area

Central sulcus

Postcentral gyrus -
primary sensory area

trunk
hand
fingers
face
lips
tongue

PARIETAL LOBE -
sensation

Wernicke's area -
speech comprehension

OCCIPITAL LOBE -
visual reception

HOMUNCULUS

FRONTAL LOBE -
personality
behavior
emotion
intellectual functions

Broca's area -
motor speech

Lateral sulcus

TEMPORAL LOBE -
hearing
taste
smell

CEREBELLUM -
motor coordination
equilibrium
balance

CEREBRAL CORTEX
Left Lateral View

© Pat Thomas, 2006.

23-1

The nervous system can be divided into two parts: central and peripheral. The **central nervous system** (CNS) includes the brain and spinal cord. The **peripheral nervous system** includes all the nerve fibers *outside* the brain and spinal cord: the 12 pairs of cranial nerves, the 31 pairs of spinal nerves, and all their branches. The peripheral nervous system carries sensory (**afferent**) messages *to* the CNS from sensory receptors, motor (**efferent**) messages *from* the CNS out to muscles and glands, and autonomic messages that govern the internal organs and blood vessels.

THE CENTRAL NERVOUS SYSTEM

Cerebral Cortex. The cerebral cortex is the outer layer of nerve cell bodies; it looks like "gray matter" because it lacks myelin. Myelin is the white insulation on the axon that increases the conduction velocity of nerve impulses.

The cerebral cortex is the center for a human's highest functions, governing thought, memory, reasoning, sensation,

and voluntary movement (Fig. 23-1). Each half of the cerebrum is a **hemisphere;** the left hemisphere is dominant in most (95%) people, including those who are left-handed.

Each hemisphere is divided into four **lobes:** frontal, parietal, temporal, and occipital. The lobes have certain areas that mediate specific functions.

- The **frontal** lobe has areas concerned with personality, behavior, emotions, and intellectual function.
- The precentral gyrus of the frontal lobe initiates voluntary movement.
- The **parietal** lobe's postcentral gyrus is the primary center for sensation.
- The **occipital** lobe is the primary visual receptor center.
- The **temporal** lobe behind the ear has the primary auditory reception center, with functions of hearing, taste, and smell.
- **Wernicke's area** in the temporal lobe is associated with language comprehension. When damaged in the person's dominant hemisphere, *receptive aphasia* results.

633

Plane of coronal section B

Corpus callosum

Thalamus

Internal capsule

Hypothalamus

Pituitary

BRAINSTEM

Midbrain
Pons
Cerebellum
Medulla
Spinal cord

Basal ganglia

Hypothalamus

A. Medial view of right hemisphere

B. Coronal section

23-2   **COMPONENTS OF THE CENTRAL NERVOUS SYSTEM**   © Pat Thomas, 2006.

The person hears sound, but it has no meaning, like hearing a foreign language.

- **Broca's area** in the frontal lobe mediates motor speech. When injured in the dominant hemisphere, *expressive aphasia* results; the person cannot talk. The person can understand language and knows what he or she wants to say but can produce only a garbled sound.

Damage to any of these specific cortical areas produces a corresponding loss of function: motor weakness, paralysis, loss of sensation, or impaired ability to understand and process language. Damage occurs when the highly specialized neurologic cells are deprived of their blood supply such as when a cerebral artery becomes occluded (ischemic stroke) or when vascular bleeding (hemorrhagic stroke) occurs.

Basal Ganglia. The basal ganglia are large bands of gray matter buried deep within the two cerebral hemispheres that form the subcortical-associated motor system (the extrapyramidal system) (Fig. 23-2). They help to initiate and coordinate movement and control automatic associated movements of the body (e.g., the arm swing alternating with the legs during walking).

Thalamus. The thalamus is the main relay station where the sensory pathways of the spinal cord, cerebellum, basal ganglia, and brainstem form **synapses** (sites of contact between two neurons) on their way to the cerebral cortex. It is an integrating center with connections that are crucial to human emotion and creativity.

Hypothalamus. The hypothalamus is a major respiratory center with basic vital functions: temperature, appetite, sex drive, heart rate, and blood pressure (BP) control; sleep center; anterior and posterior pituitary gland regulator; and coordinator of autonomic nervous system activity and stress response.

Cerebellum. The cerebellum is a coiled structure located under the occipital lobe that is concerned with motor coordination of voluntary movements, equilibrium (i.e., the postural balance of the body), and muscle tone. It does not initiate movement but coordinates and smooths it (e.g., the complex and quick coordination of many different muscles needed in playing the piano, swimming, or juggling). It is like the "automatic pilot" on an airplane in that it adjusts and corrects the voluntary movements but operates entirely below the conscious level.

Brainstem. The brainstem is the central core of the brain consisting of mostly nerve fibers. Cranial nerves III through XII originate from nuclei in the brainstem. It has three areas:

1. **Midbrain**—The most anterior part of the brainstem that still has the basic tubular structure of the spinal cord. It merges into the thalamus and hypothalamus. It contains many motor neurons and tracts.

2. **Pons**—The enlarged area containing ascending sensory and descending motor tracts. It has two respiratory centers (pneumotaxic and apneustic) that coordinate with the main respiratory center in the medulla.

3. **Medulla**—The continuation of the spinal cord in the brain that contains all ascending and descending fiber tracts. It has vital autonomic centers (respiration, heart, gastrointestinal function) and nuclei for cranial nerves VIII through XII. Pyramidal decussation (crossing of the motor fibers) occurs here (see p. 636).

Spinal Cord. The spinal cord is the long, cylindric structure of nervous tissue about as big around as your little finger. It occupies the upper two thirds of the vertebral canal from the medulla to lumbar vertebrae L1-L2. Its white matter is bundles of myelinated axons that form the main highway for ascending and descending fiber tracts that connect the brain to the spinal nerves. It mediates reflexes of posture control, urination, and pain response. Its nerve cell bodies, or gray matter, are arranged in a butterfly shape with anterior and posterior "horns."

The vertebral canal continues down beyond the spinal cord for several inches. The lumbar cistern is inside this space and is the favored spot to withdraw samples of cerebrospinal fluid (CSF).

Pathways of the CNS

Crossed representation is a notable feature of the nerve tracts; the *left* cerebral cortex receives sensory information from and controls motor function to the *right* side of the body, whereas *the right* cerebral cortex likewise interacts with the *left* side of the body. Knowledge of where the fibers cross the midline helps you interpret clinical findings.

Sensory Pathways

Millions of sensory receptors are embroidered into the skin, mucous membranes, muscles, tendons, and viscera. They monitor conscious sensation, internal organ functions, body position, and reflexes. Sensation travels in the afferent fibers in the peripheral nerve, through the posterior (dorsal) root,

and into the spinal cord. There it may take one of two routes: the anterolateral or spinothalamic tract, or the posterior (dorsal) columns (Fig. 23-3).

Spinothalamic Tract. The spinothalamic tract contains sensory fibers that transmit the sensations of pain, temperature, and crude or light touch (i.e., not precisely localized). The fibers enter the dorsal root of the spinal cord and synapse with a second sensory neuron. The second-order neuron fibers cross to the opposite side and ascend up the spinothalamic tract to the thalamus. Fibers carrying pain and temperature sensations ascend the lateral spinothalamic tract, whereas those of crude touch form the anterior spinothalamic tract. At the thalamus the fibers synapse with a third sensory neuron, which carries the message to the sensory cortex for full interpretation.

Posterior (Dorsal) Columns. These fibers conduct the sensations of position, vibration, and finely localized touch.

- **Position** (proprioception)—Without looking you know where your body parts are in space and in relation to one another.
- **Vibration**—You can feel vibrating objects
- **Finely localized touch** (stereognosis)—Without looking you can identify familiar objects by touch

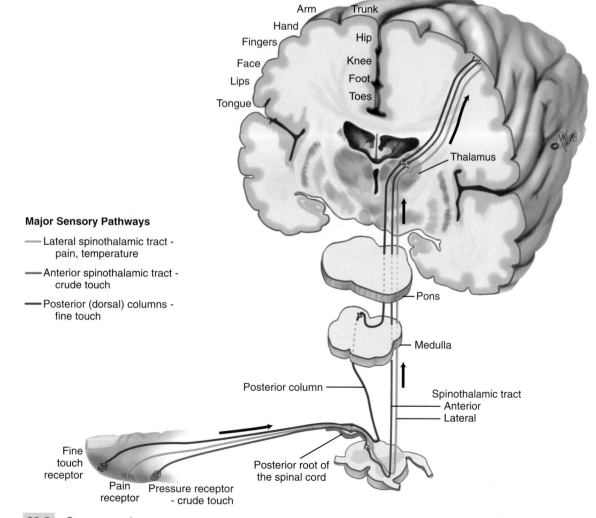

Major Sensory Pathways

— Lateral spinothalamic tract - pain, temperature

— Anterior spinothalamic tract - crude touch

— Posterior (dorsal) columns - fine touch

23-3 Sensory pathways.

© Pat Thomas, 2006.

Structure and Function

These fibers enter the dorsal root and proceed immediately up the same side of the spinal cord to the brainstem. At the medulla they synapse with a second sensory neuron and then cross. They travel to the **thalamus,** synapse again, and proceed to the sensory cortex, which localizes the sensation and makes full discrimination.

The sensory cortex is arranged in a specific pattern forming a corresponding "map" of the body (see the homunculus in Fig. 23-1). Pain in the right hand is perceived at its specific spot on the left cortex map. Some organs are absent from the brain map such as the heart, liver, or spleen. You know you have one but you have no "felt image" of it. Pain originating in these organs is referred because no felt image exists in which to have pain. Pain is felt "by proxy" by another body part that does have a felt image. For example, pain in the heart is referred to the chest, shoulder, and left arm, which were its neighbors in fetal development. Pain originating in the spleen is felt on the top of the left shoulder.

Motor Pathways

Corticospinal or Pyramidal Tract (Fig. 23-4). The area has been named *pyramidal* because it originates in pyramidal-shaped cells in the motor cortex. Motor nerve fibers originate in the motor cortex and travel to the brainstem, where they cross to the opposite or contralateral side *(pyramidal decus-sation)* and then pass down in the lateral column of the spinal cord. At each cord level they synapse with a lower motor neuron contained in the anterior horn of the spinal cord. Ten percent of corticospinal fibers do not cross, and these descend in the anterior column of the spinal cord. Corticospinal fibers mediate voluntary movement, particularly very skilled, discrete, purposeful movements such as writing.

The corticospinal tract is a newer, "higher" motor system that permits humans to have very skilled and purposeful movements. The origin of the tract in the motor cortex is arranged in a specific pattern called *somatotopic organization.* It is another body map, this one of a person, or *homunculus,* hanging "upside down" (see Fig. 23-1). Body parts are not equally represented on the map, and the homunculus looks distorted. To use political terms, it is more like an electoral map than a geographic map. That is, body parts with movements that are relatively more important to humans (e.g., the hand) occupy proportionally more space on the brain map.

Extrapyramidal Tracts. The extrapyramidal tracts include all the motor nerve fibers originating in the motor cortex, basal ganglia, brainstem, and spinal cord that are *outside* the pyramidal tract. This is a phylogenetically older, "lower," more primitive motor system. These subcortical motor fibers maintain muscle tone and control body movements, especially gross automatic movements such as walking.

Major Motor Pathways

— Corticospinal crossed tract

— Corticospinal uncrossed tract

— Extrapyramidal tracts

23-4
Motor pathways.

© Pat Thomas, 2006.

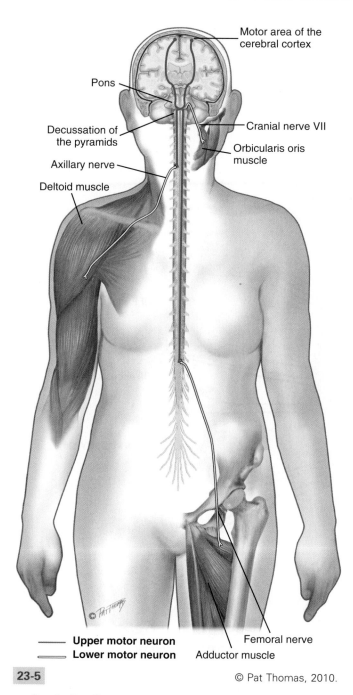

Upper motor neuron
Lower motor neuron

Motor area of the cerebral cortex
Pons
Decussation of the pyramids
Axillary nerve
Deltoid muscle
Cranial nerve VII
Orbicularis oris muscle
Femoral nerve
Adductor muscle

23-5   © Pat Thomas, 2010.

Cerebellar System. This complex motor system coordinates movement, maintains equilibrium, and helps maintain posture. The cerebellum receives information about the position of muscles and joints, the equilibrium of the body, and what kind of motor messages are being sent from the cortex to the muscles. The information is integrated, and the cerebellum uses feedback pathways to exert its control back on the cortex or down to lower motor neurons in the spinal cord. This entire process occurs on a subconscious level.

Upper and Lower Motor Neurons

Upper motor neurons (UMN) are a complex of all the descending motor fibers that can influence or modify the lower motor neurons. They are located completely within the CNS. The UMNs convey impulses from motor areas of the cerebral cortex to the lower motor neurons in the anterior

horn cells of the spinal cord (Fig. 23-5). Examples of UMNs are corticospinal, corticobulbar, and extrapyramidal tracts. Examples of UMN diseases are stroke, cerebral palsy, and multiple sclerosis.

Lower motor neurons (LMN) are located mostly in the peripheral nervous system. The cell body of the LMN is located in the anterior gray column of the spinal cord, but the nerve fiber extends from here to the muscle. The LMN is the "final common pathway" because it funnels many neural signals here and provides the final direct contact with the muscles. Any movement must be translated into action by LMN fibers. Examples of LMNs are cranial nerves and spinal nerves of the peripheral nervous system. Examples of LMN diseases are spinal cord lesions, poliomyelitis, and amyotrophic lateral sclerosis.

THE PERIPHERAL NERVOUS SYSTEM

A **nerve** is a bundle of fibers *outside* the CNS. The peripheral nerves carry input to the CNS via their sensory afferent fibers and deliver output from the CNS via the efferent fibers.

Reflex Arc

Reflexes are basic defense mechanisms of the nervous system. They are involuntary, operating below the level of conscious control and permitting a quick reaction to potentially painful or damaging situations. Reflexes also help the body maintain balance and appropriate muscle tone. There are four types of reflexes: (1) **Deep tendon reflexes** (myotatic), e.g., patellar (or knee jerk); (2) **superficial**, e.g., corneal reflex, abdominal reflex; (3) **visceral** (organic), e.g., pupillary response to light and accommodation; and (4) **pathologic** (abnormal), e.g., Babinski (or extensor plantar) reflex.

The fibers that mediate the reflex are carried by a specific spinal nerve. In the simplest reflex tapping the tendon stretches the muscle spindles in the muscle, which activates the sensory afferent nerve. The sensory afferent fibers carry the message from the receptor and travel through the dorsal root into the spinal cord (Fig. 23-6). They synapse directly in

Cell body in dorsal root ganglion
Sensory nerve
Muscle spindle
Motor nerve
Patellar tendon

23-6   REFLEX ARC

the cord with the motor neuron in the anterior horn. Motor efferent fibers leave via the ventral root and travel to the muscle, stimulating a sudden contraction.

The deep tendon (myotatic, or stretch) reflex has five components: (1) an intact sensory nerve (afferent); (2) a functional synapse in the cord; (3) an intact motor nerve fiber (efferent); (4) the neuromuscular junction; and (5) a competent muscle.

Cranial Nerves

Cranial nerves are LMNs that enter and exit the brain rather than the spinal cord (Fig. 23-7). Cranial nerves I and II extend

Cranial Nerve	Type	Function
I: Olfactory	Sensory	Smell
II: Optic	Sensory	Vision
III: Oculomotor	Mixed*	Motor—most EOM movement, opening of eyelids Parasympathetic—pupil constriction, lens shape
IV: Trochlear	Motor	Down and inward movement of eye
V: Trigeminal	Mixed	Motor—muscles of mastication Sensory—sensation of face and scalp, cornea, mucous membranes of mouth and nose
VI: Abducens	Motor	Lateral movement of eye
VII: Facial	Mixed	Motor—facial muscles, close eye, labial speech, close mouth Sensory—taste (sweet, salty, sour, bitter) on anterior two thirds of tongue Parasympathetic—saliva and tear secretion
VIII: Acoustic	Sensory	Hearing and equilibrium
IX: Glossopharyngeal	Mixed	Motor—pharynx (phonation and swallowing) Sensory—taste on posterior one third of tongue, pharynx (gag reflex) Parasympathetic—parotid gland, carotid reflex
X: Vagus	Mixed	Motor—pharynx and larynx (talking and swallowing) Sensory—general sensation from carotid body, carotid sinus, pharynx, viscera Parasympathetic—carotid reflex
XI: Spinal accessory	Motor	Movement of trapezius and sternomastoid muscles
XII: Hypoglossal	Motor	Movement of tongue

Mixed refers to a nerve carrying a combination of fibers: motor + sensory; motor + parasympathetic; or motor + sensory + parasympathetic.

23-7

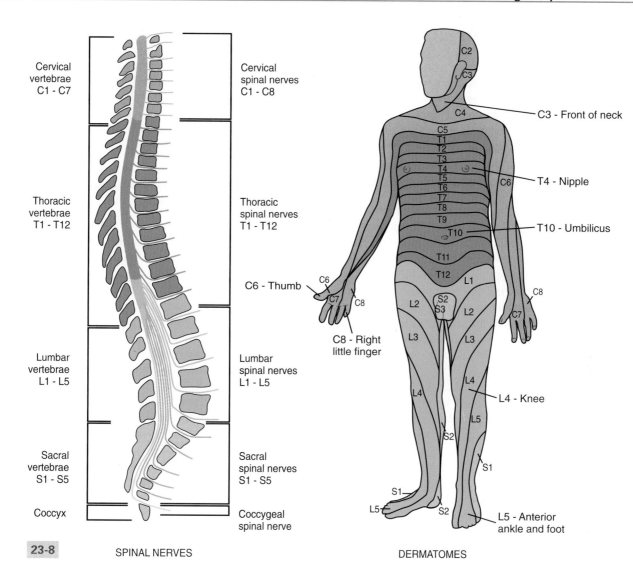

23-8 SPINAL NERVES

DERMATOMES

from the cerebrum; cranial nerves III through XII extend from the lower diencephalon and brainstem. The 12 pairs of cranial nerves supply primarily the head and neck, except the vagus nerve (Lat. *vagus,* or wanderer, as in "vagabond"), which travels to the heart, respiratory muscles, stomach, and gallbladder.

Spinal Nerves

The 31 pairs of **spinal nerves** arise from the length of the spinal cord and supply the rest of the body. They are named for the region of the spine from which they exit: 8 cervical, 12 thoracic, 5 lumbar, 5 sacral, and 1 coccygeal. They are "mixed" nerves because they contain both sensory and motor fibers. The nerves enter and exit the cord through roots—sensory afferent fibers through the posterior or dorsal roots and motor efferent fibers through the anterior or ventral roots.

The nerves exit the spinal cord in an orderly ladder. Each nerve innervates a particular segment of the body. **Dermal segmentation** is the cutaneous distribution of the various spinal nerves.

A **dermatome** is a circumscribed skin area that is supplied mainly from one spinal cord segment through a particular spinal nerve (Fig. 23-8). The dermatomes overlap, which is a form of biologic insurance, i.e., if one nerve is severed, most of the sensations can be transmitted by the one above and the one below. Do not attempt to memorize all dermatome segments; just focus on the following as useful landmarks:

- The **thumb, middle finger,** and **fifth finger** are each in the dermatomes of **C6, C7,** and **C8.**
- The **axilla** is at the level of **T1.**
- The **nipple** is at the level of **T4.**
- The **umbilicus** is at the level of **T10.**
- The **groin** is in the region of **L1.**
- The **knee** is at the level of **L4.**

Autonomic Nervous System

The peripheral nervous system is composed of cranial nerves and spinal nerves. These nerves carry fibers that can be divided functionally into two parts: somatic and autonomic. The somatic fibers innervate the skeletal (voluntary) muscles; the autonomic fibers innervate smooth (involuntary) muscles, cardiac muscle, and glands. The autonomic system mediates unconscious activity. Although a description of the autonomic system is beyond the scope of this book, its overall function is to maintain homeostasis of the body.

Structure and Function

❖ DEVELOPMENTAL COMPETENCE

Infants

The neurologic system is not completely developed at birth. Motor activity in the newborn is under the control of the spinal cord and medulla. Very little cortical control exists, and the neurons are not yet myelinated. Movements are directed primarily by primitive reflexes. As the cerebral cortex develops during the first year, it inhibits these reflexes, and they disappear at predictable times. Persistence of the primitive reflexes is an indication of CNS dysfunction.

The infant's sensory and motor development proceeds along with the gradual acquisition of myelin because myelin is needed to conduct most impulses. The process of myelinization follows a cephalocaudal and proximodistal order (head, then neck, trunk, and out to extremities). This is just the order in which we observe the infant gaining motor control (lifts head, lifts head and shoulders, rolls over, moves whole arm, uses hands, walks). As the milestones are achieved, each is more complex and coordinated. Milestones occur in an orderly sequence, although the exact age of occurrence may vary.

Sensation also is rudimentary at birth. The newborn needs a strong stimulus and then responds by crying and with whole body movements. As myelinization develops, the infant is able to localize the stimulus more precisely and make a more accurate motor response.

The Aging Adult

The aging process causes a general atrophy with a steady loss of neuron structure in the brain and spinal cord. This causes a decrease in weight and volume with a thinning of the cerebral cortex, reduced subcortical brain structures, and expansion of the ventricles.[9] Neuron loss leads many people older than 65 years to show signs that in the younger adult would be considered abnormal, such as general loss of muscle bulk; loss of muscle tone in the face, in the neck, and around the spine; decreased muscle strength; impaired fine coordination and agility; loss of vibratory sense at the ankle; decreased or absent Achilles reflex; loss of position sense at the big toe; pupillary miosis; irregular pupil shape; and decreased pupillary reflexes.

The velocity of nerve conduction decreases between 5% and 10% with aging, making the reaction time slower in some older people. An increased delay at the synapse also occurs, so the impulse takes longer to travel. As a result, touch and pain sensation, taste, and smell may be diminished.

The motor system may show a general slowing of movement. Muscle strength and agility decrease. A generalized decrease occurs in muscle bulk, which is most apparent in the dorsal hand muscles. Muscle tremors may occur in the hands, head, and jaw, along with possible repetitive facial grimacing (dyskinesias).

Aging is accompanied by a progressive decrease in cerebral blood flow and oxygen consumption. In some people this causes dizziness and a loss of balance with position change. These people need to be taught to get up slowly. Otherwise

they have an increased risk for falls and resulting injuries. In addition, older people may forget they fell, which makes it hard to diagnose the cause of the injury.

When they are in good health, aging people walk about as well as they did during their middle and younger years, except more slowly and deliberately. Some survey the ground for obstacles or uneven terrain. Some show a hesitation and a slightly wayward path.

🌐 CULTURE AND GENETICS

Genetic evidence suggests that age-related memory loss (e.g., lost car keys) is a condition distinct from early Alzheimer disease.[18] A specific gene in the hippocampal memory center produces less of a key protein in older people. Boosting the protein in aged laboratory mice reversed their memory loss and may help direct future therapy.

Stroke is an interruption of blood supply to the brain and is the fourth most common cause of death in the United States.[11] There is racial/ethnic disparity here because 6% of American Indian/Alaska natives have had a stroke, 4% of African Americans, 2.5% of Hispanics, 2.4% of Whites, and only 1.5% of Asian/Pacific Islanders. Further, African Americans, American Indian/Alaska natives (AI/AN), and Asian/Pacific Islanders die from stroke at younger ages than do Whites.[11]

There is geographic disparity too; 8 states with high stroke mortality are concentrated in the U.S. southeast region, called the *stroke belt*. Within the stroke belt even higher stroke mortality occurs in the coastal plain of North Carolina, South Carolina, and Georgia, now called the *buckle* region.[11] Stroke mortality is approximately 20% higher in the stroke belt and approximately 40% higher in the stroke buckle than in the rest of the United States. Many reasons are posited for this, but one issue is knowledge deficit of stroke risk factors, warning signs, and treatment, especially among Hispanic groups.[4] Time is crucial for stroke intervention, with only a 3-hour window from the onset of stroke symptoms until the protocol pharmaceutical intervention at a hospital emergency department (ED). Evidence shows that residents in the stroke belt were less likely to be evaluated at a hospital stroke center that is certified to evaluate and perform acute therapies for stroke.[17] This study found no disparity related to race, education, or low income.

Nationwide the burden of stroke is higher among African Americans than in Caucasians. There are differences in stroke risk factors, with African Americans having a higher prevalence of hypertension, diabetes, hyperlipidemia, peripheral vascular disease, cardiac hypertrophy, heavy alcohol use, and current cigarette smoking and physical inactivity.[6] Metabolic syndrome (obesity, hypertension, dyslipidemia, insulin resistance) is more common among Hispanics than among African Americans or Caucasians. There also are disparities in access to care, with minority groups having less use of emergency medical services, longer waiting times in the ED, and a decreased occurrence of thrombolysis therapy.[6]

SUBJECTIVE DATA

1. Headache	6. Weakness	11. Patient-centered care
2. Head injury	7. Incoordination	12. Environmental/occupational
3. Dizziness/vertigo	8. Numbness or tingling	hazards
4. Seizures	9. Difficulty swallowing	
5. Tremors	10. Difficulty speaking	

Examiner Asks

Rationale

1. **Headache.** Any unusually frequent or severe headaches?
   - When did they start? How often do they occur?
   - Where in your head do you feel the headaches? Do they seem to be associated with anything? (Headache history is discussed in Chapter 13.)

A patient who says, "This is the worst headache of my life," needs emergency referral to screen possible stroke.

2. **Head injury.** Ever had any **head injury?** Please describe.
   - What part of your head was hit?
   - Did you have a loss of consciousness? For how long?
   - Do you remember details of the event?

Concussion comes from a direct blow that causes the brain to shift rapidly back and forth inside the skull.[13]

3. **Dizziness/vertigo.** Ever feel light-headed, a swimming sensation, like feeling faint?
   - When have you noticed this? How often does it occur? Does it occur with activity, change in position?
   - Do you ever feel a sensation called **vertigo,** a rotational spinning sensation? (NOTE: Distinguish vertigo from dizziness.) Do you feel as if the room spins (objective vertigo)? Or do you feel that you are spinning (subjective vertigo)? Did this come on suddenly or gradually?

Syncope is a sudden loss of strength, a temporary loss of consciousness (a faint) caused by lack of cerebral blood flow, e.g., low BP.

True **vertigo** is rotational spinning caused by neurologic disease in the vestibular apparatus in the ear or the vestibular nuclei in the brainstem.

4. **Seizures.** Ever had convulsions? When did they start? How often do they occur?

   - Course and duration—When a seizure starts, do you have any warning sign? What type of sign?
   - Motor activity—Where in your body do the seizures begin? Do they travel through your body? On one side or both? Does your muscle tone seem tense or limp?
   - Any associated signs—Color change in face or lips, loss of consciousness (for how long), automatisms (eyelid fluttering, eye rolling, lip smacking), incontinence?
   - Postictal phase—After the seizure, are you told that you spent time sleeping or had any confusion? Do you have weakness, headache, or muscle ache?
   - Precipitating factors—Does anything seem to bring on the seizures: activity, discontinuing medication, fatigue, stress?
   - Do you take any medication?
   - Coping strategies—How have the seizures affected daily life, occupation?

Seizures occur with epilepsy, a paroxysmal disease characterized by altered or loss of consciousness, involuntary muscle movements, and sensory disturbances.

Aura is a subjective sensation that precedes a seizure; it could be auditory, visual, or motor.

5. **Tremors.** Any shakes or **tremors** in the hands or face? When did they start?
   - Do they seem to grow worse with anxiety, intention, or rest?
   - Are they relieved with rest, activity, alcohol? Do they affect daily activities?

Tremor is an involuntary shaking, vibrating, or trembling (see Table 23-5, Abnormalities in Muscle Movement, p. 681).

Examiner Asks	Rationale

6. Weakness. Any **weakness** or problem moving any body part? Is it generalized or local? Does weakness occur with any particular movement (e.g., with proximal or large muscle weakness, it is hard to get up out of a chair or reach for an object; with distal or small muscle weakness, it is hard to open a jar, write, use scissors, or walk without tripping)?

Paresis is a partial or incomplete paralysis.
Paralysis is a loss of motor function caused by a lesion in the neurologic or muscular system or loss of sensory innervation.

7. Incoordination. Any problem with **coordination?** Any problem with balance when walking? Do you list to one side? Any falling? Which way? Do your legs seem to give way? Any clumsy movement?

Dysmetria is the inability to control the distance, power, and speed of a muscular action.

8. Numbness or tingling. Any **numbness or tingling** in any body part? Does it feel like pins and needles? When did it start? Where do you feel it? Does it occur with activity?

Paresthesia is an abnormal sensation (e.g., burning, tingling).

9. Difficulty swallowing. Any problem **swallowing?** Occur with solids or liquids? Have you experienced excessive saliva, drooling?

10. Difficulty speaking. Any problem **speaking:** with forming words or with saying what you intended to say? When did you first notice this? How long did it last?

Dysarthria is difficulty forming words; *dysphasia* is difficulty with language comprehension or expression (see Table 5-2, p. 80).

11. Patient-centered care. Past history of stroke, spinal cord injury, meningitis or encephalitis, congenital defect, or alcohol use problem?

12. Environmental/occupational hazards. Are you exposed to any environmental/occupational hazards: insecticides, organic solvents, lead?
- Are you taking any medications now?
- How much alcohol do you drink? Each week? Each day?
- How about other mood-altering drugs: marijuana, cocaine, barbiturates, tranquilizers?

Review anticonvulsants and antitremor, antivertigo, and pain medication.

Additional History for Infants and Children

1. Did you (the mother) have any health problems during the pregnancy: any infections or illnesses, medications taken, toxemia, hypertension, alcohol or drug use, diabetes?

Prenatal history may affect infant's neurologic development.

2. Please tell me about this baby's birth. Was the baby at term or premature? Birth weight?
- Any birth trauma? Did the baby breathe immediately?
- Were you told the baby's Apgar scores?
- Any congenital defects?

3. Reflexes—What have you noticed about the baby's behavior? Do sucking and swallowing seem coordinated? When you touch the cheek, does the baby turn his or her head toward touch? Does the baby startle with a loud noise or shaking of crib? Does the baby grasp your finger?

4. Does the child seem to have any problem with balance? Have you noted any unexplained falling, clumsy or unsteady gait, progressive muscular weakness, problem with going up or down stairs, problem with getting up from lying position?

If it occurs, may not be noticed until starts to walk in late infancy.
Screens for muscular dystrophy.

5. Has this child had any seizures? Please describe. Did the seizure occur with a high fever? Did any loss of consciousness occur—how long? How many seizures occurred with this same illness (if occurred with high fever)?

Seizures may occur with high fever in infants and toddlers. Or they may be a sign of neurologic disease.

Examiner Asks	Rationale
6. Did this child's motor or developmental milestones seem to come at about the right age? Does he or she seem to be growing and maturing normally to you? How does his or her development compare with siblings or age-mates?	
7. Do you know if your child has had any environmental exposure to lead? When was he or she tested for lead levels?	Often tested at 1 year. Chronically elevated lead levels may cause a developmental delay or a loss of a newly acquired skill or be asymptomatic.
8. Have you been told about any learning problems in school: problems with attention span, inability to concentrate, hyperactivity?	
9. Any family history of seizure disorder, cerebral palsy, muscular dystrophy?	
10. Does your teen play sports? Which ones? (Include cheerleading.) • Ever had injury to head? What symptoms did he or she have—headache, nausea and vomiting, poor balance, blurred vision, loss of consciousness, memory loss, mental fogginess? • Screened for concussion? What did they tell you about when to return to play?	Teens are more susceptible to concussion because of thinner cranial bones, larger head-to-body ratio, immature central nervous system, and larger subarachnoid space in which brain can rattle.[13] Detailed history with evidence of direct impact helps diagnosis. If asymptomatic, gradual return to play every 24 hours in stepwise fashion: rest, light aerobics, sport-specific exercise, non-contact drills, full-contact practice, return to game play.[13]

Additional History for the Aging Adult

Examiner Asks	Rationale
1. Any problem with dizziness? Does it occur when you first sit or stand up, when you move your head, when you get up and walk just after eating? Does it occur with any of your medications? Any recent falls? • (For men) Do you ever get up at night and then feel faint while standing to urinate? • How does dizziness affect your daily activities? Are you able to drive safely and maneuver within your house safely? • Which safety modifications have you applied at home?	Diminished cerebral blood flow and vestibular response may increase risk for falls. Falls risk increases with diagnosis of stroke or dementia, gait and balance disorder, use of assistive devices, history of recent falls.[3] Micturition syncope.
2. Have you noticed any decrease in memory, change in mental function? Have you felt any confusion? Did it seem to come on suddenly or gradually?	Memory loss and cognitive decline are early indicators of Alzheimer disease and are mistaken for normal cognitive decline of aging[19] (see Table 23-2, 10 Warning Signs of Alzheimer Disease, p. 677).
3. Have you ever noticed any tremor? Is it in your hands or face? Is it worse with anxiety, activity, rest? Does it seem to be relieved with alcohol, activity, rest? Does it interfere with daily or social activities?	Senile tremor is relieved by alcohol, but this is not a recommended treatment. Assess if the person is abusing alcohol in effort to relieve tremor.
4. Have you ever had any sudden vision change, fleeting blindness? Did it occur along with weakness? Did you have any loss of consciousness?	Screen symptoms of stroke.

Subjective Data

OBJECTIVE DATA

PREPARATION

Perform a **screening neurologic examination** on seemingly well people who have no significant subjective findings from the history.[2]

1. Mental status (level of alertness, appropriateness of responses, orientation to date and place)
2. Cranial nerves (II–visual acuity, pupillary light reflex; III, IV, VI–eye movements; VII–facial strength (smile, eye closure); VIII–hearing
3. Motor function: Strength (shoulder abduction, elbow extension, wrist extension, finger abduction, hip flexion, knee flexion, ankle dorsiflexion); coordination (fine finger movements, finger to nose); gait (casual, tandem)
4. Sensation (one modality at toes can be light touch, pain/temperature, or proprioception)
5. Reflexes: Deep tendon reflexes (biceps, patellar, Achilles); plantar responses

Perform a **complete neurologic examination** on people who have neurologic concerns (e.g., headache, weakness, loss of coordination) or who have shown signs of neurologic dysfunction.

Perform a **neurologic recheck** examination on people who have neurologic deficits and require periodic assessments (e.g., hospitalized people or those in extended care), using the examination sequence beginning on p. 670.

Integrate the steps of the neurologic examination with the examination of each particular part of the body as much as you are able. For example, test cranial nerves while assessing the head and neck (recall Chapters 13 through 16) and superficial abdominal reflexes while assessing the abdomen. However, when recording your findings, consider all neurologic data as a functional unit and record them all together.

Position the person sitting up with the head at your eye level.

Normal Range of Findings	Abnormal Findings

Test Cranial Nerves

Cranial Nerve I—Olfactory Nerve

Do not test routinely. Test the sense of smell in those who report loss of smell, those with head trauma, and those with abnormal mental status and when the presence of an intracranial lesion is suspected. First assess patency by occluding one nostril at a time and asking the person to sniff. Then with the person's eyes closed, occlude one nostril and present an aromatic substance. Use familiar, conveniently obtainable, and nonnoxious smells such as coffee, toothpaste, orange, vanilla, soap, or peppermint. Alcohol wipes smell familiar and are easy to find but are irritating.

Normally a person can identify an odor on each side of the nose. Smell normally is decreased bilaterally with aging. Any asymmetry in the sense of smell is important.

One cannot test smell when air passages are occluded with upper respiratory infection or sinusitis.

Anosmia—Decrease or loss of smell occurs bilaterally with tobacco smoking, allergic rhinitis, and cocaine use.

Unilateral loss of smell in the absence of nasal disease is *neurogenic anosmia* (see Table 23-3, Abnormalities in Cranial Nerves, p. 678).

Cranial Nerve II—Optic Nerve

Test visual acuity and visual fields by confrontation (see Chapter 14).

Using the ophthalmoscope, examine the ocular fundus to determine the color, size, and shape of the optic disc (see Chapter 14).

Visual field loss (see Table 14-5, p. 318).

Papilledema with increased intracranial pressure; optic atrophy (see Table 14-9, p. 322).

Cranial Nerves III, IV, and VI—Oculomotor, Trochlear, and Abducens Nerves

Palpebral fissures are usually equal in width or nearly so.

Ptosis (drooping) occurs with myasthenia gravis, dysfunction of cranial nerve III, or Horner syndrome (see Table 14-2, p. 314).

Normal Range of Findings	Abnormal Findings

Check pupils for size, regularity, equality, direct and consensual light reaction, and accommodation (see Chapter 14).

Assess extraocular movements by the cardinal positions of gaze (see Chapter 14).

Nystagmus is a back-and-forth oscillation of the eyes. End-point nystagmus, a few beats of horizontal nystagmus at extreme lateral gaze, occurs normally. Assess any other nystagmus carefully, noting:
- Presence of nystagmus in one or both eyes.
- *Pendular* movement (oscillations move equally left to right) or *jerk* (a quick phase in one direction, then a slow phase in the other). Classify the jerk nystagmus in the direction of the quick phase.
- Amplitude. Judge whether the degree of movement is fine, medium, or coarse.
- Frequency. Is it constant or does it fade after a few beats?
- Plane of movement. Horizontal, vertical, rotary, or a combination?

Cranial Nerve V—Trigeminal Nerve

Motor Function. Assess the muscles of mastication by palpating the temporal and masseter muscles as the person clenches the teeth (Fig. 23-9). Muscles should feel equally strong on both sides. Next try to separate the jaws by pushing down on the chin; normally you cannot.

23-9

Sensory Function. With the person's eyes closed, test light touch sensation by touching a cotton wisp to these designated areas on person's face: forehead, cheeks, and chin (Fig. 23-10). Ask the person to say "Now" whenever the touch is felt. This tests all three divisions of the nerve: (1) ophthalmic, (2) maxillary, and (3) mandibular.

23-10

Abnormal Findings

Increasing intracranial pressure causes a sudden, unilateral, dilated, and nonreactive pupil.

Strabismus (deviated gaze) or limited movement (see Table 14-1, p. 312).

Nystagmus occurs with disease of the vestibular system, cerebellum, or brainstem.

Decreased strength on one or both sides.

Asymmetry in jaw movement.

Pain with clenching of teeth.

Decreased or unequal sensation. With a stroke, sensation of face and body is lost on the opposite side of the lesion.

Objective Data

Normal Range of Findings	**Abnormal Findings**

Cranial Nerve VII—Facial Nerve

Motor Function. Note mobility and facial symmetry as the person responds to these requests: smile (Fig. 23-11), frown, close eyes tightly (against your attempt to open them), lift eyebrows, show teeth, and puff cheeks (Fig. 23-12). Press the person's puffed cheeks in and note that the air should escape equally from both sides.

Muscle weakness is shown by flattening of the nasolabial fold, drooping of one side of the face, lower eyelid sagging, and escape of air from only one cheek that is pressed in.

Loss of movement and asymmetry of movement occur with both CNS lesions (e.g., stroke that affects lower face on one side) and peripheral nervous system lesions (e.g., Bell palsy that affects the upper *and* lower face on one side).

23-11   23-12

Cranial Nerve VIII—Acoustic (Vestibulocochlear) Nerve

Test hearing acuity by the ability to hear normal conversation and by the whispered voice test (see Chapter 15).

Cranial Nerves IX and X—Glossopharyngeal and Vagus Nerves

Motor Function. Depress the tongue with a tongue blade and note pharyngeal movement as the person says "ahhh" or yawns; the uvula and soft palate should rise in the midline, and the tonsillar pillars should move medially.

Touch the posterior pharyngeal wall with a tongue blade and note the gag reflex. Also note that the voice sounds smooth and not strained.

Absence or asymmetry of soft palate movement or tonsillar pillar movement. Following a stroke, dysfunction in swallowing may increase risk for aspiration.

Hoarse or brassy voice occurs with vocal cord dysfunction; nasal twang occurs with weakness of soft palate.

Cranial Nerve XI—Spinal Accessory Nerve

Examine the sternomastoid and trapezius muscles for equal size. Check equal strength by asking the person to rotate the head forcibly against resistance applied to the side of the chin (Fig. 23-13). Then ask the person to shrug the shoulders against resistance (Fig. 23-14). These movements should feel equally strong on both sides.

Atrophy.

Muscle weakness or paralysis occurs with a stroke or following injury to the peripheral nerve (e.g., surgical removal of lymph nodes).

23-13   23-14

| **Normal Range of Findings** | **Abnormal Findings** |

Cranial Nerve XII—Hypoglossal Nerve

Inspect the tongue. No wasting or tremors should be present. Note the forward thrust in the midline as the person protrudes the tongue. Also ask the person to say "light, tight, dynamite" and note that lingual speech (sounds of letters l, t, d, n) is clear and distinct.

Atrophy. Fasciculations.

Tongue deviates to side with lesions of the hypoglossal nerve (when this occurs, deviation is toward the paralyzed side).

Inspect and Palpate the Motor System

Muscles

Size. As you proceed through the examination, inspect all muscle groups for size. Compare the right side with the left. Muscle groups should be within the normal size limits for age and symmetric bilaterally. When muscles in the extremities look asymmetric, measure each in centimeters and record the difference. A difference of 1 cm or less is not significant. Note that it is difficult to assess muscle mass in very obese people.

Strength. (See Chapter 22.) Test the power of homologous muscles simultaneously. Test muscle groups of the extremities, neck, and trunk.

Atrophy—Abnormally small muscle with a wasted appearance; occurs with disuse, injury, LMN disease such as polio, diabetic neuropathy.

Hypertrophy—Increased size and strength; occurs with isometric exercise.

Paresis or weakness is diminished strength; paralysis or plegia is absence of strength.

Tone. Tone is the normal degree of tension (contraction) in voluntarily relaxed muscles. It shows as a mild resistance to passive stretch. To test muscle tone, move the extremities through a passive range of motion. First persuade the person to relax completely, to "go loose like a rag doll." Move each extremity smoothly through a full range of motion. Support the arm at the elbow and the leg at the knee (Fig. 23-15). Normally you will note a mild, even resistance to movement.

Limited range of motion.

Pain with motion.

Flaccidity—Decreased resistance, hypotonia occur with peripheral weakness.

Spasticity and rigidity—Types of increased resistance that occur with central weakness (see Table 23-4, Abnormalities in Muscle Tone, p. 679).

23-15

Normal Range of Findings	Abnormal Findings

Involuntary Movements. Normally no involuntary movements occur. If they are present, note their location, frequency, rate, and amplitude. Note if the movements can be controlled at will.

Tic, tremor, fasciculation, myoclonus, chorea, and athetosis (see Table 23-5, p. 679).

Cerebellar Function
Coordination and Skilled Movements

Rapid Alternating Movements (RAM). Ask the person to pat the knees with both hands, lift up, turn hands over, and pat the knees with the backs of the hands (Fig. 23-16). Then ask the person to do this faster. Normally this is done with equal turning and a quick, rhythmic pace.

Lack of coordination.
Slow, clumsy, and sloppy response is termed *dysdiadochokinesia* and occurs with cerebellar disease.

23-16

Alternatively ask the person to touch the thumb to each finger on the same hand, starting with the index finger; then reverse direction (Fig. 23-17). Normally this can be done quickly and accurately.

23-17

Finger-to-Finger Test. With the person's eyes open, ask that he or she use the index finger to touch your finger and then his or her own nose (Fig. 23-18). After a few times, move your finger to a different spot. The person's movement should be smooth and accurate.

Lack of coordination.
Dysmetria is clumsy movement with overshooting the mark and occurs with cerebellar disorders or acute alcohol intoxication.
Past-pointing is a constant deviation to one side.
Intention tremor when reaching to a visually directed object.

| **Normal Range of Findings** | **Abnormal Findings** |

23-18

Finger-to-Nose Test. Ask the person to close the eyes and stretch out the arms. Ask him or her to touch the tip of his or her nose with each index finger, alternating hands and increasing speed. Normally this is done with accurate and smooth movement.

Heel-to-Shin Test. Test lower-extremity coordination by asking the person, who is in a supine position, to place the heel on the opposite knee and run it down the shin from the knee to the ankle (Fig. 23-19). Normally the person moves the heel in a straight line down the shin.

Misses nose. Worsening of coordination when the eyes are closed occurs with cerebellar disease or alcohol intoxication.

Lack of coordination, heel falls off shin; occurs with cerebellar disease.

23-19

Balance Tests

Gait. Observe as the person walks 10 to 20 feet, turns, and returns to the starting point. Normally the person moves with a sense of freedom. The gait is smooth, rhythmic, and effortless; the opposing arm swing is coordinated; the turns are smooth. The step length is about 15 inches from heel to heel.

(NOTE: To minimize position changes, observe these balance tests at the end of the examination.)

Stiff, immobile posture. Staggering or reeling. Wide base of support.

Lack of arm swing or rigid arms.

Unequal rhythm of steps. Slapping of foot. Scraping of toe of shoe.

Ataxia—Uncoordinated or unsteady gait (see Table 23-7, Abnormal Gaits, p. 683).

Normal Range of Findings	Abnormal Findings

Normal Range of Findings

Ask the person to walk a straight line in a heel-to-toe fashion (tandem walking) (Fig. 23-20). This decreases the base of support and will accentuate any problem with coordination. Normally the person can walk straight and stay balanced.

Abnormal Findings

Crooked line of walk.
Widens base to maintain balance.
Staggering, reeling, loss of balance.
An ataxia that did not appear with regular gait may appear now. Inability to tandem walk is sensitive for an upper motor neuron lesion such as multiple sclerosis and for acute cerebellar dysfunction such as alcohol intoxication.

23-21   Romberg test.

23-20   Tandem walking.

You may also test for balance by asking the person to walk on his or her toes and then on the heels for a few steps. Normally plantar flexion and dorsiflexion are strong enough to permit this.

The Romberg Test. Ask the person to stand up with feet together and arms at the sides. Once in a stable position, ask him or her to close the eyes and to hold the position (Fig. 23-21). Wait about 20 seconds. Normally a person can maintain posture and balance even with the visual orienting information blocked, although slight swaying may occur. (Stand close to catch the person in case he or she falls.)

Muscle weakness in the legs prevents this.

Sways, falls, widens base of feet to avoid falling.
Positive Romberg sign is loss of balance that occurs when closing the eyes. You eliminate the advantage of orientation with the eyes, which had compensated for sensory loss. A positive Romberg sign occurs with cerebellar ataxia (multiple sclerosis, alcohol intoxication), loss of proprioception, and loss of vestibular function.

Normal Range of Findings	Abnormal Findings

Ask the person to perform a shallow knee bend or to hop in place, first on one leg and then the other (Fig. 23-22). This demonstrates normal position sense, muscle strength, and cerebellar function. Note that some individuals cannot hop because of aging or obesity. Alternatively you can ask them to rise from a chair without using the arm rests for support.

Unable to perform knee bend because of weakness in quadriceps muscle or hip extensors.

23-22

Assess the Sensory System

Ask the person to identify various sensory stimuli to test the intactness of the peripheral nerve fibers, the sensory tracts, and higher cortical discrimination.

Ensure validity of sensory system testing by making sure that the person is alert, cooperative, and comfortable and has an adequate attention span. Otherwise you may get misleading and invalid results. Testing the sensory system can be fatiguing. You may need to repeat the examination later or to break it into parts when the person is tired.

You do not need to test the entire skin surface for every sensation. Screening procedures include testing superficial pain or light touch and vibration in a few distal locations and testing stereognosis. Complete testing of the sensory system is warranted only in those with neurologic symptoms (e.g., localized pain, numbness, and tingling) or when you discover abnormalities (e.g., motor deficit). Then test all sensory modalities and cover most dermatomes of the body.

Compare sensations on symmetric parts of the body. When you find a definite decrease in sensation, map it out by systematic testing in that area. Proceed from the point of decreased sensation toward the sensitive area. By asking the person to tell you where the sensation changes, you can map the exact borders of the deficient area. Draw your results on a diagram.

Note if the topographic pattern of sensory loss is distal (i.e., over the hands and feet in a "glove and stocking" distribution) or if it is over a specific dermatome.

Objective Data

Normal Range of Findings	Abnormal Findings

Avoid asking leading questions, "Can you feel this pinprick?" This creates an expectation of how the person should feel the sensation, which is called *suggestion*. Instead, use unbiased directions, "Tell me what you feel."

The person's eyes should be closed during each of the tests. Take time to explain what will be happening and exactly how you expect the person to respond.

Spinothalamic Tract

Pain. Pain is tested by the person's ability to perceive a pinprick. Break a tongue blade lengthwise, forming a sharp point at the fractured end and a dull spot at the rounded end. Lightly apply the sharp point or the dull end to the person's body in a random, unpredictable order (Fig. 23-23). Ask the person to say "sharp" or "dull," depending on the sensation felt. (Note that the sharp edge is used to test for pain; the dull edge is used as a general test of the person's responses.)

Hypoalgesia—Decreased pain sensation.
Analgesia—Absent pain sensation.
Hyperalgesia—Increased pain sensation.

23-23

Let at least 2 seconds elapse between each stimulus to avoid *summation*. With summation, frequent consecutive stimuli are perceived as one strong stimulus. Discard tongue blade to prevent transmitting any possible infection.

Light Touch. Apply a wisp of cotton to the skin. Stretch a cotton ball to make a long end and brush it over the skin in a random order of sites and at irregular intervals (Fig. 23-24). This prevents the person from responding just from repetition. Include the arms, forearms, hands, chest, thighs, and legs. Ask the person to say "now" or "yes" when touch is felt. Compare symmetric points.

Hypoesthesia—Decreased touch sensation.
Anesthesia—Absent touch sensation.
Hyperesthesia—Increased touch sensation.

23-24

Normal Range of Findings	Abnormal Findings

Posterior (Dorsal) Column Tract

Vibration. Test the person's ability to feel vibrations of a tuning fork over bony prominences. Use a low-pitch tuning fork (128 Hz or 256 Hz) because its vibration has a slower decay. Strike the tuning fork on the heel of your hand and hold the base on a bony surface of the fingers and great toe (Fig. 23-25). Ask the person to indicate when the vibration starts and stops. If he or she feels a normal vibration or buzzing sensation on these distal areas, you may assume that proximal spots are normal and proceed no further. If no vibrations are felt, move proximally and test ulnar processes and ankles, patellae, and iliac crests. Compare the right side with the left side. If you find a deficit, note whether it is gradual or abrupt.

Unable to feel vibration. Loss of vibration sense occurs with peripheral neuropathy (e.g., diabetes and alcoholism). Often this is the first sensation lost.

Peripheral neuropathy is worse at the feet and gradually improves as you move up the leg, as opposed to a specific nerve lesion, which has a clear zone of deficit for its dermatome (see Table 23-10, Patterns of Sensory Loss, p. 686).

23-25

Position (Kinesthesia). Test the person's ability to perceive passive movements of the extremities. Move a finger or the big toe up and down and ask the person to tell you which way it is moved (Fig. 23-26). The test is done with the eyes closed; but, to be sure that it is understood, have the person watch a few trials first. Vary the order of movement up or down. Hold the digit by the sides since upward or downward pressure on the skin may provide a clue as to how it has been moved. Normally a person can detect movement of a few millimeters.

Loss of position sense.

23-26

Normal Range of Findings	Abnormal Findings

Objective Data

Tactile Discrimination (Fine Touch). The following tests also measure the discrimination ability of the sensory cortex. As a prerequisite the person needs a normal or near-normal sense of touch and position sense.

Problems with tactile discrimination occur with lesions of the sensory cortex or posterior column.

Stereognosis. Test the person's ability to recognize objects by feeling their forms, sizes, and weights. With his or her eyes closed, place a familiar object (paper clip, key, coin, cotton ball, or pencil) in the person's hand and ask him or her to identify it (Fig. 23-27). Normally a person will explore it with the fingers and correctly name it. Test a different object in each hand; testing the left hand assesses right parietal lobe functioning.

Astereognosis—Inability to identify object correctly. Occurs in sensory cortex lesions (e.g., stroke).

23-27 Stereognosis.

Graphesthesia. Graphesthesia is the ability to "read" a number by having it traced on the skin. With the person's eyes closed, use a blunt instrument to trace a single digit number or a letter on the palm (Fig. 23-28). Ask the person to tell you what it is. Graphesthesia is a good measure of sensory loss if the person cannot make the hand movements needed for stereognosis, as occurs in arthritis.

Inability to distinguish number occurs with lesions of the sensory cortex.

23-28 Graphesthesia.

Normal Range of Findings	Abnormal Findings

Two-Point Discrimination. Test the person's ability to distinguish the separation of two simultaneous pin points on the skin. Apply the two points of an opened paper clip lightly to the skin in ever-closing distances. Note the distance at which the person no longer perceives two separate points. The level of perception varies considerably with the region tested; it is most sensitive in the fingertips (2 to 8 mm) and least sensitive on the upper arms, thighs, and back (40 to 75 mm).

An increase in the distance it normally takes to identify two separate points occurs with sensory cortex lesions.

Extinction. Simultaneously touch both sides of the body at the same point. Ask the person to state how many sensations are felt and where they are. Normally both sensations are felt.

The ability to recognize only one of the stimuli occurs with sensory cortex lesion; the stimulus is extinguished on the side *opposite* the cortex lesion.

Point Location. Touch the skin and withdraw the stimulus promptly. Tell the person, "Put your finger where I touched you." You can perform this test simultaneously with light touch sensation.

With a sensory cortex lesion, the person cannot localize the sensation accurately, even though light touch sensation may be retained.

Test the Reflexes

Stretch Reflexes or Deep Tendon Reflexes (DTRs)

Measurement of the stretch reflexes reveals the intactness of the reflex arc at specific spinal levels and the normal override on the reflex of the higher cortical levels.

For an adequate response, the limb should be relaxed, and the muscle partially stretched. Stimulate the reflex by directing a short, snappy blow of the reflex hammer onto the insertion tendon of the muscle. Use a relaxed hold on the hammer.

As with the percussion technique, the action takes place at your wrist. Strike a brief, well-aimed blow and bounce up promptly; do not let the hammer rest on the tendon. Use the pointed end of the reflex hammer when aiming at a smaller target such as your thumb on the tendon site; use the flat end when the target is wider or to diffuse the impact and prevent pain.

Use just enough force to get a response. Compare right and left sides—the responses should be equal. The reflex response is graded on a 4-point scale:

4+   Very brisk, hyperactive with clonus, indicative of disease
3+   Brisker than average, may indicate disease, probably normal
2+   Average, normal
1+   Diminished, low normal, or occurs only with reinforcement
0   No response

This is a subjective scale and requires some clinical practice. Even then, the scale is not completely reliable because no standard exists to say *how* brisk a reflex should be to warrant a grade of 3+. Also, a wide range of normal exists in reflex responses. Healthy people may have diminished reflexes, or they may have brisk ones. Your best plan is to interpret DTRs *only* within the context of the rest of the neurologic examination.

Clonus is a set of rapid, rhythmic contractions of the same muscle.

Hyperreflexia is the exaggerated reflex seen when the monosynaptic reflex arc is released from the usually inhibiting influence of higher cortical levels. This occurs with upper motor neuron lesions (e.g., stroke).

Hyporeflexia, which is the absence of a reflex, is a lower motor neuron problem. It occurs with interruption of sensory afferents or destruction of motor efferents and anterior horn cells (e.g., spinal cord injury).

Normal Range of Findings	Abnormal Findings

Sometimes the reflex response fails to appear. Try further encouragement of relaxation, varying the person's position or increasing the strength of the blow. **Reinforcement** is another technique to relax the muscles and enhance the response (Fig. 23-29). Ask the person to perform an isometric exercise in a muscle group somewhat away from the one being tested. For example, to enhance a patellar reflex, ask the person to lock the fingers together and "pull as hard as you can." Then strike the tendon. To enhance a biceps response, ask the person to clench the teeth or to grasp the thigh with the opposite hand.

23-29
Reinforcement.

Biceps Reflex (C5 to C6). Support the person's forearm on yours; this position relaxes and partially flexes the person's arm. Place your thumb on the biceps tendon and strike a blow on your thumb. You can feel as well as see the normal response, which is contraction of the biceps muscle and flexion of the forearm (Fig. 23-30).

23-30
Biceps reflex.

Normal Range of Findings	Abnormal Findings

Triceps Reflex (C7 to C8). Tell the person to let the arm "just go dead" as you suspend it by holding the upper arm. Strike the triceps tendon directly just above the elbow (Fig. 23-31). The normal response is extension of the forearm. Alternatively hold the person's wrist across the chest to flex the arm at the elbow and tap the tendon.

23-31   Triceps reflex.

Brachioradialis Reflex (C5 to C6). Hold the person's thumbs to suspend the forearms in relaxation. Strike the forearm directly, about 2 to 3 cm above the radial styloid process (Fig. 23-32). The normal response is flexion and supination of the forearm.

23-32   Brachioradialis reflex.

Objective Data

Normal Range of Findings	Abnormal Findings

Quadriceps Reflex ("Knee Jerk") (L2 to L4). Let the lower legs dangle freely to flex the knee and stretch the tendons. Strike the tendon directly just below the patella (Fig. 23-33). Extension of the lower leg is the expected response. You also will palpate contraction of the quadriceps.

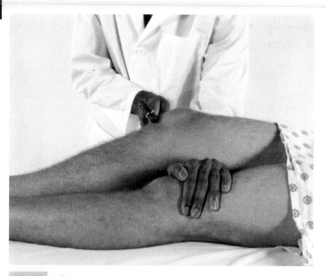

23-33 Quadriceps reflex.

For the person in the supine position, use your own arm as a lever to support the weight of one leg against the other (Fig. 23-34). This maneuver also flexes the knee.

23-34 Supine quadriceps reflex.

Achilles Reflex ("Ankle Jerk") (L5 to S2). Position the person with the knee flexed and the hip externally rotated. Hold the foot in dorsiflexion and strike the Achilles tendon directly (Fig. 23-35). Feel the normal response as the foot plantar flexes against your hand.

Objective Data

Normal Range of Findings	**Abnormal Findings**

23-35 Achilles reflex.

For the person in the supine position, flex one knee and support that lower leg against the other leg so it falls "open." Dorsiflex the foot and tap the tendon (Fig. 23-36).

23-36 Supine Achilles reflex.

Clonus. Test for clonus, particularly when the reflexes are hyperactive. Support the lower leg in one hand. With your other hand move the foot up and down a few times to relax the muscle. Then stretch the muscle by briskly dorsiflexing the foot. Hold the stretch (Fig. 23-37). With a normal response you feel no further movement. When clonus is present, you feel and see rapid, rhythmic contractions of the calf muscle and movement of the foot.

Clonus is repeated reflex muscular movements. A hyperactive reflex with sustained clonus (lasting as long as the stretch is held) occurs with UMN disease.

23-37

Normal Range of Findings	**Abnormal Findings**

Superficial (Cutaneous) Reflexes

Here the sensory receptors are in the skin rather than the muscles. The motor response is a localized muscle contraction.

Abdominal Reflexes—Upper (T8 to T10), Lower (T10 to T12). Have the person assume a supine position, with the knees slightly bent. Use the handle end of the reflex hammer, a wood applicator tip, or the end of a split tongue blade to stroke the skin. Move from each corner of the abdomen toward the midline at both the upper and lower abdominal levels (Fig. 23-38). The normal response is ipsilateral contraction of the abdominal muscle with an observed deviation of the umbilicus toward the stroke. When the abdominal wall is very obese, pull the skin to the opposite side and feel it contract toward the stimulus.

Superficial reflexes are absent with diseases of the pyramidal tract (e.g., they are absent on the contralateral side with stroke).

Abdominal reflex

Cremasteric reflex

23-38

Cremasteric Reflex (L1 to L2). This is not done routinely. On the male lightly stroke the inner aspect of the thigh with the reflex hammer or tongue blade (see Fig. 23-38). Note elevation of the ipsilateral testicle.

Absent in both UMN and LMN lesions.

Plantar Reflex (L4 to S2). Position the thigh in slight external rotation. With the reflex hammer draw a light stroke up the lateral side of the sole of the foot and inward across the ball of the foot, like an upside-down J (Fig. 23-39, *A*). The normal response is plantar flexion of the toes and inversion and flexion of the forefoot.

Except in infancy, the abnormal response is dorsiflexion of the big toe and fanning of all toes, which is a positive Babinski sign, also called "upgoing toes" (Fig. 23-39, *B*). This occurs with UMN disease of the corticospinal (or pyramidal) tract.

A   B

23-39   Plantar reflex.

Normal Range of Findings

❖ DEVELOPMENTAL COMPETENCE

Infants (Birth to 12 Months)

The neurologic system shows dramatic growth and development during the first year of life. Assessment includes noting that milestones you normally would expect for each month have indeed been achieved and that the early, more primitive reflexes are eliminated from the baby's repertory when they are supposed to be.

At birth the newborn is very alert, with the eyes open, and demonstrates strong, urgent sucking. The normal cry is loud, lusty, and even angry. The next 2 or 3 days may be spent mostly sleeping as the baby recovers from the birth process. After that the pattern of sleep and waking activity is highly variable; it depends on the baby's individual body rhythm and external stimuli.

The behavioral assessment should include your observations of the infant's spontaneous waking activity, responses to environmental stimuli, and social interaction with the parents and others.

By 2 months, the baby smiles responsively and recognizes the parent's face. Babbling occurs at 4 months, and one or two words (mama, dada) are used nonspecifically after 9 months.

The cranial nerves cannot be tested directly, but you can infer their proper functioning by the maneuvers shown in Table 23-1.

Abnormal Findings

Failure to attain a skill by expected time.

Persistence of reflex behavior beyond the normal time.

A high-pitched, shrill cry or cat-sounding screech occurs with CNS damage.

A weak, groaning cry or expiratory grunt occurs with respiratory distress.

Lethargy, hyporeactivity, hyperirritability, and parent's report of significant change in behavior all warrant referral.

TABLE 23-1 Testing Cranial Nerve Function of Infants	
CRANIAL NERVE	**RESPONSE**
II, III, IV, VI	Optical blink reflex—Shine light in open eyes, note rapid closure Size, shape, equality of pupils Regards face or close object Eyes follow movement
V	Rooting reflex, sucking reflex
VII	Facial movements (e.g., wrinkling forehead and nasolabial folds) symmetric when crying or smiling
VIII	Loud noise yields Moro reflex (until 4 mo) Acoustic blink reflex—Infant blinks in response to loud hand clap 30 cm (12 inches) from head (avoid making air current) Eyes follow direction of sound
IX, X	Swallowing, gag reflex Coordinate sucking and swallowing
XII	Pinch nose and infant's mouth opens and tongue rises in midline

Objective Data

Normal Range of Findings

The Motor System

Observe spontaneous motor activity for smoothness and symmetry. Smoothness of movement suggests proper cerebellar function, as does the coordination involved in sucking and swallowing. To screen gross- and fine-motor coordination, use the Denver II test with its age-specific developmental milestones. You also can assess movement by testing the reflexes listed in the following section. Note their smoothness of response and symmetry. Also note whether their presence or absence is appropriate for the infant's age.

Assess muscle tone by first observing resting posture. The newborn favors a flexed position; extremities are symmetrically folded inward, the hips are slightly abducted, and the fists are tightly flexed (Fig. 23-40). However, infants born by breech delivery do not have flexion in the lower extremities.

23-40

After 2 months, flexion gives way to gradual extension, beginning with the head and continuing in a cephalocaudal direction. Now is the time to check for spasticity; none should be present. Test for spasticity by flexing the infant's knees onto the abdomen and then quickly releasing them. They will unfold but not too quickly. Also gently push the head forward—the baby should comply.

The fists normally are held in tight flexion for the first 3 months. Then they open for part of the time.

A purposeful reach for an object with both hands occurs around 4 months, a transfer of an object from hand to hand at 7 months, a grasp using fingers and opposing thumb at 9 months, and a purposeful release at 10 months. Babies are normally ambidextrous for the first 18 months.

Head control is an important milestone in motor development. You can incorporate the following two movements into every infant assessment to check the muscle tone necessary for head control.

First, with the baby supine, pull to a sit holding the wrists and note head control (Fig. 23-41). The newborn will hold the head almost in the same plane as the body, and it will balance briefly when the baby reaches a sitting position and then flop forward. (Even a premature infant shows some head flexion.) At 4 months, the head stays in line with the body and does not flop.

Abnormal Findings

Delay in motor activity occurs with brain damage, mental disability, peripheral neuromuscular damage, prolonged illness, and parental neglect.

Abnormal postures:

Frog position—Hips abducted and almost flat against the table, externally rotated (normal only after breech delivery).

Opisthotonos—Head arched back, stiffness of neck, and extension of arms and legs; occurs with meningeal or brainstem irritation and kernicterus (see Table 23-11, Abnormal Postures, p. 688).

Extension of limbs may occur with intracranial hemorrhage.

Any type of continual asymmetry (e.g., asymmetry of upper limbs) occurs with brachial plexus palsy.

Spasticity is an early sign of cerebral palsy. After releasing flexed knees, legs will quickly extend and adduct, even to a "scissoring" motion when spasticity is present. The baby also often resists head flexion and extends back against your hand when spasticity is present.

Note persistent one-hand preference in baby younger than 18 months of age, which may indicate a motor deficit on the opposite side.

Because development progresses in a cephalocaudal direction, head lag is an early sign of brain damage.

After 6 months refer any baby with failure to hold head in midline when sitting.

| **Normal Range of Findings** | **Abnormal Findings** |

23-41

Second, lift up the baby in a prone position, with one hand supporting the chest (Fig. 23-42). The term newborn holds the head at an angle of 45 degrees or less from horizontal, the back is straight or slightly arched, and the elbows and knees are partly flexed.

23-42

At 3 months the baby raises the head and arches the back, as in a swan dive. This is the *Landau reflex*, which persists until 1½ years of age (Fig. 23-43).

Head lag; a limp, floppy trunk; and dangling arms and legs.

Absence of the reflex indicates motor weakness, upper motor neuron disease, or mental disability.

23-43

Objective Data

Normal Range of Findings	Abnormal Findings

Assess muscle strength by noting the strength of sucking and of spontaneous motor activity. Normally no tremors are present, and no continual overshooting of the mark occurs when reaching.

The Sensory System

You will perform very little sensory testing with infants and toddlers. The newborn normally has hypoesthesia and requires a strong stimulus to elicit a response. The baby responds to pain by crying and a general reflex withdrawal of all limbs. By 7 to 9 months, the infant can localize the stimulus and shows more specific signs of withdrawal. Other sensory modalities are not tested.

Unusually rapid withdrawal is *hyperesthesia*, which occurs with spinal cord lesions, CNS infections, increased intracranial pressure, peritonitis.

No withdrawal is decreased sensation, which occurs with decreased consciousness, mental deficiency, spinal cord or peripheral nerve lesions.

Reflexes

Infantile automatisms are reflexes that have a predictable timetable of appearance and departure. The reflexes most commonly tested are listed in the following section. For the screening examination you can just check the rooting, grasp, tonic neck, and Moro reflexes.

Rooting Reflex. Brush the infant's cheek near the mouth. Note whether he or she turns the head toward that side and opens the mouth (Fig. 23-44). Appears at birth and disappears at 3 to 4 months.

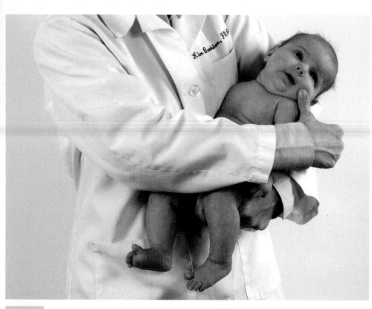

23-44

Sucking Reflex. Touch the lips and offer your gloved little finger to suck. Note strong sucking reflex. The reflex is present at birth and disappears at 10 to 12 months.

Palmar Grasp. Place the baby's head midline to ensure symmetric response. Offer your finger from the baby's ulnar side, away from the thumb. Note tight grasp of all the baby's fingers (Fig. 23-45). Sucking enhances grasp. Often you can pull baby to a sit from grasp. The reflex is present at birth, is strongest at 1 to 2 months, and disappears at 3 to 4 months.

The palmar grasp reflex is absent with brain damage and local muscle or nerve injury.

Persistence of palmar grasp reflex after 4 months of age occurs with frontal lobe lesion.

Normal Range of Findings	Abnormal Findings

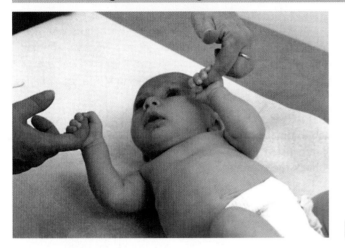

23-45

Plantar Grasp. Touch your thumb at the ball of the baby's foot. Note that the toes curl down tightly (Fig. 23-46). The reflex is present at birth and disappears at 8 to 10 months.

23-46

Babinski Reflex. Stroke your finger up the lateral edge and across the ball of the infant's foot. Note fanning of toes (positive Babinski reflex) (Fig. 23-47). The reflex is present at birth and disappears (changes to the adult response) by 24 months of age (variable).

Positive Babinski reflex after 2 or 2½ years occurs with pyramidal tract disease.

23-47

Normal Range of Findings

Abnormal Findings

Tonic Neck Reflex. With the baby supine, relaxed, or sleeping, turn the head to one side with the chin over shoulder. Note ipsilateral extension of the arm and leg and flexion of the opposite arm and leg; this is the "fencing" position. If you turn the infant's head to the opposite side, positions will reverse (Fig. 23-48). The reflex appears by 2 to 3 months, decreases at 3 to 4 months, and disappears by 4 to 6 months.

Persistence later in infancy occurs with brain damage.

23-48 Tonic neck reflex.

Moro Reflex. Startle the infant by jarring the crib, making a loud noise, or supporting the head and back in a semi-sitting position and quickly lowering the infant to 30 degrees. The baby looks as if he or she is hugging a tree: symmetric abduction and extension of the arms and legs, fanning fingers, and curling of the index finger and thumb to C-position occur. The infant then brings in both arms and legs (Fig. 23-49). The reflex is present at birth and disappears at 1 to 4 months.

Absence of the Moro reflex in the newborn or persistence after 5 months indicates severe CNS injury.

Absence of movement in just one arm occurs with fracture of the humerus or clavicle and with brachial nerve palsy.

Absence in one leg occurs with a lower spinal cord problem or a dislocated hip.

A hyperactive Moro reflex occurs with tetany or CNS infection.

23-49 Moro reflex.

Normal Range of Findings	**Abnormal Findings**

Placing Reflex. Hold the infant upright under the arms, close to a table. Let the dorsal "top" of foot touch the underside of the table. Note flexing of hip and knee, followed by extension at the hip, to place foot on table (Fig. 23-50). Reflex appears at 4 days after birth.

23-50   Placing reflex.

23-51   Stepping reflex.

Stepping Reflex. Hold the infant upright under the arms, with the feet on a flat surface. Note regular alternating steps (Fig. 23-51). The reflex disappears before voluntary walking.

Extensor thrust, or "scissoring"; crossing of lower extremities.

Preschool- and School-Age Children

Assess the child's general behavior during play activities, reaction to parent, and cooperation with parent and with you. Complete details are described in Chapter 5, Mental Status Assessment.

When testing visual fields (cranial nerve II) and cardinal positions of gaze (cranial nerves III, IV, VI), you often need to gently immobilize the head, or the child will track with the whole head. Make a game out of asking the child to imitate your funny "faces" (cranial nerve VII); thus the child has fun and you win a friend.

Much of the motor assessment can be derived from watching the child undress and dress and manipulate buttons. This indicates muscle strength, symmetry, joint range of motion, and fine-motor skills. Use the Denver II to screen gross- and fine-motor skills that are appropriate for the child's specific age. Be familiar with developmental milestones for each age.

Muscle hypertrophy or atrophy occurs with muscular dystrophy.
Muscle weakness.
Incoordination.

Objective Data

Normal Range of Findings

Note the child's gait during both walking and running. Allow for the normal wide-based gait of the toddler and the normal knock-kneed walk of the pre-schooler. Normally the child can balance on one foot for about 5 seconds by 4 years, can balance for 8 to 10 seconds at 5 years, and can hop at 4 years. Children enjoy performing these tests (Fig. 23-52).

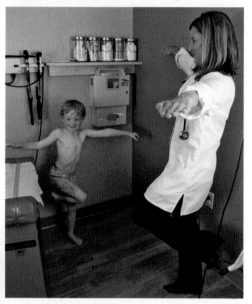

23-52

Observe the child as he or she rises from a supine position on the floor to a sitting position and then to a stand. Note the muscles of the neck, abdomen, arms, and legs. Normally the child curls up in the midline to sit up and pushes off with both hands against the floor to stand (Fig. 23-53, *A*).

A

B

23-53

Assess fine coordination by using the finger-to-nose test if you can be sure that the young child understands your directions. Demonstrate the procedure first; then ask the child to do the test with the eyes open and then with the eyes closed. Fine coordination is not fully developed until the child has reached 4 to 6 years. Consider it normal if a younger child can bring the finger to within 2 to 5 cm (1 to 2 inches) of the nose.

Abnormal Findings

Causes of motor delay are listed earlier in the infant section.

Staggering, falling.

Weakness climbing up or down stairs occurs with muscular dystrophy.

Broad-based gait beyond toddler-hood, scissor gait (see Table 23-7).

Failure to hop after 5 years of age indicates incoordination of gross-motor skill.

Weak pelvic muscles are a sign of muscular dystrophy; from the supine position the child will roll to one side, bend forward to all four extremities, plant hands on legs, and literally "climb" up himself or herself. This is *Gower's sign* (Fig. 23-53, *B*).

Failure of the finger-to-nose test with the eyes open indicates gross incoordination; failure of the test with the eyes closed indicates minor incoordination or lack of position sense.

Normal Range of Findings

Testing sensation is very unreliable in toddlers and preschoolers. You may test light touch by asking the child to close the eyes and then to point to the spot where you touch or tickle. A child younger than 6 years is not usually tested for vibration, position, stereognosis, graphesthesia, or two-point discrimination. In addition, do not test for perception of superficial pain. In children older than 6 years, you may perform sensory testing as with adults. Use a fractured tongue blade if you need to test superficial pain.

The DTRs usually are not tested in children younger than 5 years because of lack of cooperation in relaxation. When you need to test DTRs in a young child, use your finger to percuss the tendon. Use a reflex hammer only with an older child. Coax the child to relax or distract and percuss discreetly when the child is not paying attention. The knee jerk is present at birth, then the ankle jerk and brachial reflex appear, and the triceps reflex is present at 6 months.

The Aging Adult

Use the same examination as used with the younger adult. Be aware that some aging adults show a slower response to your requests, especially to those calling for coordination of movements.

Any decrease in muscle bulk is most apparent in the hand, as seen by guttering between the metacarpals. These dorsal hand muscles often look wasted, even with no apparent arthropathy. The grip strength remains relatively good.

Senile tremors occasionally occur. These benign tremors include an intention tremor of the hands, head nodding (as if saying "yes" or "no"), and tongue protrusion. *Dyskinesias* are the repetitive stereotyped movements in the jaw, lips, or tongue that may accompany senile tremors. No associated rigidity is present.

The gait may be slower and more deliberate than that in the younger person, and it may deviate slightly from a midline path.

The aging adult may have more difficulty performing rapid alternating movements (e.g., pronating and supinating the hands on the thigh).

After 65 years, loss of the sensation of vibration at the ankle malleolus is common and is usually accompanied by loss of the ankle jerk. Position sense in the big toe may be lost, although this is less common than vibration loss. Tactile sensation may be impaired. The aging person may need stronger stimuli for light touch and especially for pain.

The DTRs are less brisk. Those in the upper extremities are usually present, but the ankle jerks commonly are lost. Knee jerks may be lost, but this occurs less often. Because aging people find it difficult to relax their limbs, always use reinforcement when eliciting the DTRs.

The plantar reflex may be absent or difficult to interpret. Often you will not see a definite normal flexor response.

Neurologic Recheck

Some hospitalized people have head trauma or a neurologic deficit caused by a systemic disease process. These people must be monitored closely for any improvement or deterioration in neurologic status and for any indication of increasing intracranial pressure. Signs of increasing intracranial pressure signal impending cerebral disaster and death and require early and prompt intervention.

Abnormal Findings

Sensory loss occurs with decreased consciousness, mental deficiency, or spinal cord or peripheral nerve dysfunction.

Hyperactivity of DTRs occurs with UMN lesion, hypocalcemia, and hyperthyroidism and with muscle spasm associated with early poliomyelitis.

Decreased or absent reflexes occur with a LMN lesion, muscular dystrophy, and flaccidity or flaccid paralysis.

Clonus may occur with fatigue, but it usually indicates hyperreflexia.

Hand muscle atrophy is worsened with disuse and degenerative arthropathy.

Distinguish senile tremors from tremors of parkinsonism. The latter includes rigidity and slowness and weakness of voluntary movement.

Absence of a rhythmic reciprocal gait pattern is seen in parkinsonism and hemiparesis (see Table 23-7).

Note any difference in sensation between right and left sides, which may indicate a neurologic deficit.

Still consider a definite extensor response to be abnormal.

Normal Range of Findings	Abnormal Findings

Use an abbreviation of the neurologic examination in the following sequence:
1. Level of consciousness
2. Motor function
3. Pupillary response
4. Vital signs

Level of Consciousness. A *change* in the level of consciousness is the single most important factor in this examination. It is the earliest and most sensitive index of change in neurologic status. Note the ease of *arousal* and the state of awareness, or *orientation*. Assess orientation by asking questions about:
- Person—Own name, occupation, names of workers around person, their occupations
- Place—Where person is, nature of building, city, state
- Time—Day of week, month, year

Vary the questions during repeat assessments so the person is not merely memorizing answers. Note the quality and content of the verbal response; articulation, fluency, manner of thinking; and any deficit in language comprehension or production (see Chapter 5).

When the person is intubated and cannot speak, you have to ask questions that require a nod or shake of the head (e.g., "Is this a hospital?" "Are you at home?" "Are we in Texas?")

A person is fully alert when his or her eyes open at your approach or spontaneously; when he or she is oriented to person, place, and time; and when he or she is able to follow verbal commands appropriately.

If the person is not fully alert, increase the amount of stimulus used in this order:
1. Name called
2. Light touch on person's arm
3. Vigorous shake of shoulder
4. Pain applied (pinch nail bed, pinch trapezius muscle, rub your knuckles on the person's sternum)

Record the stimulus used and the person's response to it.

Motor Function. Check the voluntary movement of each extremity by giving the person specific commands. (This procedure also tests level of consciousness by noting the person's ability to follow commands.)

Ask the person to lift the eyebrows, frown, bare teeth. Note symmetric facial movements and bilateral nasolabial folds (cranial nerve VII).

You can check upper arm strength by checking hand grasps. Ask the person to squeeze your fingers. Offer your two fingers, one on top of the other, so a strong hand grasp does not hurt your knuckles (Fig. 23-54). Be judicious about asking the person to squeeze your hands; some people with diffuse brain damage, especially frontal lobe injury, have a grasp that is a reflex only.

A change in consciousness may be subtle. Note any decreasing level of consciousness, disorientation, memory loss, uncooperative behavior, or even complacency in a previously combative person.

Review Table 5-1, Levels of Consciousness, p. 79.

A weak grip occurs with upper and lower motor neuron disease and with local hand problems (arthritis, carpal tunnel syndrome).

23-54

Normal Range of Findings

Alternatively ask the person to lift each hand or to hold up one finger. You also can check upper-extremity strength by palmar drift. Ask the person to extend both arms forward or halfway up, palms up, eyes closed, and hold for 10 to 20 seconds (Fig. 23-55). Normally the arms stay steady with no downward drift.

23-55

Check lower extremities by asking the person to do straight leg raises. Ask the person to lift one leg at a time straight up off the bed (Fig. 23-56). Full strength allows the leg to be lifted 90 degrees. If multiple trauma, pain, or equipment precludes this motion, ask the person to push one foot at a time against the resistance in your hand, "like putting your foot on the gas pedal of your car" (Fig. 23-57).

23-56

23-57

For the person with decreased level of consciousness, note if movement occurs spontaneously and as a result of noxious stimuli such as pain or suctioning. An attempt to push away your hand after such stimuli is called *localizing* and is characterized as purposeful movement.

Pupillary Response. Note the size, shape, and symmetry of both pupils. Shine a light into each pupil, and note the direct and consensual light reflex. Both pupils should constrict briskly. (Allow for the effects of any medication that could affect pupil size and reactivity.) When recording, pupil size is best expressed in millimeters. Tape a millimeter scale onto a tongue blade and hold it next to the person's eyes for the most accurate measurement (Fig. 23-58).

Abnormal Findings

Pronator drift is a downward unilateral drift and turning in of the forearm that occurs with mild hemiparesis.

Any abnormal posturing, decorticate rigidity, or decerebrate rigidity indicates diffuse brain injury (see Table 23-11).

In a brain-injured person a sudden unilateral dilated and nonreactive pupil is ominous. Cranial nerve III runs parallel to the brainstem. When increasing intracranial pressure pushes the brainstem down (uncal herniation), it puts pressure on cranial nerve III, causing pupil dilation.

Normal Range of Findings	Abnormal Findings

23-58

Vital Signs. Measure the temperature, pulse, respiration, and BP as often as the person's condition warrants. Although they are vital to the overall assessment of the critically ill person, pulse and BP are notoriously unreliable parameters of CNS deficit. Any changes are late consequences of rising intracranial pressure.

The Glasgow Coma Scale. Because the terms describing levels of consciousness are ambiguous, the Glasgow Coma Scale (GCS) was developed as an accurate and reliable *quantitative* tool (Fig. 23-59). The GCS is a standardized, objective assessment that defines the level of consciousness by giving it a numeric value.

The Cushing reflex shows signs of increasing intracranial pressure: BP—sudden elevation with widening pulse pressure; pulse—decreased rate, slow and bounding.

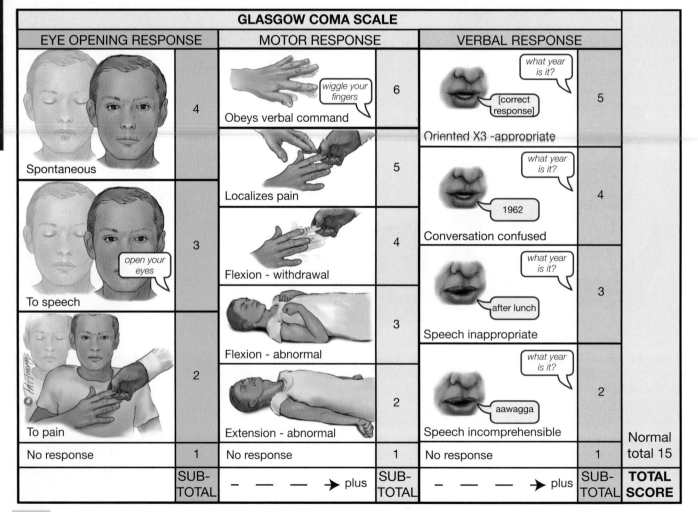

GLASGOW COMA SCALE							
EYE OPENING RESPONSE		**MOTOR RESPONSE**		**VERBAL RESPONSE**			
Spontaneous	4	Obeys verbal command *wiggle your fingers*	6	Oriented X3 -appropriate *what year is it?* [correct response]	5		
To speech *open your eyes*	3	Localizes pain	5	Conversation confused *what year is it?* 1962	4		
		Flexion - withdrawal	4	Speech inappropriate *what year is it?* after lunch	3		
To pain	2	Flexion - abnormal	3	Speech incomprehensible *what year is it?* aawagga	2		
		Extension - abnormal	2				
No response	1	No response	1	No response	1		Normal total 15
	SUB-TOTAL	— — — → plus	SUB-TOTAL	— — — → plus	SUB-TOTAL		**TOTAL SCORE**

23-59

Images © Pat Thomas, 2014.

Objective Data

Normal Range of Findings

Abnormal Findings

The scale is divided into three areas: eye opening, verbal response, and motor response. Each area is rated separately, and a number is given for the person's best response. The three numbers are added; the total score reflects the functional level of the brain. A fully alert, normal person has a score of 15, whereas a score of 7 or less reflects coma. Serial assessments can be plotted on a graph to illustrate visually whether the person is stable, improving, or deteriorating.

The GCS assesses the functional state of the brain as a whole, not of any particular site in the brain. The scale is easy to learn and master, has good interrater reliability, and enhances interprofessional communication by providing a common language.

PROMOTING A HEALTHY LIFESTYLE

Stroke Prevention

A stroke, or cerebrovascular accident (CVA), occurs when the blood flow is interrupted to a part of the brain, which is why it is often referred to as a *brain attack*. According to the National Institutes of Health (NIH), strokes are the leading cause of long-term disability and the 4th leading cause of death after heart disease and cancer. Nearly 75% of all strokes occur in people over the age of 65, and the risk of having a stroke more than doubles each decade after the age of 55.

The NINDS campaign *Know Stroke. Know the Signs. Act in Time* focuses on educating the public about the symptoms of stroke and the need to get the person with symptoms to the hospital quickly. An 8-minute video *Know Stroke* video is available, featuring experts discussing the symptoms of stroke and what to do. The video also includes stories from people who have successfully recovered from a stroke. A *Know Stroke* Community Education Kit, including a facilitator's guide and step-by-step materials for planning and conducting a stroke education event, is also available through the NINDS campaign website in English and/or Spanish: http://stroke.nih.gov/.

The most common type is an **ischemic stroke**, occurring when a blood clot blocks a blood vessel in the brain. Less common is a **hemorrhagic stroke**, which occurs when a blood vessel in the brain ruptures and causes bleeding. The symptoms and aftereffects of a stroke depend on which area of the brain is affected and to what extent. This can make a stroke difficult to diagnose. However, early recognition of symptoms and prompt treatment are essential.

Stroke symptoms usually do not hurt, which is why many people ignore them or delay seeking medical attention. Sometimes people can have a "mini-stroke" or transient ischemic attack (TIA). In these cases the stroke symptoms last only temporarily and disappear, often within an hour. Because the symptoms "go away," people too often do not report them or seek medical attention. However, a TIA is a warning sign that should not be ignored. Having a TIA should prompt people to seek medical attention to rule out the possibility of a future brain attack.

Common symptoms of stroke include **sudden**:
- Weakness or numbness in the face, arms, or legs, especially when it is on one side of the body.

- Confusion, trouble speaking or understanding.
- Changes in vision such as blurry vision or partial or complete loss of vision in one or both eyes.
- Trouble walking, dizziness, loss of balance, or coordination.
- Severe headache with no reason or explanation.

One tool that can be useful is the NIH Stroke Scale (NIHSS), a 15-item systematic assessment tool that provides a quantitative measure of stroke-related neurologic deficit. It is widely used as a clinical assessment tool to evaluate acuity and predict patient outcome. It can be downloaded directly as a pdf from http://www.ninds.nih.gov/doctors/NIH_Stroke_Scale.pdf or accessed through NIH Stroke Scale (NIHSS) International at http://www.nihstrokescale.org/.

Another tool that is particularly useful for public education is the American Heart Association and American Stroke Association **F.A.S.T.** acronym, an easy way to remember the sudden signs of stroke:
- **F** = Face drooping
- **A** = Arm weakness
- **S** = Speech difficulty
- **T** = Time to call 9-1-1

To view an effective 60-second public service announcement that shows how body language cannot only communicate a wide range of emotions but can also tell you if someone might be having a stroke, go to: http://www.youtube.com/watch?feature=player_embedded&v=wH7k5CFp4hl.

The F.A.S.T. app can be downloaded from: http://strokeassociation.org/STROKEORG/WarningSigns/Stroke-Warning-Signs-and-Symptoms_UCM_308528_SubHomePage.jsp.

References

The National Institute of Neurological Disorders and Stroke (NINDS): Stroke information page, *http://www.ninds.nih.gov/disorders/stroke/stroke.htm.*

The National Institutes of Health (NIH)/Senior Health Pages: About stroke, *http://nihseniorhealth.gov/stroke/aboutstroke/01.html.*

The American Stroke Association: *http://www.strokeassociation.org/STROKEORG/.*

Objective Data

DOCUMENTATION AND CRITICAL THINKING

Sample Charting

SUBJECTIVE

No unusually frequent or severe headaches; no head injury, dizziness or vertigo, seizures, or tremors. No weakness, numbness or tingling, or difficulty swallowing or speaking. Has no past history of stroke, spinal cord injury, meningitis, or alcohol disorder.

OBJECTIVE

Mental status: Appearance, behavior, and speech appropriate; alert and oriented to person, place, and time; recent and remote memory intact.

Cranial nerves:

II: Vision 20/20 left eye, 20/20 right eye; peripheral fields intact by confrontation; fundi normal.

III, IV, VI: EOMs intact, no ptosis or nystagmus; pupils equal, round, react to light and accommodation (PERRLA).

V: Sensation intact and equal bilaterally; jaw strength equal bilaterally.

VII: Facial muscles intact and symmetric.

VIII: Hearing—whispered words heard bilaterally.

IX, X: Swallowing intact, gag reflex present, uvula rises in midline on phonation.

XI: Shoulder shrug, head movement intact and equal bilaterally.

XII: Tongue protrudes midline, no tremors.

Motor: No atrophy, weakness, or tremors. Rapid alternating movements—finger-to-nose smoothly intact. Gait smooth and coordinated, able to tandem walk, negative Romberg.

Sensory: Pinprick, light touch, vibration intact. Stereognosis—able to identify key.

Reflexes: Normal abdominal, no Babinski sign, DTRs 2+ and = bilaterally with downgoing toes; see following drawing:

ASSESSMENT

Neurologic system intact; normal function

Clinical Case Study 1

J.T. is a 61-year-old Caucasian male carpenter with a large building firm who is admitted to the Rehabilitation Institute with a diagnosis of right hemiplegia and aphasia following a stroke (CVA) 4 weeks PTA.

SUBJECTIVE

Because of J.T.'s speech dysfunction, history provided by wife.

4 weeks PTA—Complaint of severe headache; then sudden onset of collapse and loss of consciousness while at work. Did not strike head as he fell. Transported by ambulance to Memorial Hospital where admitting physician said J.T. "probably had a stroke." Right arm and leg were limp, and he remained unconscious. Admitted to critical care unit. Regained consciousness day 3 after admission, unable to move right side, unable to speak clearly or write. Remained in ICU 4 more days until "doctors were sure heart and breathing were steady."

3 weeks PTA—Transferred to medical floor where care included physical therapy 2 ×/day and passive ROM 4 ×/day.

Now—Some improvement in right motor function. Bowel control achieved with use of commode same time each day (after breakfast). Bladder control improved. Some occasional incontinence, usually when he cannot tell people he needs to urinate.

OBJECTIVE

Mental status: Dressed in jogging suit, sitting in wheelchair, appears alert with appropriate eye contact, listening intently to history. Speech is slow, requires great effort, able to give one-word answers that are appropriate but lack normal tone. Seems to understand all language spoken to him. Follows requests appropriately, within limits of motor weakness.

Cranial nerves:

II: Acuity normal; fields by confrontation—right homonymous hemianopsia; fundi normal.

III, IV, VI: EOMs intact, no ptosis or nystagmus, PERRLA.

V: Sensation intact to pinprick and light touch. Jaw strength weak on right.

VII: Flat nasolabial fold on right, motor weakness on right lower face. Able to wrinkle forehead bilaterally but unable to smile or bare teeth on right.

VIII: Hearing intact.

IX, X: Swallowing intact, gag reflex present, uvula rises midline on phonation.

XI: Shoulder shrug, head movement weaker on right.

XII: Tongue protrudes midline; no tremors.

Sensory: Pinprick and light touch present but diminished on right arm and leg. Vibration intact. Position sense impaired on right side. Stereognosis intact.

Motor: Right hand grip weak, right arm drifts, right leg weak, unable to support weight. Spasticity in right arm and leg muscles, limited range of motion on passive motion. Unable to stand up and walk unassisted. Unable to perform finger-to-nose or heel-to-shin on right side; left side smoothly intact.

Reflexes: Hyperactive 4+ with clonus, and upgoing toes in right leg. Abdominal and cremasteric reflexes absent on right.

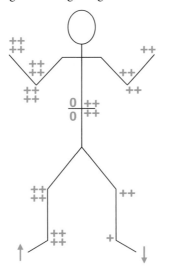

ASSESSMENT

Impaired verbal communication R/T effects of CVA
Impaired physical mobility R/T neuromuscular impairment
Disturbed body image R/T effects of loss of body function
Self-care deficits: feeding, bathing, toileting, dressing/grooming R/T muscular weakness
Disturbed sensory perception (absent right visual fields) R/T neurologic impairment
Risk for injury R/T visual field deficit

Clinical Case Study 2

L.B. is a 38-year-old premenopausal female who recently underwent treatment for breast cancer. Her treatment included a right radical mastectomy followed by chemotherapy. Her cancer is in remission, and she is in the clinic for her annual follow-up. During her course of chemotherapy L.B. described symptoms of peripheral neuropathy in her hands and feet.

SUBJECTIVE

L.B. reports difficulty walking, including balance problems for the past 6 months. "It feels like my feet and hands are burning all the time." L.B. describes episodes of sharp, shooting pain—"like an electric shock"—that occur approximately 2 to 3 times per week. No precipitating factors identified. "I kept thinking it'd get better now that I'm off chemo." Reports pain with computer use and difficulty using her cell phone because of inability to "hit the right key."

OBJECTIVE

Mental status: Dressed appropriately for weather, age, and sex. Appears alert. Crying as she relays current symptoms. Avoids eye contact.
Cranial nerves: Grossly intact.
Motor: No atrophy or tremors. Bilateral lower extremity strength 3+. Grips weak but equal. Gait smooth and coordinated. Unable to tandem walk without losing balance. Rapid alternating movement smoothly intact.
Sensory: Pinprick, light touch, and vibration intact on arms. Unable to identify pinprick, light touch, or vibration on hands to the wrists and feet to the ankles. Stereognosis—unable to identify key or coin bilaterally.
Reflexes: Normal abdominal, no Babinski sign, DTRs 2+ and equal bilaterally with downgoing toes.

ASSESSMENT

Severe chemotherapy-induced peripheral neuropathy
Risk for impaired skin integrity R/T decreased sensation in hands and feet
Risk for depression R/T severe peripheral neuropathy
Impaired physical mobility R/T sensoriperceptual impairment
Disturbed sensory perception: tactile R/T peripheral neuropathy

Clinical Case Study 3

S.S., an 11-month-old Caucasian male, is brought to the ED via ambulance after parents called 911.

SUBJECTIVE

45 minutes PTA—S.S. was crawling when he "just stiffened, collapsed on his tummy, and then his arms and legs started shaking for about 2 minutes. We tried to talk to him, but he acted 'out of it.'" Parents report that S.S. had been experiencing a "cold since yesterday but no fever until today." They deny S.S. experiencing any vomiting or diarrhea and state that he has been eating, drinking, and voiding "as usual."

OBJECTIVE

Vital signs: Temp 102.9° F (39.4° C) (rectal). Pulse 146 bpm. Resp 42/min. BP 94/56 mm Hg (resting).
General appearance: Quiet and appears drowsy but quickly awakens when touched or spoken to.
HEENT: Fontanels closed; conjunctivae clear, sclera white; bilat TMs dull red and bulging, no light reflex, no mobility on pneumatic otoscopy; no lymphadenopathy.
Neuro: All CNs intact without deficit; no atrophy, weakness, or tremors; sensory intact w/light and deep touch and vibration; DTRs 2+, Babinski +.
Cardiovascular: Regular rate and rhythm w/o abnormal heart sounds.
Respiratory: Breath sounds clear and equal bilat; unlabored

ASSESSMENT

Simple febrile seizure
Ineffective health maintenance R/T lack of knowledge regarding fever reduction
Risk for ineffective airway clearance R/T accumulation of secretions during seizure
Risk for injury R/T uncontrolled movements during seizure and falls

ABNORMAL FINDINGS

TABLE 23-2	10 Warning Signs of Alzheimer Disease (Alzheimer's Association, 2009)	
	Alzheimer Disease (AD)	**Normal Aging**
1 MEMORY LOSS	Memory loss: Forgetting recently learned information is one of the most common early signs of dementia. A person begins to forget more often and is unable to recall the information later.	Forgetting names or appointments occasionally but later remembering
2 LOSING TRACK	Difficulty performing familiar tasks: People with dementia often find it hard to plan or complete everyday tasks. Individuals may lose track of the steps involved in preparing a meal, placing a telephone call, or playing a game.	Occasionally forgetting why you came into a room or what you planned to say
3 FORGETTING WORDS	Problems with language: People with AD often forget simple words or substitute unusual words, making their speech or writing hard to understand. For example, they may be unable to find the toothbrush and instead ask for "that thing for my mouth."	Sometimes having trouble finding the right word
4 GETTING LOST	Disorientation to time and place: People with AD can become lost in their own neighborhood, forget where they are and how they got there, and not know how to get back home.	Forgetting the day of the week or where you were going
5 POOR JUDGMENT	Poor or decreased judgment: Those with AD may dress inappropriately, wearing several layers on a warm day or little clothing in the cold. They may show poor judgment such as giving away large sums of money to telemarketers.	Making a questionable or debatable decision from time to time
6 ABSTRACT FAILING	Problems with abstract thinking: Someone with AD may have unusual difficulty performing complex mental tasks such as forgetting what numbers are for and how they should be used.	Finding it challenging to balance a checkbook
7 LOSING THINGS	Misplacing things: A person with AD may put things in unusual places (e.g., an iron in the freezer or a wristwatch in the sugar bowl).	Misplacing keys or a wallet temporarily
8 MOOD SWINGS	Changes in mood or behavior: Someone with AD may show rapid mood swings—from calm to tears to anger—for no apparent reason.	Occasionally feeling sad or moody
9 PERSONALITY CHANGE	Changes in personality: The personalities of people with dementia can change dramatically. They may become extremely confused, suspicious, fearful, or dependent on a family member.	People's personalities do change somewhat with age
10 GROWING PASSIVE	Loss of initiative: A person with AD may become very passive, sitting in front of the television for hours, sleeping more than usual, or not wanting to do usual activities.	Sometimes feeling weary of work or social obligations

Adapted from Leifer, B.P. (2009). Alzheimer's disease: seeing the signs early. *J Acad Nurse Pract, 21*(11), 588-595.

Abnormal Findings

TABLE 23-3 Abnormalities in Cranial Nerves

Nerve	Test	Abnormal Findings	Possible Causes
I: Olfactory	Identify familiar odors	Anosmia	Upper respiratory infection (temporary); tobacco or cocaine use; fracture of cribriform plate or ethmoid area; frontal lobe lesion; tumor in olfactory bulb or tract
II: Optic	Visual acuity	Defect in or absent central vision	Congenital blindness; refractive error; acquired vision loss from numerous diseases (e.g., stroke, diabetes); trauma to globe or orbit (see discussion of CN III)
	Visual fields	Defect in peripheral vision, hemianopsia	
	Shine light in eye	Absent light reflex	
	Direct inspection	Papilledema	Increased intracranial pressure; glaucoma; diabetes
		Optic atrophy	
		Retinal lesions	
III: Oculomotor	Inspection	Dilated pupil, ptosis, eye turns out and slightly down	Paralysis in CN III from internal carotid aneurysm; tumor; inflammatory lesions; uncal herniation with increased intracranial pressure
	Extraocular muscle movement	Failure to move eye up, in, down	Ptosis from myasthenia gravis; oculomotor nerve palsy; Horner syndrome
	Shine light in eye	Absent light reflex	Blindness; drug influence; increased intracranial pressure; CNS injury; circulatory arrest; CNS syphilis
IV: Trochlear	Extraocular muscle movement	Failure to turn eye down or out	Fracture of orbit; brainstem tumor
V: Trigeminal	Superficial touch—three divisions	Absent touch and pain, paresthesias	Trauma; tumor; pressure from aneurysm; inflammation; sequelae of alcohol injection for trigeminal neuralgia
	Corneal reflex	No blink	
	Clench teeth	Weakness of masseter or temporalis muscles	Unilateral weakness with CN V lesion; bilateral weakness with UMN or LMN disorder
VI: Abducens	Extraocular muscle movement to right and left sides	Failure to move laterally, diplopia on lateral gaze	Brainstem tumor or trauma; fracture of orbit
VII: Facial	Wrinkle forehead, close eyes tightly	Absent or asymmetric facial movement	Bell palsy (LMN lesion) causes paralysis of entire half of face
	Smile, puff cheeks	Loss of taste	UMN lesions (stroke, tumor, inflammatory) cause paralysis of lower half of face, leaving forehead intact; other LMN causes of paralysis: swelling from ear or meningeal infections
	Identify tastes		
VIII: Acoustic	Hearing acuity	Decrease or loss of hearing	Inflammation; occluded ear canal; otosclerosis; presbycusis; drug toxicity; tumor
IX: Glossopharyngeal	Gag reflex	See CN X	
X: Vagus	Phonates "ahh"	Uvula deviates to side	Brainstem tumor; neck injury; CN X lesion
	Gag reflex	No gag reflex	Vocal cord weakness
	Note voice quality	Hoarse or brassy	Soft palate weakness
		Nasal twang	Unilateral CN X lesion
		Husky	
	Note swallowing	Dysphagia, fluids regurgitate through nose	Bilateral CN X lesion
XI: Spinal accessory	Turn head, shrug shoulders against resistance	Absent movement of sternomastoid or trapezius muscles	Neck injury, torticollis
XII: Hypoglossal	Protrude tongue	Deviates to side	LMN lesion
	Wiggle tongue from side to side	Slowed rate of movement	Bilateral UMN lesion

TABLE 23-4 Abnormalities in Muscle Tone

Condition	Description	Associated With
Flaccidity	Decreased muscle tone or *hypotonia;* muscle feels limp, soft, and flabby; muscle is weak and easily fatigued; limb feels like a rag doll	**Lower motor neuron** injury anywhere from the anterior horn cell in the spinal cord to the peripheral nerve (peripheral neuritis, poliomyelitis, Guillain-Barré syndrome); early stroke and spinal cord injury are flaccid at first
Spasticity	Increased tone or *hypertonia;* increased resistance to passive lengthening; then may suddenly give way (clasp-knife phenomenon) like a pocket knife sprung open	**Upper motor neuron** injury to corticospinal motor tract (e.g., paralysis with stroke develops spasticity days or weeks after incident)
Rigidity	Constant state of resistance (lead-pipe rigidity); resists passive movement in any direction; dystonia	Injury to extrapyramidal motor tracts (e.g., basal ganglia with parkinsonism)
Cogwheel rigidity	Type of rigidity in which the increased tone is released by degrees during passive range of motion so it feels like small, regular jerks	Parkinsonism

TABLE 23-5 Abnormalities in Muscle Movement

Paralysis

Decreased or loss of motor power caused by problem with motor nerve or muscle fibers. Causes: acute—trauma, spinal cord injury, stroke, poliomyelitis, polyneuritis, Bell palsy; chronic—muscular dystrophy, diabetic neuropathy, multiple sclerosis; episodic—myasthenia gravis.

Patterns of paralysis: *hemiplegia*—spastic or flaccid paralysis of one side (right or left) of body and extremities; *paraplegia*—symmetric paralysis of both lower extremities; *quadriplegia*—paralysis in all four extremities. *Paresis*—weakness of muscles rather than paralysis.

Fasciculation

Rapid, continuous twitching of resting muscle or part of muscle without movement of limb, which can be seen by clinicians or felt by patients. Types: fine—occurs with LMN disease, associated with atrophy and weakness; coarse—occurs with cold exposure or fatigue and is not significant.

Continued

TABLE 23-5   Abnormalities in Muscle Movement—cont'd

Myoclonus

Rapid, sudden jerk or a short series of jerks at fairly regular intervals. A hiccup is a myoclonus of diaphragm. Single myoclonic arm or leg jerk is normal when the person is falling asleep; myoclonic jerks are severe with grand mal seizures.

Tic

Involuntary, compulsive, repetitive twitching of a muscle group (e.g., wink, grimace, head movement, shoulder shrug); due to a neurologic cause (e.g., tardive dyskinesias, Tourette syndrome) or a psychogenic cause (habit tic).

Chorea

Sudden, rapid, jerky, purposeless movement involving limbs, trunk, or face. Occurs at irregular intervals, not rhythmic or repetitive, more convulsive than a tic. Some are spontaneous, and some are initiated; all are accentuated by voluntary acts. Disappears with sleep. Common with Sydenham chorea and Huntington disease.

Athetosis

Slow, twisting, writhing, continuous movement, resembling a snake or worm. Involves the distal more than the proximal part of the limb. Occurs with cerebral palsy. Disappears with sleep. "Athetoid" hand—Some fingers are flexed, and some are extended.

TABLE 23-5 Abnormalities in Muscle Movement—cont'd

Seizure Disorder (not illustrated)

A seizure is a time-limited event caused by excessive, hypersynchronous discharge of neurons in the brain. It may be from a clear provocation such as cerebral trauma, structural lesions (tumor, blood clot, infection), hyponatremia, acute alcohol withdrawal, or medication overdose. Also, epilepsy has unprovoked recurrent seizures due to cerebrovascular disease, or in 70% of patients of unknown cause. Generalized seizures involve the entire brain such as the tonic-clonic or grand mal seizure. This type of seizure has distinct phases: (1) loss of consciousness; (2) tonic phase with muscular rigidity, opening of mouth and eyes, tongue biting, and high-pitched cry; (3) clonic phase with violent muscular contractions, facial grimacing, and increased heart rate; and (4) postictal phase with deep sleeping, disorientation, and confusion.

Tremor

Involuntary contraction of opposing muscle groups. Results in rhythmic, back-and-forth movement of one or more joints. May occur at rest or with voluntary movement. All tremors disappear while sleeping. Tremors may be slow (3 to 6 per second) or rapid (10 to 20 per second).

Rest Tremor

It occurs when muscles are quiet and supported against gravity (hand in lap). Coarse and slow (3 to 6 per second); partly or completely disappears with voluntary movement (e.g., "pill rolling" tremor of parkinsonism, with thumb and opposing fingers).

Intention Tremor

Rate varies; worse with voluntary movement as in reaching toward a visually guided target. Occurs with cerebellar disease and multiple sclerosis.

Essential tremor (familial)—A type of intention tremor; most common tremor with older people. Benign (no associated disease) but causes emotional stress in business or social situations. Improves with the administration of sedatives, propranolol, or alcohol; but alcohol discouraged because of the risk for addiction.

TABLE 23-6   Ischemic and Hemorrhagic Stroke

Ischemic stroke is a sudden interruption of blood flow to the brain and accounts for 87% of all strokes. These are of two types. Thrombotic strokes result from atherosclerotic plaque formation. A vulnerable plaque ruptures, and a local thrombus forms that deprives the brain tissue in the region of crucial oxygen and glucose. Embolic strokes result from a traveling clot caused by atrial fibrillation or flutter, recent heart attack, growth around prosthetic heart valves, and endocarditis. Acute ischemic stroke symptoms include unilateral facial droop, arm drift, weakness or paralysis on one half of the body, difficulty speaking or understanding speech, confusion, loss of balance, clouding of vision.[5,8,20]

Hemorrhagic stroke results from acute rupture and bleeding from a weakened artery in the brain and accounts for 13% of all strokes. Most are intracerebral hemorrhages caused by ruptured aneurysm, arteriovenous malformation, disturbed coagulation cascade, tumor, or cocaine abuse. A subarachnoid hemorrhage is less common and is due to an aneurysm between the base of the cerebral cortex and the arachnoid layer of the meninges. Symptoms include sudden severe headache, nausea and vomiting, sudden loss of consciousness, and focal seizures.[5,20]

Images © Pat Thomas, 2014.

ABNORMAL FINDINGS
FOR ADVANCED PRACTICE

TABLE 23-7	Abnormal Gaits	
Type	Characteristic Appearance	Possible Causes
Spastic Hemiparesis	Arm is immobile against the body, with flexion of the shoulder, elbow, wrist, and fingers and adduction of shoulder; does not swing freely. Leg is stiff and extended and circumducts with each step (drags toe in a semicircle).	UMN lesion of the corticospinal tract (e.g., stroke, trauma)
Cerebellar Ataxia	Staggering, wide-based gait; difficulty with turns; uncoordinated movement with positive Romberg sign.	Alcohol or barbiturate effect on cerebellum; cerebellar tumor; multiple sclerosis
Parkinsonian (Festinating)	Posture is stooped; trunk is pitched forward; elbows, hips, and knees are flexed. Steps are short and shuffling. Hesitation to begin walking, and difficult to stop suddenly. The person holds the body rigid. Walks and turns body as one fixed unit. Difficulty with any change in direction.	Parkinsonism
Scissors	Knees cross or are in contact, like holding an orange between the thighs. The person uses short steps, and walking requires effort.	Paraparesis of legs, multiple sclerosis
Steppage or Footdrop	Slapping quality—Looks as if walking up stairs and finding no stair there. Lifts knee and foot high and slaps it down hard and flat to compensate for footdrop.	Weakness of peroneal and anterior tibial muscles; caused by LMN lesion at spinal cord (e.g., poliomyelitis)

Continued

TABLE 23-7	Abnormal Gaits—cont'd	
Type	Characteristic Appearance	Possible Causes
Waddling	Weak hip muscles—When the person takes a step, the opposite hip drops, which allows compensatory lateral movement of pelvis. Often the person also has marked lumbar lordosis and a protruding abdomen.	Hip girdle muscle weakness caused by muscular dystrophy, dislocation of hips
Short Leg	Leg length discrepancy >2.5 cm (1 inch). Vertical telescoping of affected side, which dips as person walks. Appearance of gait varies, depending on amount of accompanying muscle dysfunction.	Congenital dislocated hip; acquired shortening from disease, trauma

TABLE 23-8	Characteristics of Upper and Lower Motor Neuron Lesions	
	Upper Motor Neuron Lesion	Lower Motor Neuron Lesion
Weakness/paralysis	In muscles corresponding to distribution of damage in pyramidal tract lesion; usually in hand grip, arm extensors, leg flexors	In specific muscles served by damaged spinal segment, ventral root, or peripheral nerve
Location	Descending motor pathways that originate in motor areas of cerebral cortex and carry impulses to anterior horn cells of spinal cord	Nerve cells that originate in anterior horn of spinal cord or brainstem and carry impulses by spinal or cranial nerves to muscles, the "final common pathway"
Example	Stroke (brain attack)	Poliomyelitis, herniated intervertebral disk
Muscle tone	Increased tone; spasticity	Loss of tone; flaccidity
Bulk	May have some atrophy from disuse; otherwise normal	Atrophy (wasting), may be marked
Abnormal movements	None	Fasciculations
Reflexes	Hyperreflexia, ankle clonus; diminished or absent superficial abdominal reflexes; positive Babinski sign	Hyporeflexia or areflexia; no Babinski sign, no pathologic reflexes
Possible nursing diagnoses	Risk for contractures; impaired physical mobility	Impaired physical mobility

TABLE 23-9 Patterns of Motor System Dysfunction

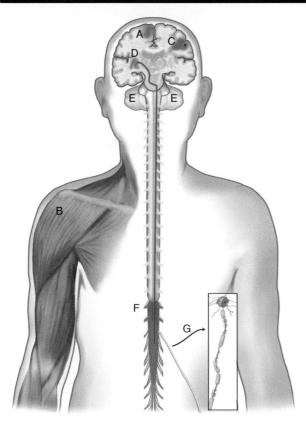

A—Cerebral palsy. Mixed group of paralytic neuromotor disorders of infancy and childhood; due to damage to cerebral cortex from a developmental defect, intrauterine meningitis or encephalitis, birth trauma, anoxia, or kernicterus.

B—Muscular dystrophy. Chronic, progressive wasting of skeletal musculature, which produces weakness, contractures, and in severe cases respiratory dysfunction and death. Onset of symptoms occurs in childhood. Many types exist; the most severe is Duchenne dystrophy, characterized by the waddling gait described in Table 23-7.

C—Hemiplegia. Damage to corticospinal tract (stroke). UMN damage occurs above the pyramidal decussation crossover; thus motor impairment is on contralateral (opposite) side. Initially flaccid when lesion is acute; later the muscles become spastic, and abnormal reflexes appear. Characteristic posture: arm—shoulder adducted, elbow flexed, wrist pronated, leg extended; face—weakness only in lower muscles. Hyperreflexia and possible clonus occur on the involved side; loss of corneal, abdominal, and cremasteric reflexes; positive Babinski and Hoffman reflexes.

D—Parkinsonism. Loss of dopamine-containing neurons in the basal ganglia with motor tract dysfunction. Cardinal symptoms are resting tremor, bradykinesia, cogwheel rigidity, loss of balance; also cognitive decline, depression, and urinary incontinence.[21] Body tends to stay immobile; facial expression is flat, staring, expressionless; excessive salivation occurs; eye blinking is reduced. Posture is stooped; equilibrium is impaired; balance is easily lost; gait is described in Table 23-7. Parkinsonian tremor; cogwheel rigidity on passive range of motion.

E—Cerebellar. A lesion in one hemisphere produces motor abnormalities on the ipsilateral side. Characterized by ataxia, lurching forward of affected side while walking; rapid alternating movements are slow and arrhythmic; finger-to-nose test reveals ataxia and tremor with overshoot or undershoot; and eyes display coarse nystagmus.

F—Paraplegia. LMN damage caused by spinal cord injury. A severe injury or complete transection initially produces "spinal shock," which is defined as no movement or reflex activity below level of lesion. Gradually deep tendon reflexes reappear and become increased; flexor spasms of legs occur; and finally extensor spasms of legs occur; these spasms lead to prevailing extensor tone.

G—Multiple sclerosis (MS). Chronic, progressive, immune-mediated disease in which axons experience inflammation, demyelination, degeneration and, finally, sclerosis. Structures most frequently involved are the optic nerve, oculomotor nerve, corticospinal tract, posterior column tract, and cerebellum. Thus symptoms include nystagmus, diplopia, extreme fatigue, weakness, spasticity, loss of balance, hyperreflexia, Babinski sign (upgoing toes). MS affects young adults in their productive years, with 32 years the average age at diagnosis.[15]

Image © Pat Thomas, 2010.

TABLE 23-10 Patterns of Sensory Loss

Type	Characteristics	Possible Causes
Peripheral Neuropathy	Loss of sensation involves all modalities. Loss is most severe distally (feet and hands); response improves as stimulus is moved proximally (glove-and-stocking anesthesia). Anesthesia zone gradually merges into a hypoesthesia zone and gradually becomes normal.	Diabetes, chronic alcoholism, nutritional deficiency
Individual Nerves or Roots	Decrease or loss of all sensory modalities. Area of sensory loss corresponds to distribution of involved nerve.	Trauma, vascular occlusion
Spinal Cord Hemisection (Brown-Séquard Syndrome)	Loss of pain and temperature, contralateral side, starting one to two segments below level of lesion. Loss of vibration and position discrimination on ipsilateral side, below level of lesion.	Meningioma, neurofibroma, cervical spondylosis, multiple sclerosis

TABLE 23-10	Patterns of Sensory Loss—cont'd	
Type	Characteristics	Possible Causes
Complete Transection of the Spinal Cord	Complete loss of *all* sensory modalities below level of lesion. Condition is associated with motor paralysis and loss of sphincter control.	Spinal cord trauma, demyelinating disorders, tumor
Thalamus	Loss of *all* sensory modalities on the face, arm, and leg on side contralateral to lesion.	Vascular occlusion
Cortex	Because pain, vibration, and crude touch are mediated by the thalamus, little loss of these sensory functions occurs with a cortex lesion. Loss of discrimination occurs on contralateral side. Loss of graphesthesia, loss of stereognosis (recognition of shapes and weights), loss of finger finding.	Cerebral cortex, parietal lobe lesion (e.g., stroke)

TABLE 23-11 Abnormal Postures

Decorticate Rigidity

Upper extremities—flexion of arm, wrist, and fingers; adduction of arm (i.e., tight against thorax). Lower extremities—extension, internal rotation, plantar flexion. This indicates hemispheric lesion of cerebral cortex.

Decerebrate Rigidity

Upper extremities stiffly extended, adducted; internal rotation, palms pronated. Lower extremities stiffly extended; plantar flexion; teeth clenched; hyperextended back. More ominous than decorticate rigidity; indicates lesion in brainstem at midbrain or upper pons.

Flaccid Quadriplegia

Complete loss of muscle tone and paralysis of all four extremities, indicating completely nonfunctional brainstem.

Opisthotonos

Prolonged arching of back, with head and heels bent backward. This indicates meningeal irritation.

Images © Pat Thomas, 2006.

TABLE 23-12 Pathologic Reflexes

Reflex	Method of Testing	Abnormal Response (Reflex is Present)	Indications
Babinski	Stroke lateral aspect and across ball of foot.	Extension of great toe, fanning of toes	Corticospinal (pyramidal) tract disease (e.g., stroke, trauma)
Oppenheim	Using heavy pressure with your thumb and index finger, stroke anterior medial tibial muscle.	Same as above	Same
Gordon	Firmly squeeze calf muscles.	Same as above	Same
Hoffmann	With patient's hand relaxed, wrist dorsiflexed, and fingers slightly flexed, sharply flick nail of distal phalanx of middle or index finger.	Clawing of fingers and thumb	Same
Kernig	In flat-lying supine position raise leg straight or flex thigh on abdomen and extend knee.	Resistance to straightening (because of hamstring spasm), pain down posterior thigh	Meningeal irritation (e.g., meningitis, infections)
Brudzinski	With one hand under neck and other hand on person's chest, sharply flex chin on chest and watch hips and knees.	Resistance and pain in neck, with flexion of hips and knees	Meningeal irritation (e.g., meningitis, infections)

TABLE 23-13   Frontal Release Signs

Reflex

Snout reflex

Snout

Method of testing
Gently percuss oral region
Abnormal response (reflex is present)
Puckers lips
Indications
Frontal lobe disease, cerebral degenerative disease (Alzheimer), amyotrophic
   sclerosis, corticobulbar lesions

Sucking reflex

Sucking

Method of testing
Touch oral region
Abnormal response (reflex is present)
Sucking movement of lips, tongue, jaw, swallowing
Indications
Same as for snout reflex

Grasp reflex

Grasp

Method of testing
Touch palm with your finger
Abnormal response (reflex is present)
Uncontrolled, forced grasping (grasp is usually last of these signs to appear;
   thus its presence indicates severe disease)
Indications
When unilateral, frontal lobe lesion on contralateral side; when bilateral,
   diffuse bifrontal lobe disease

Images © Pat Thomas, 2006.

Abnormal Findings

Summary Checklist: Neurologic Examination

Neurologic Screening Examination
1. **Mental status**
2. **Cranial nerves**
   II: Optic
   III, IV, VI: Extraocular muscles
   V: Trigeminal
   VII: Facial mobility
3. **Motor function**
   Gait and balance
   Knee flexion—hop or shallow knee
      bend

4. **Sensory function**
   Superficial pain and light touch—
      arms and legs
   Vibration—arms and legs
5. **Reflexes**
   Biceps
   Triceps
   Patellar
   Achilles

Neurologic Complete Examination
1. **Mental status**
2. **Cranial nerves II through XII**

3. **Motor system**
   Muscle size, strength, tone
   Rapid alternating movements
   Gait and balance
4. **Sensory function**
   Superficial pain and light touch
   Vibration, position sense
   Stereognosis, graphesthesia,
      two-point discrimination
5. **Reflexes**
   DTRs: Biceps, triceps,
      brachioradialis, patellar, Achilles
   Superficial: Abdominal, plantar

BIBLIOGRAPHY

1. Alzheimer's Association. (2010). *10 signs of Alzheimer's.* Available at www.alz.org/alzheimers_disease_10_signs_of_alzheimers.asp.

2. American Academy of Neurology. (2000). *Guidelines for a screening neurological exam.* Available at http://www.aan.com/uploadedFiles/4CME_and_Training/2Training/3Fellowship_Resources/5Core_Curricula/skilz.pdf.

3. American Academy of Neurology. (2008). *Assessing patients in a neurology practice for risk of falls.* Available at http://www.aan.com/Guidelines/home/GetGuidelineContent/265.

4. Biederman, D. J., Sienkiewicz, H. C, Bibeau, D. L, et al. (2012). Ethnic and racial differences of baseline stroke knowledge in a "stroke belt" community. *Health Promot Pract, 13*(1), 63-70.

5. Cook, L. K., & Clements, S. L. (2011). Emergency: Stroke recognition and management. *Am J Nurs, 111*(5), 64-69.

6. Cruz-Flores, S., Rabinstein, A., Biller, J., et al. (2011). Racial-ethnic disparities in stroke care: the American experience. *Stroke, 42*(7), 2091-2116.

7. Davis, N. J., Hendrix, C. C., & Superville, J. G. (2011). Supportive approaches for Alzheimer disease. *Nurse Pract, 36*(8), 22-29.

8. Davis, S. M., & Donnan, G. A. (2012). Secondary prevention after ischemic stroke or transient ischemic attack. *N Engl J Med, 366*(20), 1914-1922.

9. Fjell, A. M., Walhovd, K. B., & Fennema-Notestine, C. (2009). One-year brain atrophy evident in healthy aging. *J Neurosci, 29*(48), 1523-1531.

10. Futagi, Y., Toribe, Y., & Suzuki, Y. (2009). Neurological assessment of early infants. *Curr Pediatr Rev, 5*(2), 65-70.

11. Go, A. S., Mozaffarian, D., Roger, V. L., et al. (2013). Heart disease and stroke statistics—2013 update. *Circulation, 127*(1), e6-e245.

12. Hammersla, M., & Kapustin, J. F. (2012). Peripheral neuropathy: evidence based treatment of a complex disorder. *Nurse Pract, 37*(5), 32-39.

13. Jamault, V., & Duff, E. (2013). Adolescent concussions: when to return to play. *Nurse Pract, 38*(2), 16-22.

14. Leifer, B. P. (2009). Alzheimer's disease: seeing the signs early. *J Acad Nurse Pract, 21*(11), 588-595.

15. Maloni, H. W. (2013). Multiple sclerosis: managing patients in primary care. *Nurse Pract, 38*(4), 24-35.

16. Mertz, L. (2011). Meningococcal disease: early recognition is vital to patient outcomes. *Nurse Pract, 36*(7), 12-20.

17. Mullen, M. T., Judd, S., & Howard, V. J. (2013). Disparities in evaluation at certified primary stroke centers. *Stroke, 44*, 1930-1935.

18. Pavlopoulos, E., Jones, S., & Kosmidis, S., et al. (2013). Molecular mechanism for age-related memory loss. *Sci Transl Med, 5*(200), 200ra115.

19. Querfurth, H. W. (2011). Alzheimer's disease. *N Engl J Med, 362*(4), 329-344.

20. Saccomano, S. J. (2012). Ischemic stroke: the first 24 hours. *Nurse Pract, 37*(10), 12-18.

21. Shin, J. Y., & Hendrix, C. C. (2013). Management of patients with Parkinson disease. *Nurse Pract, 38*(10), 35-43.

22. Stephens, B. E., Liu, J., Lester, B., et al. (2010). Neurobehavioral assessment predicts motor outcome in preterm infants. *J Pediatr, 156*(3), 366-371.

23. Struble, L. M. (2010). Tremors: learning to stop the shakes. *Nurse Pract, 35*(6), 18-26.

24. Takao, H., Hayashi, N., & Ohtomo, K. (2012). A longitudinal study of brain volume changes in normal aging. *Eur J Radiol, 81*(10), 2801-2804.

25. Tiemstra, J. D., & Khatkhate, N. (2007). Bell's palsy: diagnosis and management. *Am Fam Physician, 76*(7), 997-1002.

26. Xu, Y., Yolton, K., & Khoury, J. (2011). Earliest appropriate time for administering neurobehavioral assessment in newborn infants. *Pediatrics, 127*(1), e69-e75.

27. Yuki, N., & Hartung, H. P. (2012). Guillain-Barré syndrome. *N Engl J Med, 366*(24), 2294-2304.

CHAPTER 24

Male Genitourinary System

ⓔ http://evolve.elsevier.com/Jarvis/

STRUCTURE AND FUNCTION

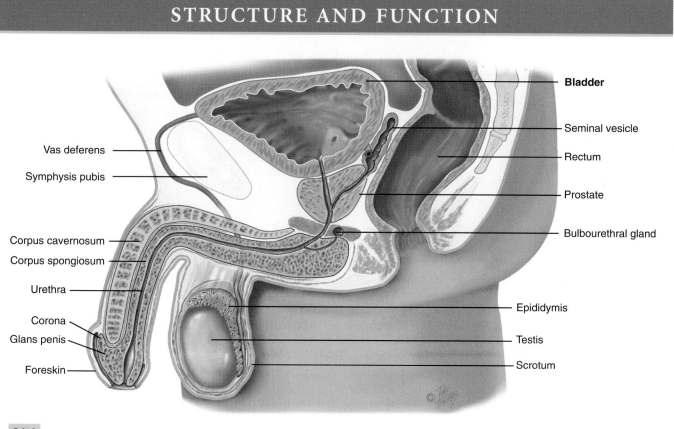

Bladder

Vas deferens

Symphysis pubis

Corpus cavernosum

Corpus spongiosum

Urethra

Corona

Glans penis

Foreskin

Seminal vesicle

Rectum

Prostate

Bulbourethral gland

Epididymis

Testis

Scrotum

24-1

© Pat Thomas, 2010.

THE MALE GENITALIA

The male genital structures include the penis and scrotum externally and the testis, epididymis, and vas deferens internally. Glandular structures accessory to the genital organs (the prostate, seminal vesicles, and bulbourethral glands) are discussed in Chapter 25.

Penis

The **penis** is composed of three cylindric columns of erectile tissue: the two corpora cavernosa on the dorsal side and the corpus spongiosum ventrally (Fig. 24-1). At the distal end of the shaft the corpus spongiosum expands into a cone of erectile tissue, the **glans.** The shoulder where the glans joins the shaft is the **corona.** The **urethra** is a conduit for both the genital and the urinary systems. It transverses the corpus spongiosum, and its meatus forms a slit at the glans tip. Over

the glans, the skin folds in and back on itself, forming a hood or flap. This is the **foreskin** or **prepuce.** Often it is surgically removed shortly after birth by circumcision. The **frenulum** is a fold of the foreskin extending from the urethral meatus ventrally.

Scrotum

The **scrotum** is a loose protective sac, which is a continuation of the abdominal wall. After adolescence the scrotal skin is deeply pigmented and has large sebaceous follicles. The scrotal wall consists of thin skin lying in folds, or **rugae,** and the underlying cremaster muscle. The **cremaster muscle** controls the size of the scrotum by responding to ambient temperature. This is to keep the testes at 3° C below abdominal temperature, the best temperature for producing sperm. When it is cold, the muscle contracts, raising the sac and bringing the testes closer to the body to absorb heat necessary

691

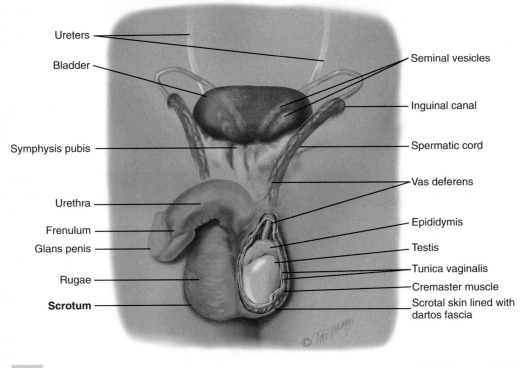

24-2   © Pat Thomas, 2010.

for sperm viability. As a result the scrotal skin looks corrugated. When it is warmer, the muscle relaxes, the scrotum lowers, and the skin looks smoother.

Inside a septum separates the sac into two halves. In each scrotal half is a **testis,** which produces sperm. The testis has a solid oval shape, which is compressed laterally and measures 4 to 5 cm long by 3 cm wide in the adult. It is suspended vertically by the spermatic cord (Fig. 24-2). The left testis is lower than the right because the left spermatic cord is longer. Each testis is covered by a double-layered membrane, the tunica vaginalis, which separates it from the scrotal wall. The two layers are lubricated by fluid so the testis can slide a little within the scrotum; this helps prevent injury.

Sperm are transported along a series of ducts. First the testis is capped by the **epididymis,** which is a markedly coiled duct system and the main storage site of sperm. It is a comma-shaped structure, curved over the top and the posterior surface of the testis. Occasionally (in 6% to 7% of males), the epididymis is anterior to the testis.

The lower part of the epididymis is continuous with a muscular duct, the **vas deferens.** This duct approximates with other vessels (arteries and veins, lymphatics, nerves) to form the **spermatic cord.** The spermatic cord ascends along the posterior border of the testis and runs through the tunnel of the inguinal canal into the abdomen. Here the vas deferens continues back and down behind the bladder, where it joins the duct of the seminal vesicle to form the **ejaculatory duct.** This duct empties into the urethra.

The **lymphatics** of the penis and scrotal surface drain into the inguinal lymph nodes, whereas those of the testes drain into the abdomen. Abdominal lymph nodes are not accessible to clinical examination.

Inguinal Area

The **inguinal area,** or groin, is the juncture of the lower abdominal wall and the thigh (Fig. 24-3). Its diagonal borders are the anterior superior iliac spine and the symphysis pubis. Between these landmarks lies the **inguinal ligament** (Poupart ligament). Superior to the ligament lies the **inguinal canal,** a narrow tunnel passing obliquely between layers of abdominal muscle. It is 4 to 6 cm long in the adult. Its openings are an internal ring, located 1 to 2 cm above the midpoint of the inguinal ligament, and an external ring, located just above and lateral to the pubis.

Inferior to the inguinal ligament is the **femoral canal.** It is a potential space located 3 cm medial to and parallel with the femoral artery. You can use the artery as a landmark to find this space.

Knowledge of these anatomic areas in the groin is useful because they are potential sites for a hernia, which is a loop of bowel protruding through a weak spot in the musculature.

❖ DEVELOPMENTAL COMPETENCE

Infants

Prenatally the testes develop in the abdominal cavity near the kidneys. During the later months of gestation the testes migrate, pushing the abdominal wall in front of them and dragging the vas deferens, blood vessels, and nerves behind. The testes descend along the inguinal canal into the scrotum before birth. At birth each testis measures 1.5 to 2 cm long and 1 cm wide. Only a slight increase in size occurs during the prepubertal years.

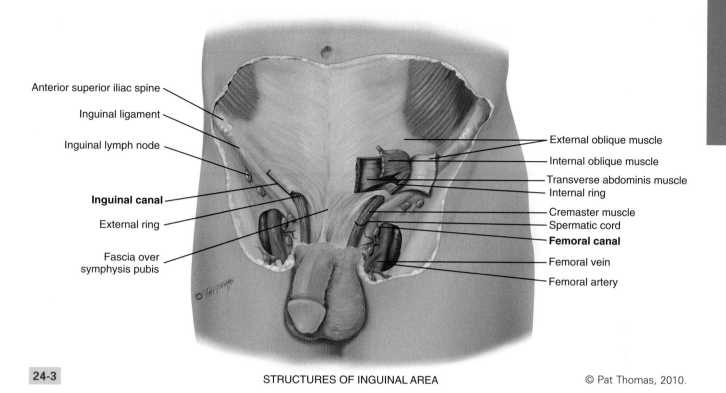

Anterior superior iliac spine

Inguinal ligament

Inguinal lymph node

Inguinal canal

External ring

Fascia over
symphysis pubis

External oblique muscle

Internal oblique muscle

Transverse abdominis muscle

Internal ring

Cremaster muscle

Spermatic cord

Femoral canal

Femoral vein

Femoral artery

24-3   STRUCTURES OF INGUINAL AREA   © Pat Thomas, 2010.

Adolescents

Signs of puberty are beginning earlier in boys than in previous U.S. studies—now at an average of age 9 for African-American boys and age 10 for Caucasians and Hispanics.[6] The first sign is enlargement of the testes. Next pubic hair appears, and then penis size increases. The stages of development are documented in Tanner's sexual maturity ratings (SMRs) (Table 24-1).

Compared to earlier studies, the onset of Tanner stage 2 (testes enlargement and pubic hair growth) is now about 2 years earlier for African-American boys and about $1\frac{1}{2}$ years earlier for Caucasians.[6] This earlier onset of puberty has also been noted in other countries. In the United States it may relate to environmental factors such as chemical exposure, diet changes, and less physical activity. Just because physical maturity occurs earlier does not mean that boys have the psychologic or emotional maturity to go with the physical changes. It is important for clinicians and parents to be aware of physical changes so they can help boys negotiate the emotions and behaviors associated with puberty.

Is the age of puberty onset associated with testicular cancer risk? Undescended testicles and familial testicular cancer are risk factors but account for less than 10% of incidence.[11] Evidence from a European study showed early puberty to have no effect on testicular cancer risk. However, later puberty was protective, especially a later age for starting shaving and a later age for voice change.[11]

Adults and Aging Adults

The older man does not experience a definite end to fertility as the woman does. The production of sperm begins to decrease around 40 years, although it continues into the 80s and 90s. Testosterone production declines after age 30 but very gradually, so resulting physical changes are not evident until later in life.

In the aging male the amount of pubic hair decreases and turns gray. Penis size decreases. Because of decreased tone of the dartos muscle, the scrotal contents hang lower, the rugae decrease, and the scrotum looks pendulous. The testes decrease in size and are less firm to palpation. Increased connective tissue is present in the tubules; thus these become thickened and produce less sperm.

In general, declining testosterone production leaves the older male with a slower and less intense sexual response, and an erection takes longer to develop and is less full or firm. Ejaculation is shorter and less forceful, and the volume of seminal fluid is less than when the man was younger. After ejaculation, rapid detumescence (return to the flaccid state) occurs, especially after 60 years.

Sexual Expression in Later Life. Chronologic age by itself should not mean a halt in sexual activity. The just-mentioned physical changes need not interfere with the libido and pleasure from sexual intercourse. The older male is capable of sexual function as long as he is in reasonably good health and has an interested, willing partner. In the absence of disease, a withdrawal from sexual activity may be caused by loss of spouse; depression; preoccupation with work; marital or family conflict; side effects of medications such as antihypertensives, psychotropics, antidepressants, antispasmodics, sedatives, tranquilizers or narcotics, and estrogens; heavy use of alcohol; lack of privacy (living with adult children or in a nursing home); economic or emotional stress; poor nutrition; or fatigue.

TABLE 24-1 Sexual Maturity Rating (SMR) in Boys

Developmental Stage	Pubic Hair	Penis	Scrotum
1	No pubic hair; fine body hair on abdomen (vellus hair) continues over pubic area	Preadolescent, size and proportion the same as during childhood	Preadolescent, size and proportion the same as during childhood
2	Few straight, slightly darker hairs at base of penis; hair is long and downy	Little or no enlargement	Testes and scrotum begin to enlarge; scrotal skin reddens and changes in texture
3	Sparse growth over entire pubis; hair is darker, coarser, and curly	Penis begins to enlarge, especially in length	Further enlarged
4	Thick growth over pubic area but not on thighs; hair coarse and curly as in adult	Penis grows in length and diameter, with development of glans	Testes almost fully grown; scrotum darker
5	Growth spread over medial thighs, although not yet up toward umbilicus; after puberty, pubic hair growth continues until the mid-20s, extending up the abdomen toward the umbilicus	Adult size and shape	Adult size and shape

Adapted from Tanner, J. M. (1962). *Growth at adolescence.* Oxford, England: Blackwell Scientific Publications.

🌐 CULTURE AND GENETICS

Circumcision. Early in pregnancy expectant parents make the decision about whether to circumcise their newborn son. Circumcision is an elective surgical procedure to remove all or part of the foreskin (prepuce) from the penis. Parents need an unbiased presentation of the risks and benefits of this procedure.

Medical benefits of male circumcision include a reduced risk of acquiring HIV infection through heterosexual contact.

However, these data come from studies in sub-Saharan Africa and may not generalize to the United States, where HIV transmission is higher among men who have sex with men. In addition to HIV, the studies in Africa found that male circumcision reduces the risk for men of acquiring genital herpes, genital ulcers, and oncogenic human papillomavirus (HPV).[17] Female partners of circumcised men have a reduced risk of acquiring HPV, bacterial vaginosis, trichomoniasis, and cervical cancer. Additional benefits of male circumcision include reduced incidence of infant urinary tract infection, phimosis and paraphimosis, and penile cancer.[1]

The American Academy of Pediatrics (AAP) states that current evidence (listed above) shows that health benefits of newborn male circumcision outweigh the risks and that all families should have access to male circumcision if they choose it.[1] The AAP further states that the procedure should be covered by insurance. Although these guidelines stop short of recommending the procedure for all newborn boys, they will influence neonatal care and how insurance companies decide to provide coverage.

Circumcision is a nontherapeutic surgical procedure with a small but possible risk for complications. Most are minor and treatable: pain, bleeding, swelling, or inadequate skin removal. Serious complications are rare and include excess bleeding, wound infection, and urinary retention.[19] Neonates certainly are capable of perceiving pain; therefore parents need to be apprised of pain-relief measures for the circumci-

sion procedure. These include dorsal penile nerve block and a lidocaine-prilocaine cream (EMLA).[1]

Kidney Disease. Chronic kidney disease (CKD) is determined by blood tests, urinalysis, and imaging studies that show decreased kidney function or kidney damage lasting 3 months or longer. This can lead progressively and irreversibly to end-stage renal disease (ESRD), when the person survives only by kidney transplant or dialysis. CKD is a global health problem. It has two main causes, hypertension and diabetes, which comprise 70% or more of patients who progress to ESRD and are undergoing dialysis.

The prevalence of diabetes and hypertension is higher in some racial groups, which reflects the high incidence of kidney failure in these groups. Compared to Whites, African Americans are almost 4 times as likely to develop kidney failure, and American Indians are 1.8 times as likely. Compared to non-Hispanics, Hispanics are almost 1.5 times more likely to develop kidney failure.[14] Also in the United States, racial and ethnic minorities are strongly associated with lower socioeconomic status (SES) and thus with poorer health outcomes.[15] Individuals in minority groups are less likely to have health insurance and have reduced access to usual sources of care. This would affect diagnosis and treatment of CKD. Even at ESRD, the multiple steps necessary to receive a kidney transplant (access to the waiting list, completing the transplant evaluation, access to transplant) would be daunting for low-income, low–health literacy, or uninsured patients.[15]

Subjective Data

SUBJECTIVE DATA

1. Frequency, urgency, and nocturia	5. Past genitourinary history	8. Sexual activity and contraceptive use
2. Dysuria	6. Penis—pain, lesion, discharge	9. Sexually transmitted infection (STI) contact
3. Hesitancy and straining	7. Scrotum, self-care behaviors, lump	
4. Urine color		

Examiner Asks	Rationale
1. Frequency, urgency, and nocturia. Urinating more often than usual?	**Frequency.** Average adult voids 5-6 times/day, varying with fluid intake, individual habits. Polyuria—Excessive quantity. Oliguria—Diminished quantity, <400 mL/ 24 hours.
• Feel as if you cannot wait to urinate? • Awaken during the night because you need to urinate? How often? Is this a recent change?	**Urgency.** **Nocturia** occurs together with frequency and urgency in urinary tract disorders. Other origins: cardiovascular, habitual, diuretic medication.
2. Dysuria. Any pain or burning with urinating?	**Dysuria.** Burning is common with acute cystitis, prostatitis, urethritis.

Subjective Data

Examiner Asks	Rationale

3. Hesitancy and straining. Any trouble starting the urine stream?
- Need to strain to start or maintain stream?
- Any change in force of stream: narrowing, becoming weaker?
- Dribbling such that you must stand closer to the toilet?
- Afterward do you still feel you need to urinate?
- Ever had any urinary tract infections?

Hesitancy.
Straining.
Loss of force and decreased caliber.
Terminal dribbling.
Sense of residual urine.
Recurrent episodes of acute cystitis.
Symptoms suggest bladder outlet obstruction from progressive benign prostate hyperplasia.

4. Urine color. Is the usual **urine** clear or discolored, cloudy, foul-smelling, bloody (Fig. 24-4)?

Cloudy in urinary tract infection.
Hematuria—A danger sign that warrants further workup.
Some color changes are temporary or harmless. However, for blood in urine or for a color change lasting longer than a day, the person should seek health care. For a complete description, see Table 24-2, Urine Color and Discolorations, p. 711.

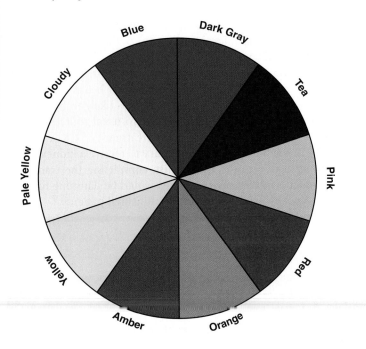

24-4

Courtesy Connie Cooper.

5. Past genitourinary history. Any difficulty controlling your urine?

Urge incontinence—Involuntary urine loss from overactive detrusor muscle in bladder.

- Accidentally urinate when you sneeze, laugh, cough, or bear down?

Stress incontinence—Involuntary urine loss with physical strain, sneezing, or coughing caused by weakness of pelvic floor.

- Any **history** of kidney disease, kidney stones, flank pain, urinary tract infections, prostate trouble?

6. Penis. Any problem with penis—**pain, lesions?**
- Any **discharge?** How much? Has it increased or decreased since start?
- The color? Any odor? Discharge associated with pain or urination?

Urethral discharge occurs with infection (see Table 24-3, Urinary Problems, p. 712).

7. Scrotum, self-care behaviors. Any problem with the scrotum or testicles?
- Any **lump** or **swelling** on testes?
- Any change in size of the scrotum? Any history of undescended testicle as infant?
- Noted any bulge or swelling in the scrotum? For how long? Ever been told you have a hernia? Any dragging, heavy feeling in scrotum?

Concern about any self-discovered mass (spermatocele, hydrocele, varicocele, rarely testicular cancer) alerts you to careful exploration during examination.

Possible hernia.

Examiner Asks	Rationale

8. **Sexual activity and contraceptive use.** Are you in a relationship involving sexual intercourse now?
   - Are aspects of sex satisfactory to you and your partner?
   - Are you satisfied with the way you and your partner communicate about sex?
   - Occasionally a man notices a change in ability to have an erection when aroused. Have you noticed any changes?*

   - Do you and your partner use a contraceptive? Which method? Is it satisfactory? Any questions about this method?
   - How many sexual partners have you had in the past 6 months?

   - What is your sexual preference—relationship with a woman, a man, both?

Questions about **sexual activity** should be routine in review of body systems for these reasons:
- Communicates that you accept individual's sexual activity and believe that it is important.
- Your comfort with discussion prompts person's interest and possibly relief that topic has been introduced.
- Establishes a database for comparisons with any future sexual activities.
- Provides opportunity to screen sexual problems.

Your questions should be objective and matter-of-fact.

Gay and bisexual men need to feel acceptance to discuss their health concerns. Men who have sex with men (MSM) are at increased risk for sexually transmitted infection (STI); psychological distress.

9. **STI contact.** Any sexual contact with a partner having an STI such as gonorrhea, herpes, HIV, chlamydia, human papilloma virus (HPV), venereal warts, syphilis?
   - When was this contact? Did you get the disease?
   - How was it treated? Any complications?
   - Do you use condoms to help prevent STIs?
   - Any questions or concerns about any of these diseases?

Additional History for Infants and Children

1. Does your child have any problem urinating? Urine stream look straight?
   - Any pain with urinating, crying, or holding the genitals?
   - Any urinary tract infection?

2. (If child older than 2 to 2½ years.) Has toilet training started? How is it progressing?
   - (If child 5 years or older.) Wet the bed at night? Is this a problem for child or for you (parents)? What have you done? How does the child feel about it?

Nocturnal enuresis—Involuntarily urinating at night after age 5 to 6 years.

3. Any problem with child's penis or scrotum: sores, swelling, discoloration?
   - Told if his testes are descended or undescended?
   - Ever had a hernia or hydrocele?
   - Swelling in his scrotum during crying or coughing?

4. (Ask directly to preschooler or young school-age child.) Has anyone ever touched your penis or in between your legs, and you did not want them to? Sometimes that happens to children, and it's not okay. They should remember that they have not been bad. They should try to tell a big person about it. Can you tell me three different big people whom you trust to whom you could talk?

Screen for sexual abuse. For prevention, teach the child that it is not okay for someone to look at or touch his private parts while telling him it is a secret. Naming three trusted adults will include someone outside the family—important, since most molestation is by a parent.

*At times, phrase your questions so that all is right for the person to acknowledge a problem.

Subjective Data

Subjective Data

Examiner Asks	Rationale

Additional History for Preadolescents and Adolescents

Ask questions that seem appropriate for boy's age, but be aware that norms vary widely. When you are in doubt, it is better to ask too many questions than to omit something. Children obtain information, often misinformation, from the media, Internet, and peers at very early ages. You may be sure that your information will be more thoughtful and accurate.

Ask direct, matter-of-fact questions. Avoid sounding judgmental.

Start with a *permission statement*. "Often boys your age experience. ..." This conveys that it is normal and all right to think or feel a certain way.

Try the *ubiquity approach*. "When did you ...?" rather than "Do you ...?" This method is less threatening because it implies that the topic is normal and unexceptional.

Do not be concerned if a boy will not discuss sexuality with you or respond to offers for information. He may not wish to let on that he needs or wants more information. You do well to "open the door." The adolescent may come back at a future time.

1. Around age 10 to 12 years, boys start to change and grow around the penis and scrotum. What changes have you noticed?

    Who can you talk to about your body changes and for sex information? How do these talks go? Do you think you get enough information? What about sex education classes at school? How about your parents? Is there a favorite teacher, nurse, doctor, minister, or counselor to whom you can talk?

2. Boys around age 12 years have a normal experience of fluid coming out of the penis at night, called nocturnal emissions, or "wet dreams." Have you had this?

    An occasional boy confuses this with a sign of STI or feels guilty.

3. Teenage boys have other normal experiences and wonder if they are the only ones who ever had them, such as having an erection at embarrassing times, having sexual fantasies, or masturbating. Also, a boy might have a thought about touching another boy's genitals and wonder if this means he might be homosexual. Would you like to talk about any of these things?

    A boy may feel guilty about experiencing these things if not informed that they are normal.

4. Often boys your age have questions about sexual activity. What questions do you have? How about things such as birth control or STIs such as gonorrhea or herpes? Any questions about these?
    - Are you dating? Someone steady? Have you had intercourse? Are you using birth control? Which kind?

    Assess level of knowledge. Many boys will not admit that they need more knowledge.

    Avoid the term "having sex." It is ambiguous, and teens can take it to mean anything from foreplay to intercourse. Use behavior-specific words.

    - Which kind of birth control did you use the *last* time you had intercourse?

    This particular question often reveals that the teen is not using any method of birth control.

5. Has a nurse or doctor ever taught you how to examine your own testicles to make sure they are healthy?

    Assess knowledge of testicular self-examination.

6. Has anyone ever touched your genitals when you did not want them to? Another boy, or an adult, even a relative? Sometimes that happens to teenagers. They should remember it is not their fault. They should tell another adult about it.

    Screen for sexual abuse.

Examiner Asks	Rationale
7. Have you had the vaccine Gardasil?	Approved in 2009 for boys and men ages 9 to 26 years for prevention of STI genital warts in men and for reducing HPV-related cervical cancer in women.

Additional History for the Aging Adult

Examiner Asks	Rationale
1. Any difficulty urinating? Any hesitancy and straining? A weakened force of stream? Any dribbling? Any incomplete emptying?	Early symptoms of enlarging prostate may be tolerated or ignored. Later symptoms are more dramatic: hematuria, urinary tract infection.
2. Do you ever leak water/urine when you don't want to? Do you use pads/tissue to catch urine in your underwear?	Incontinence is any involuntary leaking of urine.
3. Do you need to get up at night to urinate? Which medications are you taking? What fluids do you drink in the evening?	Nocturia may be caused by diuretic medication, habit, or fluid ingestion 3 hours before bedtime; coffee and alcohol especially have a diuretic effect. Fluid retention from mild heart failure or varicose veins produces nocturia because recumbency at night mobilizes fluid.
4. Is it all right to ask you about your sexual function? This is something I ask all the men. For example, it is normal for an erection to develop slowly at this age. This is not a sign of impotence, but a man might wonder if it is. • Any change in your ability to have an erection? • Wanting to have an erection is normal, and it is treatable with medication.	Excluding physical illness, an older man is fully capable of sexual function. But some assume that normal changes mean they are "old men," and they withdraw from sexual activity. The older person is not reluctant to discuss sexual activity, and most welcome the opportunity. Depressants to sexual desire and function include antihypertensives, sedatives, tranquilizers, estrogens, and alcohol. Alcohol decreases the sexual response even more dramatically in the older person.

Objective Data

OBJECTIVE DATA

PREPARATION

Position the male standing with undershorts down and appropriate draping. The examiner should be sitting. Alternatively the male may be supine for the first part of the examination and stand to check for a hernia.

It is normal for a male to feel apprehensive about having his genitalia examined, especially by a female examiner. Younger adolescents usually have more anxiety than older adolescents. But any male may have difficulty dissociating a necessary, matter-of-fact step in the physical examination from the feeling that this is an invasion of his privacy. His concerns are: modesty, fear of pain, cold hands, negative judgment, or fear of having an erection during the examination and that this would be misinterpreted by the examiner.

This normal apprehension shows in different behaviors. Many act resigned and embarrassed and avoid eye contact. An occasional man will laugh and make

EQUIPMENT NEEDED

Gloves: wear gloves during every male genitalia examination
Occasionally: glass slide for urethral specimen
Materials for cytology
Flashlight

jokes to cover embarrassment. Also, a man may refuse examination by a female and insist on a male examiner.

Take time to consider these feelings and to explore your own. It is normal for you to feel embarrassed and apprehensive too. You may worry about your age, lack of clinical experience, causing pain, or even that your movements might "cause" an erection. You need to accept these feelings and work through them so you can examine the male in a professional way. Discuss these concerns with an experienced examiner. Your demeanor is important. Your unresolved discomfort magnifies any discomfort the man may have.

Your demeanor should be *confident* and relaxed, unhurried yet businesslike. Do not discuss genitourinary history or sexual practices while you are performing the examination. This may be perceived as judgmental. Instead say, "I'm just checking for changes" and "You are normal and healthy."

Use a firm, deliberate touch, not a soft, stroking one. If an erection does occur, say, "This is only a normal physiologic response to touch, just as when the pupil constricts in response to bright light." Proceed with the rest of the examination.

Normal Range of Findings	Abnormal Findings

Inspect and Palpate the Penis

The skin normally looks wrinkled, hairless, and without lesions. The dorsal vein may be apparent (Fig. 24-5).

24-5

The glans looks smooth and without lesions. Ask the uncircumcised male to retract the foreskin, or you retract it. It should move easily. Some cheesy smegma may have collected under the foreskin. After inspection slide the foreskin back to the original position.

The urethral meatus is positioned just about centrally.

At the base of the penis, pubic hair distribution is consistent with age. Hair is without pest inhabitants.

Abnormal Findings

Inflammation.
Lesions: nodules, solitary ulcer (chancre), grouped vesicles or superficial ulcers, wartlike papules (see Table 24-4, Male Genital Lesions, p. 713).

Inflammation. Lesions on glans or corona.
Phimosis—Narrowed opening of prepuce so cannot retract the foreskin.
Paraphimosis—Painful constriction of glans by retracted foreskin.
Hypospadias—Ventral location of meatus. **Epispadias**—Dorsal location of meatus (see Table 24-5, Penis Abnormalities, p. 714).
Pubic lice or nits can be seen with the unaided eye. Excoriated skin usually accompanies.

Normal Range of Findings

Compress the glans anteroposteriorly between your thumb and forefinger (Fig. 24-6). The meatus edge should appear pink, smooth, and without discharge.

24-6

If you note urethral discharge, collect a smear for microscopic examination and a culture. If no discharge shows but the person gives a history of it, ask him to milk the shaft of the penis. This should produce a drop of discharge.

Palpate the shaft of the penis between your thumb and first two fingers. Normally it feels smooth, semifirm, and nontender.

Inspect and Palpate the Scrotum

Inspect the scrotum as the male holds the penis out of the way. Alternatively you hold the penis out of the way with the back of your hand (Fig. 24-7). Scrotal size varies with ambient room temperature. Asymmetry is normal, with the left scrotal half usually lower than the right.

Abnormal Findings

Stricture—Narrowed opening.

Edges that are red, everted, edematous, along with purulent discharge, suggest urethritis (see Table 24-3, p. 712).

Nodule or induration.
Tenderness.

Scrotal swelling (edema) may be taut and pitting. This occurs with heart failure, renal failure, or local inflammation.
Lesions.

Objective Data

Normal Range of Findings

Spread rugae out between your fingers. Lift the sac to inspect the posterior surface. Normally no scrotal lesions are present, except for the commonly found sebaceous cysts. These are yellowish, 1-cm nodules and are firm, nontender, and often multiple.

Palpate gently each scrotal half between your thumb and first two fingers (Fig. 24-8). The scrotal contents should slide easily. Testes normally feel oval, firm and rubbery, smooth, and equal bilaterally and are freely movable and slightly tender to moderate pressure. Each epididymis normally feels discrete, softer than the testis, smooth, and nontender.

24-8

Palpate each spermatic cord between your thumb and forefinger along its length from the epididymis up to the external inguinal ring (Fig. 24-9, *A*). You should feel a smooth, nontender cord.

Abnormal Findings

Inflammation.

Absent testis—May be a temporary migration or true cryptorchidism (see Table 24-6, Scrotum Abnormalities, p. 716).

Atrophied testes—Small and soft.

Fixed testes.

Nodules on testes or epididymides warrant ultrasound imaging.

Marked tenderness.

An indurated, swollen, and tender epididymis indicates epididymitis.

Thickened cord.

Soft, swollen, and tortuous cord—See the discussion of varicocele (Fig. 24-9, *B*).

A

24-9, A

B

24-9, B   Varicocele. (Lemmi & Lemmi, 2011.)

Objective Data

Normal Range of Findings	Abnormal Findings

Normally no other scrotal contents are present. If you do find a mass, note:
- Any tenderness?
- Is the mass distal or proximal to testis?
- Can you place your fingers over it?
- Does it reduce when the person lies down?
- Can you auscultate bowel sounds over it?

Abnormalities in the scrotum: hernia, tumor, orchitis, epididymitis, hydrocele, spermatocele, varicocele (see Table 24-6, Scrotum Abnormalities, p. 717).

Transillumination. Perform this maneuver only if you note a swelling or mass. Darken the room. Shine a strong flashlight from behind the scrotal contents. Normal scrotal contents do not transilluminate.

Serous fluid does transilluminate and shows as a red glow (e.g., hydrocele or spermatocele). Solid tissue and blood do not transilluminate (e.g., hernia, epididymitis, or tumor) (see Table 24-6).

Inspect and Palpate for Hernia

Inspect the inguinal region for a bulge as the person stands and as he strains down. Normally none is present.

Bulge at external inguinal ring or femoral canal. (A hernia may be present but easily reduced and may appear only intermittently with an increase in intra-abdominal pressure.)

Palpate the inguinal canal (Fig. 24-10). For the right side, ask the male to shift his weight onto the left (unexamined) leg. Place your right index finger low on the right scrotal half so you carry as much skin as possible as you proceed. Palpate up the length of the spermatic cord, invaginating the scrotal skin as you go, to the external inguinal ring. It feels like a triangular slitlike opening. If positioned properly, it will admit your finger; gently insert it into the canal and ask the man to "bear down." Normally you feel no change. Repeat the procedure on the left side.

Palpable herniating mass bumps your fingertip or pushes against the side of your finger (see Table 24-7, Inguinal and Femoral Hernias, p. 719).

External inguinal ring

24-10

Place your right hand upright on the man's right upper thigh, remembering the acronym NAVEL (*N*erve, *A*rtery, *V*ein, *E*mpty space, *L*ymphatics). Locate the femoral *A*rtery pulse with your index finger; the empty space will be under your 4th finger. Ask the man to bear down and palpate the femoral area for a bulge. Normally you feel none. Change sides, using your left hand for the man's left side.

Objective Data

Normal Range of Findings	Abnormal Findings

Palpate Inguinal Lymph Nodes

Palpate the horizontal chain along the groin inferior to the inguinal ligament and the vertical chain along the upper inner thigh.

It is normal to palpate an isolated node on occasion; it then feels small (<1 cm), soft, discrete, and movable (Fig. 24-11).

Enlarged, hard, matted, fixed nodes.

24-11

Self-Care—Testicular Self-Examination (TSE)

Encourage self-care by teaching every male (from 13 to 14 years old through adulthood) how to examine his own testicles. The overall incidence of testicular cancer is rare, accounting for about 8000 new cases annually. It is rare before 15 years, but it occurs most often between 15 and 35 years. It is associated with a history of cryptorchidism.

Some groups consider teaching TSE controversial because the harms of causing anxiety and unwarranted medical costs[8] exceed the benefits of selective detection of a relatively rare lesion. However, testicular cancer has no early symptoms. When detected early and treated before metastasis, the cure rate is almost 100%. Therefore include the teaching but adjust your message to emphasize familiarity with the young man's own body rather than only cancer detection as the goal.

Early detection is enhanced if the male is familiar with his normal consistency. Points to include during health teaching are:

- **T** = timing, once a month
- **S** = shower, warm water relaxes scrotal sac
- **E** = examine, check for changes, report changes immediately

Normal Range of Findings	Abnormal Findings

Phrase your teaching something like this (Fig. 24-12):

24-12

A good time to examine the testicles is during the shower or bath, when your hands are warm and soapy and the scrotum is warm. Cold hands stimulate a muscle (cremasteric) reflex, retracting the scrotal contents. The procedure is simple. Hold the scrotum in the palm of your hand and gently feel each testicle using your thumb and first two fingers. If it hurts, you are using too much pressure. The testicle is egg shaped and movable. It feels rubbery with a smooth surface, like a peeled hard-boiled egg. The epididymis is on top and behind the testicle; it feels a bit softer. The spermatic cord feels like thick, straight strands of string. Abnormal lumps are very rare and usually not worrisome. But, if you ever notice a firm, painless lump; a hard area; or an overall enlarged testicle, call your provider for a further check.

Assess Urinary Function

A urinalysis shows a color of pale yellow to amber caused by the presence of urochrome pigments. Normal urine is clear and slightly acidic with a pH range of 4.5 to 8.0. Specific gravity measures the concentration of urine, from very dilute at 1.003 to concentrated at 1.030. There is little or no protein, no glucose, and fewer than 5 red blood cells (RBCs) or white blood cells (WBCs) per high-powered field in the microscope.

Cloudiness suggests presence of WBCs, bacteria, casts. Certain drugs or foods can change urine color (see Table 24-2). Proteinuria indicates glomerular disease in the nephron. Glycosuria suggests hyperglycemia occurring with diabetes. Increased WBCs occur with urinary tract infection (UTI); increased RBCs occur with UTI, glomerulonephritis, renal calculi, trauma, and cancer.

Serum analysis of kidney function is measured with creatinine, an end-product of muscle metabolism. Normal levels range from 0.7 to 1.5 mg/dL and are fairly constant from day to day. Blood urea nitrogen (BUN) measures urea, an end-product of protein metabolism. It measures 10 to 20 mg/dL and rises with a decrease in fluid volume or an increase in protein intake.

Creatinine measures glomerular filtration rate (GFR). The GFR is the product of filtration pressure in the glomeruli, normally 125 mL/min. When the GFR decreases by half, the serum creatinine level doubles, indicating decreased kidney function. The BUN rises with decreased kidney function but is less specific.

Objective Data

Normal Range of Findings	Abnormal Findings

❖ DEVELOPMENTAL COMPETENCE

Infants and Children

For an infant or a toddler, perform this procedure right after the abdominal examination. In a preschool-age to young school-age child (3 to 8 years), leave underpants on until just before the examination. In an older school-age child or adolescent, offer an extra drape, as with the adult. Reassure child and parents of normal findings.

Inspect the penis and scrotum. Penis size is usually small in infants (2 to 3 cm) (Fig. 24-13) and in young boys until puberty. In the obese boy the penis looks even smaller because of folds of skin covering the base.

Rarely a very small penis may be an enlarged clitoris in a genetically female infant. Newborns with ambiguous genitalia need prompt evaluation to determine the appropriate sex of rearing.[10]

Redness, swelling, lesions.
Discharge.

24-13

In the circumcised infant the glans looks smooth, with the meatus centered at the tip. While the child wears diapers, the meatus may become ulcerated from ammonia irritation. This is more common in circumcised infants.

Hypospadias, epispadias (see Table 24-5). Stricture—Narrowed opening.

Occasionally ulceration may produce a stricture, shown by a pinpoint meatus and a narrow stream. This increases the risk for urine obstruction.

If possible, observe the newborn's first voiding to assess strength and direction of stream.

Poor stream is significant because it may indicate a stricture or neurogenic bladder.

If uncircumcised, the foreskin is normally tight during the first 3 months and should *not* be retracted because of the risk of tearing the adhesions attaching the foreskin to the shaft. This leads to scarring; most adhesions resolve spontaneously by age 2 to 4 months, and the foreskin can be retracted gently to check the glans and meatus.[1] It should return to its original position easily.

Phimosis—Unable to retract the foreskin.

Paraphimosis—The foreskin cannot be slipped forward once it is retracted.

Dirt and smegma collecting under foreskin.

The scrotum looks pink in light-skinned infants and dark brown in dark-skinned infants. Rugae are well formed in the full-term infant. Size varies with ambient temperature, but overall the infant's scrotum looks large in relation to the penis. No bulges, either constant or intermittent, are present.

Palpate the scrotum and testes. The cremasteric reflex is strong in the infant, pulling the testes up into the inguinal canal and abdomen from exposure to cold, touch, exercise, or emotion. Take care not to elicit the reflex: (1) keep your hands warm and palpate from the external inguinal ring down, and (2) block the inguinal canals with the thumb and forefinger of your other hand to prevent the testes from retracting (Fig. 24-14).

Objective Data

Normal Range of Findings	Abnormal Findings

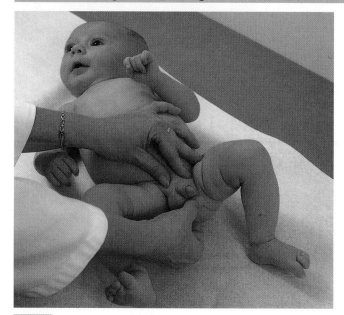

24-14

Normally the testes are descended and equal in size bilaterally (1.5 to 2 cm until puberty). It is important to document that you have palpated the testes. Once palpated, they are considered descended, even if they have retracted momentarily at the next visit.

If the scrotal halves feel empty, search for the testes along the inguinal canal and try to milk them down. Ask the toddler or child to squat with the knees flexed up; this pressure may force the testes down. Or have the young child sit cross-legged to relax the reflex (Fig. 24-15).

Cryptorchidism—Undescended testes (those that have never descended). Undescended testes are common in premature infants. They occur in 3% to 4% of term infants, although most have descended by 3 months of age. Age at which child should be referred differs among physicians (see Table 24-6).

Migratory testes (physiologic cryptorchidism) are common because of the strength of the cremasteric reflex and the small mass of the prepubertal testes. Note that the affected side has a normally developed scrotum (with true cryptorchidism, the scrotum is atrophic) and that the testis can be milked down. These testes descend at puberty and are normal.

Palpate the epididymis and spermatic cord as described in the adult section. A common scrotal finding in the boy younger than 2 years is a **hydrocele,** or fluid in the scrotum. It appears as a large scrotum and transilluminates as a faint pink glow. It usually disappears spontaneously.

Inspect the inguinal area for a bulge. If you do not see a bulge but the parent gives a positive history of one, try to elicit it by increasing intra-abdominal pressure. Ask the boy to hold his breath and strain down, or have him blow up a balloon.

If a hernia is suspected, palpate the inguinal area. Use your little finger to reach the external inguinal ring.

24-15

A hydrocele is a cystic collection of serous fluid in the tunica vaginalis, surrounding the testis. (See Table 24-6.)

Normal Range of Findings	Abnormal Findings

The Adolescent

The adolescent shows a wide variation in normal development of the genitals. Using the SMR charts, note: (1) enlargement of the testes and scrotum; (2) pubic hair growth; (3) darkening of scrotal color; (4) roughening of scrotal skin; (5) increase in penis length and width; and (6) axillary hair growth.

Be familiar with the normal sequence of growth.

The Aging Adult

In the older male you may note thinner, graying pubic hair and the decreased size of the penis. The size of the testes may be decreased and may feel less firm. The scrotal sac is pendulous with less rugae. The scrotal skin may become excoriated if the man continually sits on it.

PROMOTING A HEALTHY LIFESTYLE

Prostate Cancer

The discussion of prostate health and the examination of the prostate gland (see Chapter 25) are unique aspects of male health. Discussions about changes in urinary elimination patterns and sexual activity, including ejaculation, often provide the early signs and symptoms of prostatic changes that may indicate a need for further studies and workup.

The prostate gland goes through two main periods of growth. The first occurs early in puberty, and the second begins after age 25 years. Although the prostate continues to grow during a man's life, the enlargement rarely causes symptoms before age 40 years. However, more than half of men in their 60s and as many as 90% of men in their 70s have some symptoms. The gradual enlargement is expected in aging and is *benign prostatic hypertrophy* (BPH). By itself BPH does not raise an individual's risk for prostate cancer, yet the symptoms of BPH and prostate cancer are very similar, including hesitant, interrupted, or weak urinary stream; urinary urgency; leaking or dribbling; and increased frequency, especially at night.

Careful history taking is important for identifying at-risk men. Two groups at increased risk for prostate cancer are African-American men and men whose first-degree relatives had prostate cancer. In African-American men prostate cancer tends to start younger and grow faster than in men of other racial/ethnic groups. Men who have a first-degree relative (father, brother, or son) who have had prostate cancer have a 2- to 3-times higher risk of the disease than those without a family history. The risk for men who have three or more family members with prostate cancer is about 10 times. Also important is the age at diagnosis; the younger a man's relative(s) were at diagnosis, the greater is his risk for developing it.

Prostate cancer is detected with a screening *prostate-specific antigen* (PSA) blood test and/or a *digital rectal examination* (DRE).

- **PSA** is a substance made by the normal prostate gland. When prostate cancer develops, the PSA level increases.

However, benign or noncancerous enlargement of the prostate (BPH), age, and prostatitis can also cause the PSA to increase. Ejaculation causes a temporary increase in PSA levels, and men need to be instructed to abstain from ejaculation for 2 days before PSA testing. In addition, some medications, such as finasteride (Proscar) or dutasteride (Avodart), falsely lower PSA levels.

- **DRE** involves a gloved, lubricated finger being inserted into the rectum. The prostate gland is located just in front of the rectum, making it possible to palpate the surface of the gland manually for bumps or hard areas that may be a developing cancer. Although it is less effective than the PSA blood test in finding prostate cancer, it can sometimes find cancers in men who have normal PSA levels.

However, the U.S. Preventive Services Task Force recently issued an updated *Recommendation Statement on PSA Screening* (May, 2012) with or without the addition of a DRE or other screening tests. It concluded that the expected harms of PSA screening are greater than the potential benefit. Screening tests are able to detect cancer, but it is not clear whether this earlier detection and treatment leads to any change in the natural history and outcome of the disease. This is quite a shift in thinking. Accordingly the Centers for Disease Control and Prevention (CDC) incorporated the Task Force recommendations into its *Talking with Your Patients About Screening for Prostate Cancer* guide. The guide encourages health care professionals to have open conversations with patients who have questions about prostate cancer and/or screening: http://www.uspreventiveservicestaskforce.org/prostatecancerscreening/prostatecancerscript.pdf.

References

The Centers for Disease Control and Prevention (CDC) Prostate Cancer: http://www.cdc.gov/cancer/prostate/index.htm.

DOCUMENTATION AND CRITICAL THINKING

Sample Charting

SUBJECTIVE

Urinates 4 or 5 times/day, clear, straw-colored. No nocturia, dysuria, or hesitancy. No pain, lesions, or discharge from penis. Does not do testicular self-examination. No history of genitourinary disease. Sexually active in a monogamous relationship. Sexual life satisfactory to self and partner. Uses birth control via barrier method (partner uses diaphragm). No known STI contact.

OBJECTIVE

No lesions, inflammation, or discharge from penis. Scrotum—testes descended, symmetric, no masses. No inguinal hernia.

ASSESSMENT

Genital structures normal and healthy

Case Study 1

H.P. is a 75-year-old Caucasian retired college professor. Past medical history includes prostatectomy 2 weeks PTA due to severe benign prostatic hypertrophy; also hypertension, type 2 diabetes, and COPD.

SUBJECTIVE

H.P. presents to the emergency department in severe pain, rated at 10/10. "My balls hurt so bad I can't walk straight." Reports urinary frequency and "pink" urine. Low-grade fever for 24 hours.

OBJECTIVE

Vital signs: Temp 100.4° F (38° C). Pulse 118 bpm, regular. Resp 18/min. BP 146/88 mm Hg, right arm, sitting.
Inspection: Scrotum appears reddened and enlarged.
Palpation: Extreme tenderness with palpation. Epididymis enlarged bilaterally. Difficult to identify testicles. Scrotal skin edematous. No discharge.
Laboratory data: White blood cell count 15,000/mcL with a left shift; *E. coli* in urine

ASSESSMENT

Epididymitis
Acute pain R/T swelling and inflammatory process

Clinical Case Study 2

R.C. is a 19-year-old Caucasian male student who 2 days PTA noted acute onset of painful urination, frequency, and urgency. Noted some thick penile discharge.

SUBJECTIVE

States has no side pain, no abdominal pain, no fever, and no genital skin rash. R.C. is concerned that he has an STI because of an episode of unprotected intercourse with a new partner 6 days PTA. Has no known allergies.

OBJECTIVE

Vital signs: Temp 98.6° F (37° C). Pulse 72 bpm. Resp 16/min. No lesions or inflammation around penis or scrotum. Urethral meatus has mild edema with purulent urethral discharge. No pain on palpation of genitalia. Testes symmetric with no masses. No lymphadenopathy.

Documentation and Critical Thinking

ASSESSMENT

Urethral discharge

Deficient knowledge about STI prevention R/T lack of information recall

J.T. is a 13-year-old Caucasian male who presents to the ED with abdominal pain, nausea, and testicular pain.

SUBJECTIVE

4 hours PTA: J.T. was in summer camp playing basketball when pain to groin "came on all of a sudden." Reports pain began in left testicle but now radiates to entire scrotum (10 on 1-10 pain scale). Rest and scrotal support do not provide relief.

OBJECTIVE

Vital signs: Temp 97.9° F (36.6° C) (oral). Pulse 72 bpm. Resp 16/min. BP 119/70 mm Hg (standing).

General appearance: Bent over, anxious, grimacing, and guarding stomach and genital area.

Abdomen: BS active in all 4 quadrants; nausea; denies vomiting and/or pain on palpation.

Genitourinary: Red, warm, edematous scrotum w/pain on palpation. L testicle especially painful, elevated and lying transversely; cremasteric reflex absent on L side; no pelvic lymphadenopathy; denies sexual history

ASSESSMENT

Testicular (left) torsion

Acute pain R/T injury agent (physical)

Impaired tissue perfusion R/T impaired blood flow to the testicle

ABNORMAL FINDINGS

TABLE 24-2 Urine Color and Discolorations

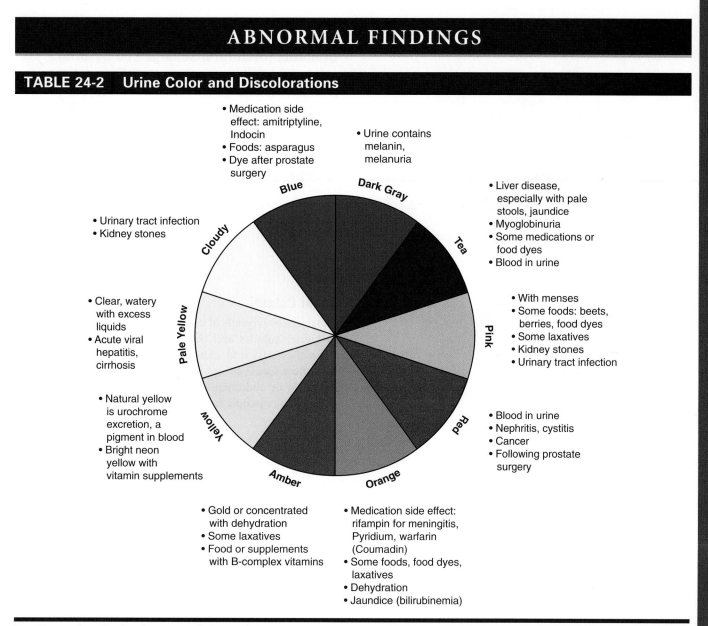

• Medication side effect: amitriptyline, Indocin
• Foods: asparagus
• Dye after prostate surgery

• Urine contains melanin, melanuria

• Urinary tract infection
• Kidney stones

• Liver disease, especially with pale stools, jaundice
• Myoglobinuria
• Some medications or food dyes
• Blood in urine

• Clear, watery with excess liquids
• Acute viral hepatitis, cirrhosis

• With menses
• Some foods: beets, berries, food dyes
• Some laxatives
• Kidney stones
• Urinary tract infection

• Natural yellow is urochrome excretion, a pigment in blood
• Bright neon yellow with vitamin supplements

• Blood in urine
• Nephritis, cystitis
• Cancer
• Following prostate surgery

• Gold or concentrated with dehydration
• Some laxatives
• Food or supplements with B-complex vitamins

• Medication side effect: rifampin for meningitis, Pyridium, warfarin (Coumadin)
• Some foods, food dyes, laxatives
• Dehydration
• Jaundice (bilirubinemia)

Blue / Dark Gray / Tea / Cloudy / Pink / Pale Yellow / Red / Yellow / Orange / Amber

See Illustration Credits for source information.

TABLE 24-3   Urinary Problems

◀ Urethritis (Urethral Discharge and Dysuria)

Infection of urethra causes painful, burning urination or pruritus. Meatus edges are reddened, everted, and swollen with purulent discharge. Urine is cloudy with discharge and mucus shreds. Cause determined by culture: (1) gonococcal urethritis has thick, profuse, yellow or gray-brown discharge; (2) nonspecific urethritis (NSU) may have similar discharge but often has scanty, mucoid discharge. Of these, about 50% are caused by chlamydia infection. The cause is important to differentiate because antibiotic treatment is different.

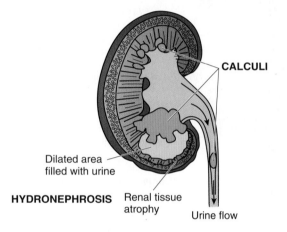

CALCULI

Dilated area
filled with urine

HYDRONEPHROSIS   Renal tissue
atrophy

Urine flow

◀ Renal Calculi

Renal stones (crystals of calcium oxalate or uric acid) form in kidney tubules and then migrate and become urgent when they pass into ureter, become lodged, and obstruct urine flow. Cause abrupt severe flank pain with radiation to the groin or abdomen, nausea and vomiting, restlessness, gross or microscopic hematuria.

Acute Urinary Retention (not illustrated)

Abrupt inability to pass urine with bladder distention and lower abdominal pain. Much more common in men due to bladder outlet obstruction such as benign prostatic hyperplasia (BPH) (see Chapter 25). Must catheterize to relieve acute discomfort; then manage underlying problem.

Urethral Stricture (not illustrated)

Pinpoint, constricted opening at meatus or inside along urethra. Occurs congenitally or secondary to urethral injury. Gradual decrease in force and caliber of urine stream is most common symptom. Shaft feels indurated along ventral aspect at site of stricture.

See Illustration Credits for source information.

ABNORMAL FINDINGS
FOR ADVANCED PRACTICE

TABLE 24-4 Male Genital Lesions

Tinea Cruris

A fungal infection in the crural fold, not extending to scrotum, occurring in postpubertal males ("jock itch") after sweating or wearing layers of occlusive clothing. It forms a red-brown half-moon shape with well-defined borders.

Genital Herpes—HSV-2 Infection

Clusters of small vesicles with surrounding erythema, which are often painful and erupt on the glans, foreskin, or anus. These rupture to form superficial ulcers. May have mild tingling before outbreak or shooting pain in buttock or leg. A STI, the initial infection lasts 7 to 10 days and is treated with oral acyclovir. The virus remains dormant indefinitely; recurrent infections last 3 to 10 days with milder symptoms.

◀ ### Genital Warts

Soft, pointed, moist, fleshy, painless papules may be single or multiple in a cauliflower-like patch. Color may be gray, pale yellow, or pink in White males and black or translucent gray-black in Black males. They occur on shaft of penis, behind corona, or around the anus where they may grow into large, grapelike clusters.

These are caused by the human papillomavirus (HPV) and are one of the most common STIs. The HPV infection is correlated with early onset of sexual activity, infrequent use of contraception, and multiple sexual partners.

The vaccine Gardasil is indicated for prevention of genital warts; as of October 2009 it is approved for boys and men ages 9-26 years. It also reduces HPV-related disease in women, such as cervical cancer.[13]

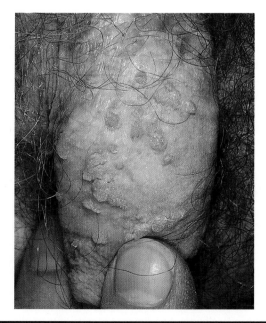

Continued

TABLE 24-4 Male Genital Lesions

Syphilitic Chancre

Begins within 2 to 4 weeks of infection as a small, solitary, silvery papule that erodes to a red, round or oval, superficial ulcer with a yellowish serous discharge. Palpation reveals a nontender indurated base that can be lifted like a button between the thumb and the finger. Lymph nodes enlarge early but are nontender. This is an STI easily treated with penicillin G; but untreated it leads to cardiac and neurologic problems and blindness. Almost eradicated in the United States in 1957; epidemics recur cyclically every 7 to 10 years.

Carcinoma

Begins as red, raised, warty growth or as an ulcer with watery discharge. As it grows, may necrose and slough. Usually painless. Almost always on glans or inner lip of foreskin and following chronic inflammation. Enlarged lymph nodes are common.

See Illustration Credits for source information.

TABLE 24-5 Penis Abnormalities

◀ Hypospadias

Urethral meatus opens on the ventral (under) side of glans or shaft or at the penoscrotal junction. A groove extends from the meatus to the normal location at the tip. This congenital defect is important to recognize at birth. The newborn should not be circumcised because surgical correction may need to use foreskin tissue to extend urethral length.

Priapism (not illustrated)

Prolonged painful erection of penis without sexual stimulation and unrelieved by intercourse or masturbation, most common in men in 30s and 40s. A rare condition but when lasting 4 hours or longer can cause ischemia of penis, fibrosis of tissue, erectile dysfunction. Can occur as a side effect of some medications and street drugs; with sickle-cell trait or disease; with leukemia in which increased numbers of white blood cells produce engorgement; with malignancy; from local trauma; or as a result of spinal cord injuries with autonomic nervous system dysfunction.

TABLE 24-5   Penis Abnormalities—cont'd

Phimosis

Nonretractable foreskin forming a pointy tip with a tiny orifice. Foreskin is advanced and so tight that it is impossible to retract over glans. May be congenital or acquired from adhesions secondary to infection. Poor hygiene leads to retained dirt and smegma, which increases risk for inflammation, calculus formation, obstructive uropathy.

Paraphimosis

Foreskin is retracted and fixed. Once retracted behind glans, a tight or inflamed foreskin cannot return to its original position. Constriction impedes circulation, so glans swells. A medical emergency; the constricting band prevents venous and lymphatic return from the glans and compromises arterial circulation.

Peyronie Disease

Hard, nontender, subcutaneous plaques palpated on dorsal or lateral surface of penis. May be single or multiple and asymmetric. They are associated with painful bending of the penis during erection. Plaques are fibrosis of covering of corpora cavernosa. Usually occurs after 45 years. Its cause is trauma to the erect penis (e.g., unexpected change in angle during intercourse). More common in men with diabetes, gout, and Dupuytren contracture of the palm.

Epispadias

Meatus opens on the dorsal (upper) side of glans or shaft above a broad, spadelike penis. Rare; less common than hypospadias but more disabling because of associated urinary incontinence and separation of pubic bones.

TABLE 24-6 Scrotum Abnormalities

Disorder	Clinical Findings	Discussion
Absent Testis, Cryptorchidism 	S: Empty scrotal half O: Inspection—In true maldescent, atrophic scrotum on affected side Palpation—No testis A: Absent testis	True cryptorchidism—Testes that have never descended. Incidence at birth is 3% to 4%; one half of these descend in first month. Incidence with premature infants is 30%; in the adult, 0.7% to 0.8%. True undescended testes have a histologic change by 6 years, causing decreased spermatogenesis and infertility. Also increases risk for testicular cancer.
Small Testis 	S: (None) O: Palpation—Small and soft (rarely may be firm) A: Small testis	Small and soft (<3.5 cm) indicates atrophy as with cirrhosis or hypopituitarism, following estrogen therapy, or as a sequelae of orchitis. Small and firm (<2 cm) occurs with Klinefelter's syndrome (hypogonadism).
Testicular Torsion	S: Excruciating unilateral pain in testicle of sudden onset, often during sleep or following trauma; may also have lower abdominal pain, nausea and vomiting, no fever O: Inspection—Red, swollen scrotum, one testis (usually left) higher owing to rotation and shortening Palpation—Cord feels thick, swollen, tender; epididymis may be anterior; cremasteric reflex absent on side of torsion	Sudden twisting of spermatic cord. Occurs in late childhood, early adolescence; rare after age 20 years. Torsion usually on left side; faulty anchoring of testis on wall of scrotum allows testis to rotate. The anterior testis rotates medially toward the other testis. Blood supply is cut off, resulting in ischemia and engorgement. An emergency requiring surgery; testis can become gangrenous in a few hours.
Epididymitis 	S: Severe pain of sudden onset in scrotum, relieved by elevation (positive Prehn sign); also rapid swelling, fever O: Inspection—Enlarged scrotum; reddened Palpation—Exquisitely tender; epididymis enlarged, indurated; hard to distinguish from testis. Overlying scrotal skin may be thick and edematous Laboratory—White blood cells and bacteria in urine A: Tender swelling of epididymis	Acute infection of epididymis commonly caused by prostatitis; after prostatectomy because of trauma of urethral instrumentation; or from chlamydia, gonorrhea, or other bacterial infection. Often difficult to distinguish between epididymitis and testicular torsion.

TABLE 24-6	Scrotum Abnormalities—cont'd	
Disorder	*Clinical Findings*	*Discussion*
Varicocele 	S: Dull pain; constant pulling or dragging feeling; or may be asymptomatic O: Inspection—Usually no sign; or bluish color through light scrotal skin Palpation—When standing, feel soft, irregular mass posterior to and above testis; collapses when supine, refills when upright; feels distinctive, like a "bag of worms" Testis on side of varicocele may be smaller due to impaired circulation A: Soft mass on spermatic cord	A varicocele is dilated, tortuous varicose veins in the spermatic cord caused by incompetent valves, which permit reflux of blood; 90% left-sided, perhaps because left spermatic vein is longer and inserts at a right angle into left renal vein. Occurs in 15% by age 15 years.[10] Screen at early adolescence; obtain scrotal ultrasound; early treatment important to prevent potential infertility when an adult.
Spermatocele 	S: Painless, usually found on examination O: Inspection—Does transilluminate higher in the scrotum than a hydrocele, and the sperm may fluoresce Palpation—Round, freely movable mass lying above and behind testis; if large, feels like a third testis A: Free cystic mass on epididymis	Retention cyst in epididymis; cause unclear but may be obstruction of tubules. Filled with thin, milky fluid that contains sperm. Most spermatoceles are small (<1 cm); occasionally they may be larger and mistaken for hydrocele.
Early Testicular Tumor 	S: Painless, found on examination; may have history of undescended testicle or familial testicular cancer. O: Palpation—Firm nodule or harder-than-normal section of testicle; testicular swelling occurs in most A: Solitary nodule	Most testicular tumors occur between ages 18 and 35; practically all are malignant. More common in Whites; must biopsy to confirm. Most important risk factor is undescended testis, even those surgically corrected. Early detection important in prognosis, but practice of testicular self-examination is low.
Diffuse Tumor 	S: Enlarging testis (most common symptom). When enlarges, has feel of increased weight O: Inspection—Enlarged, does not transilluminate Palpation—Enlarged, smooth, ovoid, firm Important—Firm palpation does *not* cause usual sickening discomfort as with normal testis A: Nontender swelling of testis	Diffuse tumor maintains shape of testis.

TABLE 24-6   Scrotum Abnormalities—cont'd

Disorder	Clinical Findings	Discussion
Hydrocele	S: Painless swelling, although person may complain of weight and bulk in scrotum O: Inspection—Enlarged mass does transilluminate with a pink or red glow (in contrast to a hernia) Palpation—Nontender mass; able to get fingers above mass (in contrast to scrotal hernia) A: Nontender swelling of testis	Cystic. Circumscribed collection of serous fluid in tunica vaginalis surrounding testis. May occur following epididymitis, trauma, hernia, tumor of testis, or spontaneously in the newborn. Usually resolves during first year; if large or enlarging, may need surgical decompression.
Scrotal Hernia	S: Swelling, may have pain with straining O: Inspection—Enlarged, may reduce when supine, does not transilluminate Palpation—Soft, mushy mass; palpating fingers cannot get above mass. Mass is distinct from testicle that is normal A: Nontender swelling of scrotum	Scrotal hernia usually caused by indirect inguinal hernia (see Table 24-7). Requires surgery. Teach patient or boy's parents signs of incarcerated hernia; proceed to ED if these occur before planned surgery.[10]
Orchitis	S: Acute or moderate pain of sudden onset, swollen testis, feeling of weight, fever O: Inspection—Enlarged, edematous, reddened; does not transilluminate Palpation—Swollen, congested, tense, and tender; hard to distinguish testis from epididymis A: Tender swelling of testis	Acute inflammation of testis. Most common cause is mumps; can occur with any infectious disease. May have associated hydrocele that does transilluminate.
Scrotal Edema	S: Tenderness O: Inspection—Enlarged, may be reddened (with local irritation) Palpation—Taut with pitting. Probably unable to feel scrotal contents A: Scrotal edema	Accompanies marked edema in lower half of body (e.g., congestive heart failure, renal failure, and portal vein obstruction). Occurs with local inflammation: epididymitis, torsion of spermatic cord. Also, obstruction of inguinal lymphatics produces lymphedema of scrotum.

S, Subjective data; *O,* objective data; *A,* assessment.

Images © Pat Thomas, 2006.

TABLE 24-7   Inguinal and Femoral Hernias

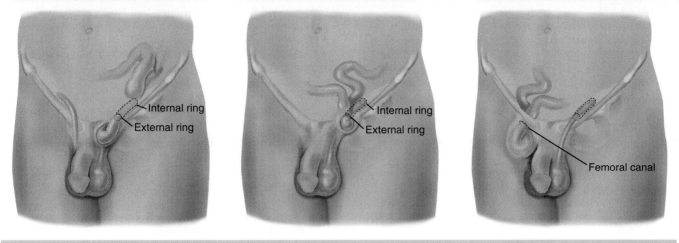

	Indirect Inguinal	Direct Inguinal	Femoral
Course	Sac herniates through internal inguinal ring; can remain in canal or pass into scrotum	Directly behind and through external inguinal ring, above inguinal ligament; rarely enters scrotum	Through femoral ring and canal, below inguinal ligament, more often on right side
Clinical Symptoms and Signs	Pain with straining; soft swelling that increases with increased intra-abdominal pressure; may decrease when lying down	Usually painless; round swelling close to the pubis in area of internal inguinal ring; easily reduced when supine*	Pain may be severe; may become strangulated
Frequency	Most common; 60% of all hernias More common in infants <1 year and males 16 to 20 years of age	Less common; occurs most often in men older than 40 years, rare in women	Least common, 4% of all hernias; more common in women
Cause	Congenital or acquired	Acquired weakness; brought on by heavy lifting, muscle atrophy, obesity, chronic cough, or ascites	Acquired; due to increased abdominal pressure, muscle weakness, or frequent stooping

Images © Pat Thomas, 2006.

*Reducible—Contents will return to abdominal cavity by lying down or gentle pressure. **Incarcerated**—Herniated bowel cannot be returned to abdominal cavity. **Strangulated**—Blood supply to hernia is shut off. Accompanied by nausea, vomiting, and tenderness.

Abnormal Findings

Summary Checklist: Male Genitalia Examination

1. Inspect and palpate the penis.
2. Inspect and palpate the scrotum.
3. If a mass exists, transilluminate it.
4. Palpate for an inguinal hernia.
5. Palpate the inguinal lymph nodes.

BIBLIOGRAPHY

1. American Academy of Pediatrics. (2012). Male circumcision. *Pediatrics, 130*(3), e756-e785.
2. Baer, J. T. (2012). Testosterone replacement therapy to improve health in older males. *Nurse Pract, 37*(8), 39-44.
3. Reference deleted in proofs.
4. Bradway, C., & Rodgers, J. (2009). Evaluation and management of genitourinary emergencies. *Nurse Pract, 34*(5), 37-44.

5. Guzzo, T. J., & Drach, G. W. (2011). Major urologic problems in geriatrics: assessment and management. *Med Clin North Am, 95,* 253-264.

6. Herman-Giddens, M. E., Steffes, J., Harris, D., et al. (2012). Secondary sexual characteristics in boys. *Pediatrics, 130*(5), e1058-e1068.

7. Hoffman, R.M. (2011). Screening for prostate cancer. *N Engl J Med, 365*(21), 2013-2019.

8. Joffe, A. (2009). Should we teach testicular self-exam? *Contemp Pediatr, 26,* 50-52.

9. Koyle, M. A., & Shifrin, D. (2012). Issues in febrile urinary tract infection management. *Pediatr Clin North Am, 59*(4), 909-922.

10. Lambert, S. M. (2012). Pediatric urological emergencies. *Pediatr Clin North Am, 59*(4), 965-976.

11. Maule, M., Malavassi, J. L., & Richiardi, L. (2012). Age at puberty and risk of testicular cancer. *Intern J Androl, 35*(6), 828-834.

12. Merriman, L. S., Herrel, L., & Kirsch, A. J. (2012). Inguinal and genital anomalies. *Pediatr Clin North Am, 59*(4), 769-781.

13. Nandwani, M. C. R. (2010). Men's knowledge of the human papillomavirus vaccine. *Nurse Pract, 35*(11), 32-39.

14. National Kidney Disease Education Program. (2013). *Race, ethnicity and kidney disease.* http://nkdep.nih.gov/learn/are-you-at-risk/race-ethnicity.shtml.

15. Patzer, R. E., & McClellan, W. M. (2012). Influence of race, ethnicity and socioeconomic status on kidney disease. *Nature Rev Nephrol, 8*(9), 533-541.

16. Sarma, A. V., & Wei, J. T. (2012). Benign prostatic hyperplasia and lower urinary tract symptoms. *N Engl J Med, 367*(3), 248-256.

17. Tobian, A. A., & Gray, R. H. (2011). The medical benefits of male circumcision. *JAMA, 306*(13), 1479-1480.

18. Wampler, S. M., & Llanes, M. (2010). Common scrotal and testicular problems. *Primary Care Clin Office Pract, 37*(3), 613-626.

19. Weiss, H. A., Larke, N., Halperin, D., et al. (2010). Complications of circumcision in male neonates, infants, and children. *BMC Urol, 10*(1), 2.

20. Zoltick, B. H. (2011). Shedding light on testicular cancer. *Nurse Pract, 36*(7), 32-39.

CHAPTER 25

Anus, Rectum, and Prostate

STRUCTURE AND FUNCTION

Labels, top to bottom, right side:
- Sigmoid colon
- Rectosigmoid junction
- Rectum
- Valves of Houston
- Rectal ampulla
- Levator ani muscle
- Anorectal junction
- Internal sphincter
- External sphincter

Labels, left side:
- Peritoneum
- Anal canal — Anal column, Anal valve, Anal crypt
- Intersphincteric groove

25-1

ANUS AND RECTUM

The **anal canal** is the outlet of the gastrointestinal (GI) tract; it is about 3.8 cm long in the adult. It is lined with modified skin (having no hair or sebaceous glands) that merges with rectal mucosa at the anorectal junction.

The anal canal is surrounded by two concentric layers of muscle, the **sphincters** (Fig. 25-1). The internal sphincter is under involuntary control by the autonomic nervous system. The external sphincter surrounds the internal sphincter but also has a small section overriding the tip of the internal sphincter at the opening. It is under voluntary control. Except for the passing of feces and gas, the sphincters keep the anal canal tightly closed. The **intersphincteric groove** separates the internal and external sphincters and is palpable.

The **anal columns** (or columns of Morgagni) are folds of mucosa. These extend vertically down from the rectum and end in the **anorectal junction** (also called the *mucocutaneous junction, pectinate,* or *dentate line*). This junction is not palpable, but it is visible on proctoscopy. Each anal column

721

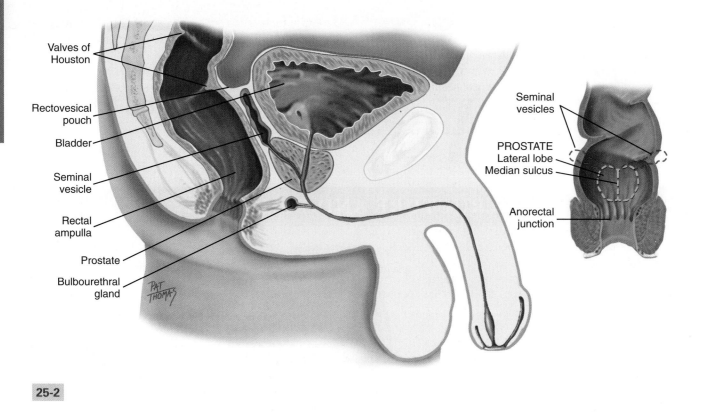

Valves of Houston

Rectovesical pouch

Bladder

Seminal vesicle

Rectal ampulla

Prostate

Bulbourethral gland

Seminal vesicles

PROSTATE
Lateral lobe
Median sulcus

Anorectal junction

25-2

contains an artery and a vein. Under conditions of chronic increased venous pressure, the vein may enlarge, forming a hemorrhoid. At the lower end of each column is a small crescent fold of mucous membrane, the **anal valve.** The space above the anal valve (between the columns) is a small recess, the **anal crypt.**

The anal canal slants forward toward the umbilicus, forming a distinct right angle with the rectum, which rests back in the hollow of the sacrum (Fig. 25-2). Although the rectum contains only autonomic nerves, numerous somatic sensory nerves are present in the anal canal and external skin; therefore a person feels sharp pain from any trauma to the anal area.

The **rectum,** which is 12 cm long, is the distal portion of the large intestine. It extends from the sigmoid colon, at the level of the 3rd sacral vertebra, and ends at the anal canal. Just above the anal canal the rectum dilates and turns posteriorly, forming the rectal ampulla. The rectal interior has 3 semilunar transverse folds called the **valves of Houston.** These cross one-half the circumference of the rectal lumen. Their function is unclear, but they may serve to hold feces as the flatus passes. The lowest is within reach of palpation, usually on the person's left side, and must not be mistaken for an intrarectal mass.

Peritoneal Reflection. The peritoneum covers only the upper two thirds of the rectum. In the male the anterior part of the peritoneum reflects down to within 7.5 cm of the anal opening, forming the **rectovesical pouch** (see Fig. 25-2) and then covers the bladder. In the female this is termed the **recto-uterine pouch** and extends down to within 5.5 cm of the anal opening.

PROSTATE

In the male the **prostate gland** lies in front of the anterior wall of the rectum and 2 cm behind the symphysis pubis. It surrounds the bladder neck and urethra and has 15 to 30 ducts that open into the urethra. The prostate secretes a thin, milky, alkaline fluid that helps sperm viability. It is a bilobed structure with a round or heart shape. It measures 2.5 cm long and 4 cm in diameter. The two lateral lobes are separated by a shallow groove called the **median sulcus.**

The two **seminal vesicles** project like rabbit ears above the prostate. They secrete a fluid that is rich in fructose, which nourishes the sperm and contains prostaglandins. The two **bulbourethral** (Cowper) glands are each the size of a pea and are located inferior to the prostate on either side of the urethra (also see Fig. 25-5). They secrete a clear, viscid mucus.

Regional Structures

In the female the uterine cervix lies in front of the anterior rectal wall and may be palpated through it.

The combined length of the anal canal and the rectum is about 16 cm in the adult. The average length of the examining finger is from 6 cm to 10 cm, bringing many rectal structures within reach.

The sigmoid colon is named from its S-shaped course in the pelvic cavity. It extends from the iliac flexure of the descending colon and ends at the rectum. It is 40 cm long and is accessible to examination only through the colonoscope. The flexible fiberoptic scope in current use provides a view of the entire mucosal surface of the sigmoid and the colon.

❖ DEVELOPMENTAL COMPETENCE

The first stool passed by the newborn is dark green meconium and occurs within 24 to 48 hours of birth, indicating anal patency. From that time on the infant usually has a stool after each feeding. This response to eating is a wave of peristalsis called the *gastrocolic reflex*. It continues throughout life, although children and adults usually produce no more than one or two stools per day.

The infant passes stools by reflex. Voluntary control of the external anal sphincter cannot occur until the nerves supplying the area have become fully myelinated, usually around 1½ to 2 years of age. Toilet training usually starts after age 2 years.

At male puberty the prostate gland undergoes a very rapid increase to more than twice its prepubertal size. During young adulthood its size remains fairly constant.

The prostate gland commonly starts to enlarge during the middle adult years, but this is not cancer. This **benign prostatic hypertrophy (BPH)** is present in 1 of 10 males at the age of 40 years and grows larger with age. It is thought that the hypertrophy is caused by hormonal imbalance that leads to the proliferation of benign adenomas. These gradually impede urine output because they obstruct the urethra.

🌐 CULTURE AND GENETICS

Prostate cancer (PC) is the most frequently diagnosed cancer in men. It is more common in North America and northwestern Europe and less common in Central and South America, Africa, and Asia. The incidence of PC is 70% higher for African-American men than for Whites; African-American men are more likely to be diagnosed at an advanced stage of the disease, and mortality rates are 2 times higher for African-American men than for White men.[1]

The risk factors include increasing age, African-American and African-Jamaican ancestry, and family history.[1] Men with one first-degree relative (father or brother) with a history of PC are 2 to 3 times more likely to develop PC. Genetic factors contribute some risk: men with BRCA2 mutations have increased risk for developing a more aggressive form of PC and at a younger age.

Environmental factors may account for more risk than genetics because migration studies show that men of Asian and African heritage who live in the United States have a higher risk for PC than their counterparts living in Asia and Africa. Environmental factors include diet, a potentially modifiable risk factor. Diets high in red and processed meat, animal and saturated fats, and dairy products may increase risk,[1,16] whereas diets high in fiber, fruits, and vegetables may lower risk.[17] Obesity may increase risk of aggressive PC.[1]

Of the men who have PC, those more likely to have an advanced disease at diagnosis include men who were uninsured or Medicaid-insured and men of racial/ethnic minority groups.[10] This may be due to lack of access to preventive PSA screening and barriers to evaluation. This has implications for screening and culturally appropriate health education. Screening guidelines were updated in 2010.[1] Men at average risk for PC should receive health information about benefits and risks of PC tests at 50 years; at higher risk (African American and positive family history) at 45 years; and at very high risk (multiple family members with PC) at 40 years. Screening includes the blood test for prostate-specific antigen (PSA) and a physical examination (i.e., a digital rectal examination [DRE]).[14]

Colorectal cancer has a racial variation as well. The incidence rates are almost 20% higher for African-American women and men than for Whites, and the mortality rates are almost 50% higher for African Americans than for Whites.[8] This may be due to differences in access to care or quality of care.[24] Because colorectal cancer can largely be prevented by removal of adenomatous polyps, guidelines for average-risk adults start at age 50 years and include health teaching about options for screening. Options include a colonoscopy every 10 years with bowel preparation and conscious sedation and an annual fecal immunochemical test (FIT).[4,25,27]

SUBJECTIVE DATA

1. Usual bowel routine
2. Change in bowel habits
3. Rectal bleeding, blood in the stool
4. Medications (laxatives, stool softeners, iron)
5. Rectal conditions (pruritus, hemorrhoids, fissure, fistula)
6. Family history
7. Patient-centered care (diet of high-fiber foods, most recent examinations)

Examiner Asks	Rationale
1. **Usual bowel routine.** Bowels move regularly? How often? Usual color? Hard or soft? • Any straining at stool, incomplete evacuation, urge to have bowel movement but nothing comes? • Eat breakfast? (This increases colon motility and prompts a bowel movement in many.) • Pain while passing a bowel movement?	Rome III criteria for constipation include: ≤ 3 stools/week, straining, lumpy or hard stools, and incomplete evacuation. Risks for constipation: older age, women, inactivity, low-calorie or low-fiber diet, low income or educational level.[15] **Dyschezia.** Pain due to local condition (hemorrhoid, fissure) or constipation.

Subjective Data

Examiner Asks	Rationale
2. **Change in bowel habits.** Any **change** in usual **bowel habits?** Loose stools or diarrhea? When did it start? Is the diarrhea associated with nausea and vomiting, abdominal pain, something you ate recently?	Diarrhea occurs with gastroenteritis, colitis, irritable colon syndrome. Epidemiologic risks include: visit to child-care center, eating raw shellfish, undercooked meat or eggs, swimming in contaminated water, physical contact with other sick people.[3] Consider food poisoning.
• Eaten at a restaurant recently? Anyone else in your group or family have the same symptoms? • Traveled to a developing country during the past 6 months?	Consider parasitic or bacterial infection. *E. coli* is the most frequent cause of traveler's diarrhea.
3. **Rectal bleeding, blood in the stool.** Ever had black or bloody stools? When did you first notice blood in the stools? What is the color—bright red or dark red–black? How much blood: spotting on the toilet paper or outright passing of blood with the stool? Do the bloody stools have a particular smell?	**Melena.** Black stools may be tarry due to occult blood (melena) from GI bleeding or nontarry from ingestion of iron medications. Red blood in stools occurs with GI bleeding or local bleeding around the anus and with colon and rectal cancer.
• Ever had clay-colored stools? • Ever had mucus or pus in stool?	Clay color indicates absent bile pigment, as with biliary cirrhosis, gallstones, alcoholic or viral hepatitis.
• Frothy stool?	**Steatorrhea** is excessive fat in the stool, from malabsorption of fat as in celiac disease, cystic fibrosis, chronic pancreatitis, Crohn disease.
• Need to pass gas frequently?	Flatulence occurs with some medications, nutritional supplements, Crohn disease, certain foods.
4. **Medications.** Which **medications** do you take—prescription and over-the-counter? Laxatives or stool softeners? Which ones? How often? Iron pills? Do you ever use enemas to move your bowels? How often?	
5. **Rectal conditions.** Any problems in rectal area: itching, pain or burning, hemorrhoids? How do you treat these? Any hemorrhoid preparations? Ever had a fissure or fistula? How was it treated? • Ever had a problem controlling your bowels?	Pruritus. Fecal incontinence is leaking of solid or liquid stool involuntarily. Mucoid discharge and soiled underwear occur with prolapsed hemorrhoids.
6. **Family history.** Any **family history:** polyps or cancer in colon or rectum, inflammatory bowel disease, prostate cancer?	Risk factors for colon cancer, rectal cancer, prostate cancer.
7. **Patient-centered care.** What is the usual amount of **high-fiber foods** in your daily diet: cereals, apples or other fruits, vegetables, whole-grain breads? How many glasses of water do you drink each day?	High-fiber foods of the soluble type (beans, prunes, barley, carrots, broccoli, cabbage) lower cholesterol levels, whereas insoluble fiber foods (cereals, wheat germ) reduce risk for colon cancer. Also, fiber foods fight obesity, stabilize blood sugar, and help some GI disorders.

Examiner Asks	Rationale
• Date of last: digital rectal examination, stool blood test, colonoscopy, prostate-specific antigen blood test (for men).	Early detection for cancer: DRE performed annually after age 50 years; fecal occult blood test annually after age 50 years; sigmoidoscopy every 5 years or colonoscopy every 10 years after age 50 years in average-risk adults, age 45 years for African Americans[20]; information about PSA blood test annually for men older than 50 years or African-American men beginning at age 45 years.[1]

Additional History for Infants and Children

1. Have you ever noticed any irritation in your child's anal area: redness, raised skin, frequent itching?	In children, pinworms are a common cause of intense itching and irritated anal skin.
2. How are your child's bowel movements (BMs)? Frequency? Any problems? Any pain or straining with BM?	Assess usual stooling pattern. Constipation is decrease in BM frequency, with difficult passing of very hard, dry stools. **Encopresis** is persistent passing of stools into clothing in a child older than 4 years, at which age continence would be expected.

OBJECTIVE DATA

PREPARATION

Perform a rectal examination on all adults and particularly those in middle and late years. Help the person assume one of the following positions (Fig. 25-3):

Examine the male in the left lateral decubitus or standing position. Instruct the standing male to rest his elbows on the exam table and point his toes together; this relaxes the regional muscles, making it easier to spread the buttocks.

Place the female in the lithotomy position if examining genitalia as well; use the left lateral decubitus position for the rectal area alone.

EQUIPMENT NEEDED

Penlight
Lubricating jelly
Gloves
Fecal occult blood test container

Left lateral

Lithotomy

Standing

25-3   Positions for rectal examination.

Normal Range of Findings	Abnormal Findings

Inspect the Perianal Area

Spread the buttocks wide apart with both gloved hands and observe the perianal region. The anus normally looks moist and hairless, with coarse, folded skin that is more pigmented than the perianal skin. The anal opening is tightly closed. No lesions are present.

Inspect the sacrococcygeal area. Normally it appears smooth and even.

Instruct the person to hold the breath and bear down by performing a Valsalva maneuver. No break in skin integrity or protrusion through the anal opening should be present. Describe any abnormality in clock-face terms, with the 12 o'clock position as the anterior point toward the symphysis pubis and the 6 o'clock position toward the coccyx.

Palpate the Anus and Rectum

Drop lubricating jelly onto your gloved index finger. Instruct the person that palpation is not painful but may feel like needing to move the bowels. Ask the man to take a deep breath and hold it. Place the pad of your index finger gently against the anal verge (Fig. 25-4). You will feel the sphincter tighten and then relax. As it relaxes ask the man to exhale and flex the tip of your finger and slowly insert it into the anal canal in a direction toward the umbilicus. *Never* approach the anus at right angles with your index finger extended. Such a jabbing motion does not promote sphincter relaxation and is painful.

Abnormal Findings

Inflammation. Lesions or scars.

Linear split—Fissure.

Flabby skin sac—Hemorrhoid. Shiny blue skin sac—Thrombosed hemorrhoid.

Small round opening in anal area—Fistula (see Table 25-1, Anal Region Abnormalities, p. 732).

Inflammation or tenderness, swelling, tuft of hair, or dimple at tip of coccyx may indicate pilonidal cyst (see Table 25-1).

Appearance of fissure or hemorrhoids.

Circular red doughnut of tissue—Rectal prolapse.

25-4

Normal Range of Findings

Rotate your examining finger to palpate the entire muscular ring. The canal should feel smooth and even. Note the intersphincteric groove circling the canal wall. To assess tone, ask the person to tighten the muscle. The sphincter should tighten evenly around your finger with no pain to the person.

Use a bidigital palpation with your thumb against the perianal tissue (Fig. 25-5). Press your examining finger toward it. This maneuver highlights any swelling or tenderness and helps assess the bulbourethral glands.

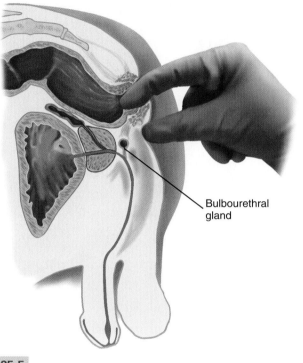

Bulbourethral gland

25-5

Above the anal canal the rectum turns posteriorly, following the curve of the coccyx and sacrum. Insert your finger farther and explore all around the rectal wall. It normally feels smooth with no nodularity. Promptly report any mass you discover for further examination.

Prostate Gland. On the anterior wall in the male, note the elastic, bulging prostate gland (Fig. 25-6). Find the median sulcus and palpate the entire prostate in a systematic manner, but note that only the superior and part of the lateral surfaces are accessible to examination. Press *into* the gland at each location because when a nodule occurs, it will not project into the rectal lumen. The surface should feel smooth and muscular; search for any distinct nodule or diffuse firmness. Note these characteristics:

Abnormal Findings

Decreased tone.
Increased tone occurs with inflammation and anxiety.
Tenderness.

Internal hemorrhoid above anorectal junction is not palpable unless thrombosed.

A soft, slightly movable mass may be a polyp.

A firm or hard mass with irregular shape or rolled edges may signify carcinoma (see Table 25-2, Rectum Abnormalities, p. 734).

Objective Data

Normal Range of Findings	Abnormal Findings

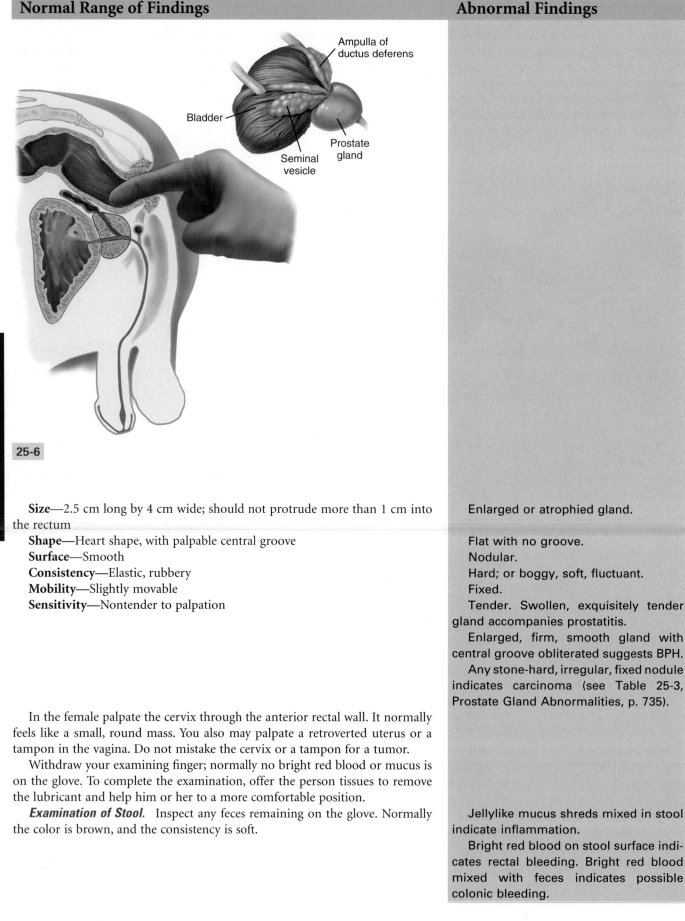

25-6

Size—2.5 cm long by 4 cm wide; should not protrude more than 1 cm into the rectum

Shape—Heart shape, with palpable central groove
Surface—Smooth
Consistency—Elastic, rubbery
Mobility—Slightly movable
Sensitivity—Nontender to palpation

In the female palpate the cervix through the anterior rectal wall. It normally feels like a small, round mass. You also may palpate a retroverted uterus or a tampon in the vagina. Do not mistake the cervix or a tampon for a tumor.

Withdraw your examining finger; normally no bright red blood or mucus is on the glove. To complete the examination, offer the person tissues to remove the lubricant and help him or her to a more comfortable position.

Examination of Stool. Inspect any feces remaining on the glove. Normally the color is brown, and the consistency is soft.

Abnormal Findings

Enlarged or atrophied gland.

Flat with no groove.
Nodular.
Hard; or boggy, soft, fluctuant.
Fixed.
Tender. Swollen, exquisitely tender gland accompanies prostatitis.
Enlarged, firm, smooth gland with central groove obliterated suggests BPH.
Any stone-hard, irregular, fixed nodule indicates carcinoma (see Table 25-3, Prostate Gland Abnormalities, p. 735).

Jellylike mucus shreds mixed in stool indicate inflammation.
Bright red blood on stool surface indicates rectal bleeding. Bright red blood mixed with feces indicates possible colonic bleeding.

Normal Range of Findings	**Abnormal Findings**

Test any stool on the glove for **occult blood**. A negative response is normal. If the stool is *Hematest* positive, it indicates occult blood. The fecal immunochemical test (FIT) is newer and can be used without the diet or medication restrictions of the older guaiac-based tests. There are two types of FITs: liquid-based tests that store the stool sample in a hemoglobin stabilizing buffer, and dry-slide cards that are analyzed manually.[7]

Enhance self-care by providing the average-risk patient an at-home collection kit to screen for asymptomatic colorectal cancer and precancerous lesions (high-risk adenomas). A patient collects the stool specimen at home and mails it to the laboratory. Evidence shows that the newer fecal immunochemical test is easier and requires only one stool sample. It detects antibodies specific for human hemoglobin and is sensitive to invasive cancers and precancerous lesions.[7]

Black tarry stool with distinct malodor indicates upper GI bleeding with blood partially digested. (Must lose more than 50 mL from upper GI tract to be considered melena.)

Black stool—Also occurs with ingesting iron or bismuth preparations.

Gray, tan stool—Absent bile pigment (e.g., obstructive jaundice).

Pale yellow, greasy stool—Increased fat content (steatorrhea), as occurs with malabsorption syndrome.

Occult bleeding usually indicates cancer of the colon.

❖ DEVELOPMENTAL COMPETENCE

Infants and Children

For the newborn, hold the feet with one hand and flex the knees up onto the abdomen. Note the presence of the anus. Confirm a patent rectum and anus by noting the first meconium stool passed within 24 to 48 hours of birth. To assess sphincter tone, check the *anal reflex*. Gently stroke the anal area and note a quick contraction of the sphincter.

Imperforate anus.

For each infant and child, note that the buttocks are firm and rounded with no masses or lesions. Recall that the *mongolian spot* is a common variation of hyperpigmentation in Black, American Indian, Mediterranean, and Asian newborns (see Chapter 12).

Flattened buttocks in cystic fibrosis or celiac syndrome.

Coccygeal mass. Meningocele (sac containing meninges that protrude through a defect in the bony spine).

Tuft of hair or pilonidal dimple.

The perianal skin is free of lesions. However, diaper rash is common in children younger than 1 year and is exhibited as a generalized reddened area with papules or vesicles.

Pustules indicate secondary infection of diaper rash.

Signs of physical or sexual abuse (e.g., anal abrasions, perianal tears).

Fissure—Common cause of constipation or rectal bleeding in child. (Painful, so the child does not defecate.)

Omit palpation unless the history or symptoms warrant. When internal palpation is needed, position the infant or child on the back with the legs flexed and gently insert a gloved, well-lubricated finger into the rectum. Your 5th finger usually is long enough, and its smaller size is more comfortable for the infant or child. However, you may need to use the index finger because of its better control and increased tactile sensitivity. On withdrawing the finger, scant bleeding or protruding rectal mucosa may occur.

Inspect the perianal region of the school-age child and adolescent during examination of the genitalia. Internal palpation is not performed routinely.

The Aging Adult

As an aging person performs the Valsalva maneuver, you may note relaxation of the perianal musculature and decreased sphincter control. Otherwise the full examination proceeds as that described earlier for the younger adult.

Objective Data

DOCUMENTATION AND CRITICAL THINKING

Sample Charting

SUBJECTIVE

Has one BM daily, soft, brown, no pain, no change in bowel routine. On no medications. Has no history of pruritus, hemorrhoids, fissure, or fistula. Diet includes 1 to 2 servings daily each of fresh fruits and vegetables but no whole-grain cereals or breads.

OBJECTIVE

No fissure, hemorrhoids, fistula, or skin lesions in perianal area. Sphincter tone good; no prolapse. Rectal walls smooth; no masses or tenderness. Prostate not enlarged; no masses or tenderness. Stool brown; Hematest negative.

ASSESSMENT

Rectal structures intact; no palpable lesions

Clinical Case Study 1

D.R. is a 55-year-old Caucasian male. Employed as a database analyst. No personal or family history of GI disease or colon cancer. Personal history of obesity (BMI 42.5); low-fiber, high-fat diet; hypertension; recent knee replacement. Medications include antihypertensive agent and hydrocodone prn for knee pain.

SUBJECTIVE

D.R. presents with inability to sit without pain, constipation, and "bleeding when I wipe." Last bowel movement 1 day PTA. D.R. reports stool was difficult to expel.

OBJECTIVE

Abdomen: Rounded appearance. Bowel sounds present. Tympany predominates. Dull over LLQ. Firm, nontender LLQ. No organomegaly.

Rectal: Skin sac indicative of hemorrhoid located at 6 o'clock. Grade IV thrombosed hemorrhoids located at 12 o'clock and 2 o'clock. Sphincter tone good. Rectal walls smooth; no masses. Reports tenderness with rectal exam. No stool present.

ASSESSMENT

Thrombosed hemorrhoids R/T constipation and straining to defecate
Acute pain R/T hemorrhoids and constipation
Constipation R/T narcotic use and low-fiber diet
Alteration in bowel elimination: Constipation R/T decreased gastrointestinal mobility

Clinical Case Study 2

C.M. is a 62-year-old African-American male with COPD for 15 years who today has "diarrhea for 3 days."

SUBJECTIVE

7 days PTA—C.M. seen at this agency for acute respiratory infection that was diagnosed as acute bronchitis and treated with oral ampicillin. Took medication as directed.
3 days PTA—Symptoms of respiratory infection improved. Ingesting usual diet. Onset of 4-5 loose, unformed brown stools a day. No abdominal pain or cramping. No nausea.
Now—Diarrhea continues. No blood or mucus noticed in stool. No new foods or restaurant food in past 3 days. Wife not ill.

OBJECTIVE

Vital signs: Temp 98.6° F (37° C). Pulse 88 bpm. Resp 18/min. BP 142/82 mm Hg.
Respiratory: Respirations unlabored. Barrel chest. Hyperresonant to percussion. Lung sounds clear but diminished. No crackles or rhonchi today.
Abdomen: Flat. Bowel sounds present. No organomegaly or tenderness to palpation.
Rectal: No lesions in perianal area. Sphincter tone good. Rectal walls smooth; no masses or tenderness. Prostate smooth and firm, no median sulcus palpable, no masses or tenderness. Stool brown; Hematest negative.

ASSESSMENT

Diarrhea R/T effects of antibiotic medication

Clinical Case Study 3

S.D. is a 7-year-old Caucasian female who presents early in the morning to the clinic with her mother for a back-to-school checkup.

SUBJECTIVE

S.D. mentions that she has trouble sleeping at night and that "the hole in her bottom itches real bad."
7 days PTA—S.D. began reporting the itching to her anus but denies any abdominal cramping, bloating, bleeding, diarrhea, nausea or vomiting. "It really itches down there when I'm sleeping."

OBJECTIVE

Abdomen: Bowel sounds present; no tenderness to palpation.
Rectal: Anus is swollen and moist w/abrasions; microscopic tape test reveals translucent eggs that are approximately 55 μm in diameter.

ASSESSMENT

Pinworms
Impaired comfort R/T infestation causing itching
Impaired skin integrity R/T inflammation caused by itching
Disturbed sleep pattern R/T interruptions

ABNORMAL FINDINGS

TABLE 25-1 Anal Region Abnormalities

Fistula

Indurated cord

Pilonidal Cyst or Sinus

A hair-containing cyst or sinus located in the midline over the coccyx or lower sacrum. Often opens as a dimple with visible tuft of hair and possibly an erythematous halo. Or may appear as a palpable cyst. When advanced, has a palpable sinus tract. Although a congenital disorder, it is first diagnosed between 15 and 30 years.

Sinus tract

Anorectal Fistula

A chronically inflamed GI tract (Crohn disease, local irradiation) creates an abnormal passage from inner anus or rectum out to skin surrounding anus. May result from a local abscess. The red, raised tract opening may drain serosanguineous or purulent matter when pressure is applied. Bidigital palpation may reveal an indurated cord. May heal with warm bath, high-fiber diet, and analgesics.

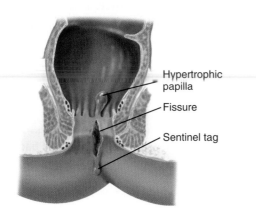

Hypertrophic papilla

Fissure

Sentinel tag

Internal hemorrhoid

Thrombosed external hemorrhoid

Fissure

An exquisitely painful longitudinal tear in the superficial mucosa at the anal margin. Most (>90%) occur in the posterior midline area. Pain is described as passing "shards of glass"; may have bright red blood in the stool.[9] A resulting spasm in the sphincters makes the area painful to examine. Inspection shows a recent fissure as having sharp edges and a chronic fissure as indurated and accompanied by a papule of skin, *sentinel tag,* on the anal margin below or a polyp above. Fissures may be caused by trauma (passing a large hard stool) or from irritant diarrheal stools. Treat with stool softeners, fiber, warm soaking baths, topical analgesics. Healing may be enhanced with topical nitroglycerin ointment or Botox injection.[9]

Hemorrhoids

These painless, flabby papules are caused by a varicose vein. An *external hemorrhoid* starts below the anorectal junction and is covered by anal skin. When *thrombosed,* it contains clotted blood and becomes a painful, swollen, shiny blue mass that itches and bleeds with defecation. When it resolves, it leaves a painless, flabby skin sac around the anal orifice. An *internal hemorrhoid* starts above the anorectal junction and is covered by mucous membrane. When the person performs a Valsalva maneuver, it may appear as a red mucosal mass. All hemorrhoids result from increased portal venous pressure: as occurs with straining at stool, chronic constipation, pregnancy, obesity, chronic liver disease, or the low-fiber diet common in Western society.

TABLE 25-1   Anal Region Abnormalities—cont'd

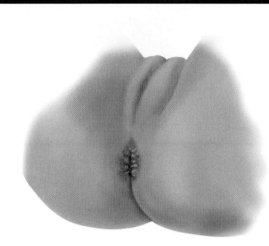

Rectal Prolapse

The complete rectal mucous membrane protrudes through the anus, appearing as a moist red doughnut with radiating lines. When prolapse is incomplete, only the mucosa bulges. When complete, it includes the anal sphincters. Occurs following a Valsalva maneuver such as straining at stool or with exercise. Caused by weakened pelvic support muscles and requires surgery.

Pruritus Ani

Intense perianal itching is caused by pinworm infection in children and institutionalized adults and by prolapsed hemorrhoids, anal fissure, dermatitis, chronic diarrhea, poor hygiene, perfume or dye irritants, systemic diseases such as diabetes mellitus or inflammatory bowel disease.[9] Inspection shows red, raised, thickened excoriated skin around the anus. The area is swollen and moist; with a fungal infection it appears dull grayish pink. Treat the underlying cause; encourage good hygiene, use of topical steroid cream.

TABLE 25-2   Rectum Abnormalities

Submucosal

Perianal   Ischiorectal

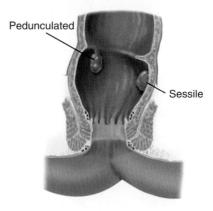

Pedunculated

Sessile

Abscess

A localized cavity of pus from infection in a pararectal space. Infection usually extends from an anal crypt. Characterized by persistent throbbing rectal pain. Termed by the space it occupies (e.g., a perianal abscess is superficial around the anal skin) and appears red, hot, swollen, indurated, and tender. An ischiorectal abscess is deep and tender to bidigital palpation; occurs laterally between the anus and ischial tuberosity and is rare. Must be drained before it worsens or develops sepsis.

Rectal Polyp

A protruding growth from the rectal mucous membrane that is fairly common. The polyp may be *pedunculated* (on a stalk) or *sessile* (a mound on the surface, close to the mucosal wall). The soft nodule is difficult to palpate. Colonoscopy and biopsy are needed to screen for a malignant growth. Removal of adenomatous polyps has been shown to prevent deaths from colorectal cancer.[27]

Rolled-edge neoplasm

Fecal Impaction

A complete colon blockage by hard, desiccated immovable stool in the rectum, which presents as constipation or overflow incontinence. Results from decreased bowel motility as in hospitalized older adults and people with spinal cord injuries; also with low-fiber diet, hypothyroidism, opiate use.[9] Abdominal palpation or DRE reveals mass. Treat with laxatives, enemas, suppositories. Community-dwelling older adults are at risk, especially those with dementia who cannot communicate. Use extreme caution in treating this group.[6]

Carcinoma

A malignant neoplasm in the rectum is asymptomatic; thus the importance of routine DRE. An early lesion may be a single firm nodule. You may palpate an ulcerated center with rolled edges. As the lesion grows it has an irregular cauliflower shape and is fixed and stone-hard. Refer a person with any rectal lesion for cancer screening. Suggest screening guidelines: careful family history, fecal occult blood tests annually, and colonoscopy every 10 years, starting at age 50 years for those at average risk.[20]

ABNORMAL FINDINGS
FOR ADVANCED PRACTICE

TABLE 25-3   Prostate Gland Abnormalities

Benign Prostatic Hypertrophy (BPH)

S: Urinary frequency, urgency, hesitancy, straining to urinate, weak stream, intermittent stream, sensation of incomplete emptying, nocturia.

O: A symmetric nontender enlargement; commonly occurs in males beginning in the middle years. The prostate surface feels smooth, rubbery, or firm (like the consistency of the nose), with the median sulcus obliterated.

Prostatitis

S: Fever, chills, malaise, urinary frequency and urgency, dysuria, urethral discharge; dull, aching pain in perineal and rectal area.

O: An exquisitely tender enlargement is *acute* inflammation, yielding a swollen, slightly asymmetric gland.

With a chronic inflammation the signs can vary from tender enlargement with a boggy feel to isolated firm areas caused by fibrosis. Or the gland may feel normal.

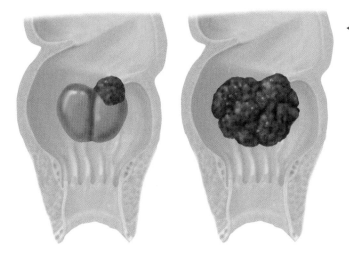

◀ Carcinoma

S: Frequency, nocturia, hematuria, weak stream, hesitancy, pain or burning on urination; continuous pain in lower back, pelvis, thighs.

O: A malignant neoplasm often starts as a single hard nodule on the posterior surface, producing asymmetry and a change in consistency. As it invades normal tissue, multiple hard nodules appear, or the entire gland feels stone-hard and fixed. The median sulcus is obliterated.

S, Subjective data; *O*, objective data.

Summary Checklist: Anus, Rectum, and Prostate Examination

1. **Inspect anus** and perianal area.
2. Inspect during Valsalva maneuver.
3. **Palpate anal canal** and rectum on all adults.
4. **Test stool** for occult blood.

BIBLIOGRAPHY

1. American Cancer Society. (2013). *Cancer facts & figures 2013*. Atlanta: American Cancer Society.
2. Atassi, K. (2012). Strategies to increase colorectal cancer screening. *Nurse Pract, 37*(7), 21-26.
2a. Bill-Axelson, A., Holmberg, L., Ruutu, M., et al. (2014). Radical prostatectomy or watchful waiting in early prostate cancer. *N Engl J Med, 370*(10), 932-942.
3. Blush, R. R., & Matzo, M. (2012). Acute infectious diarrhea. *Am J Nurs, 112*(8), 65-68.
4. Byers, T. (2011). Examining stools for colon cancer prevention. *Cancer Prev Res, 4*(10), 1531-1533.
5. Chien, D., & Bradway, C. (2010). Acquired fecal incontinence in community-dwelling adults. *Nurse Pract, 35*(1), 14-22.
6. Craft, L., & Prahlow, J. A. (2011). From fecal impaction to colon perforation. *Am J Nurs, 111*(8), 38-43.
7. Daly, J. (2012). Fecal immunochemical tests for colorectal cancer screening. *Am J Nurs, 112*(10), 67-69.
8. Edwards, B. K., Ward, E., Kohler, B. A., et al. (2010). Colorectal cancer trends and impact of interventions (risk factors, screening, and treatment) to reduce future rates. *Cancer, 116*(3), 544-573.
9. Fargo, M. V., & Latimer, K. M. (2012). Evaluation and management of common anorectal conditions. *Am Fam Physician, 85*(6), 624-630.
10. Fedewa, S. A., Etzioni, R., Flanders, W. D., et al. (2010). Association of insurance and race/ethnicity with disease severity among men diagnosed with prostate cancer. *Cancer Epidemiol Biomarkers Prev, 19*(10), 2437-2444.
11. Fried, R. G. (2010). Performing digital rectal examination can detect cancers. *Am Fam Physician, 31*(9), 1073.
12. Greene, M. D. (2009). Diagnosis and management of HPV-related anal dysplasia. *Nurse Pract, 34*(5), 45-51.
13. Heijnsdijk, E. A., Wever, E. M., Auvinen, A., et al. (2012). Quality-of-life effects of prostate-specific antigen screening. *N Engl J Med, 367*(7), 595-605.
14. Hoffman, R. M. (2011). Screening for prostate cancer. *N Engl J Med, 365*(21), 2013-2019.
15. Jamshed, N., Lee, Z. E., & Olden, K. W. (2011). Diagnostic approach to chronic constipation in adults. *Am Fam Physician, 84*(3), 299.
16. Kristal, A. R., Arnold, K. B., Neuhouser, M. L., et al. (2010). Diet, supplement use, and prostate cancer risk. *Am J Epidemiol, 172*(5), 566-577.
17. Lewis, J. E., Soler-Vilá, H., Clark, P. E., et al. (2009). Intake of plant foods and associated nutrients in prostate cancer risk. *Nutr Cancer, 61*(2), 216-224.
18. Mounsey, A. L., Halladay, J., & Sadiq, T. S. (2011). Hemorrhoids. *Am Fam Physician, 84*(2), 204-210.
19. Nishihara, R., Wu, K., Lochhead, P., et al. (2013). Long-term colorectal-cancer incidence and mortality after lower endoscopy. *N Engl J Med, 369*(12), 1095-1105.
20. Qaseem, A., Denberg, T. D., Hopkins, R. H., et al. (2012). Screening for colorectal cancer. *Ann Intern Med, 156*(5), 378-386.
21. Quintero, E., Castells, A., Bujanda, L., et al. (2012). Colonoscopy versus fecal immunochemical testing in colorectal-cancer screening. *N Engl J Med, 366*(8), 697-706.
22. Ross, A. G., Olds, G. R., Cripps, A. W., et al. (2013). Enteropathogens and chronic illness in returning travelers. *N Engl J Med, 368*(19), 1817-1825.
23. Schröder, F. H. (2011). Stratifying risk—the U.S. Preventive Services Task Force and prostate-cancer screening. *N Engl J Med, 365*(21), 1953-1955.
24. Soneji, S., Iyer, S. S., Armstrong, K., et al. (2010). Racial disparities in stage-specific colorectal cancer mortality: 1960–2005. *J Information, 100*(10), 1912-1916.
25. Vart, G., Banzi, R., & Minozzi, S. (2012). Comparing participation rates between immunochemical and guaiac faecal occult blood tests. *Prev Med, 55*(2), 87-92.
26. Wallace, M., Bailey, D. E., & Brion, J. (2009). Shedding light on prostate cancer. *Nurse Pract, 34*(10), 25-34.
27. Zauber, A. G., Winawer, S. J., O'Brien, M. J., et al. (2012). Colonoscopic polypectomy and long-term prevention of colorectal-cancer deaths. *N Engl J Med, 366*(8), 687-696.

CHAPTER 26

Female Genitourinary System

STRUCTURE AND FUNCTION

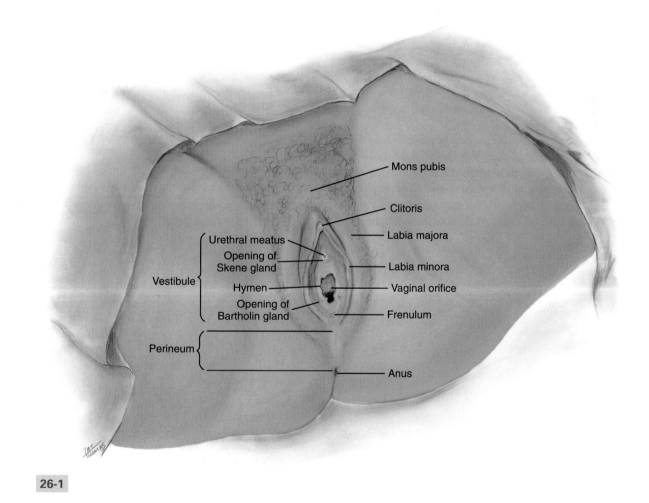

- Mons pubis
- Clitoris
- Labia majora
- Labia minora
- Vaginal orifice
- Frenulum
- Anus

Urethral meatus
Opening of Skene gland
Vestibule
Hymen
Opening of Bartholin gland
Perineum

26-1

EXTERNAL GENITALIA

The external genitalia are called the **vulva,** or pudendum (Fig. 26-1). The **mons pubis** is a round, firm pad of adipose tissue covering the symphysis pubis. After puberty it is covered with hair in the pattern of an inverted triangle. The **labia majora** are two rounded folds of adipose tissue extending from the mons pubis down and around to the perineum. After puberty hair covers the outer surfaces of the labia, whereas the inner folds are smooth and moist and contain sebaceous follicles.

Inside the labia majora are two smaller, darker folds of skin, the **labia minora.** These are joined anteriorly at the clitoris where they form a hood, or prepuce. The labia minora are joined posteriorly by a transverse fold, the **frenulum,** or fourchette. The **clitoris** is a small, pea-shaped erectile body, homologous with the male penis and highly sensitive to tactile stimulation.

The labial structures encircle a boat-shaped space, or cleft, termed the **vestibule.** Within it are numerous openings. The **urethral meatus** appears as a dimple 2.5 cm posterior to the clitoris. Surrounding the urethral meatus are the tiny, multiple **paraurethral (Skene) glands.** Their ducts are not visible but open posterior to the urethra at the 5 and 7 o'clock positions.

The **vaginal orifice** is posterior to the urethral meatus. It appears either as a thin median slit or a large opening with irregular edges, depending on the presentation of the membranous **hymen.** The hymen is a thin, circular or crescent-shaped fold that may cover part of the vaginal orifice or may be absent completely. On either side and posterior to the vaginal orifice are two **vestibular (Bartholin) glands,** which secrete a clear lubricating mucus during intercourse. Their ducts are not visible but open in the groove between the labia minora and the hymen.

INTERNAL GENITALIA

The internal genitalia include the **vagina,** a flattened, tubular canal extending from the orifice up and backward into the pelvis (Fig. 26-2). It is 9 cm long and sits between the rectum posteriorly and the bladder and urethra anteriorly. Its walls are in thick transverse folds, or **rugae,** enabling the vagina to dilate widely during childbirth.

At the end of the canal, the uterine **cervix** projects into the vagina. In the nulliparous female the cervix appears as a smooth doughnut shape with a small circular hole, or **os.** After childbirth the os is slightly enlarged and irregular. The cervical epithelium is of two distinct types. The vagina and cervix are covered with smooth, pink, stratified squamous epithelium. Inside the os the endocervical canal is lined with columnar epithelium that looks red and rough. The point where these two tissues meet is the **squamocolumnar junction** and is not visible.

A continuous recess is present around the cervix, termed the **anterior fornix** in front and the **posterior fornix** in back. Behind the posterior fornix another deep recess is formed by the peritoneum. It dips down between the rectum and cervix to form the **rectouterine pouch,** or **cul-de-sac of Douglas.**

The **uterus** is a pear-shaped, thick-walled, muscular organ. It is flattened anteroposteriorly, measuring 5.5 to 8 cm long by 3.5 to 4 cm wide and 2 to 2.5 cm thick. It is freely movable, not fixed, and usually tilts forward and superior to the bladder (a position labeled as *anteverted* and *anteflexed,* see p. 756).

The **fallopian tubes** are two pliable, trumpet-shaped tubes, 10 cm in length, extending from the uterine fundus laterally to the brim of the pelvis. There they curve posteriorly, their fimbriated ends located near the **ovaries.** The two ovaries are located one on each side of the uterus at the level of the anterior superior iliac spine. Each is oval shaped, 3 cm long by 2 cm wide by 1 cm thick, and serves to develop ova (eggs) and the female hormones.

◈ DEVELOPMENTAL COMPETENCE

Infants and Adolescents

At birth the external genitalia are engorged because of the presence of maternal estrogen. The structures recede in a few weeks, remaining small until puberty. The ovaries are located

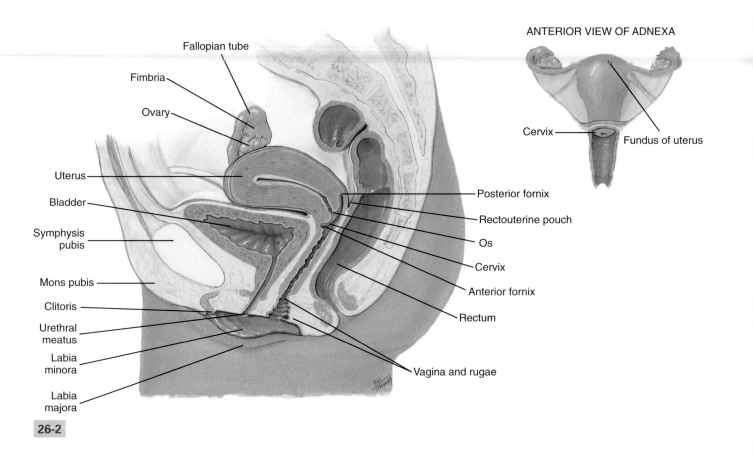

ANTERIOR VIEW OF ADNEXA

Cervix — Fundus of uterus

Fallopian tube
Fimbria
Ovary
Uterus
Bladder
Symphysis pubis
Mons pubis
Clitoris
Urethral meatus
Labia minora
Labia majora

Posterior fornix
Rectouterine pouch
Os
Cervix
Anterior fornix
Rectum
Vagina and rugae

26-2

TABLE 26-1	Sexual Maturity Rating (SMR) in Girls

Stage 1 Preadolescent. No pubic hair. Mons and labia covered with fine vellus hair as on abdomen.

Stage 2 Growth sparse and mostly on labia. Long, downy hair, slightly pigmented, straight or only slightly curly.

Stage 3 Growth sparse and spreading over mons pubis. Hair is darker, coarser, curlier.

Stage 4 Hair is adult in type but over smaller area; none on medial thigh.

Stage 5 Adult in type and pattern; inverse triangle. Also on medial thigh surface.

Adapted from Tanner, J.M. (1962). *Growth at adolescence.* Oxford, England: Blackwell Scientific.

in the abdomen during childhood. The uterus is small with a straight axis and no anteflexion.

At puberty estrogens stimulate the growth of cells in the reproductive tract and the development of secondary sex characteristics. The first signs of puberty are breast development (thelarche) and pubic hair development, beginning between the ages of 8 to 10 years (mean = 11.6 years).[26] Puberty culminates with the first menstrual cycle (menarche) just after the peak of growth velocity. Irregularity of the menstrual cycle is common during adolescence because of the occasional failure to ovulate. With menarche the uterine body flexes on the cervix. The ovaries now are in the pelvic cavity.

Tanner's table on the 5 stages of pubic hair development (sexual maturity rating [SMR]) is helpful in teaching girls the expected sequence of sexual development (Table 26-1). These data were developed on Caucasian girls and may not generalize to all racial groups, i.e., mature Asian women normally have fine, sparse pubic hair.

Data from NHANES III found that African-American and Mexican-American girls had pubic hair and achieved menarche at younger ages than White girls.[39] The mean age at onset of pubic hair and menarche was 9.5 and 12.1 years for African-American girls, 10.3 and 12.2 years for Mexican-American girls, and 10.5 and 12.7 years for White girls. Thus African-American girls on average enter puberty first, followed by Mexican-American and then White girls.[26,39]

During the past 4 decades the prevalence of overweight and obesity in U.S. children has more than tripled,[24] with African-American, Hispanic, and Native American girls at especially high risk. Evidence shows that increased weight and body mass index (BMI) contribute to earlier pubertal development, with a median age of menarche occurring 5.4 months earlier in obese preteen girls than in girls with normal BMI.[26] African-American girls enter puberty before Caucasian and Hispanic girls, but it is not clear if obesity alone contributes to this earlier onset or if genetic or environmental factors contribute as well.[24]

The Pregnant Woman

A complete discussion of the pregnant woman follows in Chapter 30. In summary, shortly after the first missed menstrual period the genitalia show signs of the growing fetus. The cervix softens (*Goodell sign*) at 4 to 6 weeks, and the vaginal mucosa and cervix look cyanotic (*Chadwick sign*) at 8 to 12 weeks. These changes occur because of increased vascularity and edema of the cervix and hypertrophy and hyperplasia of the cervical glands. The isthmus of the uterus softens (*Hegar sign*) at 6 to 8 weeks.

The greatest change is in the uterus itself. The nonpregnant uterus has a flattened pear shape. Its early growth encroaches on the space occupied by the bladder, producing the symptom of urinary frequency. By 10 to 12 weeks' gestation, the uterus becomes globular in shape and is too large to stay in the pelvis. At 20 to 24 weeks, the uterus has an oval shape. It rises almost to the liver, displacing the intestines superiorly and laterally.

Cervical and vaginal secretions increase during pregnancy and are thick, white, and more acidic because of *Lactobacillus acidophilus,* which changes glycogen into lactic acid. The acidic pH keeps pathogenic bacteria from multiplying in the vagina, but the increase in glycogen increases the risk for candidiasis (commonly called a *yeast infection*) during pregnancy.

The Aging Woman

In contrast to the slowly declining hormones in the aging male, the female's hormonal milieu decreases rapidly. *Menopause* is cessation of the menses. Usually this occurs around 48 to 51 years, although a wide variation of age from 35 to 60 years exists. The stage of menopause includes the preceding 1 to 2 years of decline in ovarian function, shown by irregular menses that gradually become farther apart and produce a lighter flow. Ovaries stop producing progesterone and estrogen. Because cells in the reproductive tract are estrogen dependent, decreased estrogen levels during menopause bring dramatic physical changes.

The uterus shrinks in size because of decreased myometrium. The ovaries atrophy to 1 to 2 cm and are not palpable after menopause. Ovulation still may occur sporadically after menopause. The sacral ligaments relax, and the pelvic musculature weakens; thus the uterus droops. The cervix shrinks and looks paler with a thick, glistening epithelium.

The vagina becomes shorter, narrower, and less elastic. Without sexual activity the vagina atrophies to one-half its former length and width. The vaginal epithelium atrophies, becoming thinner, drier, and itchy. This results in a fragile mucosal surface that is at risk for bleeding and vaginitis. Decreased vaginal secretions leave the vagina dry and at risk for irritation and pain with intercourse (dyspareunia). The vaginal pH becomes more alkaline, and glycogen content decreases from the decreased estrogen. These factors also increase the risk for vaginitis because they create a suitable medium for pathogens.

Externally the mons pubis looks smaller because the fat pad atrophies. The labia and clitoris gradually decrease in size. Pubic hair becomes thin and sparse.

Declining estrogen levels produce some physiologic changes in the female sexual response cycle: reduced amount of vaginal secretion and lubrication during excitement; shorter duration of orgasm; and rapid resolution. However, these changes do not affect sexual pleasure and function. As with the male, the older female is capable of sexual expression and function given reasonably good health and an interested partner. Aging women greatly outnumber their male counterparts, and aging women are more likely to be single, whereas males their same age are more likely to be married.

CULTURE AND GENETICS

During the past 35 years the use of the Papanicolaou (Pap) screening test in the United States has decreased rates of cervical cancer by 51% in Caucasians and 70% in African Americans.[1] However, the absolute incidence still is higher in African-American women, perhaps because of decreased follow-up and treatment after abnormal screening tests. Another point is that the Pap test screens the subtype of squamous cervical cancer better than it does the adeno subtype; adenocarcinomas now account for 25% of invasive cervical cancer. Thus human papilloma virus (HPV) testing and HPV vaccination must be prioritized to control this subtype of cervical cancer.[1] Vaccines now are approved to prevent the most common HPV infections, and routine HPV vaccination is recommended for all girls ages 11 and 12 years and even at 9 years.[12]

Female *genital mutilation,* or "cutting," is an invasive surgical procedure performed on girls before puberty. It is practiced within Aboriginal, Christian, and Muslim families who have immigrated to the United States from western and southern Asia, the Middle East, and large areas of Africa. It is a social custom, not a religious practice. This procedure involves removal, partial or total, of the clitoris and is believed to inhibit sexual pleasure. However the procedure can cause death, sterility, infection, and psychological trauma[3] and is outlawed in the United States.

SUBJECTIVE DATA

1. Menstrual history	5. Acute pelvic pain	9. Sexual activity
2. Obstetric history	6. Urinary symptoms	10. Contraceptive use
3. Menopause	7. Vaginal discharge	11. Sexually transmitted infection
4. Patient-centered care	8. Past history	(STI) contact

Examiner Asks	Rationale

1. Menstrual history. Tell me about your menstrual periods:
 	
  • Date of your last menstrual period?
  • Age at first period?
	Menstrual history is usually nonthreatening; thus it is a good place to start.
	LMP—Last menstrual period.
	Menarche—Mean age at onset at 12 to 13 years; delayed onset suggests endocrine or underweight problem.

Examiner Asks	Rationale
• How often are your periods?	Cycle—Normally every 28 days; varies from 18 to 45 days.
	Amenorrhea—Absent menses.
• How many days does your period last?	Duration—Average 3 to 7 days.
• Usual amount of flow: light, medium, heavy? How many pads or tampons do you use each day or hour?	Menorrhagia—Heavy menses.
• Any clotting?	Clotting indicates heavy flow or vaginal pooling.
• Any pain or cramps before or during period? How do you treat it? Interfere with daily activities? Any other associated symptoms: bloating, breast tenderness, moodiness? Any spotting between periods?	**Dysmenorrhea** responds to ibuprofen because it works on uterine smooth muscle.
2. **Obstetric history**. Have you ever been pregnant?	
• How many times?	Gravida—Number of pregnancies.
• How many babies have you had?	Para—Number of births.
• Any miscarriage or abortion?	Abortions—Interrupted pregnancies, including elective abortions and spontaneous miscarriages.
• For each pregnancy describe: duration, any complication, labor and delivery, baby's sex, birth weight, condition.	
• Do you think you may be pregnant now? What symptoms have you noticed?	
3. **Menopause**. Have your periods slowed down or stopped?	**Menopause**, cessation of menstruation.
• Any associated symptoms of menopause (e.g., hot flashes, night sweats, numbness and tingling, headache, palpitations, drenching sweats, mood swings, vaginal dryness, itching)? Any treatment?	Perimenopausal period from 40 to 55 years has hormone shifts, resulting in vasomotor instability.
• If hormone replacement therapy (HRT), how much? How is it working? Any side effects?	Side effects of HRT include fluid retention, breast pain, vaginal bleeding, and cardiovascular and breast cancer risk. Selected women with severe vasomotor symptoms may choose HRT but at the lowest effective dose for the shortest time.[27]
• How do you feel about going through menopause?	Although a normal life stage, reaction varies from acceptance to feelings of loss.
4. **Patient-centered care**. How often do you have a gynecologic checkup?	Although Pap tests save lives, cervical cancer is rare in young women. In 2012 new recommendations are: (1) no Pap tests for women under age 21 years, regardless of sexual activity; (2) Pap test interval of 3 years for women ages 21-30 years; (3) HPV and Pap "co-testing" every 5 years for women ages 30 to 65 years.[4,23,33]
• Last Pap test? Results?	Pap testing should begin at 21 years, no matter the age of sexual debut or history.[16]
5. **Acute pelvic pain**. Any pain in the lower abdomen or pelvis? When did it start? Constant or come and go? Associated with periods? On a scale of 1 to 10, with 10 being the strongest, how would you rate your pain?	Acute pain lasts <3 months. Consider urgent conditions: pelvic inflammatory disease (PID), appendicitis, ruptured ovarian cysts, ovarian torsion, which need transvaginal ultrasound imaging.[17]

Examiner Asks	Rationale
6. Urinary symptoms. Any problems with urinating? Frequently and small amounts?	Most women will not bring up urinary incontinence (UI). Important to ask because UI can decrease quality of life, limit activities, and increase falls and fracture risk.[15,35]
• Cannot wait to urinate?	Urgency.
• Any burning or pain on urinating?	Dysuria.
• Awaken during night to urinate?	Nocturia.
• Blood in the urine?	Hematuria occurs with urinary tract infection (UTI) and kidney disease.
• Urine dark, cloudy, foul smelling?	Bile in urine or UTI.
• Any difficulty controlling urine or wetting yourself?	**Urge incontinence**—Involuntary urine loss from overactive detrusor muscle in bladder.
• Urinate with a sneeze, laugh, cough, bearing down?	**Stress incontinence**—Involuntary urine loss with physical strain, sneezing, or coughing.
7. Vaginal discharge. Any unusual **vaginal discharge?** Increased amount?	Normal discharge is small, clear or cloudy, and always nonirritating.
• Character or color: white, yellow-green, gray, curdlike, foul smelling?	Suggests vaginal infection; character of discharge often suggests causative organism (see Table 26-5, p. 768).
• When did it begin?	Acute versus chronic problem.
• Is the discharge associated with vaginal itching, rash, pain with intercourse?	Rash is result of irritation from discharge. Dyspareunia occurs with vaginitis of any cause.
• Taking any medications?	Oral contraceptives increase glycogen content of vaginal epithelium, providing fertile medium for some organisms. Broad-spectrum antibiotics alter balance of normal flora.
• Family history of diabetes?	Diabetes increases glycogen content.
• In which part of your menstrual cycle are you now?	Menses, postpartum, menopause have a more alkaline vaginal pH.
• Use a vaginal douche? How often?	Frequent douching alters pH.
• Use feminine hygiene spray?	Spray has risk for contact dermatitis.
• Wear nonventilating underpants, pantyhose?	Local irritation.
• Treated the discharge with anything? Result?	
8. Past history. Any other problems in the genital area? Sores or lesions—now or in the past? How were they treated? Any abdominal pain?	
• Any past surgery on uterus, ovaries, vagina?	Assess feelings. Some fear loss of sexual response after hysterectomy, which may affect intimate relationships.
9. Sexual activity. Often women have a question about their **sexual relationship** and how it affects their health. Do you?	Begin with open-ended question to assess individual needs. Include appropriate questions as a routine.
• Are you in a relationship involving sex now?	
• Are aspects of sex satisfactory to you and your partner?	Communicates that you accept individual's sexual activity and believe that it is important.
• Satisfied with the way you and partner communicate about sex?	
• Satisfied with your ability to respond sexually?	Your comfort with discussion prompts person's interest and possibly relief that the topic has been introduced.
• Do you have more than one sexual partner?	

Examiner Asks	Rationale

Establishes a database for comparison with any future sexual activities.

Provides opportunity to screen sexual problems.

The practice environment must be welcoming and respectful of lesbians and bisexual women to discuss their health concerns.

• What is your sexual preference: relationship with a man, with a woman, both?

10. Contraceptive use. Currently planning a pregnancy or avoiding pregnancy?
• Do you and your partner use a **contraceptive?** Which method? Is it satisfactory? Do you have any questions about method?
• Which methods have you used in the past? Have you and partner discussed having children?
• Have you ever had any problems becoming pregnant?

Assess smoking history. Oral contraceptives, together with cigarette smoking, increase the risk for vascular problems.

Infertility is considered after 1 year of unprotected sexual intercourse without conceiving.

11. STI contact. Any sexual contact with partner having an STI such as gonorrhea, herpes, HIV/AIDS, chlamydial infection, venereal warts, syphilis? When? How was it treated? Were there any complications?
• Any precautions to reduce risk for STIs? Use condoms at each episode of sexual intercourse?

A STI includes all conditions that can be transmitted during intimate sexual contact with an infected partner.

Additional History for Infants and Children

1. Does your child have any problem urinating? Pain with urinating, crying, holding genitals? UTI?
   • (If the child is older than 2 to 2½ years) Has toilet training started? How is it progressing?
   • Does the child wet bed at night? Is this a problem for child or you (parents)? What have you (parents) done?

2. Problem with genital area: itching, rash, vaginal discharge?

Occurs with poor perineal hygiene or insertion of foreign body into vagina.

3. (To child) Has anyone ever touched you in between your legs when you did not want them to? Sometimes that happens to children. They should remember that they have not been bad. They should try to tell a big person about it. Can you tell me three different big people you trust whom you could talk to?

Screen for sexual abuse (see Chapter 7). For prevention, teach the child that it is not okay for someone to look at or touch her private parts while telling her it is a secret. Naming three trusted adults will include someone outside the family—important because most molestation is by a parent.

Additional History for Preadolescents and Adolescents

Assess sexual growth and development and sexual behavior. First:
• Ask questions that seem appropriate for girl's age, but norms vary widely. Children obtain information, often misinformation, from the media and from peers at surprisingly early ages. You can be sure your information will be more thoughtful and accurate.
• Ask direct, matter-of-fact questions. Avoid sounding judgmental.
• Start with a *permission statement*: "Often girls your age experience …." This conveys that it is normal to think or feel a certain way.
• Try the open-ended question: "When did you …?" rather than "Do you …?" This is less threatening because it implies that the topic is normal and unexceptional.

Examiner Asks	Rationale
1. Around age 9 or 10 years, girls start to develop breasts and pubic hair. Have you ever seen charts and pictures of normal growth patterns for girls? Let us go over these now.	
2. Have your periods started? How did you feel? Were you ready or surprised?	Assess attitude of girl and parents. Note inadequate preparation or attitude of distaste.
3. To whom in your family do you talk about your body changes and sex information? How do these talks go? Do you think you get enough information? What about sex education classes at school? Is there a teacher, a nurse or doctor, a minister, a counselor to whom you can talk? Often girls your age have questions about sexual activity. Do you have questions? Are you dating? Someone steady? Do you and your boyfriend have intercourse? Are you using condoms? What kind of protection did you use the last time you had sex?	Avoid the term "sexually active," which is ambiguous. Also, a Pap test is not needed to safely prescribe oral contraceptives; just weight, BP, and health history. Requiring a pelvic exam for asymptomatic teens is a barrier to access for some teens.[13,16]
4. Has anyone ever talked to you about sexually transmitted infections such as chlamydia, herpes, gonorrhea, or HIV/AIDS?	Teach STI risk reduction.
5. Have you and your parents discussed the human papillomavirus (HPV) vaccine (Gardasil, Cervarix)? It is recommended before girls become sexually active.	HPV is the most common STI in the United States. The HPV vaccines are approved for girls and women ages 9 to 26 for prevention of the most common types of cervical cancer.[4]
6. Sometimes a person touches a girl in a way that she does not want them to. Has that ever happened to you? If that happens, the girl should remember that it is not her fault. She should tell another adult about it.	Screen for sexual abuse.

Additional History for the Aging Adult

1. After menopause, noted any vaginal bleeding?	Postmenopausal bleeding warrants pelvic exam, transvaginal ultrasonography, and referral.
2. Any vaginal itching, discharge, pain with intercourse?	Associated with atrophic vaginitis.
3. Any pressure in genital area, loss of urine with cough or sneeze, back pain, or constipation?	Occurs with weakened pelvic musculature and uterine prolapse.
4. Are you in a relationship involving sex now? Are aspects of sex satisfactory to you and your partner? Is there adequate privacy for a sexual relationship?	

Objective Data (side tab)

OBJECTIVE DATA

PREPARATION

Assemble the equipment before helping the woman into position. Arrange within easy reach. Familiarize yourself with the vaginal speculum before the examination. Practice opening and closing the blades, locking them into position, and releasing them. Try both metal and plastic types. Note that the plastic

EQUIPMENT NEEDED

Gloves
Gooseneck lamp with a strong light
Vaginal speculum of appropriate size
(Fig. 26-3):

speculum locks and unlocks with a resounding click that can be alarming to the uninformed woman.

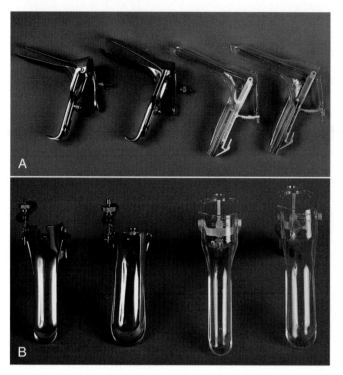

26-3

Graves speculum for most adult women, available in varying lengths and widths
Pederson speculum, narrow blades for young or postmenopausal women with narrowed introitus
Large cotton-tipped applicators (rectal swabs)
Materials for cytologic study:
Cytobrush and liquid-based cytology vial
Glass slide with frosted end, Ayre spatula, spray fixative for convention cytology
Specimen container for gonorrhea culture (GC)/chlamydia
Small bottles of normal saline, potassium hydroxide (KOH), and acetic acid (white vinegar)
Water-based lubricant
Roll of pH test tape

POSITION

Initially the woman should be sitting. An equal-status position is important to establish trust and rapport before the vaginal examination.

For the examination, place the woman in the lithotomy position with the examiner sitting on a stool. Help the woman into supine position with feet in stirrups and knees apart, and

26-4

buttocks at edge of examining table (Fig. 26-4). Ask the woman to lift her hips as you guide them to the edge of the table. Some women prefer to wear their shoes or socks. Or you can place an examination glove over each of the stirrups to warm the stirrups and keep her feet from slipping.

Place her arms at her sides or across the chest, not over the head, because this position only tightens the abdominal muscles. Be sure to push down the drape between the woman's legs and elevate her head to a 45-degree angle so you can see her face. The 45-degree table angle also helps locate internal structures.

The lithotomy position leaves many women feeling helpless and vulnerable. Indeed, many women tolerate the pelvic examination because they consider it basic for health care, yet they find it embarrassing and uncomfortable. Previous examinations may have been painful, or the previous examiner's attitude hurried and patronizing.

The examination need not be this way. You can help the woman relax, decrease her anxiety, and retain a sense of control by using these measures:

- Have her empty the bladder before the examination.
- Position the examination table so her perineum is not exposed to an inadvertent open door.
- Ask if she would like a friend, family member, or chaperone to be present. Position this person by the woman's head to maintain privacy.
- Elevate her head and shoulders to a semisitting position to maintain eye contact.
- Place the stirrups so the legs are not abducted too far.
- Explain each step in the examination before you do it.

- Assure the woman she can say "stop" at any point should she feel any discomfort.
- Use a gentle, firm touch and gradual movements.
- Communicate throughout the examination. Maintain a dialogue to share information.
- Use the techniques of the *educational* or *mirror pelvic examination* (Fig. 26-5). This has some modifications in attitude, position, and communication. First the woman is considered an active participant, one who is interested in learning and sharing decisions about her own health care. She holds a mirror between her legs, above the examiner's hands. She can see all you are doing and has a full view of her genitalia.

26-5

The mirror works well for teaching normal anatomy and its relationship to sexual behavior. Even women who are in a sexual relationship or who have had children may be surprisingly uninformed about their own anatomy. You will find that the woman's enthusiasm on seeing her own cervix is rewarding too. The mirror pelvic examination also works well when abnormalities arise because the woman can see the rationale for treatment and monitor progress at the next appointment. She is more willing to comply with treatment when she shares in the decision.

<table>
<tr><td>

Normal Range of Findings

</td><td>

Abnormal Findings

</td></tr>
<tr><td>

External Genitalia

Inspection

NOTE:
- Skin color is even; labia minora are a darker pink (Fig. 26-6).

26-6

- Hair distribution is in the usual female pattern of inverted triangle, although it normally may trail up the abdomen toward the umbilicus.

- Labia majora normally are symmetric, plump, and well formed. In the nulliparous woman labia meet in the midline; after a vaginal delivery the labia are gaping and slightly shriveled.

</td><td>

Note any pigmented nevus or lesion that the woman cannot see. Refer any suspicious lesion for biopsy.

Consider delayed puberty if no pubic hair or breast development has occurred by age 13 years.
Nits or lice at the base of pubic hair.
Swelling.

</td></tr>
</table>

Objective Data

Normal Range of Findings	Abnormal Findings

- No lesions should be present, except for occasional sebaceous cysts. These are yellowish, 1-cm nodules that are firm, nontender, and often multiple.

With your gloved hand separate the labia majora to inspect:

- Clitoris (Fig. 26-7).

Excoriation, nodules, rash, or lesions (see Table 26-2, External Genitalia Abnormalities, p. 764).

26-7

- Labia minora are dark pink and moist, usually symmetric.
- Urethral opening appears stellate or slitlike and is midline.
- Vaginal opening, or introitus, may appear as a narrow vertical slit or as a larger opening.
- Perineum is smooth. A well-healed episiotomy scar, midline or mediolateral, may be present after a vaginal birth.
- Anus has coarse skin of increased pigmentation (see Chapter 25 for assessment).

Inflammation or lesions.
Polyp.
Foul-smelling, irritating discharge.

Palpation

Assess the urethra and Skene glands (Fig. 26-8). Dip your gloved finger in a bowl of warm water to lubricate. Then insert your index finger into the vagina, and gently milk the urethra by applying pressure up and out. This procedure should produce no pain. If any discharge appears at 11 o'clock and 1 o'clock positions, culture it.

Tenderness.
Induration along urethra.
Urethral discharge.

26-8

Normal Range of Findings	Abnormal Findings

Objective Data

Assess Bartholin glands. Palpate the posterior parts of the labia majora with your index finger in the vagina and your thumb outside at 5 and 7 o'clock positions (Fig. 26-9). Normally the labia feel soft and homogeneous.

Swelling (see Table 26-2).
Induration.
Pain with palpation.
Erythema around or discharge from duct opening.

26-9

Assess the support of pelvic musculature by using these maneuvers:
1. Palpate the perineum. Normally it feels thick, smooth, and muscular in the nulliparous woman and thin and rigid in the multiparous woman.
2. Using your index and middle fingers, separate the vaginal orifice and ask the woman to strain down. Normally no bulging of vaginal walls or urinary incontinence occurs.

Tenderness.
Paper-thin perineum.

Bulging of the vaginal wall indicates cystocele, rectocele, or uterine prolapse (see Table 26-3, Pelvic Musculature Abnormalities, p. 766).
Urinary incontinence.

Internal Genitalia

Speculum Examination

Select the proper-size speculum. Warm and lubricate it under warm running water. Regarding Pap test cytology, evidence shows that applying a small amount (dime size) of water-soluble gel lubricant on the outer blades increases patient comfort and does not obscure interpretation of conventional or liquid-based cytology).[32,37] Further, women in the No Gel groups of two research studies reported significantly higher pain scores than did women in the Gel groups.

A good technique is to dedicate one hand to the patient and the other hand to picking up equipment in the room. For example, hold the speculum in your left hand (the equipment hand), with the index and middle fingers surrounding the blades and your thumb under the thumbscrew. This prevents the blades from opening painfully during insertion. With your right index and middle fingers (the patient hand), push the introitus down and open to relax the pubococcygeal muscle (Fig. 26-10). Tilt the width of the blades obliquely and insert the speculum past your right fingers, applying any pressure *downward*. This avoids pressure on the sensitive urethra above it.

Normal Range of Findings	Abnormal Findings

26-10

Ease insertion by asking the woman to bear down. This method relaxes the perineal muscles and opens the introitus. (With experience you can combine speculum insertion with assessing the support of the vaginal muscles.) As the blades pass your right fingers, withdraw your fingers. Now move the speculum to your right hand and turn the width of the blades horizontally. Continue to insert in a 45-degree angle *downward* toward the small of the woman's back (Fig. 26-11). This matches the natural slope of the vagina.

26-11

Normal Range of Findings	Abnormal Findings

After the blades are fully inserted, open them by squeezing the handles together (Fig. 26-12). The cervix should be in full view. Sometimes this does not occur (especially with beginning examiners) because the blades are angled above the location of the cervix. Try closing the blades, withdrawing about halfway, and reinserting in a more *downward* plane. Then slowly sweep upward. Once you have the cervix in full view, lock the blades open by tightening the thumbscrew.

26-12

Inspect the Cervix and Its Os

NOTE:

- **Color.** Normally the cervical mucosa is pink and even (Fig. 26-13, *A*). During the 2nd month of pregnancy it looks blue (Chadwick sign), and after menopause it is pale.

  Redness, inflammation.
  Pallor with anemia.
  Cyanotic other than with pregnancy (see Table 26-4, Cervix Abnormalities, p. 766).

- **Position.** Midline, either anterior or posterior. Projects 1 to 3 cm into the vagina.

  Lateral position may be due to adhesion or tumor. Projection of more than 3 cm may be a prolapse.

- **Size.** Diameter is 2.5 cm (1 inch).

  Hypertrophy of more than 4 cm occurs with inflammation or tumor.

- **Os.** This is small and round in the nulliparous woman. In the parous woman it is a horizontal, irregular slit and also may show healed lacerations on the sides (see Fig. 26-13, *A* and *B*).

- **Surface.** This is normally smooth, but **cervical eversion,** or ectropion, may occur normally after vaginal deliveries (Fig. 26-13, *B*). The endocervical canal is everted or "rolled out." It looks like a red, beefy halo inside the pink cervix surrounding the os. It is difficult to distinguish this normal variation from an abnormal condition (e.g., erosion or carcinoma), and biopsy may be needed.

  Surface reddened, granular, and asymmetric, particularly around os.
  Friable, bleeds easily.
  Any lesions: white patch on cervix; strawberry spot.

Normal Range of Findings

Abnormal Findings

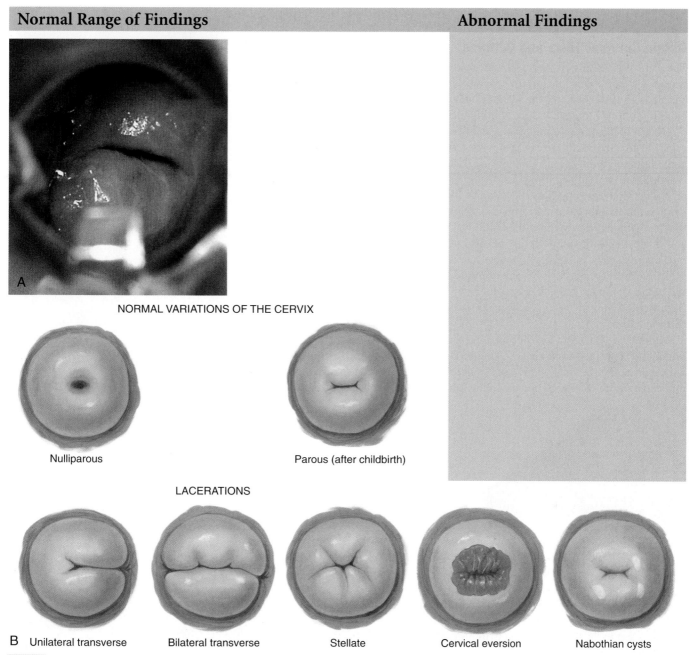

NORMAL VARIATIONS OF THE CERVIX

Nulliparous

Parous (after childbirth)

LACERATIONS

B   Unilateral transverse   Bilateral transverse   Stellate   Cervical eversion   Nabothian cysts

26-13

Nabothian cysts are benign growths that commonly appear on the cervix after childbirth. They are small, smooth, yellow nodules that may be single or multiple. Less than 1 cm, they are retention cysts caused by obstruction of cervical glands.

- **Note the cervical secretions.** Depending on the day of the menstrual cycle, secretions may be clear and thin, or thick, opaque, and stringy. Always they are odorless and nonirritating.

If secretions are copious, swab the area with a thick-tipped rectal swab. This method sponges away secretions, and you have a better view of the structures.

Refer any suspicious red, white, or pigmented lesion for biopsy (see Erosion and Cervical Cancer sections in Table 26-4).

Cervical polyp—Bright red growth protruding from the os (see Table 26-4).

Foul-smelling, irritating, with yellow, green, white, or gray discharge (see Table 26-5, Vulvovaginal Inflammations, p. 768).

Normal Range of Findings	Abnormal Findings

Obtain Cervical Tests and Cultures

The Pap test screens for cervical cancer and not for endometrial or ovarian cancer. Do not obtain during the woman's menses or if a heavy infectious discharge is present. Instruct the woman not to douche, have intercourse, or put anything into the vagina within 24 hours before collecting the specimens.

Obtain the Pap test before other specimens so you will not disrupt or remove cells. Most U.S. clinics have changed from conventional cytology collection using glass slides to liquid-based cytology vials. Using liquid-based cytology, the cervical specimens are dipped into a vial with preservative rather than being smeared on a slide. Conventional glass slides can be "unsatisfactory" because of obscuring by blood, inflammation, or clumped distribution of cells. Thus evidence shows that just stirring the cells into the liquid vial results in fewer unsatisfactory tests and is more sensitive in detecting cervical neoplasia.[6] Using liquid-based cytology, microscopic evaluation is made clearer by the uniform spread of epithelial cells in a thin layer. After cytology examination, pathologists can further study the liquid remnant, such as testing for high-risk HPV types. Whichever collection method you are using, collect the cellular specimens from the following three locations.

Vaginal Pool. Gently rub the blunt end of an Ayre spatula over the vaginal wall under and lateral to the cervix (Fig. 26-14). Dip the specimen into a liquid vial or wipe it on a glass slide. If the mucosa is very dry (as in a postmenopausal woman), moisten a sterile swab with normal saline solution to collect this specimen.

26-14

Cervical Scrape (Fig. 26-15). Use a cytobrush or insert the bifid end of the Ayre spatula into the vagina with the more pointed bump into the cervical os. Rotate it 360 to 720 degrees, using firm pressure. The rounded cervix fits snugly into the spatula's groove. The spatula scrapes the surface of the squamocolumnar junction (SCJ) and cervix as you turn the instrument. Dip into a liquid vial or spread the specimen from both sides of the spatula onto a glass slide. Use a single stroke to thin out the specimen, not a back-and-forth motion. This specimen is important for the adolescent whose endocervical cells have not yet migrated into the endocervical canal.

26-15

Objective Data

Normal Range of Findings	Abnormal Findings

Endocervical Specimen (Fig. 26-16). Insert a cytobrush (instead of a cotton applicator) into the os. A cytobrush gives a higher yield of endocervical cells at the SCJ and is safe for use during pregnancy. The woman may feel a slight pinch with the brush, and scant bleeding may occur. For this reason collect the endocervical specimen last so bleeding will not obscure cytologic evaluation.

SCJ

T zone

26-16

Rotate the brush 720 degrees in ONE direction in the endocervical canal, either clockwise or counterclockwise. Then stir the cytobrush gently into the liquid vial. Or rotate it gently on a slide to deposit all the cells. Rotate in the opposite direction from the one in which you obtained the specimen. Avoid leaving a thick specimen that would be hard to read under the microscope. Immediately (within 2 seconds) spray the slide with fixative to avoid drying.

For the woman after hysterectomy whose cervix has been removed, collect a scrape from the end of the vagina and a vaginal pool.

Label the frosted ends of the slides or the vial with the woman's name. Send specimens to the laboratory with the following necessary data:

- Date of specimen
- Woman's date of birth
- Date of last menstrual period
- Any hormone medication
- If pregnant, estimated date of delivery

- Known infections
- Prior surgery or radiation
- Prior abnormal cytology
- Abnormal findings on physical examination

These data are important for accurate interpretation (e.g., a specimen may be interpreted as positive unless the laboratory technicians know that the woman has had prior radiation treatment).

To screen for STIs and if you note any abnormal vaginal discharge, obtain the GC/chlamydia culture. Insert a sterile cotton applicator into the os, rotate it 360 degrees, and leave it in place 10 to 20 seconds for complete saturation. Insert into labeled container.

Occasionally you will need the following samples:

Saline Mount, or "Wet Prep." Spread a sample of the discharge onto a glass slide and add one drop of normal saline solution and a coverslip.

KOH Prep. To a sample of the discharge on a glass slide, add one drop of potassium hydroxide and a coverslip.

Anal Culture. Insert a sterile cotton swab into the anal canal about 1 cm. Rotate it and move it side to side. Leave in place 10 to 20 seconds. If the swab collects feces, discard it and begin again. Insert into specimen container.

Objective Data

Objective Data

Normal Range of Findings	Abnormal Findings

Acetic Acid Wash. Acetic acid (white vinegar) screens for asymptomatic HPV, which causes genital warts and cervical cancer. After all other specimens are gathered, soak a thick-tipped cotton rectal swab with acetic acid and "paint" the cervix. Acetic acid dissolves mucus and temporarily causes intracellular dehydration and coagulation of protein. A normal response (indicating no HPV infection) is no change in the cervical epithelium.

Rapid acetowhitening or blanching, especially with irregular borders, suggests HPV infection (see Table 26-2).

Inspect the Vaginal Wall

Loosen the thumbscrew but continue to hold the speculum blades open. Slowly withdraw the speculum, rotating it as you go, to fully inspect the vaginal wall. Normally the wall looks pink, deeply rugated, moist and smooth, and free of inflammation or lesions. Normal discharge is thin and clear or opaque and stringy but always odorless.

Inflammation or lesions.
Leukoplakia appears as spot of dried white paint.
Vaginal discharge: thick, white, and curdlike with candidiasis; profuse, watery, gray-green, and frothy with trichomoniasis; or any gray, green-yellow, white, or foul-smelling discharge (see Table 26-5).

When the blade ends are near the vaginal opening, let them close, but be careful not to pinch the mucosa or catch any hairs. Turn the blades obliquely to avoid stretching the opening. Place the metal speculum in a basin to be cleaned later and soaked in a sterilizing and disinfecting solution; discard the plastic variety. Discard your gloves and wash hands.

Bimanual Examination

Rise to a stand and have the woman remain in lithotomy position. Drop lubricant onto the first two fingers of your gloved intravaginal hand (Fig. 26-17).

Assume the "obstetric" position with the first two fingers extended, the last two flexed onto the palm, and the thumb abducted. Insert your fingers into the vagina, with any pressure directed posteriorly. Wait until the vaginal walls relax and then insert your fingers fully.

26-17

You will use both hands to palpate the internal genitalia to assess their location, size, and mobility and to screen for any tenderness or mass. One hand is on the abdomen while the other hand (often the dominant, more sensitive hand) inserts two fingers into the vagina (Fig. 26-18). It does not matter which you choose as the intravaginal hand; try each way and settle on the most comfortable method for you.

Normal Range of Findings	**Abnormal Findings**

26-18 Bimanual examination.

Palpate the vaginal wall. Normally it feels smooth and has no area of induration or tenderness.

Cervix. Locate the cervix in the midline, often near the anterior vaginal wall. The cervix points in the opposite direction of the fundus of the uterus. Palpate with the palmar surface of the fingers. Note these characteristics of a normal cervix:

- **Consistency**—Feels smooth and firm, as the consistency of the tip of the nose. It softens and feels velvety at 5 to 6 weeks of pregnancy (Goodell sign).
- **Contour**—Evenly rounded.
- **Mobility**—With a finger on either side, move the cervix gently from side to side. Normally this produces no pain (Fig. 26-19).

Palpate all around the fornices; the wall should feel smooth.

Nodule.
Tenderness.

Hard with malignancy.
Nodular.
Irregular.
Immobile with malignancy.
Painful with inflammation, pelvic inflammatory disease (PID), ectopic pregnancy.

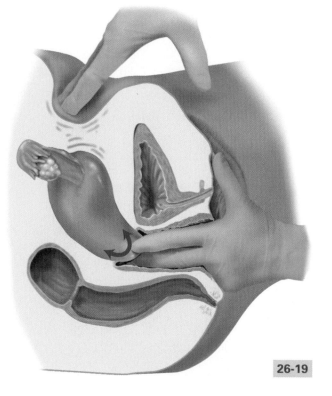

26-19

Objective Data

Normal Range of Findings

Next use your abdominal hand to push the pelvic organs closer for your intravaginal fingers to palpate. Place your hand midway between the umbilicus and the symphysis; push down in a slow, firm manner, fingers together and slightly flexed. Brace the elbow of your pelvic arm against your hip and keep it horizontal. The woman must be relaxed.

Uterus. With your intravaginal fingers in the anterior fornix, assess the uterus. Determine the position, or *version*, of the uterus (Fig. 26-20). This compares the long axis of the uterus with the long axis of the body. In many women the uterus is anteverted; you palpate it at the level of the pubis with the cervix pointing posteriorly. Two other positions occur normally (midposition and retroverted); two aspects of flexion also occur, in which the long axis of the uterus is not straight but is flexed.

Anteverted

Midposition

Anteflexed

Retroflexed

Retroverted

26-20

Abnormal Findings

Normal Range of Findings

Palpate the uterine wall with your fingers in the fornices. Normally it feels firm and smooth, with the contour of the fundus rounded. It softens during pregnancy. Bounce the uterus gently between your abdominal and intravaginal hand. It should be freely movable and nontender.

Adnexa. Move both hands to the right to explore the adnexa. Place your abdominal hand on the lower quadrant just inside the anterior iliac spine and your intravaginal fingers in the lateral fornix (Fig. 26-21). Push the abdominal hand in and try to capture the ovary. Often you cannot feel it. When you can, it normally feels smooth, firm, and almond-shaped and is highly movable, sliding through the fingers. It is slightly sensitive but not painful. The fallopian tube is not palpable normally. No other mass or pulsation should be felt.

26-21

A note of caution—normal adnexal structures often are not palpable. Be careful not to mistake an abnormality for a normal structure. To be safe, consider abnormal any mass that you cannot *positively* identify and refer the woman for further study.

Move to the left to palpate the other side. Then, withdraw your hand and check secretions on the fingers before discarding the glove. Normal secretions are clear or cloudy and odorless.

Abnormal Findings

If the retroverted uterus is fixed and immobile, there may be endometriosis or PID adhering it.

Enlarged uterus (see Table 26-6, Uterine Enlargement, p. 769).

Lateral displacement.

Nodular mass. Irregular, asymmetric uterus.

Fixed and immobile.

Tenderness.

Enlarged adnexa. Nodules or mass in adnexa.

Immobile.

Markedly tender (see Table 26-7, Adnexal Enlargement, p. 771).

Pulsation or palpable fallopian tube suggests ectopic pregnancy; this warrants immediate referral.

Objective Data

Normal Range of Findings	Abnormal Findings

Rectovaginal Examination

Use this technique to assess the rectovaginal septum, posterior uterine wall, cul-de-sac, and rectum. Change gloves to avoid spreading any possible infection. Lubricate the first two fingers. Instruct the woman that this may feel uncomfortable and will mimic the feeling of moving her bowels. Ask her to bear down as you insert your index finger into the vagina and your middle finger gently into the rectum (Fig. 26-22).

Uterus retroflexed

RECTOVAGINAL PALPATION

26-22

While pushing with the abdominal hand, repeat the steps of the bimanual examination. Try to keep the intravaginal finger on the cervix so the intrarectal finger does not mistake the cervix for a mass. Note:

- Rectovaginal septum should feel smooth, thin, firm, and pliable.
- Rectovaginal pouch, or cul-de-sac, is a potential space and usually not palpated.
- Uterine wall and fundus feel firm and smooth.

Rotate the intrarectal finger to check the rectal wall and anal sphincter tone. (See Chapter 25 for assessment of anus and rectum.) Check your gloved finger as you withdraw; test any adherent stool for occult blood.

Use tissues to wipe the area and help her up. Remind her to slide her hips back from the edge before sitting up so she will not fall.

Nodular or thickened.

Normal Range of Findings	Abnormal Findings

✦ DEVELOPMENTAL COMPETENCE

Infants and Children

Preparation

- **Infant**—Place on examination table.
- **Toddler/preschooler**—Place on parent's lap.
  - Frog-leg position—Hips flexed, soles of feet together and up to bottom.
  - Preschool child may want to separate her own labia.
  - No drapes—The young girl wants to see what you are doing.
- **School-age child**—Place on examination table, frog-leg position, no drapes.

During childhood a routine screening is limited to inspection of the external genitalia to determine that (1) the structures are intact, (2) the vagina is present, and (3) the hymen is patent (open).

The newborn's genitalia are somewhat engorged. The labia majora are swollen, the labia minora are prominent and protrude beyond the labia majora, the clitoris looks relatively large, and the hymen appears thick. Because of transient engorgement, the vaginal opening is more difficult to see now than it will be later. Place your thumbs on the labia majora. Push laterally while pushing the perineum down and try to note the vaginal opening above the hymenal ring. Do not palpate the clitoris because it is very sensitive.

A sanguineous vaginal discharge or leukorrhea (mucoid discharge) is normal during the first few weeks because of the maternal estrogen effect. (This also may cause transient breast engorgement and secretion.) During the early weeks the genital engorgement resolves, and the labia minora atrophy and remain small until puberty (Fig. 26-23).

Ambiguous genitalia are rare but are suggested by a markedly enlarged clitoris, fusion of the labia (resembling scrotum), and palpable mass in fused labia (resembling testes) (see Table 26-8, Pediatric Genitalia Abnormalities, p. 773).

Imperforate hymen warrants referral.

Lesions, rash.

26-23

Between the ages of 2 months and 7 years, the labia majora are flat, the labia minora are thin, the clitoris is relatively small, and the hymen is tissue-paper thin. Normally no irritation or foul-smelling discharge is present.

In the young school-age girl (7 to 10 years), the mons pubis thickens, the labia majora thicken, and the labia minora become slightly rounded. Pubic hair

Poor perineal hygiene.

Pest inhabitants. Excoriations.

During and after toddler age, foul-smelling discharge occurs with lodging of foreign body, pinworms, or infection.

Absence of pubic hair by 13 years indicates delayed puberty.

Objective Data

Normal Range of Findings	Abnormal Findings

appears beginning around age 11 years, although sparse pubic hair may occur as early as age 8 years. Normally the hymen is perforate.

> Amenorrhea in adolescent, together with bluish and bulging hymen, indicates imperforate hymen and warrants referral.

Almost always in these age-groups an external examination will suffice. If needed, an internal pelvic examination is best performed by a pediatric gynecologist using specialized instruments.

The Adolescent

The adolescent girl has special needs during the genitalia examination. Examine her alone, without the mother present. Assure her of privacy and confidentiality. Allow plenty of time for health education and discussion of pubertal progress. Assess her growth velocity and menstrual history, and use the SMR charts to teach breast and pubic hair development. Assure her that increased vaginal fluid (physiologic *leukorrhea*) is normal because of the estrogen effect.

Perform a pelvic examination when the history suggests abnormal vaginal discharge, missed periods and a positive pregnancy test, or at 21 years of age. Start Pap tests at age 21 years. Although the techniques of the examination are listed in the adult section, you will need to provide additional time and psychological support for the adolescent having her first pelvic examination.

> Because the STI rates are higher among adolescents than other age-groups, screen for STIs (1) with history of multiple sexual partners; (2) with previous STI treatment; (3) chlamydia and gonorrhea screening annually for sexually active adolescents; and (4) syphilis screening for teens who trade sex for drugs or money, use IV drugs, or live in a high-prevalence neighborhood.[16]

The experience of the first pelvic examination determines how the adolescent will approach future care. Your accepting attitude and gentle, unhurried approach are important. You have a unique teaching opportunity here. Take the time to teach, using the girl's own body as illustration. Your frank discussion of anatomy and sexual behavior communicates that these topics are acceptable to discuss and not taboo with health care providers. This affirms the girl's self-concept.

During the bimanual examination note that the adnexa are not palpable in the adolescent.

> Pelvic or adnexal mass.

The Pregnant Woman

Depending on the week of gestation of the pregnancy, inspection shows the enlarging abdomen (see Fig. 30-2 on p. 808). The height of the fundus ascends gradually as the fetus grows.

The external genitalia show hyperemia of the perineum and vulva because of increased vascularity. Internally the walls of the vagina appear violet or blue (Chadwick sign) because of hyperemia. The vaginal walls are deeply rugated, and the vaginal mucosa thickens. The cervix looks blue, feels velvety, and feels softer than in the nonpregnant state, making it a bit more difficult to differentiate from the vaginal walls.

During bimanual examination the isthmus of the uterus feels softer and is more easily compressed between your two hands (Hegar sign). The fundus balloons between your two hands; it feels connected to, but distinct from, the cervix because the isthmus is so soft.

Search the adnexal area carefully during early pregnancy. Normally the adnexal structures are not palpable.

> An ectopic pregnancy has serious consequences (see Table 26-7).

The Aging Adult

Natural lubrication is decreased; to avoid a painful examination, take care to lubricate instruments and the examining hand adequately. Use the Pedersen

Normal Range of Findings	**Abnormal Findings**

speculum (rather than the Graves) because its narrower, flatter blades are more comfortable in women with vaginal stenosis or dryness.

Menopause and the resulting decrease in estrogen production cause numerous physical changes. Pubic hair gradually decreases, becoming thin and sparse in later years. The skin is thinner, and fat deposits decrease, leaving the mons pubis smaller and the labia flatter with a hanging appearance. Clitoris size also decreases after age 60 years.

Internally the rugae of the vaginal walls decrease, and the walls look pale pink because of the thinned epithelium. The cervix shrinks and looks pale and glistening. It may retract, appearing to be flush with the vaginal wall. In some it is hard to distinguish the cervix from the surrounding vaginal mucosa. Or the cervix may protrude into the vagina if the uterus has prolapsed.

With the bimanual examination you may need to insert only one gloved finger if vaginal stenosis exists. The uterus feels smaller and firmer, and the ovaries are not palpable normally.

Be aware that older women may have special needs and will appreciate the following plans of care: for those with arthritis, taking a mild analgesic or anti-inflammatory before the appointment may ease joint pain in positioning; schedule appointment times when joint pain or stiffness is at its least; allow extra time for positioning and "unpositioning" after the examination; and be careful to maintain dignity and privacy.

Women ages 65+ years should stop cervical cancer screening if they have ≥3 consecutive negative Pap tests or ≥2 consecutive negative HPV and Pap tests within the last 10 years.[4] Also, women with a total hysterectomy should stop cervical cancer screening.[4]

Abnormal Findings:

Refer any suspicious red, white, or pigmented lesion for biopsy.

Vaginal atrophy increases the risk for infection and trauma.

Refer any mass for prompt evaluation.

PROMOTING A HEALTHY LIFESTYLE

HPV Vaccine

In June 2006 the Advisory Committee on Immunization Practices (ACIP) voted to recommend the first vaccine developed to prevent cervical cancer. This represents one of the most important advances in women's health. But it is also important for men and boys. The vaccine targets human papilloma virus (HPV), which is not only the most common STI but is also the virus associated with most cases (96% to 99%) of cervical cancer, 90% to 93% of anal cancers, and 36% to 40% of penile cancers (Thomas & Snell, 2013). HPV is spread by skin-to-skin contact, and those who become infected with it often do not know they have it because the virus usually does not cause any symptoms.

The CDC recommends the HPV vaccination for girls AND boys at age 11 or 12 years. The HPV vaccine series includes 3 separate injections over a 6-month period. The second dose is given 1 to 2 months after the first dose, and the third dose is given 6 months after the first dose. Two vaccines, Cervarix (HPV types 16, 18) and Gardasil (HPV types 6, 11, 16, 18), protect against cervical cancers in women. Gardasil also protects against genital warts and other cancers such as anal cancer. Both vaccines are available for females; however, only Gardasil is available for males. According to Thomas & Snell (2013), the benefit of the HPV vaccine in boys has been overlooked in the initial marketing efforts. They cite that vaccinating boys and men can help to prevent more than 5 million cases of genital warts and 40,000 cancer-related deaths over the next century (p. 165).

HPV vaccines offer the best protection to girls AND boys who receive all 3 vaccine doses and have time to develop an immune response before being sexually active with another person. The vaccine can be administered at the same visit as other age-appropriate vaccines such as the Tdap, Td, and hepatitis B vaccines. To increase vaccination rates, Thomas and Snell (2013) recommend using family-centered strategies to increase parents' and teens' knowledge of HPV vaccines and to address any misconceptions and misinformation.

References

Thomas, T.L., & Snell, S. (2013). Vaccinate boys with the HPV vaccine? Really? J Spec Pediatr Nurs, 18, 165-169.

CDC has multiple resources for clinicians, including HPV vaccines, http://www.cdc.gov/hpv/vaccine.html, and

HPV vaccine information for clinicians—fact sheet, http://www.cdc.gov/std/hpv/STDFact-HPV-vaccine-hcp.htm, and for the public, http://www.cdc.gov/std/HPV/STDFact-HPV.htm.

SUBJECTIVE

Menarche age 12 years, cycle usually q 28 days, duration 5 days, flow moderate, no dysmenorrhea, LMP April 3. Grav 0/Para 0/Ab 0. Gyne checkup and last Pap test 1 year PTA, negative.

No urinary problems, no irritating or foul-smelling vaginal discharge, no sores or lesions, no history pelvic surgery. Satisfied with sexual relationship with husband, uses vaginal diaphragm for birth control, no plans for pregnancy at this time. Not aware of any STI contact to herself or husband.

OBJECTIVE

External genitalia: No swelling, lesions, or discharge. No urethral swelling or discharge.
Internal: Vaginal walls have no bulging or lesions; cervix pink with no lesions. Scant clear mucoid discharge.
Bimanual: No pain on moving cervix; uterus anteflexed and anteverted, no enlargement or irregularity.
Adnexa: Ovaries not enlarged.
Rectal: No hemorrhoids, fissures, or lesions; no masses or tenderness; stool brown with guaiac test negative.

ASSESSMENT

Genital structures intact and appear healthy

Clinical Case Study 1

J.K., 27-year-old Caucasian married woman with type 1 diabetes, Grav 0/Para 0/Ab 0. Presents at clinic with "urinary burning, vaginal itching, and curdy discharge × 4 days."

SUBJECTIVE

4 to 5 days PTA—Noted burning on urination; intense vaginal itching; thick, white, "smelly" discharge. Warm water douche—no relief. Intercourse is painful.

No previous history of vaginal infection, urinary tract infection, or pelvic surgery. Type 1 diabetes since age 12, well managed with insulin and diet, HbA1c is <6.5%. Monogamous sexual relationship, has used low-estrogen birth control pills for 3 years with no side effects.

OBJECTIVE

Vulva and vagina erythematous and edematous. Thick, white, curdlike discharge clinging to vaginal walls. Cervix pink, no lesions.
Bimanual examination: No pain on palpating cervix, uterus not enlarged, ovaries not enlarged.
Specimens: Pap test, GC/chlamydia to lab. Vaginal pH <4.5. KOH prep shows mycelia and spores of *Candida albicans.*

ASSESSMENT

Candida albicans vaginitis
Pain R/T infectious process

Clinical Case Study 2

B.L., 17-year-old Caucasian female high school student, comes to clinic for oral contraceptives.

SUBJECTIVE

Menarche 12 years, cycle q 30 days, duration 6 days, mild cramps relieved by naproxen. LMP March 10. No dysuria, vaginal discharge, vaginal itching. Relationship involving intercourse with one boyfriend for 8 months PTA. Thinks he has other sexual contacts. For birth control boyfriend uses condoms "sometimes." Wants to start birth control pills. Never had pelvic examination. Never had teaching about breast self-examination or STIs except AIDS. Smokes cigarettes, ½ PPD; started age 11 years. Has not had HPV vaccines.

OBJECTIVE

Breasts: Symmetric, no lesions or discharge. Palpation reveals no mass or tenderness.
External genitalia: No redness, lesions, or discharge.
Internal genitalia: Vaginal walls and cervix pink with no lesions or discharge. GC/chlamydia specimens obtained.
Bimanual: No tenderness to palpation. Uterus anteverted with no enlargement; ovaries not enlarged.
Specimens: GC/chlamydia, to lab.

ASSESSMENT

Breast and pelvic structures appear healthy
Deficient knowledge regarding breast self-examination, birth control measures, STI prevention, cigarette smoking R/T lack of exposure

Clinical Case Study 3

K.B. is a 65-year-old African-American female, retired elementary school teacher. Takes multivitamins daily. No prescription medications. No significant past medical history.

SUBJECTIVE

Menarche age 14 years, cycle q30 days. Menopause at age 60. Gyne checkups yearly. Last Pap test negative. Grav 2/ Para 2/ Ab 0. No urinary problems. No history of STIs. Monogamous relationship for 45 years. Husband recently cleared for sexual activity post myocardial infarction. After resumption of sexual activity, K.B. noticed bloody vaginal discharge. Dyspareunia. Vaginal itching. Not aware of any STI contact in self or husband.

OBJECTIVE

External genitalia: Thin, gray pubic hair. Labia appear flat and hanging. No lesions, swelling, or discharge.
Internal: Vaginal walls pale pink. Cervix pale pink, retracted, flush with vaginal wall. Abraded areas on posterior vaginal wall. Bloody, mucoid discharge. Tenderness reported during exam.
Bimanual: No pain with cervical movement. Unable to palpate ovaries. Uterus small, firm.
Rectal: No hemorrhoids, fissures, or tenderness. Stool brown, guaiac test negative.

ASSESSMENT

Atrophic vaginitis
Sexual dysfunction R/T pain during intercourse
Risk for infection R/T chronic estrogen deficiency

Clinical Case Study 4

C.P. is a 9-year-old Latina female who is being seen at the clinic today for vulva pain.

SUBJECTIVE

1 day PTA—States, "My foot slipped off the pedal while I was riding my brother's bike, and I fell." Reports pain localized to vulva. Denies menarche and/or urinary problems.

OBJECTIVE

External genitalia: Swelling and ecchymosis noted to labia majora; no lacerations, no rash, no lesions, and no vaginal discharge; no urethral swelling or discharge; internal and bimanual exam deferred at this time.

ASSESSMENT

Genital structures intact
Acute pain R/T physical trauma (of falling off bike)

ABNORMAL FINDINGS
FOR ADVANCED PRACTICE

TABLE 26-2 **External Genitalia Abnormalities**

Pediculosis Pubis (Crab Lice)

S: Severe perineal itching.

O: Excoriations and erythematous areas. May see little dark spots (lice are small), nits (eggs) adherent to pubic hair near roots. Usually localized in pubic hair, occasionally in eyebrows or eyelashes.

Herpes Simplex Virus—Type 2 (Herpes Genitalis)

S: Episodes of local pain, dysuria, fever.

O: This STI often presents as clusters of small, shallow vesicles with surrounding erythema; erupts on genital areas and inner thigh. Also inguinal adenopathy, edema. Vesicles on labia rupture in 1 to 3 days, leaving painful ulcers. Initial infection lasts 7 to 10 days. Virus remains dormant indefinitely; recurrent infections last 3 to 10 days with milder symptoms.

Syphilitic Chancre

O: This STI begins as a small, solitary silvery papule that erodes to a red, round or oval, superficial ulcer with a yellowish serous discharge. Palpation—Nontender indurated base; can be lifted like a button between thumb and finger. Nontender inguinal lymphadenopathy. May go unnoticed; resolves spontaneously. But secondary syphilis follows: fever, lymphadenopathy, mucocutaneous red rash, sore throat.

Red Rash—Contact Dermatitis

S: History of skin contact with allergenic substance in environment, intense pruritus.

O: Primary lesion—Red, swollen vesicles. Then may have weeping of lesions, crusts, scales, thickening of skin, excoriations from scratching. May result from reaction to feminine hygiene spray or synthetic underclothing.

TABLE 26-2   External Genitalia Abnormalities—cont'd

Human Papillomavirus Genital Warts

S: Painless warty growths; may be unnoticed by woman.

O: Pink or flesh-colored, soft, pointed, moist, warty papules. Single or multiple in a cauliflower-like patch. Occur around vulva, introitus, anus, vagina, cervix. (NOTE: Advanced case shown here.) HPV infection is the most common STI, especially in adolescents. Risk factors: early age at menarche and multiple sexual partners. Genital warts are less common than cervical lesions but must be treated with topical medication or surgical removal. Abstain from sex while warts are present.

Abscess of Bartholin Gland

S: Local pain; can be severe.

O: Overlying skin red, shiny, and hot. Posterior part of labia swollen; palpable fluctuant mass and tenderness. (Compare with wrinkled skin on the other, normal side.) Mucosa shows red spot at site of duct opening. Requires incision and drainage, antibiotic therapy.

Urethritis

Urethritis

S: Inflammation of urethra presents as dysuria, burning sensation.

O: Palpation of anterior vaginal wall shows erythema, tenderness, induration along urethra, purulent discharge from meatus. Caused by *Neisseria gonorrhoeae*, chlamydia, or staphylococcus infection.

Urethral Caruncle

S: Tender, pain with urination, urinary frequency, hematuria, dyspareunia, or asymptomatic.

O: Small, deep red, benign mass protruding from meatus; usually secondary to urethritis or skenitis; lesion may bleed on contact. More common in postmenopausal women.

S, Subjective data; *O,* objective data.
See Illustration Credits for source information.

TABLE 26-3   Pelvic Musculature Abnormalities

Cystocele

S: Feeling of pressure in vagina, stress incontinence.

O: With straining, note introitus widening and the presence of a soft, round *anterior* bulge. The bladder, covered by vaginal mucosa, prolapses into the vagina.

Rectocele

S: Feeling of pressure in vagina, possibly constipation.

O: With straining, note introitus widening and the presence of a soft, round bulge from *posterior*. Here, part of the rectum, covered by vaginal mucosa, prolapses into the vagina.

Uterine Prolapse

O: With straining or standing, uterus protrudes into vagina. Nontender, nonfluctuant, smooth hemisphere; may cause a broad-based gait. Prolapse is graded: 1st degree, cervix appears at introitus with straining; 2nd degree, cervix bulges outside introitus with straining; 3rd degree (in this case), whole uterus protrudes even without straining—essentially uterus is inside out.

S, Subjective data; *O,* objective data.
See Illustration Credits for source information.

TABLE 26-4   Cervix Abnormalities

Bluish Cervix—Cyanosis

O: Bluish discoloration of the mucosa occurs normally in pregnancy (Chadwick sign at 6 to 8 weeks' gestation) and with any other condition causing hypoxia or venous congestion (e.g., heart failure, pelvic tumor).

Erosion

O: Cervical lips inflamed and eroded. Reddened granular surface is superficial inflammation, with no ulceration (loss of tissue). Usually secondary to purulent or mucopurulent cervical discharge. Biopsy needed to distinguish erosion from carcinoma; cannot rely on inspection.

TABLE 26-4 Cervix Abnormalities—cont'd

Human Papillomavirus (HPV, Condylomata)

O: Virus can appear in various forms when affecting cervical epithelium. Here warty growth appears as abnormal thickened white epithelium. Visibility of lesion is enhanced by acetic acid (vinegar) wash, which dissolves mucus and temporarily causes intracellular dehydration and coagulation of protein. Must be treated or may progress to cervical cancer (see Cervical Cancer).

Polyp

S: May have mucoid discharge or bleeding.

O: Bright red, soft, pedunculated growth emerges from os. It is benign, but this must be determined by biopsy. May be lined with squamous or columnar epithelium.

Diethylstilbestrol (DES) Syndrome

S: Prenatal exposure to DES causes rare tumor and cervical and vaginal abnormalities not apparent until adolescence. DES was given to some pregnant women from 1940 to 1970.

O: Red, granular patches of columnar epithelium extend beyond normal squamocolumnar junction onto cervix and into fornices (vaginal adenosis). Cervical abnormalities: circular groove, transverse ridge, protuberant anterior lip, "cockscomb" formation. Structural abnormalities cause infertility, ectopic pregnancy, spontaneous abortion, and preterm labor.

Cervical Cancer

S: Bleeding between menstrual periods, after sex, after menopause; unusual vaginal discharge.

O: Chronic ulcer and induration are early signs of carcinoma, although the lesion may or may not show on the exocervix. (Here lesion is around the external os.)

Diagnosed by Pap test and biopsy. Almost always caused by persistent HPV infection. Risk factors are early age at first intercourse, multiple sex partners, cigarette smoking, undetected HPV. Prevention lies in HPV vaccines and early detection.

S, Subjective data; *O,* objective data.
See Illustration Credits for source information.

TABLE 26-5 Vulvovaginal Inflammations

Atrophic Vaginitis

S: Postmenopausal vaginal itching, dryness, burning sensation, dyspareunia, mucoid discharge (may be flecked with blood), postcoital bleeding. Symptoms occur gradually due to thinning of epithelial layers.

O: Pale, dry mucosa with abraded areas that bleed easily, decreased rugae; may have bloody discharge. Decrease in usual shiny vaginal secretions. Vagina may be shortened and narrowed; cervix may be less protuberant.[25] Estrogen normally keeps tissues thick, moist, rugated, and glycogen rich; so loss of estrogen creates signs and increases risk for trauma and infection.

Candidiasis (Moniliasis)

S: Intense pruritus; thick, whitish, clumpy discharge.

O: Vulva and vagina are erythematous and edematous. Discharge is usually thick, white, curdy, "like cottage cheese," not malodorous. Microscopic examination of discharge on KOH wet mount shows branched hyphae.

Causes: Recent use of antibiotics, some oral contraceptives, uncontrolled or undiagnosed diabetes, douching that disrupts normal flora balance, wearing tight or nylon underwear, pregnancy with increased glycogen, more alkaline vaginal pH as in menses, postpartum, or menopause.

Trichomoniasis

S: Pruritus, watery and often malodorous vaginal discharge, urinary frequency, terminal dysuria, itching. Symptoms are worse during menstruation when the pH is optimal for organism's growth.

O: Vulva may be erythematous. Vagina diffusely red; granular; occasionally with red, raised papules and petechiae ("strawberry" appearance). Frothy, yellow-green, foul-smelling discharge. Vaginal pH >4.5. Microscopic examination of saline wet mount specimen shows characteristic flagellated cells.

Bacterial Vaginosis (*Gardnerella vaginalis, Haemophilus vaginalis,* or Nonspecific Vaginitis)

S: Profuse discharge, "constant wetness" with "foul, fishy, rotten" odor.

O: Thin, creamy, gray-white, malodorous discharge. No inflammation on vaginal wall or cervix because this is a surface parasite. Vaginal pH >4.5. Microscopic view of saline wet mount specimen shows typical "clue cells" (epithelial cells with stippled borders). Sniff for fishy odor after adding KOH to slide ("whiff test"). These signs are termed *Amsel criteria.*

TABLE 26-5   Vulvovaginal Inflammations—cont'd

Chlamydia

S: Minimal or no symptoms. May have urinary frequency, dysuria, vaginal discharge, postcoital bleeding.

O: May have yellow or green mucopurulent discharge, friable cervix, cervical motion tenderness. Signs are subtle, easily mistaken for gonorrhea. If untreated or mistreated, chlamydia can ascend to cause PID and result in infertility. A common STI; the highest prevalence is among sexually active adolescents. Urine chlamydia testing using nucleic acid amplification tests (NAAT) is a noninvasive method to screen. Use a single urine specimen to detect both pregnancy and chlamydia.

Gonorrhea

S: Variable: Vaginal discharge, dysuria, abnormal uterine bleeding, abscess in Bartholin or Skene glands; 95% of cases are asymptomatic.

O: Often no signs are apparent. May have purulent vaginal discharge. Diagnose by positive culture of organism. If the condition is untreated, it may progress to acute salpingitis, PID. Treat with antibiotics and retest in 3 to 6 months.

S, Subjective data; *O,* objective data.
See Illustration Credits for source information.

TABLE 26-6   Uterine Enlargement

◄ Pregnancy

Obviously a normal condition, pregnancy is included here for comparison.

S: Amenorrhea, fatigue, breast engorgement, nausea, change in food tolerance, weight gain.

O: Early signs—Cyanosis of vaginal mucosa and cervix (Chadwick sign). Palpation—Soft consistency of cervix, enlarging uterus with compressible fundus and isthmus (Hegar sign at 10 to 12 weeks).

Continued

TABLE 26-6 Uterine Enlargement—cont'd

◀ Myomas (Leiomyomas, Uterine Fibroids)

S: Varies, depending on size and location. Often no symptoms. Symptoms that occur include vague discomfort, bloating, heaviness, pelvic pressure, dyspareunia, urinary frequency, backache, or excessive uterine bleeding and anemia if myoma disturbs endometrium.

O: Uterus irregularly enlarged; firm; mobile; and nodular with hard, painless nodules in the uterine wall. Heavy bleeding produces anemia.

These benign tumors are common; by age 50 years 70% of White women and >80% of Black women will have at least one.[7] Myomas are estrogen dependent; after menopause the lesions regress but do not disappear. Surgery may be indicated.

Carcinoma of the Endometrium

S: Abnormal and intermenstrual bleeding before menopause; postmenopausal bleeding or mucosanguineous discharge. Pain and weight loss occur late in the disease.

O: Uterus may be enlarged.

The Pap test is rarely effective in detecting endometrial cancer. Women with abnormal vaginal bleeding or at high risk should have an endometrial tissue sample. Risk factors are early menarche, late menopause, history of infertility, failure to ovulate, tamoxifen, unopposed estrogen therapy (which continually stimulates the endometrium, causing hyperplasia), and obesity (which increases endogenous estrogen).

Endometriosis

S: Cyclic or chronic pelvic pain, occurring as dysmenorrhea or dyspareunia, low backache. May have irregular uterine bleeding, hypermenorrhea, or be asymptomatic.

O: Uterus fixed, tender to movement. Small, firm nodular masses tender to palpation on posterior aspect of fundus, uterosacral ligaments, ovaries, sigmoid colon. Ovaries often enlarged.

Masses are aberrant growths of endometrial tissue scattered throughout pelvis, probably transplanted tissue by retrograde menstruation. Ectopic tissue responds to hormone stimulation; builds up between periods, sloughs during menstruation. May cause infertility from pelvic adhesions, tubal obstruction, decreased ovarian function.

S, Subjective data; *O,* objective data.

TABLE 26-7   Adnexal Enlargement

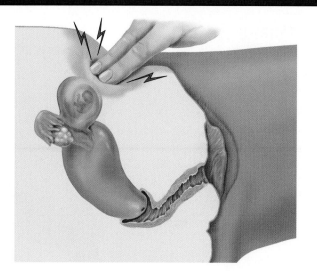

Fallopian Tube Mass—Acute Salpingitis (PID)

S: Sudden fever >38°C or 100.4°F, suprapubic pain and tenderness.

O: Acute—Rigid, boardlike lower abdominal musculature. May have purulent discharge from cervix. Movement of uterus and cervix causes intense pain. Pain in lateral fornices and adnexa. Bilateral adnexal masses difficult to palpate because of pain and muscle spasm. Chronic—Bilateral, tender, fixed adnexal masses.

Complications include ectopic pregnancy, infertility, and reinfection. PID usually caused by *Neisseria gonorrhoeae* and *Chlamydia trachomatis.*

Fallopian Tube Mass—Ectopic Pregnancy

S: Abdominal or pelvic pain, vaginal spotting or new-onset bleeding, although < half of women with ectopic pregnancy have these classic symptoms; positive urine pregnancy test.

O: Softening of cervix and fundus; movement of cervix and uterus cause pain; palpable tender, round, mobile swelling, lateral to uterus. Late signs may indicate rupture: decreased BP, tachycardia, diaphoresis, shock; regard as emergency. Transvaginal sonography crucial for all suspected ectopic pregnancies.[10]

This is an implanted fertilized ovum in the distal part of the fallopian tube; incidence may be 2.6% of all pregnancies.[10] Crucial to identify before fallopian tube ruptures and fatal hemorrhage ensues. This is leading cause of first-trimester pregnancy-related death.[10]

Continued

TABLE 26-7 Adnexal Enlargement—cont'd

Fluctuant Ovarian Mass—Ovarian Cyst

S: Usually asymptomatic.

O: Smooth, round, fluctuant, mobile, nontender mass on ovary. Some cysts resolve spontaneously within 60 days but must be followed closely.

Solid Ovarian Mass—Ovarian Cancer

S: May have abdominal pain, pelvic pain, increased abdominal size, bloating, nonspecific GI symptoms or may be asymptomatic.

O: May or may not palpate solid tumor on ovary. Heavy, solid, fixed, poorly defined mass suggests malignancy; benign mass may feel mobile and solid.

Biopsy necessary to distinguish. The Pap test does not detect ovarian cancer. Screening with serum CA 125 test is done but is not specific. Transvaginal ultrasonography may detect at an earlier stage in women at high risk for ovarian cancer.

S, Subjective data; *O*, objective data.

TABLE 26-8   Pediatric Genitalia Abnormalities

Ambiguous Genitalia

Female pseudohermaphroditism is a congenital anomaly resulting from hyperplasia of the adrenal glands, which exposes the female fetus to excess amounts of androgens. This causes masculinized external genitalia, here shown as enlargement of the clitoris and fusion of the labia. *Ambiguous* means that the enlarged clitoris here may look like a small penis with hypospadias and the fused labia look like an incompletely formed scrotum with absent testes. Other forms of intersexual conditions occur, and the family must be referred for diagnostic evaluation.

Vulvovaginitis in Child

This is acute, nonspecific vulvovaginitis.
Causes in the prepubertal child include infection from a respiratory or bowel pathogen, STI, presence of a foreign body, or *Candida albicans* in a child with diabetes.

See Illustration Credits for source information.

Abnormal Findings

Summary Checklist: Female Genitalia Examination

1. **Inspect external genitalia.**
2. **Palpate labia,** Skene and Bartholin glands.
3. Using **vaginal speculum,** inspect cervix and vagina.
4. Obtain **specimens** for cytologic study.
5. Perform **bimanual examination:** cervix, uterus, adnexa.
6. Perform **rectovaginal** examination.
7. **Test stool** for occult blood.

BIBLIOGRAPHY

1. Adegoke, O., Kulasingam, S., & Virnig, B. (2012). Cervical cancer trends in the United States: a 35-year population-based analysis. *J Women's Health, 21*(10), 1031-1037.
2. Ahonen, K. A. (2010). Polycystic ovary syndrome: recognize and intervene early. *Nurse Pract, 35*(9), 49-52.
3. American Academy of Pediatrics. (2010). Policy statement—Ritual genital cutting of female minors. *Pediatrics 126*(1), 191.
4. American Cancer Society. (2013). *Cancer facts & figures 2013.* Atlanta: American Cancer Society.
5. Ball, V., & Johnson, W. (2009). How to evaluate vaginal bleeding and discharge. *Emerg Med, April,* 27-48.
6. Beerman, H., van Dorst, E. B. L., Kuenen-Boumeester, V., et al. (2009). Superior performance of liquid-based versus conventional cytology in a population-based

cervical cancer screening program. *Gynecol Oncol,* *112*(3), 572-576.

7. Bulun, S. E. (2013). Uterine fibroids. *N Engl J Med, 369*(14), 1344-1355.

8. Burke, E. (2011). Female genital mutilation. *Nurse Pract, 36*(4), 45-50.

9. Champion, J. D., & Collins, J. L. (2012). Reducing STI screening, treatment, and counseling. *Nurse Pract, 37*(4), 40-46.

10. Crochet, J. R., Bastian, L. A., & Chireau, M. V. (2013). Does this woman have an ectopic pregnancy? *JAMA 309*(16):1722-1729.

11. Daley, A. M. (2011). Providing adolescent-friendly HPV education. *Nurse Pract, 36*(11), 35-40.

12. DeSantis, C., Naishadham, D., & Jemal, A. (2013). Cancer statistics for African Americans, (2013). *CA: Cancer J Clin, 63*(3), 151-166.

13. Henderson, J. T., Sawaya, G. F., Blum, M., et al. (2010). Pelvic examinations and access to oral hormonal contraception. *Obstet Gynecol, 116*(6), 1257-1264.

14. Kessenich, C. R., & Cronin, K. (2013). Minimizing unnecessary colposcopies and biopsies. *Nurse Pract, 38*(4), 11-13.

15. Keyock, K. L., & Newman, D. K. (2011). Understanding stress urinary incontinence. *Nurse Pract, 36*(10), 24-36.

16. Kostas-Polston, E. A., Johnson-Mallard, V., & Berman, N. R. (2012). HPV & age-appropriate cervical cancer prevention for adolescents. *Nurse Pract, 37*(6), 30-38.

17. Kruszka, P. S., & Kruszka, S. J. (2010). Evaluation of acute pelvic pain in women. *Am Fam Physician, 82*(2), 141-147.

18. Lea, J. S., & Lin, K. Y. (2012). Cervical cancer. *Obst Gynecol Clin North Am 30*, 233-253.

19. Reference deleted in proofs.

20. Lowe, N. K., & Ryan-Wenger, N. A. (2012). Uncomplicated UTIs in women. *Nurse Pract, 37*(5), 41-48.

21. Mayor, M. T., Roett, M. A., & Uduhiri, K. A. (2012). Diagnosis and management of gonococcal infections. *Am Fam Physician, 86*(10), 931-938.

22. McCloskey, C. R. (2010). Updated office testing skills for vaginal infections. *Nurse Pract, 35*(2), 46-52.

23. Morbidity and Mortality Weekly Report. (2013). Cervical cancer screening among women aged 18-30 years—United States, 2000-2010. *MMWR, 61*(51-52), 1038-1042.

24. Ramnitz, M. S., & Lodish, M. B. (2013). Racial disparities in pubertal development. *Semin Reprod Medicine, 31*(5), 333-339.

25. Reimer, A., & Johnson, L. (2011). Atrophic vaginitis signs, symptoms, and better outcomes. *Nurse Pract, 36*(1), 22-28.

26. Rosenfield, R. L., Lipton, R. B., & Drum, M. L. (2009). Thelarche, pubarche, and menarche attainment in children with normal and elevated body mass index. *Pediatrics, 123*(1), 84-88.

27. Roush, K. (2011). Menopausal hormone therapy: what we know now. *Am J Nurs 111*(6), 38-47.

28. Roush, K. (2012). Managing menopausal symptoms. *Am J Nurs, 112*(6), 28-35.

29. Schiffman, M., & Solomon, D. (2013). Cervical cancer screening with human papillomavirus and cytologic cotesting. *N Engl J Med, 369*(24), 2324-2331.

30. Schrager, S., Falleroni, J., & Edgoose, J. (2013). Evaluation and treatment of endometriosis. *Am Fam Physician, 87*(2), 107-113.

31. Sheaves, C. (2013). Advances in endometriosis treatment. *Nurse Pract, 38*(5), 42-47.

32. Simavli, S., Kaygusuz, I., Kınay, T., et al. (2014). The role of gel application in decreasing pain during speculum examination and its effects on Papanicolaou smear results. *Arch Gynecol Obstet, 289*(4), 809-815.

33. Smith, R. A., Brooks, D., & Cokkinides, V., et al. (2013). Cancer screening in the United States, 2013. *CA: Cancer J Clin, 63*(2), 88-105.

34. Thomas, M. C. (2011). Treatment options for dysfunctional uterine bleeding. *Nurse Pract, 36*(8), 14-20.

35. Townsend, M. K., Curhan, G. C., Resnick, N. M., et al. (2011). Rates of remission, improvement, and progression of urinary incontinence in Asian, black, and white women. *Am J Nurs 111*(4), 26-33.

36. Twiss, J. J. (2013). A new look at abnormal uterine bleeding. *Nurse Pract, 38*(12), 23-30.

37. Uygur, D., Guler, T., Yayci, E., et al. (2012). Association of speculum lubrication with pain and Papanicolaou test accuracy. *J Am Board Fam Med, 25*(6), 798-804.

38. Wisnieski, D. M. (2013). Promoting healthy sexual behavior in adolescents. *Am J Nurs, 113*(6), 67-70.

39. Wu, T., Mendola, P., & Buck, G. M. (2002). Ethnic differences in the presence of secondary sex characteristics and menarche among U.S. girls: the NHANES III, 1988-1994. *Pediatrics, 110*, 752-757.

CHAPTER 27

The Complete Health Assessment: Adult

The choreography of the complete history and physical examination is the art of arranging all the separate steps you have learned so far into a fluid whole. Your first examination may seem awkward and contrived; you may have to pause and think of what comes next rather than just gather data. Repeated rehearsals will make the choreography smoother. You will come to the point at which the procedure flows naturally; and even if you forget a step, you will be able to insert it gracefully into the next logical place.

The following examination sequence is one suggested route. It is intended to minimize the number of position changes for the patient and for you. With experience you may wish to adapt this and arrange a sequence that feels natural for you.

A complete examination is performed at a patient's first entry in an outpatient setting or initial admission to the hospital. Perform all the steps listed here for a complete examination. With experience you will learn to strike a balance between which steps you must retain to be thorough and which corners you may safely cut when time is pressing. The steps for the follow-up hospital assessment are described in Chapter 29.

Have all equipment prepared and accessible before the examination. Review Chapter 8 for the list of necessary equipment, the setting, the patient's emotional state, your demeanor, and the preparation of the patient considering his or her age.

Sequence	Selected Photos

The patient walks into the room, sits; the examiner sits facing the patient; the patient remains in street clothes. (NOTE: Position changes are in **bold** lines.)

The Health History

Collect the history, complete or limited as visit warrants. While obtaining the history and throughout the examination, note data on the person's general appearance.

General Appearance

1. Appears stated age
2. Level of consciousness
3. Skin color
4. Nutritional status
5. Posture and position comfortably erect
6. Obvious physical deformities
7. Mobility
   Gait
   Use of assistive devices
   Range of motion (ROM) of joints
   No involuntary movement
   Able to rise from a seated position easily
8. Facial expression
9. Mood and affect
10. Speech: articulation, pattern, content appropriate, native language
11. Hearing
12. Personal hygiene

Measurement

1. Weight
2. Height
3. Waist circumference
4. Compute body mass index
5. Vision using Snellen eye chart

Ask the person to empty the bladder (save specimen, if needed), to disrobe except for underpants, and to put on a gown. The person **sits with legs dangling** off the side of the bed or table; you stand in front of the person.

Sequence	Selected Photos

Skin

1. Examine both hands and inspect the nails.
2. For the rest of the examination, examine the skin with the corresponding regional examination.

Vital Signs

1. Radial pulse
2. Respirations
3. Blood pressure (BP) in arm(s)
4. BP in lower leg; compute ankle/brachial index (if indicated)
5. Temperature (if indicated)

Head and Face

1. Inspect and palpate scalp, hair, and cranium.
2. Inspect face: expression, symmetry (cranial nerve VII).
3. Palpate the temporal artery, then the temporomandibular joint as the person opens and closes the mouth.
4. Palpate the maxillary sinuses and the frontal sinuses.

Eyes

1. Test visual fields by confrontation (cranial nerve II).
2. Test extraocular muscles: corneal light reflex, six cardinal positions of gaze (cranial nerves III, IV, VI).
3. Inspect external eye structures.
4. Inspect conjunctivae, sclerae, corneas, irides.*
5. Test pupil: size, response to light, and accommodation.

Darken room.
6. Using an ophthalmoscope, inspect ocular fundus: red reflex, disc, vessels, and retinal background.

Ears

1. Inspect the external ear: position and alignment, skin condition, and auditory meatus.
2. Move auricle and push tragus for tenderness.
3. With an otoscope, inspect the canal, then the tympanic membrane for color, position, landmarks, and integrity.
4. Test hearing: whispered voice test.

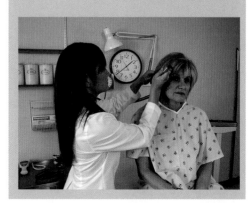

*This is the plural form of iris.

Objective Data

Sequence	Selected Photos

Nose

1. Inspect the external nose: symmetry, lesions.
2. Inspect facial symmetry (cranial nerve VII).
3. Test the patency of each nostril.
4. With a speculum, inspect the nares: nasal mucosa, septum, and turbinates.

Mouth and Throat

1. With a penlight inspect the mouth: buccal mucosa, teeth and gums, tongue, floor of mouth, palate, and uvula.
2. Grade tonsils if present.
3. Note mobility of uvula as the person phonates "ahh" and test gag reflex (cranial nerves IX, X).
4. Ask the person to stick out the tongue (cranial nerve XII).
5. With a gloved hand, bimanually palpate the mouth, if indicated.

Neck

1. Inspect the neck: symmetry, lumps, and pulsations.
2. Palpate the cervical lymph nodes.
3. Inspect and palpate the carotid pulse, one side at a time. If indicated, listen for carotid bruits.
4. Palpate the trachea in midline.
5. Test ROM and muscle strength against your resistance: head forward and back, head turned to each side, and shoulder shrug (cranial nerve XI).

Step behind the person, taking your stethoscope, ruler, and marking pen with you.
6. Palpate thyroid gland, posterior approach.

Open the person's gown to expose all of the back for examination of the thorax, but leave gown on shoulders and anterior chest.

Chest, Posterior and Lateral

1. Inspect the posterior chest: configuration of the thoracic cage, skin characteristics, and symmetry of shoulders and muscles.
2. Palpate: symmetric expansion; tactile fremitus; lumps or tenderness.
3. Palpate length of spinous processes.
4. Percuss over all lung fields; percuss diaphragmatic excursion.
5. Percuss costovertebral angle, noting tenderness.
6. Auscultate breath sounds, comparing side to side in upper and lower lung fields; note any adventitious sounds.

Objective Data

Sequence	Selected Photos

Move around to face the patient; the patient remains sitting. For a female breast examination, ask permission to lift gown to drape on the shoulders, exposing the anterior chest; for a male, lower the gown to the lap.

Chest, Anterior

1. Inspect: respirations and skin characteristics.
2. Palpate: tactile fremitus, lumps, or tenderness.
3. Percuss anterior lung fields.
4. Auscultate breath sounds, comparing side to side in upper and lateral lung fields.

Heart

1. Ask the person to lean forward and exhale briefly; auscultate cardiac base for any murmurs.

Upper Extremities

1. Test ROM and muscle strength of hands, wrists, arms, and shoulders.
2. Palpate the epitrochlear nodes.
3. Palpate temperature, capillary refill.
4. Compare radial and brachial pulses.

Female Breasts

1. Inspect for symmetry, mobility, and dimpling as the woman lifts arms over the head, pushes the hands on the hips, and leans forward.
2. Inspect supraclavicular and infraclavicular areas.

Help the woman to **lie supine with head at a flat** to 30-degree angle. Stand at the person's *right* side. Drape the gown up across shoulders and place an extra sheet across lower abdomen.
3. Palpate each breast, lifting the same-side arm up over head. Include the tail of Spence and areola.
4. Palpate each nipple for discharge.
5. Support the person's arm and palpate the axilla and regional lymph nodes.
6. Teach breast self-examination.

Male Breasts

1. Inspect and palpate while palpating the anterior chest wall.
2. Supporting each arm, palpate the axilla and regional nodes.

Neck Vessels

1. Inspect each side of neck for a jugular venous pulse, turning the person's head slightly to the other side.
2. Estimate jugular venous pressure, if indicated.

Objective Data

Sequence	Selected Photos

Heart

1. Inspect the precordium for any pulsations or heave (lift).
2. Palpate the apical impulse and note the location.
3. Palpate the precordium for any abnormal thrill.
4. Auscultate apical rate and rhythm.
5. Auscultate with the diaphragm of the stethoscope to study heart sounds, inching from the apex up to the base, or vice versa.
6. Auscultate the heart sounds with the bell of the stethoscope, again inching through all locations.
7. Turn the person over to the left side while again auscultating the apex with the bell.

The person should be **supine,** with the bed or table flat; arrange drapes to expose the abdomen from the chest to the pubis.

Abdomen

1. Inspect: contour, symmetry, skin characteristics, umbilicus, and pulsations.
2. Auscultate bowel sounds.
3. Auscultate for vascular sounds over the aorta, renal arteries, iliac and femoral arteries.
4. Percuss all quadrants.
5. Percuss height of the liver span in the right midclavicular line.
6. Percuss the location of the spleen.

7. Palpate: light palpation in all quadrants, then deep palpation in all quadrants.
8. Palpate for liver, spleen, and kidneys.
9. Palpate aortic pulsation if indicated.

Inguinal Area

1. Palpate each groin for the femoral pulse and the inguinal nodes. Lift the drape to expose the legs.

Sequence	Selected Photos

Lower Extremities

1. Inspect: symmetry, skin characteristics, and hair distribution.
2. Palpate pulses: popliteal, posterior tibial, dorsalis pedis.
3. Palpate for temperature and pretibial edema.
4. Separate toes and inspect.
5. Test ROM and muscle strength of hips, knees, ankles, and feet.

Ask the person to **sit up and to dangle** the legs off the bed or table. Keep the gown on and the drape over the lap.

Musculoskeletal

1. Note muscle strength as person sits up.

Neurologic

1. Test sensation in selected areas on face, arms, hands, legs, and feet: superficial pain, light touch, and vibration.
2. Test position sense of finger, one hand.
3. Test stereognosis, using a familiar object.
4. Test cerebellar function of the upper extremities using finger-to-nose test or rapid–alternating movements test.

5. Elicit deep tendon reflexes: biceps, triceps, brachioradialis.

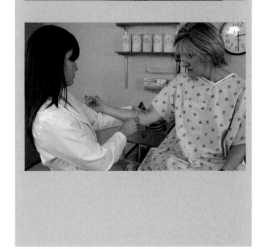

Objective Data

Sequence	**Selected Photos**

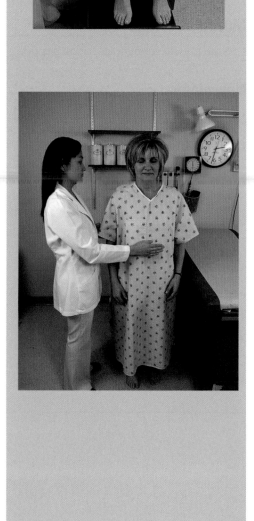

6. Test the cerebellar function of the lower extremities by asking the person to run each heel down the opposite shin.
7. Elicit deep tendon reflexes: patellar and Achilles.
8. Test the Babinski reflex.

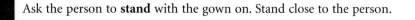

Ask the person to **stand** with the gown on. Stand close to the person.

Lower Extremities

1. Inspect legs for varicose veins.

Musculoskeletal

1. Ask the person **to walk** across the room in his or her regular walk, turn, and then walk back toward you in heel-to-toe fashion.
2. Ask the person to walk on the toes for a few steps, then to walk on the heels for a few steps.
3. Stand close and check Romberg sign.

Objective Data

Sequence	Selected Photos

4. Ask the person to hold the edge of the bed and perform a shallow knee bend, one for each leg.
5. Stand behind and check the spine as the person touches the toes.
6. Stabilize the pelvis and test the ROM of the spine as the person hyperextends, rotates, and laterally bends.

For the male patient, sit on a stool in front of him. The person stands.

Male Genitalia

1. Inspect the penis and scrotum.
2. Palpate the scrotal contents. If a mass exists, transilluminate.
3. Check for inguinal hernia.
4. Teach testicular self-examination.

For an adult male, ask him to bend over the examination table, supporting the torso with forearms on the table. Assist the bedfast male to a left lateral position with the right leg drawn up.

Male Rectum

1. Inspect the perianal area.
2. With a gloved lubricated finger, palpate the rectal walls and prostate gland.
3. Save a stool specimen for an occult blood test.

Assist the female back to the examination table and help her assume **the lithotomy position**. Drape her appropriately. You sit on a stool at the foot of the table for the speculum examination and then stand for the bimanual examination.

Objective Data

Sequence	Selected Photos

Female Genitalia

1. Inspect the perineal and perianal areas.
2. With a vaginal speculum inspect the cervix and vaginal walls.
3. Procure specimens.
4. Perform a bimanual examination: cervix, uterus, and adnexa.
5. Continue the bimanual examination, checking the rectum and rectovaginal walls.
6. Save a stool specimen for an occult blood test.
7. Provide tissues for the female to wipe the perineal area and help her up to a **sitting position**.

Tell the patient that you are finished with the examination and that you will leave the room as he or she gets dressed. Return to discuss the examination and further plans and to answer any questions. Thank the person for his or her time.

For the hospitalized person, return the bed and any room equipment to their original position. Make sure that the call light and telephone are within easy reach.

DOCUMENTATION AND CRITICAL THINKING

Recording the Data

Record the data from the history and physical examination as soon after the event as possible. Memory fades as the day develops, especially when you are responsible for the care of more than one person.

It is difficult to strike a balance between recording too much and too little data. It is important to remember that from a legal perspective, if it is not documented, it was not done. Data important for the diagnosis and treatment of the person's health should be recorded, as well as data that contribute to your decision-making process. This includes charting relevant normal or negative findings.

On the other hand, a listing of every assessment parameter described in this text yields an unwieldy, unworkable record. One way to keep your record complete yet succinct is to study your writing style. Use short, clear phrases. Avoid redundant introductory phrases such as "The patient states that...." Avoid redundant descriptions such as "No inguinal, femoral, or umbilical hernias." Just write, "No hernias."

Use simple line drawings to describe your findings. You do not need artistic talent; draw a simple sketch of a tympanic membrane, breast, abdomen, or cervix and mark your findings on it. A clear picture is worth many words.

Study the following complete history and physical examination for a sample write-up. Note the many health problems emerging through this history and examination.

Health History

BIOGRAPHIC DATA

Name: Ellen K.	Birth date: 1/18/
Address: 123 Center St.	Birthplace: Springfield
Marital Status: Single	Race: Caucasian

Ellen K. is a 23-year-old single Caucasian female cashier at a tavern, currently unemployed for 6 months.

Source. Ellen, seems reliable.

Reason for Seeking Care. "I'm coming in for alcohol treatment."

History of Present Illness. First alcoholic drink, age 16. First intoxication, age 17, drinking 1 or 2 times per week, a 6-pack per occasion. Attending high school classes every day, but grades slipping from A–B+ average to C– average. At age 20 drinking 2 times per week, 6 to 9 beers per occasion. At age 22 drinking 2 times per week, a 12-pack per occasion, and occasionally a 6-pack the next day to "help with the hangover." During this year experienced blackouts, failed attempts to cut down on drinking, was physically sick the morning after drinking, and was unable to stop drinking once started. Also incurred three driving-under-the-influence (DUI) legal offenses. Last DUI 1 month PTA; last alcohol use just before DUI, 18 beers that occasion. Abstinent since that time.

PAST HEALTH

Childhood Illnesses. Chickenpox at age 6. No measles, mumps, croup, pertussis. No rheumatic fever, scarlet fever, or polio. Received childhood vaccinations recommended at that time. No HPV vaccine series.

Accidents. (1) Auto accident, age 12; father driving; Ellen thrown from car, right leg crushed. Hospitalized at Memorial; surgery for leg pinning to repair multiple compound fractures. (2) Auto accident, age 21; not wearing seat belt, head hit dashboard, no loss of consciousness, treated and released at Memorial Hospital ED. (3) Auto accident, age 23; "car hit median strip," no injuries, not seen at hospital.

Chronic Illnesses. None.

Hospitalizations. Age 12, Memorial Hospital, surgery to repair right leg as described; Dr. M.J. Carlson, surgeon.

Obstetric History. Gravida 0/Para 0/Abortion 0.

Immunizations. Childhood immunizations up-to-date. Last tetanus "probably high school." No TB skin test.

Last Examinations. Annual pelvic examinations at health department since age 15, told "normal and healthy." High school sports physical as sophomore. Last dental examination as high school junior; last vision test for driver's license age 16; never had ECG, chest x-ray study.

Allergies. No known allergies.

Current Medications. Birth control pills, low-estrogen type, 1/day, for 5 years. No other prescription or over-the-counter medications.

FAMILY HISTORY

Ellen is second youngest child, parents divorced 8 years, father has chronic alcoholism. See family genogram that follows.

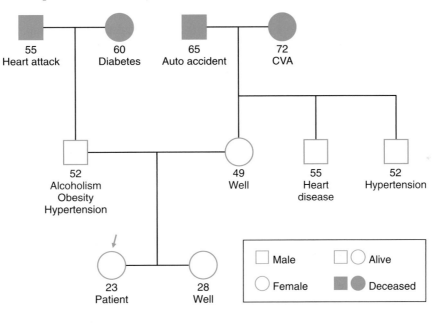

REVIEW OF SYSTEMS

General Health. Reports usual health "OK." No recent weight change; no fatigue, weakness, fever, sweats.

Skin. No change in skin color, pigmentation, or nevi. No pruritus, rash, lesions. Has bruise now over right eye; struck by boyfriend 1 week PTA. No history of skin disease. Hair: No loss, change in texture. Nails: no change.
Self-care: Stays in sun "as much as I can." No use of sunscreen. Goes to tanning beds at hair salon twice/week during winter.

Head. No unusually frequent or severe headaches; no head injury, dizziness, syncope, or vertigo.

Eyes. No difficulty with vision or double vision. No eye pain, inflammation, discharge, lesions. No history of glaucoma or cataracts. Wears no corrective lenses.

Ears. No hearing loss or difficulty. No earaches; no infections now or as child; no discharge, tinnitus, or vertigo.
Self-care: No exposure to environmental noise; cleans ears with washcloth.

Nose. No discharge; has 2 or 3 colds per year; no sinus pain, nasal obstruction, epistaxis, or allergy.

Mouth and Throat. No mouth pain, bleeding gums, toothache, sores or lesions in mouth, dysphagia, hoarseness, or sore throat. Has tonsils. Self-care: Brushes teeth twice/day, no flossing.

Neck. No pain, limitation of motion, lumps, or swollen glands.

Breasts. No pain, lump, nipple discharge, rash, swelling, or trauma. No history of breast disease in self, mother, or sister. No surgery. Self-care: Does not do breast self-examination.

Respiratory. No history of lung disease; no chest pain with breathing; no wheezing or shortness of breath. Colds sometimes "go to my chest"; treats with over-the-counter cough medicine and aspirin. Occasional early-morning cough, nonproductive. Smokes cigarettes 2 PPD × 2 years; prior use 1 PPD × 4 years. Pack years = 8. Never tried to quit. Works in poorly ventilated tavern.

Cardiovascular. No chest pain, palpitation, cyanosis, fatigue, dyspnea with exertion, orthopnea, paroxysmal nocturnal dyspnea, nocturia, edema. No history of heart murmur, hypertension, coronary artery disease, or anemia.

Peripheral Vascular. No pain, numbness or tingling, or swelling in legs. No coldness, discoloration, varicose veins, infections, or ulcers. Legs are unequal in length as sequelae of accident age 12. Self-care: Usual work as cashier involves standing for 8-hour shifts; no support hose.

Gastrointestinal. Appetite good with no recent change. No food intolerance, heartburn, indigestion, pain in abdomen, nausea, or vomiting. No history of ulcers, liver or gallbladder disease, jaundice, appendicitis, or colitis. Bowel movement 1/day, soft, brown; no rectal bleeding or pain. Self-care: No use of vitamins, antacids, laxatives. Diet recall—see Functional Assessment.

Urinary. No dysuria, frequency, urgency, nocturia, hesitancy, or straining. No pain in flank, groin, suprapubic region. Urine color yellow; no history of kidney disease.

Genitalia. Menarche age 11. Last menstrual period April 18. Cycle usually q 28 days, duration 2 to 4 days, flow small amount, no dysmenorrhea. No vaginal itching, discharge, sores, or lesions.

Sexual health. In relationship now that includes intercourse. This boyfriend has been her only sexual partner for 2 years; had one other partner before that. Uses birth control pills to prevent pregnancy; partner uses no condoms. Concerned that boyfriend may be having sex with other women but has not confronted him. Not aware of any STI contact. Never been tested for HIV/AIDS. History of sexual abuse by father from ages 12 to 16 years; abuse did not include vaginal or anal intercourse. Ellen is unwilling to discuss further at this time.

Musculoskeletal. No history of arthritis, gout. No joint pain, stiffness, swelling, deformity, or limitation of motion. No muscle pain or weakness. Bone trauma at age 12; has sequela of unequal leg lengths, right leg shorter, walks with limp.

Self-care: No walking or running for sport or exercise "because of leg." Able to stand as cashier. Uses lift pad in right shoe to equalize leg length.

Neurologic. No history of seizure disorder, stroke, fainting. Has had blackouts with alcohol use. No weakness, tremor, paralysis, problems with coordination, difficulty speaking or swallowing. No numbness or tingling. Not aware of memory problem, nervousness or mood change, depression. Had counseling for sexual abuse in the past. Denies any suicidal ideation or intent during adolescent years or now.

Hematologic. No bleeding problems in skin; no excessive bruising. Not aware of exposure to toxins, never had blood transfusion, never used needles to shoot drugs.

Endocrine. Paternal grandmother with diabetes. No increase in hunger, thirst, or urination; no problems with hot or cold environments; no change in skin or appetite; no nervousness.

FUNCTIONAL ASSESSMENT

Self-Concept. Graduated from high school. Trained "on-the-job" as bartender; also worked as cashier in tavern. Unemployed now, on public aid, does not perceive she has enough money for daily living. Lives with older sister. Raised as Presbyterian, believes in God; does not attend church. Believes self to be "honest, dependable." Believes limitations are "smoking, weight, drinking."

Activity-Exercise. Typical day: Arises 9 AM; light chores or TV; spends day looking for work, running errands, with friends; bedtime at 11 PM. No sustained physical exercise. Believes self able to perform all ADLs; limp poses no problem in bathing, dressing, cooking, household tasks, mobility, driving a car, or work as cashier. No mobility aids. Hobbies are fishing, boating, snowmobiling; however, currently has no finances to engage in most of these.

Sleep-Rest. Bedtime 11 PM. Sleeps 8 to 9 hours. No sleep aids.

Nutrition. 24-hour recall: Breakfast—none; lunch—bologna sandwich, chips, diet soda; dinner—hamburger, French fries, coffee; snacks—peanuts, pretzels, potato chips, "bar food." This menu is typical of most days. Eats lunch at home alone. Most dinners at fast-food restaurants or in tavern. Shares household grocery expenses and cooking chores with sister. No food intolerances.

Alcohol. See History of Present Illness. Denies use of illicit drugs. Cigarettes: Smokes 2 PPD × 2 years; prior use 1 PPD × 4 years. Never tried to quit. Boyfriend smokes cigarettes.

Interpersonal Relationships. Describes family life growing up as chaotic. Father physically abusive toward mother and sexually abusive toward Ellen. Parents divorced because of father's continual drinking. Few support systems currently. Estranged from mother; "Didn't believe me about my father." Father estranged from entire family. Gets along "OK" with sister. Relationship with boyfriend chaotic; has hit her twice in the past. Ellen has never pressed legal charges. No close women friends. Most friends are "drinking buddies" at tavern.

Coping and Stress Management. Believes housing adequate, adequate heat and utilities, and neighborhood safe. Believes home has no safety hazards. Does not use seat belts. No travel outside 60 miles of hometown.

Identifies current stresses to be drinking, legal problems with DUIs, unemployment, financial worries. Considers her drinking to be problematic.

PERCEPTION OF HEALTH

Identifies alcohol as a health problem for herself; feels motivated for treatment. Never been interested in physical health and own body before; "Now I think it's time I learned." Expects health care providers to "Help me with my drinking. I don't know beyond that." Expects to stay at this agency for 6 weeks; "Then I don't know what."

Physical Examination

MEASUREMENT

Height: 163 cm (5′4″). Weight: 68.6 kg (151 lbs). Waist circumference: 32 inches. BMI: 26.
BP: 142/100 mm Hg right arm, sitting. 140/96 mm Hg right arm, lying. 138/98 mm Hg left arm, lying.
Temp: 98.6° F (37° C). Pulse 76 bpm, regular. Resp 16/min, unlabored.

General Survey. Ellen K. is a 23-year-old Caucasian female, not currently under the influence of alcohol or other drugs, who articulates clearly, ambulates without difficulty, and is in no distress.

HEAD-TO-TOE EXAMINATION

Skin. Uniformly tan-pink in color, warm, dry, intact; turgor good. No lesions, birthmarks, edema. Resolving 2-cm yellow-green hematoma present over right eye; no swelling; ocular structures not involved. Hair: Normal distribution and texture; no pest inhabitants. Nails: No clubbing, biting, or discolorations. Nail beds: Pink and firm with prompt capillary refill.

Head. Normocephalic, no lesions, lumps, scaling, parasites, or tenderness. Face: Symmetric, no weakness, no involuntary movements.

Eyes. Acuity by Snellen chart: right eye 20/20; left eye 20/20−1. Visual fields full by confrontation. EOMs intact; no nystagmus. No ptosis, lid lag, discharge, or crusting. Corneal light reflex symmetric; no strabismus. Conjunctivae clear. Sclerae white; no lesion or redness. Pupils: 3 mm resting, 2 mm constricted, and = bilaterally. PERRLA.

Fundi: Discs flat with sharp margins. Vessels present in all quadrants without crossing defects. Background has even color, no hemorrhage or exudates.

Ears. Pinna: No mass, lesions, scaling, discharge, or tenderness to palpation. Canals clear. Tympanic membrane: pearly gray, landmarks intact, no perforation. Whispered words heard bilaterally.

Nose. No deformities or tenderness to palpation. Nares patent. Mucosa pink; no lesions. Septum midline; no perforation. No sinus tenderness.

Mouth. Mucosa and gingivae pink; no lesions or bleeding. Right lower 1st molar missing; multiple dark spots on most teeth; gums receding on lower incisors. Tongue symmetric, protrudes midline, no tremor. Pharynx pink; no exudate. Uvula rises midline on phonation. Tonsils 1+. Gag reflex present.

Neck. Neck supple with full ROM. Symmetric; no masses, tenderness, lymphadenopathy. Trachea midline. Thyroid nonpalpable, not tender. Jugular veins flat @45 degrees. Carotid arteries 2+ and = bilaterally; no bruits.

Spine and Back. Normal spinal profile; no scoliosis. No tenderness over spine; no CVA tenderness.

Thorax and Lungs. AP < transverse diameter. Chest expansion symmetric. Tactile fremitus equal bilaterally. Lung fields resonant. Diaphragmatic excursion 4 cm and = bilaterally. Breath sounds diminished. Expiratory wheeze in posterior chest at both bases, scattered rhonchi in posterior chest at both bases; do not clear with coughing.

Breasts. Symmetric; no retraction, discharge, or lesions. Contour and consistency firm and homogeneous. No masses or tenderness; no lymphadenopathy.

Heart. Precordium: no abnormal pulsations, no heaves. Apical impulse at 5th ICS in left MCL, no thrills. S_1–S_2 are not diminished or accentuated, no S_3 or S_4. Systolic murmur, grade 2/6, loudest at left lower sternal border; no radiation; present supine and sitting.

Abdomen. Flat, symmetric. Skin smooth with no lesions, scars, or striae. Bowel sounds present; no bruits. Tympany predominates in all quadrants. Liver span 7 cm in right MCL. Abdomen soft; no organomegaly; no masses or tenderness; no inguinal lymphadenopathy.

Extremities. Color tan-pink; no redness, cyanosis, lesions other than surgical scar. Scar right lower leg, anterior, 28 cm × 2 cm wide, well healed. No edema, varicosities. No calf tenderness. All peripheral pulses present, 2+ and = bilaterally. Asymmetric leg length—right leg 3 cm shorter than left.

Musculoskeletal. Temporomandibular joint: no slipping or crepitation. Neck: Full ROM, no pain. Vertebral column: No tenderness; no deformity or curvature; full extension, lateral bending, rotation. Arms symmetric, legs measure as described, extremities have full ROM, no pain or crepitation. Muscle strength: Able to maintain flexion against resistance and without tenderness.

Neurologic. Mental status: Appearance, behavior, speech appropriate. Alert and oriented to person, place, time. Thought coherent. Remote and recent memories intact. Cranial nerves II through XII intact. Sensory: Pinprick, light touch, vibration intact. Stereognosis: Able to identify key. Motor: No atrophy, weakness, or tremors. Gait: Has limp, able to tandem walk with shoes on. Negative Romberg sign. Cerebellar: Finger-to-nose smoothly intact. DTRs: See *stick gram*.

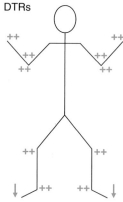

Genitalia. External genitalia: No lesion, discharge. Internal genitalia: Vaginal walls pink; no lesion. Cervix: Pink; nulliparous os; no lesions; small amount nonodorous clear discharge. Specimens for Pap test, GC/chlamydia, trichomoniasis, moniliasis obtained. Swabbing mucosa with acetic acid shows no acetowhitening.

Bimanual: No pain on moving cervix; uterus midline; no enlargement, masses, or tenderness. Adnexa—ovaries not enlarged, no tenderness. Anus—no hemorrhoids, fissures, or lesions. Rectal wall intact; no masses or tenderness. Stool soft, brown; hematest negative.

ASSESSMENT

Alcohol dependence, severe, with physiologic dependence
Nicotine dependence with physiologic dependence
Hypertension, stage I
Systolic heart murmur
Ineffective airway clearance R/T tracheobronchial secretions and obstruction
Right orbital contusion (resolving)
Overweight by about 10 lbs
Dental: missing tooth, probable caries
Risk for trauma
Self-care deficit: oral hygiene R/T lack of motivation
Deficient knowledge about alcoholism disease process, treatment options, support systems R/T lack of exposure
Deficient knowledge about balanced diet R/T lack of exposure and substance abuse
Dysfunctional family processes: alcoholism
Chronic low self-esteem R/T effects of alcoholism, sexual abuse, physical abuse

Documentation and Critical Thinking

CHAPTER 28

The Complete Physical Assessment: Infant, Child, and Adolescent

Sequence	Selected Photos

The Neonate and Infant

Review Chapter 8 for the steps on preparation and positioning and on developmental principles of the infant. The 1- and 5-minute Apgar results will give important data on the neonate's immediate response to extrauterine life. The following sequence will expand these data. You may reorder this sequence as the infant's sleep and wakefulness state or physical condition warrants.

The infant is **supine** on a warming or examination table with an overhead heating element. The infant may be nude except for a diaper over a boy.*

Vital Signs

Note pulse, respirations, and temperature.

Measurement

Weight, length, and head circumference are measured and plotted on growth curves for the infant's age.

General Appearance

1. Body symmetry, spontaneous position, flexion of head and extremities, and spontaneous movement.
2. Skin color and characteristics; any obvious deformities.
3. Symmetry and positioning of the facial features.
4. Alert, responsive affect.
5. Strong, lusty cry.

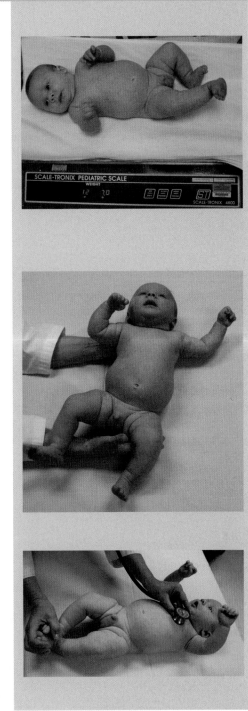

Chest and Heart

1. Inspect the skin condition over the chest and abdomen, chest configuration, and nipples and breast tissue.
2. Note movement of the abdomen with respirations, and note any chest retraction.
3. Palpate apical impulse and note its location; chest wall for thrills; tactile fremitus if the infant is crying.
4. Auscultate breath sounds, heart sounds in all locations, and bowel sounds in the abdomen and chest.

*Note: I took the diaper off this boy so you could see his body position and symmetry.

Sequence	**Selected Photos**

Abdomen

1. Inspect the shape of the abdomen and skin condition.
2. Inspect the umbilicus; count vessels; note condition of cord or stump, any hernia.
3. Palpate skin turgor.
4. Palpate lightly for muscle tone, liver, spleen tip, and bladder.
5. Palpate deeply for kidneys, any mass.
6. Palpate femoral pulses, inguinal lymph nodes.
7. Percuss all quadrants.

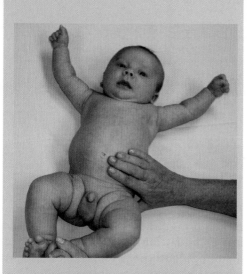

Head and Face

1. Note molding after delivery, any swelling on cranium, bulging of fontanel with crying or at rest.
2. Palpate fontanels, suture lines, and any swellings.
3. Inspect positioning and symmetry of facial features at rest and while the infant is crying.

To open the neonate's eyes, support the head and shoulders and gently lower the baby backward or ask the parent to hold the baby over his or her shoulder while you stand behind the parent.

Eyes

1. Inspect the lids (edematous in the neonate), palpebral slant, conjunctivae, any nystagmus, and any discharge.
2. Using a penlight, elicit the pupillary reflex, blink reflex, and corneal light reflex; assess tracking of moving light.
3. Using an ophthalmoscope, elicit the red reflex.

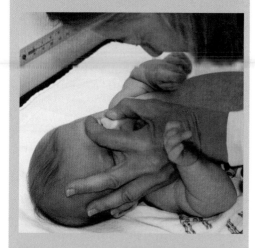

Ears

1. Inspect size, shape, alignment of auricles, patency of auditory canals, any extra skin tags or pits.
2. Note the startle reflex in response to a loud noise.
3. Palpate flexible auricles.
(Defer otoscopic examination until the end of the complete examination.)

Sequence	Selected Photos

Nose

1. Determine the patency of the nares.
2. Note the nasal discharge, sneezing, and any flaring with respirations.

Mouth and Throat

1. Inspect the lips and gums, high-arched intact palate, buccal mucosa, tongue size, and frenulum of tongue; note absent or minimal salivation in neonate.
2. Note the rooting reflex.
3. Insert a gloved little finger, note the sucking reflex, and palpate the palate.

Neck

1. Lift the shoulders and let the head lag to inspect the neck: note midline trachea, any skinfolds, and any lumps.
2. Palpate the lymph nodes, the thyroid, and any masses.
3. While the infant is supine, elicit the tonic neck reflex; note a supple neck with movement.

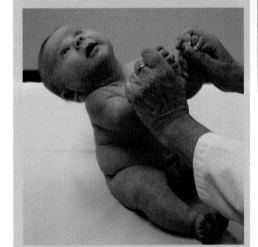

Upper Extremities

1. Inspect and manipulate, noting ROM, muscle tone, and absence of scarf sign (elbow should not reach midline).
2. Count fingers, count palmar creases, and note color of hands and nail beds.
3. Place your thumbs in the infant's palms to note the grasp reflex; then wrap your hands around infant's hands to pull up and note the head lag.

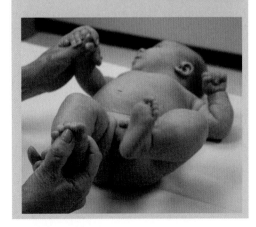

Lower Extremities

1. Inspect and manipulate the legs and feet, noting ROM, muscle tone, and skin condition.
2. Note alignment of feet and toes, look for flat soles, and count toes; note any syndactyly.
3. Test Ortolani sign for hip stability.
4. Check plantar grasp reflex (present until 8 to 10 months).
5. Check Babinski → fanning of toes until 24 months.

Objective Data

Sequence	**Selected Photos**

Genitalia

1. *Females.* Inspect labia and clitoris (edematous in the newborn), vernix caseosa between labia, and patent vagina.
2. *Males.* Inspect position of urethral meatus (do not retract foreskin), strength of urine stream if possible, and rugae on scrotum.
3. Palpate the testes in the scrotum.

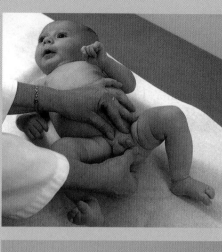

Lift the infant under the axillae and hold him or her facing you at eye level.

Neuromuscular

1. Note shoulder muscle tone and the infant's ability to stay in your hands without slipping.
2. Rotate the neonate slowly side to side; note the doll's eye reflex.
3. Turn the infant around so his or her back is to you; elicit the stepping reflex and the placing reflex against the edge of the examination table.

Turn the infant over and hold him or her prone in your hands, or place the infant prone on the examination table.

Spine and Rectum

1. Inspect the length of the spine, trunk incurvation reflex, and symmetry of gluteal folds.
2. Inspect intact skin; note any sinus openings, protrusions, or tufts of hair.
3. Note patent anal opening. Check for passage of meconium stool during the first 24 to 48 hours.

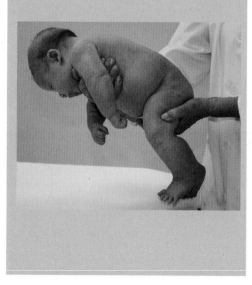

| **Sequence** | **Selected Photos** |

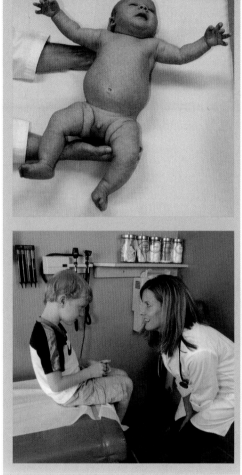

Final Procedures

1. With an otoscope, inspect the auditory canals and tympanic membranes.
2. Elicit the Moro reflex by letting the infant's head and trunk drop back a short way, jarring crib sides, or making a loud noise.

The Young Child

Review the developmental considerations in preparing for an examination of the young child in Chapter 8. The preschool child displays developing initiative and takes on tasks independently. This child is cooperative, helpful, and easy to involve. However, he or she fears any body injury and may recoil from invasive procedures (e.g., tongue blade, otoscope). The young school child is developing industry. During the examination the child is cooperative and interested in learning about the body.

The Health History

1. Collect the history, including developmental data.
2. During the history note data on general appearance.

General Appearance

1. Note child's ability to amuse himself or herself while the parent speaks.
2. Note parent and child interaction.
3. Note gross- and fine-motor skills as the child plays with toys.

Gradually focus on and involve yourself with the child, at first in a "play" period.
4. Evaluate developmental milestones by using a Denver II test: gait, jumping, hopping, standing on one foot, building a tower, and throwing a ball.
5. Evaluate posture while the child is sitting and standing. Evaluate alignment of the legs and feet while the child is walking.
6. Evaluate speech acquisition.
7. Evaluate vision, hearing ability.
8. Evaluate social interaction.

Objective Data

Sequence	Selected Photos

The preschooler and young school child are willing to undress. Leave shorts and underpants on until the genital examination. Talk to the child and explain the steps in the examination. Use games. Have the child blow on the pinwheel as you listen to lung sounds. The pinwheel can go home as a present. The young child usually feels comfortable on the examination table. With the schoolchild, talk about school, family, friends, music, sports. Demonstrate equipment to this curious child.

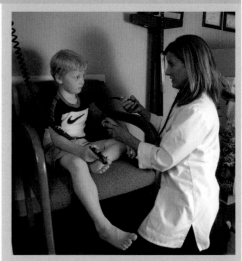

Measurement

Height, weight, temperature, blood pressure.

Upper Extremities

1. Inspect arms and hands for alignment, skin condition; inspect fingers and note palmar creases.
2. Palpate and count the radial pulse.
3. Test biceps and triceps reflexes with a reflex hammer.

Head, Face, and Neck

1. Inspect the size and shape of the head and symmetry of facies.
2. Palpate the cervical lymph nodes, trachea, and thyroid gland.

Objective Data

Sequence	Selected Photos

Eyes

1. Inspect the external structures. Note any palpebral slant.
2. With a penlight, test the corneal light and pupillary light reflexes.
3. Direct a moving penlight for cardinal positions of gaze.
4. If indicated, perform the cover test, covering the eye with your thumb in a young child or using an index card.
5. Inspect conjunctivae and sclerae.
6. With an ophthalmoscope, check the red reflex. Inspect the fundus as much as possible.

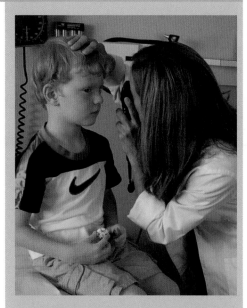

Nose

1. Inspect the external nose and skin condition.
2. With a penlight, inspect the nares for foreign body, mucosa, septum, and turbinates.

Mouth and Throat

1. With a penlight, inspect the mouth, buccal mucosa, teeth and gums, tongue, palate, and uvula in midline. Use a tongue blade as the last resort.

Ears

1. Inspect and palpate the auricles. Note any discharge from the auditory meatus. Check for any foreign body.
2. With an otoscope, inspect the ear canals and tympanic membranes. Gain cooperation by encouraging the child to handle the equipment or to look in the parent's ear as you hold the otoscope. Inspect the canal, then the tympanic membrane for color, position, landmarks, and integrity.

Objective Data

Sequence	Selected Photos

Thorax and Breath Sounds

1. Inspect the posterior chest: configuration, skin characteristics, symmetry of shoulders and muscles.
2. Palpate for lumps or tenderness, length of spinous processes.
3. Percuss over lung fields.
4. Auscultate breath sounds, comparing side to side in upper and lower lung fields; note any adventitious sounds.

Chest and Heart

1. Inspect size, shape, and configuration of chest cage. Assess respiratory movement.
2. Inspect pulsations on the precordium. Note nipple and breast development.
3. Palpate apical impulse and note location, chest wall for thrills, any tactile fremitus.
4. Auscultate breath sounds and heart sounds in all locations, count respiratory rate and heart rate.
5. Listen to S_1 and S_2 across the precordium; note any murmurs.

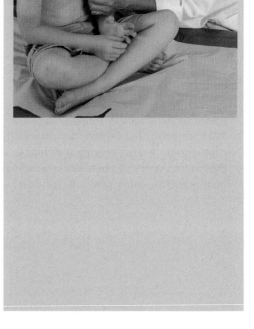

Sequence	Selected Photos

Abdomen

1. Inspect shape of abdomen, skin condition, and periumbilical area.
2. Auscultate bowel sounds.
3. Palpate skin turgor, muscle tone, liver edge, spleen, kidneys, and any masses.
4. Palpate the femoral pulses. Compare strength with radial pulses.
5. Palpate inguinal lymph nodes.

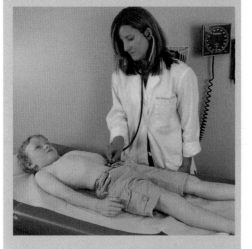

Genitalia

1. Inspect the external genitalia.
2. On males palpate the scrotum for testes. If masses are present, transilluminate.

Lower Extremities

1. Note alignment of legs and skin condition.
2. Note alignment of feet. Inspect toes and longitudinal arch.
3. Check range of motion of hips, knees, ankles.
4. Palpate the dorsalis pedis pulse.
5. Gain cooperation with reflex hammer. Elicit plantar, Achilles, and patellar reflexes.

Examining Young Children

The examination is rewarding and fun. At the end you will have made a new friend.

Objective Data

Sequence	Selected Photos

The Adolescent

The sequence for the examination is the head-to-toe format described in the adult section. Recall that the major task of adolescence is developing a self-identity. The adolescent is increasingly self-conscious and introspective. For a well-person exam, keep the adolescent in street clothes and work around them.

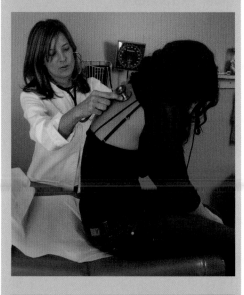

Position Sitting Up

Proceed with the head, eyes, ears, neck, and thoracic exam with the adolescent upright at the edge of the exam table.

Position Supine

Conduct the cardiac, abdomen, and lower extremity examination next.

For the inguinal area place a drape over the lower abdomen and ask the adolescent to unzip and lower the jeans under the drape. Pant legs can be pulled up to examine the lower legs and feet.

CHAPTER 29

Bedside Assessment and Electronic Health Recording

In a hospital setting the patient does not require a complete head-to-toe physical examination during every 24-hour stay. He or she *does* require a consistent specialized examination at least every 8 hours that focuses on certain parameters. Note that some measurements such as daily weights, abdominal girth, or the circumference of a limb must be taken very carefully. The utility of such measurements depends entirely on the consistency of the procedure from nurse to nurse.

Also remember that many assessments must be done frequently throughout the course of a shift. This chapter outlines the initial assessment that will allow you to get to know your patient. As you perform this sequence, take note of anything that will need continuous monitoring, such as an abnormal blood pressure or pulse oximetry reading, or abnormal or adventitious breath sounds. If there is no protocol in place for a particular assessment situation, then decide for yourself how often you need to check on the person's status; it is very easy to be distracted by ringing bells and alarms as the shift progresses, but your own judgment about a patient's needs is just as important.

The need for multiple assessments of each patient highlights the need for efficiency in the hospital setting. Your assessments must be thorough and accurate, yet you must be able to complete them rapidly without seeming hurried.

The basic assessment applies to adults in medical, surgical, and cardiac step-down care areas. Each assessment must then be specialized to each adult, and the findings must be integrated into your complete knowledge base regarding the patient. This includes what you read in the chart, what you hear in report, and the results of any laboratory tests and diagnostic imaging that are available.

Sequence	Selected Photos

Help the person into bed. The patient is in bed with the bed at a comfortable level for the examiner.

The Health History

On your way into the room, verify that any necessary markers or flags are in place at the doorway regarding conditions such as isolation precautions, latex allergies, or fall precautions. Once in the room, introduce yourself as the patient's nurse for the next 8 (or 12) hours.

Make direct eye contact, and do not allow yourself to be distracted by intravenous (IV) pumps or other equipment as you ask how he or she is feeling and how he or she spent the previous shift. Refer to what you have heard from the previous shift in the process of your own questioning; this alleviates the person's frustration at answering the same questions every time with a new staff member. Assess for pain: "Are you currently having any pain or discomfort?" You should know when the last pain medication was given and what physician orders are written. Determine if further dosing is needed or if you need to contact the physician. Knowing the written orders, confirm settings on the patient-controlled analgesia (PCA) pump or epidural setting if in place. Confirm IV solution hanging matches orders for rate and type.

Sequence

Selected Photos

Wash your hands in the patient's presence. Offer water as a courtesy but also note the physical data this gives you: the person's ability to hear, to follow directions, to cross the midline, and especially, to swallow. As you collect this and subsequent history, note data on the General Appearance in the following list. Complete your initial overview by verifying that the correct name band has been applied to the wrist.

General Appearance

1. Facial expression: Appropriate to the situation.
2. Body position: Relaxed and comfortable or tense, in pain.
3. Level of consciousness: Alert and oriented, attentive to your questions, responds appropriately.
4. Skin color: Even tone consistent with racial heritage.
5. Nutritional status: Weight appears in healthy range, fat distribution even, hydration appears healthy.
6. Speech: Articulation clear and understandable, pattern fluent and even, content appropriate.
7. Hearing: Responses and facial expression consistent with what you have said.
8. Personal hygiene: Ability to attend to hair, makeup, shaving.

Measurement

1. Measure baseline vital signs (VS) now: Temperature, pulse, respirations, blood pressure (BP). Note which arm to avoid for BP because of surgery, IV access. Collect and document VS more frequently if patient is unstable or if patient condition changes. Know that VS are the ultimate responsibility of the nurse—the nursing assistant is not responsible for interpretation.
2. Pulse oximetry—Maintain ≥92%. Check oxygen use at least first 24 hours after surgery or as ordered. May need to monitor continuously if patient is lethargic or on a PCA or epidural.
3. Rate pain level on a 1-to-10 scale at this and every subsequent visit or VS measure. Note patient's ability to tolerate pain.
4. If pain medication given, note response in 15 minutes for IV administration or 1 hour for oral dosing.

Sequence	Selected Photos

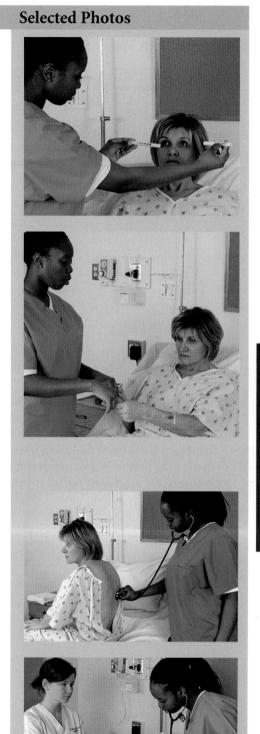

Neurologic System

1. Eyes open spontaneously to name.
2. Motor response is strong and equal bilaterally.
3. Verbal response makes sense; speech is clear and articulate.
4. Pupil size in mm and reaction, R and L.
5. Muscle strength, R and L upper, using hand grips.
6. Muscle strength, R and L lower, pushing feet against your palms.
7. Any ptosis, facial droop.
8. Sensation (omit unless indicated).
9. Communication.
10. Ability to swallow.

Respiratory System

1. Oxygen by mask, nasal prongs, check fitting.
2. Note FIo_2.
3. Respiratory effort.
4. Auscultate breath sounds, comparing side to side:
   Posterior lobes: Left upper, right upper, left lower, right lower.
   NOTE: If patient is unable to sit up, have another nurse hold patient side to side.
   Anterior lobes: Right upper, left upper, right middle and lower, left lower.
5. Cough and deep breathe. Any mucus? Check color and amount.
6. Incentive spirometer if ordered—Encourage patient to use every hour for 10 inspirations. If pulse oximetry percentage or respiratory rate drops, encourage use every 15 minutes.

Objective Data

Sequence	Selected Photos

Cardiovascular System

1. Auscultate rhythm at apex: Regular, irregular? (Do NOT listen over gown.)
2. Check apical pulse against radial pulse, noting perfusion of all beats.
3. Assess heart sounds in all auscultatory areas: First with diaphragm, repeat with bell.
4. Check capillary refill for prompt return.

5. Check pretibial edema.
6. Palpate posterior tibial pulse, right and left.
7. Palpate dorsalis pedis pulse, right and left.
   NOTE: Be prepared to assess pulses in the lower extremities by Doppler imaging if you cannot find them by palpation.
8. Verify that the proper IV solution is hanging and flowing at the proper rate according to the physician's orders and your own assessment of the patient's needs.

Skin

1. Note skin color, consistent with person's racial or ethnic heritage.
2. Palpate skin temperature; expect warm and dry.
3. Pinch up a fold of skin under the clavicle or on the forearm to note mobility and turgor.
4. Note skin integrity, any lesions, and the condition of any dressings. Note any bleeding or infection, but do not change dressing until after physical examination.
5. Date IV site, and note surrounding skin condition.
6. Complete any standardized scales used to quantify the risk for skin breakdown.
7. Verify that any air loss or pressure loss surfaces being used are properly applied and operating at the correct settings.

Objective Data

Sequence	Selected Photos

Abdomen

1. Assess contour of abdomen: Flat, rounded, protuberant.
2. Listen to bowel sounds in all four quadrants.
3. Check any drainage tube placement for color and amount of drainage and insertion site integrity.
4. Inquire whether passing flatus or stool.
5. Knowing diet orders, determine if patient is tolerating ice chips, liquids, solids. Order correct diet as it is advanced. Note if patient is at high risk for nutrition deficit.

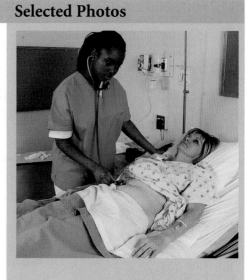

Genitourinary

1. Inquire whether voiding regularly. NOTE: Needs to void within 4 to 6 hours after surgery.
2. Check urine for color, clarity.
3. If Foley catheter in place, check color, quantity, clarity of urine with every VS check.
4. If urine output is below the expected amount, perform a bladder scan according to agency protocol. Is the problem in the production of urine or its retention?

Activity

1. Know activity orders; if on bed rest, head of bed should be ≥15 degrees. Is patient at high risk for skin breakdown?
2. Sequential compression devices (SCDs), thromboembolic disease (TED) hose, foot pumps need to be hooked up and turned on. Must be on patient 22 out of 24 hours to be effective.
3. If ambulatory, assist patient to sitting up level and move to chair.
4. Note any assistance needed, how tolerates movement, distance walked to chair, ability to turn.
5. Assess need for any ambulatory aid or equipment.
6. Complete any standardized scales used to quantify the patient's risk for falling.
7. Initiate or continue appropriate Plan of Care. Check if any core measures apply, such as heart failure. Implement core measures as appropriate.
8. Complete initial assessment to document into computer when finished.
9. Note examination findings requiring immediate attention:
   - High or low BP (≤90 or ≥160 mm Hg systolic)
   - High or low temperature (≤97° or ≥100° F)
   - High or low heart rate (≤60 or ≥90 bpm)
   - High or low respirations (≤12 or ≥28/min)
   - O₂ saturations ≤92%
   - Low or no urine output (≤30 mL/hr or ≤240 mL/8 hr)
   - Dark amber or bloody urine (except for urology patients)
   - Postop nausea and/or vomiting
   - Surgical pain not controlled with medication. Any other unusual pain such as chest pain
   - Bleeding
   - Altered level of consciousness (LOC), confusion, or difficult to arouse
   - Sudden restlessness and/or anxiety

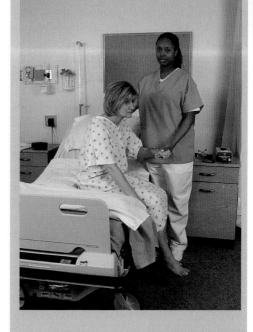

Objective Data

ELECTRONIC HEALTH RECORDING

(Potter, Perry, Stockert, Hall, 2015.)

The use of technology at the bedside extends far beyond the standard equipment. Most hospitals or clinics use a basic or a comprehensive electronic health record (EHR) system. EHRs replace the paper medical record, placing all relevant patient information in an easily accessible electronic system. EHRs do not include billing and scheduling systems, but focus instead on patient information. The Institute of Medicine report, *Crossing the Quality Chasm,* identified the importance of EHRs, which is the ability to access a lifetime of data to treat patients with chronic illness. Traditional medical records may be in a variety of locations, limiting availability; and poor penmanship can make older medical records illegible.

The federal government encourages the adoption and meaningful use of EHRs through the Health Information Technology for Economic and Clinical Health Act of 2009. The use of EHRs has increased steadily since 2008, with a threefold increase of basic EHR adoption from 2009 to 2012.[2] Basic EHR adoption includes use of the EHR in at least one clinical unit, whereas comprehensive adoption requires each function (e.g., clinical notes, medication records, consultation requests, nursing orders, and laboratory results) to be adopted by all clinical units. EHR adoption is more prevalent among larger community and academic medical centers. Rural hospital use of EHR systems has increased, but resource and infrastructure constraints have limited adoption. By the end of 2013, 89% of rural hospitals planned to adopt EHRs for meaningful use.

Patient Safety

The meaningful use of EHRs, which include physician order entry and clinical decision support, may increase patient safety and quality care. EHRs allow all providers, regardless of geographic location, to access the health information, place orders, and receive timely patient status updates. No longer does a provider have to be on the clinical unit to retrieve test results, vital signs, or the most recent nurse's or physician's note. Because of the recent adoption and increased use of EHRs, few research studies exist that identify their overall benefits.[7] As more ambulatory clinics and hospitals adopt comprehensive EHR use, research will continue as to the overall benefit of the automated system.

EHRs are being used to meet The Joint Commission National Patient Safety Goals. The use of computer physician order entry (CPOE) has decreased transcription and prescribing errors.[1] Well-designed EHR systems can notify providers of potential medication interactions, dosage adjustments for renal patients or advanced age, and additional required testing (e.g., laboratory tests). Nurses can benefit from EHR use in medication administration through the use of bar-code scanners, which identify both the patient and the medication. Checklists built into EHR systems can help clinicians identify health care–associated infections or patients at risk for these infections. Checklists have also been used successfully for depression and suicide screening.[11] Although no system is perfect, a well-designed EHR system can increase patient safety when successfully integrated into the workflow of a clinic or hospital. An EHR that is not carefully implemented with usability in mind can lead to unintended consequences, including risks to patient safety.[10] As EHR use becomes the standard of care, more research is needed to determine the specific factors that contribute to patient safety and increased quality of care.

USING SBAR FOR STAFF COMMUNICATION

Throughout this text we have used the SOAP acronym (**S**ubjective, **O**bjective, **A**ssessment, **P**lan) to organize assessment findings into written or charted communication. Now we turn to organizing assessment data for *verbal* communication (e.g., calls to physicians, nursing shift reports, patient transfers to other units). For all these verbal reports we use the SBAR framework: **S**ituation, **B**ackground, **A**ssessment, **R**ecommendation.

SBAR was first developed in the U.S. military to standardize communication and prevent misunderstandings. In the hospital, communications errors contribute to most sentinel events that are reported.[13] Thus SBAR is used at health care facilities all over the country to improve verbal communication and reduce medical errors.[14] SBAR is a standardized framework to transmit important in-the-moment information. Using SBAR will keep your message concise and focused on the immediate problem yet give your colleague enough information to grasp the current situation and make a decision. To formulate your verbal message, use these four points:

Situation. What is happening right now? Why are you calling? State your name, your unit, patient's name, room number, patient's problem, when it happened or when it started, how severe it is.

Background. Do not recite the patient's full history since admission. Do state the data pertinent to this moment's problem: admitting diagnosis, when admitted, and appropriate immediate assessment data (e.g., vital signs, pulse oximetry, change in mental status, allergies, current medications, IV fluids, laboratory results).

Assessment. What do YOU think is happening in regard to the current problem? If you do not know, at least state which body system you think is involved. How severe is the problem?

Recommendation. What do you want the physician to do to improve the patient's situation? Here you offer probable solutions. Order more pain medication? Come and assess the patient?

Review the following examples of SBAR communication.

Situation 1

S: This is Bill on the Oncology Unit. I'm calling about Daniel Meyers in room 8417. He is refusing all oral medications as of now.

B: Daniel is a 59 y.o. male with multiple myeloma. He was admitted for an autologous stem cell transplant and received chemotherapy 10 days ago. Now he is 5 days' post auto transplant. Vital signs are stable, alert, and oriented; IVs are dextrose 5% water. As of 1 hour ago, he is feeling extreme nausea and vomiting, refusing all food and oral meds.

A: I think the chemo he had pre-transplant is hitting him now. His uncontrolled nausea isn't going away in next few days.

R: I'm concerned that he cannot stay hydrated and he needs his meds. I need you to please change the IV rate and change all scheduled oral meds to IV. I also think we need to add an additional PRN antiemetic. If he continues to refuse food, we may have to consider starting him on TPN/lipids.

Situation 2

S: This is Andrea. I'm the nurse taking care of Max Goodson in 6443. His condition has changed, and his most recent vital signs show a significant drop in blood pressure.

B: Max is 40 years old with a history of alcoholism. He was admitted through the ED last night with abdominal pain and a suspected GI bleed. His BPs have been running in the 130s/80s. He just had a large amount of liquid maroon stool and reported feeling dizzy. I rechecked his vitals; his BP is 88/50, and heart rate is 104.

A: I'm worried that his GI bleed is getting worse.

R: Will you order a STAT complete blood count and place an order to transfuse red blood cells if his hemoglobin is below 8 g? Also can you please come and assess? I think we may need to drop an NG tube and lavage him.

BIBLIOGRAPHY

1. Abramson, E. L., Barron, Y., Quaresimo, J., et al. (2011). Electronic prescribing within an electronic health record reduces ambulatory prescribing errors. *TJC J Qual Patient Safety, 37*, 470-478.

2. Charles, D., King, J., Patel, V., et al. (2013). *Adoption of electronic health record systems among U.S. non-federal acute care hospitals: 2008-2012*. ONC Data Brief, no 9. Washington, D.C.: Office of the National Coordinator for Health Information Technology.

3. Gallagher, L. A. (2013). Accessing and sharing data to avoid security risks. *Nurse Pract, 38*(5), 8-11.

4. Garnica, M.P. (2011). CPOE: an essential tool for evidence-based practice. *Nurse Pract, 36*(5), 12-15.

5. Institute of Medicine. (2001). *Crossing the quality chasm: a new health system for the 21st century*. Washington, D.C.: National Academies Press.

6. Institute of Medicine. (2011). *Health IT and patient safety: building safer systems for better care*. Washington, D.C.: National Academies Press.

7. Kelley, T. F., Brandon, D. H., & Docherty, S. L. (2011). Electronic nursing documentation as a strategy to improve quality of patient care. *J Nurs Scholarsh, 43*(2), 154-162.

8. Klein, C. A. Electronic health records 101. (2011). *Nurse Pract, 36*(1), 15-18.

9. McBride, S., Delaney, J. M., & Tietze, M. (2012). Health information technology and nursing. *Am J Nurs 112*(8), 36-43.

10. Middleton, B., Bloomrosen, M., Dente, M. A., et al. (2013). Enhancing patient safety and quality of care by improving the usability of electronic health record systems. *J Am Med Inform Assoc 20*, e2-e8.

11. Radecki, R. P., & Sittig, D. F. (2011). Application of electronic health records to the Joint Commission's 2011 national patient safety goals. *JAMA, 306*, 92-93.

12. Sittig, D. F., & Singh, H. (2012). Electronic health records and national patient-safety goals. *N Engl J Med, 367*(19), 1854-1859.

13. The Joint Commission. (2008). *Hand-off communications: standardized approach*. Accessed July 15, 2010, from www.jointcommission.org/AccreditationAmbulatoryCare/Standards/09_FAQs/NPSG/Communication/NPSG.02.05.01/.

14. Thomas, C. M., Bertram, E., & Johnson, D. (2009). The SBAR communication technique. *Nurse Educ, 34*(4), 176-180.

CHAPTER 30

The Pregnant Woman

STRUCTURE AND FUNCTION

30-1

THE ENDOCRINE PLACENTA

So much happens inside the pregnant uterus before the new family can feel fetal movements (Fig. 30-1).

When the fertilized ovum enters the uterus, it is called the **blastocyst** and continues to divide, differentiate, and grow rapidly. Specialized cells in the blastocyst produce human chorionic gonadotropin (hCG), which stimulates the corpus luteum to continue making progesterone. The blastocyst implants into the wall of the uterus, which may cause a small amount of vaginal bleeding. A specialized layer of cells becomes the **placenta,** which produces progesterone to support the pregnancy at 7 weeks and takes over this function completely from the corpus luteum at about 10 weeks.

The placenta functions as an endocrine organ and produces several hormones. These hormones help in the growth and maintenance of the fetus, and they direct changes in the woman's body to prepare for birth and lactation. The hCG stimulates the rise in progesterone during pregnancy, supports the corpus luteum, supports deep implantation of the placenta into the uterine wall, and helps maintain viability of the fetus.[20] Progesterone maintains the endometrium around the fetus, increases the alveoli in the breast, and keeps the uterus in a quiescent state. Estrogen stimulates the duct formation in the breasts, increases the weight of the uterus, and increases certain receptors in the uterus that are important at birth.

The average length of pregnancy is 280 days from the first day of the last menstrual period (LMP), which is equal to 40 weeks, 10 lunar months, or 9 calendar months. Note that this includes the 2 weeks when the follicle was maturing but before conception actually occurred. Pregnancy is divided into three trimesters: (1) the first 12 weeks, (2) from 13 to 27 weeks, and (3) from 28 weeks to delivery.

A woman who is pregnant for the first time is called a **primigravida.** After she delivers she is called a **primipara.** The **multigravida** is a pregnant woman who has previously been pregnant; she is a **multipara** after delivery. Any pregnant woman might be called a *gravida.* Commonly used abbreviations are G (gravida), P (para), T (term), PT (preterm deliveries), A (abortion—missed, therapeutic, voluntary), L (living children). It may be written as G5 T3 PT0 A2 L3.

CHANGES DURING NORMAL PREGNANCY

Pregnancy is diagnosed by three types of signs and symptoms. **Presumptive signs** are those that the woman experiences such as amenorrhea, breast tenderness, nausea, fatigue, and increased urinary frequency. **Probable signs** are those detected by the examiner such as an enlarged uterus. **Positive signs** of pregnancy are those that are direct evidence of the fetus such as the auscultation of fetal heart tones (FHTs) or positive cardiac activity on ultrasound (US).

807

First Trimester

After the blastocyst (developing fertilized ovum) implants in the uterus, the serum hCG becomes positive when it is first detectable in maternal serum at approximately 8 to 11 days after conception.

The following menstrual period is missed, and then hCG can be detected in the urine. Breast tingling and tenderness begin as the rising estrogen levels promote mammary growth and development of the ductal system; progesterone stimulates both the alveolar system and the mammary growth. More than half of all pregnant women have nausea and vomiting. The cause is unclear but may involve the hormonal changes of pregnancy, low blood sugar, gastric overloading, slowed peristalsis, and an enlarging uterus. Fatigue is common and may be related to the initial fall in metabolic rate that occurs in early pregnancy.[21]

Estrogen and possibly progesterone cause hypertrophy of the uterine muscle cells, and uterine blood vessels and lymphatics enlarge. The uterus becomes globular in shape and compresses the bladder, which results in urinary frequency.

Early first-trimester blood pressures (BP) reflect prepregnancy values. In the 7th gestational week BP begins to drop until midpregnancy as a result of falling peripheral vascular resistance. Systemic vascular resistance decreases from the vasodilatory effect of progesterone and prostaglandins and possibly because of the low resistance of the placental bed.[8] The BP gradually returns to the nonpregnant baseline by term.

At the end of 9 weeks the embryonic period ends, and the fetal period begins, at which time major structures are present.[21] FHTs can be heard by Doppler US between 9 and 12 weeks. The uterus may be palpated just above the symphysis pubis at about 12 weeks. See Fig. 30-2 for growth of the uterine fundus during the first trimester.

Second Trimester

After weeks 12 to 16, the nausea, vomiting, fatigue, and urinary frequency of the first trimester improve. The woman recognizes fetal movement ("quickening") at approximately 18 to 20 weeks (the multigravida earlier). Breast enlargement continues, and **colostrum,** the precursor of milk, may be expressed from the nipples. Colostrum is yellow in color and contains more minerals and protein but less sugar and fat than mature milk. It also contains antibodies, which are protective for the newborn during its first days of life until mature milk production begins.[9]

The areolae and nipples darken because estrogen and progesterone have a melanocyte-stimulating effect, and melanocyte-stimulating hormone levels escalate from the 2nd month of pregnancy until delivery. For the same reason the midline of the abdominal skin becomes pigmented and is called the **linea nigra.** You may note **striae gravidarum** ("stretch marks") on the breast, abdomen, and areas of weight gain.

During the second trimester systolic BP may be 2 to 8 mm Hg lower, and diastolic BP 5 to 15 mm Hg lower than

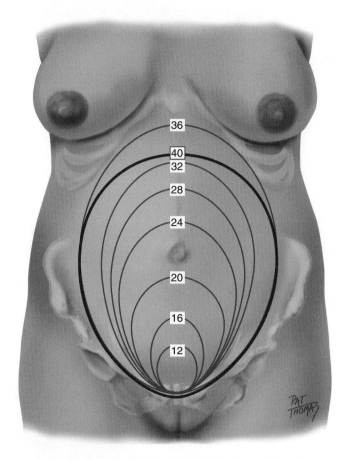

HEIGHT OF FUNDUS AT WEEKS OF GESTATION

30-2

prepregnancy levels.[9] This drop is most pronounced at 20 weeks and may cause symptoms of dizziness and faintness, particularly after rising quickly. Stomach displacement from the enlarging uterus and altered esophageal sphincter and gastric tone as a result of progesterone predispose the woman to heartburn. Intestines are also displaced by the growing uterus, and tone and motility are decreased because of the action of progesterone, often causing constipation. The gallbladder, possibly resulting from the action of progesterone on its smooth muscle, empties sluggishly and may become distended. The stasis of bile, together with the increased cholesterol saturation of pregnancy, predisposes some women to gallstone formation.

Progesterone and, to a lesser degree, estrogen cause increased respiratory effort during pregnancy by increasing tidal volume. Hemoglobin, and therefore oxygen-carrying capacity, also increase. Increased tidal volume causes a slight drop in partial pressure of arterial carbon dioxide ($Paco_2$), causing the woman to occasionally have dyspnea.[9]

With the rise of hCG in the first trimester, there is a transient decrease in thyroid-stimulating hormone (TSH) levels between 8 and 14 weeks' gestation. Plasma iodine levels decrease, allowing a transient increase in thyroid gland size in approximately 15% of pregnant women.

Cutaneous blood flow is augmented during pregnancy, caused by decreased vascular resistance, presumably helping to dissipate heat generated by increased metabolism. Gums may hypertrophy and bleed easily. This condition is called **gingivitis** or **epulis of pregnancy** because of growth of the capillaries of the gums.[9] For the same reason nosebleeds may occur more frequently than usual.

FHTs are audible by fetoscope (as opposed to Doppler imaging) at approximately 17 to 19 weeks. The fetal outline is palpable through the abdominal wall at approximately 20 weeks. Fig. 30-2 illustrates the growth of the uterine fundus during the second trimester.

Third Trimester

Blood volume, which increased rapidly during the 2nd trimester, peaks in the middle of the 3rd trimester at approximately 45% greater than the prepregnancy level and plateaus thereafter. This volume is greater in multiple gestations.[8] Erythrocyte mass increases by 20% to 30% (caused by an increase in erythropoiesis and mediated by progesterone, estrogen, and placental chorionic somatomammotropin). However, plasma volume increases slightly more, causing a slight hemodilution and a small drop in hematocrit. BP slowly rises again to approximately the prepregnancy level.[9]

Uterine enlargement causes the diaphragm to rise and the shape of the rib cage to widen at the base. Decreased space for lung expansion may cause a sense of shortness of breath. The rising diaphragm displaces the heart up and to the left. Cardiac output, stroke volume, and force of contraction are increased. The pulse rate rises 15 to 20 beats/min.[8] Because of the increase in blood volume, a functional systolic murmur, grade 2/6 or less, can be heard in more than 95% of pregnant women.[8]

Edema of the lower extremities may occur as a result of the enlarging fetus impeding venous return and from lower colloid osmotic pressure. The edema worsens with dependency, such as prolonged standing. Varicosities, which have a familial tendency, may form or enlarge from progesterone-induced vascular relaxation. Also causing varicosities is the engorgement caused by the weight of the full uterus compressing the inferior vena cava and the vessels of the pelvic area, resulting in venous congestion in the legs, vulva, and rectum. Hemorrhoids are varicosities of the rectum that are worsened by constipation, which occurs from relaxation of the large bowel by progesterone.

Progressive lordosis (an inward curvature of the lumbar spine) occurs to compensate for the shifting center of balance caused by the anteriorly enlarging uterus, predisposing the woman to backaches (Fig. 30-3). Slumping of the shoulders and anterior flexion of the neck from the increasing weight of the breasts may cause aching and numbness of the arms and hands as a result of compression of the median and ulnar nerves in the arm,[21] commonly referred to as *carpal tunnel syndrome.*

Approximately 2 weeks before going into labor, the primigravida experiences engagement (also called *lightening* or *dropping),* when the fetal head moves down into the pelvis (Fig. 30-4). Symptoms include a lower-appearing and smaller-measuring fundus, urinary frequency, increased vaginal

30-3

secretions from increased pelvic congestion, and increased lung capacity. In the multigravida the fetus may move down at any time in late pregnancy or often not until labor. In preparation for labor the cervix begins to thin (efface) and open (dilate). A thick **mucous plug,** formed in the cervix as a mechanical barrier during pregnancy, is expelled at variable times before or during labor. Between 37 and 42 weeks the pregnancy is considered *term.* After 42 weeks the pregnancy is considered *postterm.*

Determining Weeks of Gestation

The expected date of delivery, or EDD, being 280 days from the first day of the LMP, may be calculated by using **Nägele's rule**, that is, determine the first day of the last normal

30-4

menstrual period (normal in timing, length, premenstrual symptoms, and amount of flow and cramping). Using the first day of the LMP, add 7 days, and subtract 3 months. This date is the EDD. This date can then be used with a pregnancy wheel on which the EDD arrow is set; the present date will be pointing to the present week's gestation. The number of weeks of gestation also is estimated by physical examination, by measurement of the hCG, and most accurately by ultrasound (US) +/−2 to 3 days.

❖ DEVELOPMENTAL COMPETENCE

The number of teen pregnancies in the United States has decreased 42% since 1990, primarily because of improved contraceptive use. However, each year about 750,000 teens ages 15 to 19 years become pregnant. Two thirds of these teen pregnancies occur in older teens ages 18 to 19 years; and 82% of teen pregnancies are unplanned.[13] African-American and Latina teens have the highest rate of pregnancies; however, the pregnancy rate among African-American teens decreased 48% since 1990.[13] Many of these pregnancies pose serious medical risks for both mother and fetus such as toxemia and low-birth-weight infants; it is unclear whether these risks are the result of biologic or social factors, prolonged labor, or postpartum complications.

Other risks for the pregnant adolescent are psychosocial. This young woman is at risk for the downward cycle of poverty beginning with an incomplete education, failure to limit family size, and continuing with failure to establish a vocation and become independent. She may be unprepared emotionally to be a mother. Her social situation may be stressful. She may not have the support of her family, her partner, or his family. Medical risks for the pregnant adolescent are generally related to poverty, inadequate nutrition, substance abuse, and sometimes sexually transmitted infections (STI), poor health before pregnancy, and emotional and physical abuse from her partner, family, and peers.

On the other hand, many Generation X-ers have delayed childbearing, and since the advent of assisted fertility, more women older than 35 years are now becoming pregnant. Women after age 35 years are often more prepared emotionally and financially to parent; however, they are more at risk for infertility and age-related anomalies. Fertility declines with advancing maternal age because of a decrease in the number and health of eggs to be ovulated, a decrease in ovulation, endometriosis, and early-onset menopause.

The risk for Down syndrome increases from about 1 in 1250 at age 25 to 1 in 1000 at age 30, 1 in 400 at age 35, 1 in 100 at age 40, and 1 in 30 at age 45.[25] Women ages 35 years and older or with a history of a genetic abnormality are offered genetic counseling and the options of prenatal diagnostic screening tests. Two invasive prenatal diagnostic options are chorionic villi sampling (CVS) performed between weeks 11 and 13 and amniocentesis between weeks 15 and 20 in which a small amount of amniotic fluid is removed to analyze genetic makeup. Both are associated with a small risk for complications and miscarriage. Noninvasive tests include US nuchal translucency that measures the clear space in the tissues of the back of the baby's neck. Prenatal screening may include a fetal anatomy US during the second trimester and maternal serum marker screening. All these should be an informed choice after pretest counseling.

Because the incidence of chronic diseases increases with age, women older than 35 years who are pregnant may have medical complications such as diabetes, obesity, and hypertension.[9] The increased incidence of hypertension causes an increase in placental abruption and preeclampsia. Hypertension in turn increases intrauterine growth restriction (IUGR). More women of advanced maternal age have placenta previa, placental abruption, uterine rupture, and cesarean deliveries. They have more spontaneous abortions, in part because of the increase in genetically abnormal embryos.

🌐 CULTURE AND GENETICS

Genetic disorders are diseases or defects that the baby inherits from the genes or chromosomes of one or both parents. As mentioned previously, the risk of having certain chromosomal disorders such as Down syndrome increases as a woman ages. Or, parents may be carriers of genetic defects: cystic fibrosis is an inherited disorder of respiratory and gastrointestinal sequelae; Jews of Eastern European descent may have risk of having children with Tay-Sachs, a metabolic disorder; African-American parents may pass sickle cell anemia on to a child. Also, a pregnant woman may be exposed to toxins such as alcohol or cigarette smoke that increase risk of birth defects. It is beyond our scope here to describe all aspects of genetic counseling. There are many options for prenatal testing either before or after conception. It is important that the parents have an informed choice about whether to pursue such testing and that their choice be respected.

Although the rate of teenage pregnancies has decreased in the United States, racial disparities exist, with a rate of 51.5/1000 African-American teens versus 23.5/1000 White teens.[15] Racial differences in obesity also exist; 25.4% of African-American teens and 15.4% of White teens are overweight or obese. Evidence shows that, when pregnant teens are also obese, different mother and baby outcomes exist based on race.[14] Postpartum hemorrhage occurred almost 2 times as often in Black obese teens than in Black normal-weight teens; this did not occur in White obese teens. Both White and Black obese teens had increased risk of gestational hypertension, and infant complications increased in overweight or obese White teenagers.[14] With the obesity epidemic increasing in the United States, it is important to help pregnant teens find healthy food sources and safe physical activity.

Outcomes among pregnant women with gestational diabetes also differ by race and ethnicity.[27] One large California study showed a high prevalence of gestational diabetes among

Asian (10%) and Hispanic (6.9%) women, yet they were the least likely to have adverse perinatal outcomes. Black women had higher risk of preeclampsia, neonatal hypoglycemia, and preterm delivery <37 weeks' gestation, whereas Asian women had lower risk of cesarean delivery, large-for–gestational age babies, and neonatal respiratory distress syndrome.[27] Explanations may include sociocultural differences that affect glycemic control, genetic variability, access to quantity and quality of prenatal care, and sociocultural support structures and traditions.[27]

SUBJECTIVE DATA

1. Menstrual history
2. Gynecologic history
3. Obstetric history
4. Current pregnancy
5. Medical history
6. Review of systems
7. Nutritional history
8. Environment/hazards

Examiner Asks	Rationale
1. Menstrual history • When was the first day of your last menstrual period (LMP) that was normal in timing, premenstrual symptoms, length, amount of flow, cramping? • Number of days in cycle? Certainty of LMP?	Using Nägele's rule, calculate the expected date of delivery (EDD) with this date. With a pregnancy wheel, determine the current number of weeks of gestation. LMP may be uncertain because of hormone contraceptives or irregular menses.
2. Gynecologic history • Ever had surgery of the cervix (colposcopy, biopsy, loop electrosurgical excision [LEEP] procedure)? Uterus? Fallopian tubes?	Cervical surgery may increase the risk for cervical insufficiency, preterm cervical dilation, and preterm delivery. Uterine surgery increases the risk for uterine rupture during pregnancy and labor.
• Pap tests: Any history of abnormal? Tested for HPV?	Because more women delay childbearing, there may be an increase in gynecologic cancers during pregnancy.
• Any history of genital herpes, gonorrhea, chlamydia, syphilis, pelvic inflammatory disease (PID)?	STIs increase the risk for premature rupture of membranes, preterm labor/preterm delivery (PTL/PTD), postpartum maternal and fetal infections, or birth defects (herpes).
• Have you been tested for HIV? When? What was the result? Ever had a blood transfusion? Used a needle to take street drugs? Had a sexual partner who had any HIV risk factors?	HIV screening *must* be offered to all pregnant women to decrease the risk for transmission to the fetus. Breastfeeding is contraindicated for the HIV-positive mother because the virus is in the breast milk.
• What is your sexual preference?	Woman with same-sex partner may use assisted reproduction; thus important to support this couple.
• Have you had a mammogram, breast biopsy, breast surgery?	As U.S. women delay childbearing, incidence of breast cancer may increase, posing difficult treatment options.
3. Obstetric history* • Number of times pregnant? Number of term or preterm deliveries? Preterm labor? Number of spontaneous miscarriages, elective abortions, or ectopic pregnancies? • How were previous pregnancies and deliveries for you?	An obstetric history helps guide prenatal care. The subjective quality of previous experiences affects current pregnancy.

*This information is recorded best in a grid format. See sample forms in the Laboratory Manual. It is separated here to include the rationale.

Subjective Data

Examiner Asks	Rationale
• Ever had a cesarean section? If so, what was the indication? What type of uterine incision was made? Have you ever had a vaginal birth after a cesarean section (VBAC)?	The vertical, or "classical," incision has increased risk for rupture and mandates that all deliveries be by cesarean birth. The "low transverse" or horizontal incision carries a low risk, and subsequent deliveries may be vaginal. Note that the direction of the skin scar does not necessarily tell how the uterus was incised.
4. Current pregnancy • Was the pregnancy planned? How do you feel about it? How does the baby's father or your partner feel about the pregnancy? Other family members?	The woman may need help in gathering her support group. Inviting significant others to future visits affirms their importance and supports involvement.
• Experienced any vaginal bleeding? When? How much? What color? Accompanied by any pain? Occurs after sex? (Affirm here that sex is safe during pregnancy.)	Vaginal bleeding may indicate threatened abortion, cervicitis, or ectopic pregnancy in 1st trimester and must be investigated. However, a friable cervix may bleed harmlessly after sex and not hurt the fetus.
• How have you been feeling?	Breast tenderness or fatigue. Nausea and vomiting usually begin between weeks 4 and 5, peak between weeks 8 and 12, and resolve. Persistent and severe nausea and vomiting are hyperemesis.
• Experienced abdominal pain? When? Where in your abdomen? Accompanied by vaginal bleeding?	Common causes in early pregnancy are spontaneous abortion, ectopic pregnancy, urinary tract infection (UTI), and round ligament discomfort. Late pregnancy causes are premature labor, placental abruption, and HELLP syndrome (see Table 30-1, Preeclampsia, p. 826).
• Experiencing any edema? Where and under what circumstances?	In the 3rd trimester differentiate the normal weight-dependent edema of pregnancy from the edema of preeclampsia.
• How does the baby move on a daily basis?	Fetal movement is an excellent indicator of fetal health. In the third trimester clinicians assign women to count fetal movements.
• What are your plans for breastfeeding this baby?	Arrange reading, classes, and other support for the woman who is breastfeeding for the first time or the woman with an unsuccessful earlier experience.
5. Medical history • Do you take any prescribed, over-the-counter, or herbal medications?	Screen all medications to establish safety during pregnancy.
• Do you have allergies to medications or foods? If so, which type of reaction? Latex?	Prevents prescribing error.
• Ever had German measles (rubella)?	This disease is highly teratogenic, especially in 1st trimester. Instruct the woman who has not had rubella to avoid small children who are ill.
• Ever had chickenpox?	Rarely varicella causes congenital anomalies. The nonimmune woman should avoid exposure.

Examiner Asks	Rationale
• Do you smoke cigarettes? How many? For how many years? Ever tried to quit? Drink any alcohol? How many times per week? Use any street drugs?	Explain the danger of these substances in pregnancy. Smoking increases the risk for ectopic pregnancy, spontaneous abortion, low birth weight, prematurity, preterm premature rupture of membranes, pregnancy-induced HTN, placental abruption, and sudden infant death syndrome. Alcohol increases the risk to the fetus for fetal alcohol syndrome (see Table 13-2, p. 274). Cocaine use is associated with congenital anomalies, a fourfold increased risk for abruptio placentae, and fetal addiction. Narcotic-addicted infants may have developmental delays or behavioral disturbances. Refer to a counseling/support program and periodic toxicology screening. Refer to a smoking-cessation program.
• Do you have a regular exercise program? Which type?	Regular exercise in pregnancy may reduce risk for pregnancy-induced HTN.
• Has your vitamin D level been checked?	Vitamin D is essential for maternal response to the calcium demands of the fetus for growth and bone development. Daily vitamin D supplementation is recommended during pregnancy.[35]
6. Review of systems • Your weight before pregnancy? (Calculate BMI). • When did you last see the dentist? Need any dental work?	Baseline needed to evaluate changes. Gums may be puffy or bleed easily in pregnancy, predisposing caries. Poor dental hygiene can lead to PTD, low-birth-weight babies, and neonatal death. Dental care is important part of prenatal care.
• Have you had HTN or kidney disease?	Renal disease or HTN increases risk for preeclampsia.
• Do you have diabetes? On oral hypoglycemics, insulin injection, or insulin pump? Did you have diabetes during a previous pregnancy?	Diabetes is carefully managed during pregnancy to avoid serious complications such as a macrosomic infant and cesarean delivery. Consider early screening and nutritional interventions.
• Have you had UTIs?	The hormonal milieu of pregnancy predisposes the woman to UTIs. Pregnancy may mask their symptoms. A serious UTI may irritate the uterus, threatening preterm labor. Educate the woman in measures to prevent UTIs.
• Have you had depression or any other mental disorder?	Increases risk for pregnancy and postpartum depression. Help her to prepare a support network. Counseling helps navigate the developmental challenges of becoming a mother.
• Do you feel safe in your relationship or home environment?	Intimate partner violence may escalate during pregnancy.

Examiner Asks	Rationale
• Are you in a relationship with someone who physically or emotionally abuses or threatens you?	Most women will not freely offer this information. You must ask these questions at the appropriate time and in a nonthreatening manner.
• Has anyone forced you to have sexual activities against your will?	Incest or other abuse increases risk for dysfunctional labor and cesarean delivery.
7. Nutritional history • Do you follow a special diet? Are you vegetarian? Eat fish? What types? Teach her to avoid sea fish (swordfish, mackerel) because of mercury concentration. Also teach her to avoid raw eggs, soft cheeses, and unpasteurized dairy foods and sliced meats from delicatessens because of risk of *Listeria, Salmonella,* and toxoplasmosis.	A special diet may have nutritional risk. Help achieve adequate nutrition within the confines of her diet. Refer to dietitian.
• Any food intolerance? Or food craving? Taking prenatal vitamins, folic acid, iron?	A food intolerance, such as lactose intolerance limiting calcium intake, might affect the woman's and fetus's nutrition.
8. Environment/hazards • What is your occupation? What are the physical demands of the work? Are you exposed to any strong odors, chemicals, radiation, or other harmful substances? Or potentially harmful physical contact?	Hazards? Possible teratogenic exposures? The woman who is rubella nonimmune may be advised not to continue working in a daycare center. Suitability for pregnancy? The woman whose job requires long hours of standing may be disabled early if signs of PTL occur.
• Do you consider your food and housing adequate?	Refer for state and federal programs to help with food, housing, or other needs.
• How do you wear your seatbelt when driving?	For maternal and fetal safety, instruct the woman to place the lap belt below the uterus and to use the shoulder strap.

OBJECTIVE DATA

PREPARATION

The initial examination for pregnancy is often a woman's first pelvic examination, and many women are extremely anxious. Alternatively the woman may not know for certain whether she is pregnant, and she may be anxious about the findings. Verbally prepare the woman for what will happen during the examination before touching her. Save the pelvic examination for last; by that time the woman will be more comfortable with your gentle, informing manner. Communicate all findings as you go along to demonstrate your respectful affirmation of her control and responsibility in her own health and health care and that of her child.

Ask the woman to empty her bladder before the examination, reserving a clean-catch specimen for dipping for protein and glucose and for urinalysis, if required. Before the examination weigh her on the office scale and compute the BMI. Provide the woman with an escort or chaperone during examinations.

Give the woman a gown and drape. Begin the examination with the woman sitting on the exam table, wearing the gown, her lap covered by a drape.

EQUIPMENT NEEDED

Stethoscope, BP cuff
Centimeter measuring tape
Doppler fetal heart rate (FHR) monitor and gel
Reflex hammer
Urine collection containers
Dipsticks for checking urine for glucose and protein
Equipment needed for pelvic examination as noted in Chapter 26.

Help her lie down for the breast, abdominal, and extremity examination. Use the lithotomy position for the pelvic examination (see Chapter 26). Help her to a seated position to check her BP. In the 2nd and 3rd trimesters keep her back elevated to a 30- or 45-degree angle. This increases comfort by avoiding the compression of the descending aorta and inferior vena cava by the pregnant uterus.

Normal Range of Findings	Abnormal Findings

General Survey

Observe the woman's state of nourishment; a healthy BMI is 19 to 25. Note her grooming, posture, mood, and affect, which reflect her mental state. Throughout the examination observe her maturity and ability to attend and learn so you can plan your teaching of the information that she needs to successfully complete a healthy pregnancy.

Undernourished or obese. A 1st-trimester weight loss of ≥5% prepregnancy weight is worrisome and may indicate hyperemesis gravidarum.

Poor grooming, a slumped posture, and a flat affect may be signs of depression and risk for postpartum depression. Poor grooming may reflect a lack of resources and need for a social service referral.

Skin

Note any scars (particularly those of previous cesarean delivery). Many women have skin changes, such as acne or skin tags, during pregnancy that may spontaneously resolve after the pregnancy. Vascular spiders may be present on the upper body. Some women have **chloasma**, known as the *mask of pregnancy*, which is a butterfly-shaped pigmentation of the face. Note the presence of the **linea nigra**, a hyperpigmented line that begins at the sternal notch and extends down the abdomen through the umbilicus to the pubis (Fig. 30-5). Also note **striae**, or stretch marks, in areas of weight gain, particularly on the abdomen and breasts of multiparous women. These marks are bright red when they first form, but they will shrink and lighten to a silvery color (in the lightly pigmented woman) after the pregnancy.

Multiple bruises suggest physical abuse.

Note any facial edema after 20 weeks' gestation, which may signal preeclampsia.

Tracks (scars along easily accessed veins) may indicate IV drug use.

Complaints of nasal irritation, nasal crusting, nasal stuffiness, or recurrent nosebleeds may indicate drug inhaling.

Note any suspicious nevi or lesions (see Chapter 12). It is uncommon for nevi to enlarge or darken just because of pregnancy.

30-5

PUPPP (*p*ruritic *u*rticarial *p*apules and *p*laques of *p*regnancy) is the most common pruritic skin rash during pregnancy, more common in White and nulliparous women. It has an intensely pruritic erythematous eruption that appears late in pregnancy in the abdomen and thighs. The incidence is about 1 in 200 pregnancies but increases to 8 in 200 with multiple fetuses.[9]

Normal Range of Findings	Abnormal Findings

Mouth

Mucous membranes should be dark pink and moist. Gum hypertrophy (surface looks smooth, and stippling disappears) may occur normally during pregnancy (pregnancy gingivitis). Bleeding gums may be from estrogen stimulation, which causes increased vascularity and fragility.

Pale mucous membranes indicate anemia.

Poor dental hygiene during pregnancy may lead to PTD or low-birth-weight infants.

Neck

The thyroid may be palpable and feel full but smooth during the normal pregnancy of a euthyroid woman. It is stimulated by hCG.

Solitary nodules indicate neoplasm; multiple nodules usually indicate inflammation or a multinodular goiter. Significant diffuse enlargement occurs with hyperthyroidism, thyroiditis, and hypothyroidism.

Breasts

The breasts are enlarged (Fig. 30-6), perhaps with resulting striae, and may be very tender. The areolae and nipples enlarge and darken in pigmentation, the nipples become more erect, and "secondary areolae" (mottling around the areolae) may develop. The blood vessels of the breasts enlarge and may shine blue through a seemingly more translucent than usual chest wall. When auscultating, blood flow through these blood vessels can be heard and may be mistaken for a cardiac murmur. This sound is called the *mammary souffle* (SOO-FL). Montgomery's tubercles, located around the areolae and responsible for skin integrity of the areolae, enlarge. Colostrum, a thick yellow fluid, may be expressed from the nipples.

30-6 (Black, Ambros-Rudolph, Edwards, Lynch, 2008.)

Some nipples are flattened or inverted, which are common variations of normal. These can be corrected easily during pregnancy or with proper postpartum latching-on techniques. Take this opportunity in the examination to assure the pregnant woman that her breasts are "perfect breasts for breastfeeding."

Objective Data

Normal Range of Findings	Abnormal Findings

The breast tissue feels nodular as the mammary alveoli hypertrophy. Take this opportunity to teach or reinforce breast self-examination (BSE). The woman should expect changes in the breast tissue during the pregnancy. Because of the lack of menses, instruct her to perform BSE periodically during her pregnancy.

Note any abnormal mass within the breast and refer for US. US of the breast(s) is used in lieu of mammograms during pregnancy and lactation.

Heart

Later in pregnancy you can palpate the apical impulse left of the midclavicular line and up to the 4th intercostal space because of the growing fetus. The pregnant woman often has a functional, soft, blowing systolic murmur that occurs as a result of increased volume. The murmur requires no treatment and will resolve after pregnancy.

Note any other murmur and refer. Valvular disease may need prophylactic antibiotics at delivery. Pregnancy places a large hemodynamic burden on the heart, and the woman with cardiac disease is managed closely.

Lungs

The lungs are clear bilaterally to auscultation with no crackles or wheezing. Shortness of breath is common in the 3rd trimester from pressure on the diaphragm from the enlarged uterus.

Women with asthma exacerbations during pregnancy may have expiratory (and possibly inspiratory) wheeze.
Note any signs of respiratory infection: dyspnea, crackles, congested cough.

Peripheral Vascular

The legs may show diffuse, symmetric, bilateral pitting edema, particularly in the 3rd trimester and if the examination is occurring later in the day when the woman has been on her feet. Varicose veins in the legs are common in the 3rd trimester.

Edema, together with increased BP and proteinuria, is a sign of preeclampsia. Edema and pain in one leg occur with deep vein thrombosis (DVT) and warrant Doppler studies. Carefully evaluate any redness or red, hot, tender swelling to rule out phlebitis. Varicosities increase the risk for thrombophlebitis; she should not wear restrictive clothing or sit without moving legs for a long period. Varicosities will worsen with the weight and volume of pregnancy; support hose help minimize them.

Neurologic

Using the reflex hammer, check the biceps, patellar, and ankle deep tendon reflexes (DTRs). Normally these are 1+ and 2+ and equal bilaterally.

Brisk or greater than 2+ DTRs and clonus may be associated with elevated BP and cerebral edema in the preeclamptic woman.

Inspect and Palpate the Abdomen

Observe the shape and contours of the abdomen to discern signs of fetal position. As the woman lifts her head, you may see the **diastasis recti,** the separation of the abdominal muscles, which occurs during pregnancy, with the muscles returning together after pregnancy with abdominal exercise. When palpating, note the abdominal muscle tone, which grows more relaxed with each subsequent pregnancy. Note any tenderness; the uterus is normally nontender.

Objective Data

The fundus should be palpable abdominally from 12 weeks' gestation. Use the side of your hand and begin palpating centrally on the abdomen higher than you expect the uterus to be. Palpate down until you feel the fundus (the top of the uterus). Alternatively stand at the woman's right side facing her head (Fig. 30-7). Place the palm of your right hand on the curve of the uterus in the left lower quadrant and your left palm on the curve of the uterus in the right lower quadrant. Moving from hand to hand, allowing the curve of the uterus to guide you, "walk" your hands to where they meet centrally at the fundus.

30-7

Note the fundal location by landmarks and fingerbreadths, as described in Fig. 30-2. Note that individual women's variations in location of landmarks and examiner's variations in fingerbreadths make this measurement inexact. It is more accurate to use the centimeter measuring tape and measure the height of the fundus in centimeters from the superior border of the symphysis to the fundus (Fig. 30-8). After 20 weeks the number of centimeters should approximate the number of weeks of gestation in a woman with healthy body size and a singleton pregnancy. Beginning at 20 weeks you may feel fetal movement.

A lagging fundal height ≥2 cm may indicate intrauterine growth restriction (IUGR), transverse lie, or oblique presentation of the fetus.

A fundal height >4 cm than expected occurs with multiple fetuses, excess amniotic fluid, or uterine myoma.

Both conditions warrant US.

30-8

Leopold Maneuvers

In the 3rd trimester perform Leopold maneuvers to determine fetal lie, presentation, attitude, position, variety, and engagement. **Fetal lie** is the orientation of the fetal spine to the maternal spine and may be longitudinal, transverse, or oblique. **Presentation** describes the part of the fetus that is entering the pelvis first (i.e., vertex [head], breech, foot). **Attitude,** the position of fetal parts in

Normal Range of Findings	**Abnormal Findings**

relation to one another, may be flexed, military (straight), or extended. **Position** designates the location of a fetal part to the right or left of the maternal pelvis. **Variety** is the location of the fetal back to the anterior, lateral, or posterior part of the maternal pelvis. **Engagement** occurs when the widest diameter of the presenting part has descended into the pelvic inlet—specifically to the imagined plane at the level of the ischial spines.

Leopold's first maneuver is performed by facing the gravida's head and placing your fingertips around the top of the fundus (Fig. 30-9). Note its size, consistency, and shape. Imagine which fetal part is in the fundus. The breech feels large and firm. Because it is attached to the fetus at the waist, moving it between the thumb and fingers of the hand results in moving it slowly and with difficulty. In contrast, the fetal head feels large, round, and hard. When it is ballotted, it feels hard as you push it away and hard again as it bobs back against your fingers in an "answer." Note that the "bobbing" or "ballotting" sensation of the movement occurs because the head is attached at the neck and moves easily. If there is no part in the fundus, the fetus is in the transverse lie.

30-9   Leopold's first maneuver.

For **Leopold's second maneuver,** move your hands to the sides of the uterus (Fig. 30-10). Note whether small parts or a long, firm surface is palpable on the woman's left or right side. The long, firm surface is the back. Note whether the back is anterior, lateral, or out of reach (posterior). The small parts, or limbs, indicate a posterior position when they are palpable all over the abdomen.

30-10   Leopold's second maneuver.

Normal Range of Findings

In **Leopold's third maneuver,** also called *Pawlik's maneuver,* ask the woman to bend her knees up slightly for comfort (Fig. 30-11). Grasp the lower abdomen just above the symphysis pubis between the thumb and fingers of one hand to determine which part of the fetus is there. If the presenting part is beginning to engage, it will feel "fixed." With this maneuver alone, it may be difficult to differentiate the shoulder from the vertex.

30-11 Leopold's third maneuver.

The **fourth maneuver** helps to determine engagement and, in the vertex presentation, to differentiate shoulder from vertex (Fig. 30-12). The woman's knees are still bent. Facing her feet, place your palms, with fingers pointing toward the feet, on either side of the lower abdomen. Pressing your fingers firmly, move slowly down toward the pelvic inlet. If your fingers meet, the presenting part is not engaged. If your fingers diverge at the pelvic rim, meeting a hard prominence on one side, this prominence is the occiput. This indicates that the vertex is presenting with a deflexed head (the face presenting). If your fingers meet hard prominences on both sides, the vertex is engaged in either a military or a flexed position. If your fingers come to the pelvic brim diverged but with no prominences palpable, the vertex is "dipping" into the pelvis or is engaged. In this case the firm object felt above the symphysis pubis in the third maneuver is the shoulder.

30-12 Leopold's fourth maneuver.

Abnormal Findings

Normal Range of Findings	Abnormal Findings

Auscultate the Fetal Heart Tones

FHTs are a positive sign of pregnancy. They can be heard by Doppler US at 8 to 10 weeks' gestation. They are auscultated best over the back of the fetus. After identifying the position of the fetus, use the heart tones to confirm your findings. Count the FHTs for 6 seconds and multiply by 10 to obtain the rate (Fig. 30-13). The normal rate is between 110 and 160 beats/min. Spontaneous accelerations of FHTs indicate fetal well-being.

If no FHTs are heard by Doppler by 12 weeks, verify fetal cardiac activity with US.

Further investigate any FHTs that are <110/minute or >160/minute or are irregular.

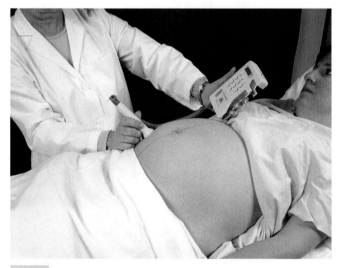

30-13

Differentiate the FHTs from the slower rate of the maternal pulse and the uterine souffle (the soft, swishing sound of the placenta receiving the pulse of maternal arterial blood) by palpating the mother's pulse while you listen.

All the abdominal findings are of interest to the woman; share them with her. Often she will want to listen to FHTs with her significant others.

Pelvic Examination

Genitalia

Use the procedure for the pelvic examination described in Chapter 26. The enlargement of the labia minora is common in multiparous women. Labial varicosities may be present. The perineum may be scarred from a previous episiotomy or from lacerations. Note any hemorrhoids. Note any lesions on the symphysis pubis, labia, or perianal area.

Lesions may indicate an infection, condyloma, or genital herpes infection.

Speculum Examination

When examining the vagina, you may see **Chadwick sign,** the bluish, purplish discoloration and congested look of the vaginal wall and cervix from increased vascularity and engorgement (Fig. 30-14). Note the vaginal discharge. Vaginal discharge in pregnancy may be heavier in amount but should be similar in description to the woman's nonpregnant discharge and should not be associated with itching, burning, or an unusual odor (except that occasionally chapping of the vaginal area may be seen because of excessive moisture). Perform a wet mount or culture of the discharge when you are uncertain of its normalcy.

Many cervical infections or STIs are asymptomatic. Any cervical secretions that are purulent or mucopurulent (chlamydia or gonorrhea); yellow or green frothy (trichomoniasis); thin, white, gray, or milky, with a "fishy" odor (bacterial vaginosis); or thick, white, and clumpy (candidiasis) should be treated appropriately during the pregnancy.

Objective Data

Normal Range of Findings	Abnormal Findings

30-14 Chadwick sign. (Apgar, Brotzman, Spitzer, 2008.)

Note whether the cervix appears open. Note whether it is the smooth, round cervix with a dotlike external os of the nulliparous woman or the irregular multiparous cervix with an external os that appears more like a crooked line, the result of cervical dilation in a previous pregnancy. A friable cervix bleeds easily when touched with a cotton swab, cytobrush, or speculum because of increased vascularity. Advise the woman that small spotting may occur.

If you suspect cervicitis, obtain cultures.

Bimanual Examination

As described in Chapter 26, palpate the uterus between your internal and external hands. Note its position. The pregnant uterus may be rotated toward the right side as it rises out of the pelvis because of the presence of the descending colon on the left. This is called **dextrorotation.** Also, you may note **Hegar sign,** when the enlarged uterus bends forward on its softened isthmus between the 4th and 6th weeks of pregnancy.

Note the size and consistency of the uterus. In a singleton pregnancy the 6-week gestation uterus may seem only slightly enlarged and softened. The 8-week gestation uterus is approximately the size of an avocado, approximately 7 to 8 cm across the fundus. The 10-week gestation uterus is about the size of a grapefruit and may reach to the pelvic brim, but it is narrow and does not fill the pelvis from side to side; the 12-week gestation uterus will fill the pelvis. After 12 weeks the uterus is sized from the abdomen. The multigravida uterus may be larger initially, and early sizing of this uterus may be less reliable for dating.

Uterine fibroids (leiomyomas) may also be felt during a bimanual examination.

Softening of the cervix is called **Goodell sign.** When examining the cervix, note its position (anterior, midposition, or posterior), degree of effacement (or thinning, expressed in percentages assuming a ≥2-cm–long cervix initially), dilation (opening, expressed in centimeters), consistency (soft or firm), and the station of the presenting part (centimeters above or below the ischial plane) (Fig. 30-15).

A shortened cervix is <2 cm and is associated with preterm labor or possible cervical insufficiency.

Normal Range of Findings	**Abnormal Findings**

Cavity of cervix with mucous plug

Internal os

External os

A

Dilating, effacing cervix

External os

B

5 cm
4
3
2
1
0 cm
+1
+2
+3
+4
+5 cm

Ischial spine

C

30-15 **A,** Cervix before labor. **B,** Cervix begins to efface and dilate. **C,** Station height of presenting part in relation to ischial spines.

The ovaries rise with the growing uterus. Always examine the adnexa to rule out the presence of a mass such as an ectopic pregnancy.

> Adnexal enlargement and pain with palpation occur with ectopic pregnancy or ovarian mass.

To determine tone, ask the woman to squeeze your fingers as they rest in the vagina. Take this opportunity to teach the Kegel exercise, the squeezing of the vagina, which the woman can do to prepare for and recover from birth. (The woman can also identify the exercise of these muscles by stopping the flow of urine midstream, although she should do this only once and should usually let urine flow freely.) Direct the woman to squeeze slowly to a peak at the count of eight and then release slowly to the count of eight. You can prescribe this exercise to be performed 50 to 100 times a day.

Blood Pressure

After the examination take the BP when the woman is the most relaxed, in the semi-Fowler or upright position. Recheck an elevated pressure.

> Chronic HTN: a documented stage 1 HTN before pregnancy or a persistent elevation of ≥140/90 mm Hg on two occasions more than 24 hours apart before the 20th week of gestation.[9]

Routine Laboratory and Radiologic Imaging Studies

At the first prenatal visit order a routine prenatal panel: a complete blood cell count, serology, rubella antibodies, HIV and hepatitis B screening, blood type and Rhesus factor, and antibody screening. Some providers screen for herpes simplex viruses I and II, thyroid function, and vitamin D level. Sickle-cell, cystic fibrosis, or thalassemia screening may be indicated. For some populations, a PPD/tine test may be indicated to rule out active tuberculosis or exposure to the disease. Obtain a Pap test with HPV screen at the initial visit along with cervical STI cultures.

Objective Data

Normal Range of Findings	Abnormal Findings
Collect a clean-catch urinalysis at the initial prenatal visit to rule out cystitis. At each prenatal visit check the urine for protein and glucose. A clean-catch specimen is ideal for this dip because a random specimen may include vaginal secretions, which contain protein, skewing the results. For women with active substance abuse, check a urine toxicology screen.	

Collect a clean-catch urinalysis at the initial prenatal visit to rule out cystitis. At each prenatal visit check the urine for protein and glucose. A clean-catch specimen is ideal for this dip because a random specimen may include vaginal secretions, which contain protein, skewing the results. For women with active substance abuse, check a urine toxicology screen.

The standard of care for US examinations is to have an US for fetal anatomic survey around 18 to 20 weeks of gestation.[1] The US is helpful in showing the age of the fetus, location of the placenta, fetal position, often the sex of the fetus, and the number of fetuses, and it may screen for certain birth defects. A cervical length measurement is recommended at 18 to 22 weeks, which can be useful to predict preterm birth. The maternal serum alpha-fetoprotein or "quad" screening is offered but is optional. Fetal nuchal translucency screening is offered as well but is optional.

Antepartum fetal testing helps improve the perinatal outcome by decreasing stillbirth and long-term neurologic impairments (of the fetus). This testing consists of monitoring fetal growth, amniotic fluid volume, biophysical profiling, and other potential fetal/maternal markers using ultrasonography. Fetal testing (nonstress test [NST] or contraction stress test [CST]) using electronic fetal monitors to graph and audibly hear the fetal heart rate and determine uterine activity is indicated for some conditions. The mother begins fetal movement counting at 28 weeks, which gives a good indication of fetal well-being.

DOCUMENTATION AND CRITICAL THINKING

Clinical Case Study 1

R.G. is a 27-year-old Latina woman, gravida 2 para 1, who presents with her husband and daughter for her first prenatal visit.

SUBJECTIVE

R.G. is a full-time homemaker who completed 2 years of college. Last normal menstrual period (LNMP) was April 4 of this year (certain of date), with an expected date of delivery (EDD) of January 11 of next year, making her 10 weeks' gestation today. Her obstetric history includes a normal spontaneous vaginal delivery (NSVD) 3 years ago of a viable 7 lb, 12 oz female infant after an 8-hour labor without anesthesia, with a midline episiotomy. No complications of pregnancy, delivery, or the postpartum. She breastfed her daughter, Ana, for 1 year. Present pregnancy was planned, and R.G. and her husband are pleased. R.G. is having breast tenderness and nausea on occasion, which resolves with crackers. No past medical or surgical conditions are present. She denies allergies. Family history is significant only for diet-controlled adult-onset diabetes in two maternal aunts.

OBJECTIVE

General: Appears well nourished and is carefully groomed. English is second language, and R.G. is fluent.
Skin: Light tan in color; surface smooth with no lesions; small tattoo noted on left forearm.
Mouth: Good dentition and oral hygiene. Oral mucosa pink; no gum hypertrophy. Thyroid gland small and smooth.
Chest: Expansion equal, respirations effortless. Lung sounds clear bilaterally with no adventitious sounds. No CVA tenderness.
Heart: Rate 76 bpm, regular rhythm; S_1 and S_2 are normal, not accentuated or diminished, with soft, blowing systolic murmur Gr 2/6 at 2nd left interspace.
Breasts: Tender, without masses; with supple, everted nipples; no lesions. Breast self-exam reviewed.
Abdomen: No masses; bowel sounds present. No hepatosplenomegaly. Fundus nonpalpable. No inguinal lymphadenopathy noted.

Extremities: No varicosities, redness, or edema. Homan sign negative. DTRs 2+ and equal bilaterally. BP 110/68 mm Hg, sitting.

Pelvic: Bartholin, urethra, and Skene glands negative for discharge. Vagina: pink, with white, creamy, nonodorous discharge. Cervix: pink, closed, multiparous, 2 cm long, firm.

Uterus: 10-week size, consistent with dates, nontender, dextrorotated. FHTs heard with Doppler, rate 140s.

ASSESSMENT

Viable intrauterine pregnancy 10 weeks by good dates, size = dates.

R.G. and husband happy with pregnancy; she feels well.

Clinical Case Study 2

K.A. is a 30-year-old Ethiopian woman, gravida 9 para 7, who presents with an interpreter and her eldest daughter for her first prenatal visit.

SUBJECTIVE

K.A. is a full-time homemaker and runs a daycare facility within her home. She immigrated to the U.S. 5 years PTA with her husband and children. Her husband is employed. She lives in a one-bedroom apartment with her family. Her last menstrual period was May 28th of this year, with an EDD of March 5th of next year, making her 11 weeks' gestation today. She is a poor historian for her deliveries in Ethiopia other than one child "died in childbirth." She delivered her last child vaginally here in the U.S. without complications after 5 hours of labor. She is unsure of the baby's weight. She had a female circumcision as a child. She is having nausea with occasional vomiting, has breast tenderness, and 1 week ago experienced "pink" vaginal spotting, unrelated to intercourse. She is unsure of her family history. Both parents and all but one of her 7 siblings are deceased. This pregnancy is unexpected but okay. She is concerned about transportation to her appointments because her husband works days and she does not drive.

OBJECTIVE

General: Appears well nourished and is carefully groomed. English is 2nd language, but she understands some. Daughter who is present with her mom is well groomed and speaks English.

Skin: Dark tan in color, surface smooth, small scarring on left arm and both legs. No lesions or tattoos.

Mouth: Poor dentition. Oral mucosa pink, some gum hypertrophy. Thyroid gland small and smooth.

Chest: Expansion equal, respiration effortless. Lung sounds clear bilaterally with no adventitious sounds. No CVA tenderness.

Heart: Rate 84 bpm, regular rhythm. S_1 and S_2 are normal, not accentuated or diminished, with soft, blowing systolic murmur Gr 2/6 at 2nd left interspace.

Breasts: Tender, no masses or lesions, large everted nipples. No drainage present. Breast self-exam reviewed.

Abdomen: No masses; bowel sounds present in four quadrants. No hepatomegaly or splenomegaly. Fundus nonpalpable. No inguinal lymphadenopathy noted. No healed incision(s) noted.

Extremities: No lower extremity varicosities, edema, or redness noted. 1+ DTRs. BP 124/76 mm Hg.

Pelvic: Female circumcision present without infibulated scarring. Bartholin, urethra, and Skene glands negative for discharge. Vagina pink, with white, creamy, nonodorous discharge. Cervix pink, nonfriable, closed, and approximately 3 cm long and soft. Vaginal wall muscles lax. No evidence of a cystocele or rectocele.

Uterus: Approximately 11-week size and nontender. Dextrorotated. FHTs not heard with Doppler. Confirmed on ultrasound along with dating.

ASSESSMENT

Intrauterine pregnancy at 11 weeks' gestation by ultrasound today with positive fetal cardiac activity. Size = dates.

Aware of potential language and cultural issues. Via clinic interpreter understands advised prenatal testing, clinic routine, and warning signs and symptoms in pregnancy.

Physical examination normal and healthy.

ABNORMAL FINDINGS
FOR ADVANCED PRACTICE

TABLE 30-1 Preeclampsia

Preeclampsia is a condition specific to pregnancy that is rarely seen before 20 weeks' gestation except in the presence of a molar (gestational trophoblastic) pregnancy. It occurs in 3% to 10% of pregnancies.

Preeclampsia seems to be a culmination of maternal, placental, and fetal factors, including: (1) placenta implanted with abnormal trophoblastic invasion; (2) immunologic intolerance among maternal, placental, and fetal tissues; (3) cardiovascular or inflammatory changes; (4) genetic factors.[9]

Predisposing factors include preeclampsia in a previous pregnancy, multifetal gestation, chronic hypertension, obesity, age 35 years or older, and African-American race.[9]

The classic symptoms of preeclampsia are hypertension and proteinuria. Hypertension is a systolic BP of ≥140 mm Hg or higher or a diastolic BP of ≥90 mm Hg that occurs after 20 weeks' gestation in a woman with previously normal blood pressure.

The BP should be compared with the woman's 1st prenatal BP (first trimester). Hypertension is necessary for the diagnosis of preeclampsia, but preeclampsia may be seen without the edema or proteinuria.

Onset and worsening symptoms may be sudden. Subjective signs may include headaches and visual changes (spots, blurring, or flashing lights) caused by cerebral edema or right upper quadrant/epigastric pain from liver enlargement, where it becomes enlarged, necrotic, and hemorrhagic. Liver enzyme levels become elevated. Hematocrit usually increases, and the platelets drop. Serum creatinine and blood urea nitrogen elevate. Hemolysis occurs at least in part as a result of vasospasm.

A serious variant of preeclampsia, the **HELLP** syndrome, involves **H**emolysis, **E**levated **L**iver enzymes, and **L**ow **P**latelets and represents an ominous clinical picture.

Untreated preeclampsia may progress to eclampsia, which is manifested by generalized tonic-clonic seizures. Eclampsia may develop as late as 10 days' postpartum.

Before the syndrome becomes clinically manifested, it is affecting the placenta through vasospasm and a series of small infarctions. The capacity of the placenta to deliver oxygen and nutrients may be seriously diminished, and fetal growth may be restricted.

See Illustration Credits for source information.

TABLE 30-2 Fetal Size Inconsistent with Dates

Size Small for Dates	Fundal height measures smaller than expected for dates.
Inaccuracy of Dates	Conception may have occurred later than originally thought. Reconsider the woman's menstrual history; sexual history; contraceptive use; early pregnancy testing; early sizing of the uterus; US results; timing of pregnancy symptoms, including the date of quickening; and the fundal height measurements. If, after this review, the expected date of delivery (EDD) is correct, further investigation is required.
Preterm Labor	Contractions causing cervical change at <37 weeks' gestation. Other than delivery, preterm labor is the leading cause of hospital admission during pregnancy. Risk factors for preterm birth include vaginal bleeding in early pregnancy, cigarette smoking, low maternal weight gain, illicit drug use, young or advanced maternal age, poverty, strenuous working conditions, psychological factors (depression, anxiety, chronic stress), African-American or African-Caribbean race, prior preterm delivery, and intrauterine infection.[9]
Size Large for Dates	Fundal height measures larger than expected for dates.
Inaccuracy of Dates	Review the same findings as listed previously.
Multiple Fetuses	The frequency of multiple fetuses increases with advanced maternal age and is enhanced by the increasing use of fertility drugs. The uterus enlarges where the fundal height may be beyond the calculated/expected gestational age. US examination confirms the diagnosis.
Leiomyoma (Myoma or "Fibroids")	These are preexisting benign tumors of the uterine wall, which then are stimulated to enlarge by the estrogen levels of pregnancy. Myomata may be located anywhere in the uterine wall (see Table 26-6, p. 770). When they grow in the outer uterine wall, the myometrium, they may affect the clinician's judgment of where the fundus of the uterus should be measured. A myoma may grow just underneath the endometrial surface into the uterine cavity, displacing the fetus or preventing its descent into the pelvis.
Fetal Macrosomia	

This is a condition in which the infant's weight is beyond 4000 g or 4500 g, regardless of the gestational age. Less than 9% of all live-born infants in the United States weighed more than 4000 g.[9] Risk factors associated with macrosomia include obesity, diabetes (gestational and type 2), postterm gestation, multiparity, large size of parents, advanced maternal age, previous macrosomic baby, and racial/ethnic factors.[9] Birth risks to the mother include labor abnormalities, an increased incidence for cesarean delivery, bladder trauma, and vaginal tissue trauma. Fetal risks include birth trauma such as fractured clavicle and brachial plexus nerve damage from shoulder dystocia, depressed Apgar scores, extended hospitalizations, and possible fetal mortality.

See Illustration Credits for source information.

TABLE 30-3 Malpresentations

Vertex (for comparison)

Footling breech

Transverse lie and
shoulder presentation

Brow presentation

Complete breech

Frank breech

Face presentation

Compound presentation

Malpresentations may be detected by the hands of an experienced examiner, confirmed by the FHT location, and further confirmed by ultrasound. Before 34 weeks' gestation, any position is normal. The vertex presentation is desirable thereafter because spontaneous turning becomes less likely as the fetus grows in proportion to the amount of space and fluid in the uterus and pelvis.

Summary Checklist: The Pregnant Woman

1. Collect history.
2. Determine EDD and current number of weeks of gestation.
3. Instruct the woman to undress and empty her bladder, saving her urine to dip it for protein and glucose or culture if 1st visit.
4. Measure weight.
5. Perform a physical examination, starting with general survey.
6. Inspect skin for pigment changes, scars.
7. Check oral mucous membranes.
8. Palpate thyroid gland.
9. Inspect breast changes and palpate for masses.
10. Auscultate breath sounds, heart sounds, heart rate, and any murmurs.
11. Check lower extremities for edema, varicosities, and reflexes.
12. The abdomen: Measure fundal height, perform Leopold's maneuvers, auscultate FHTs.
13. The pelvic examination: Note signs of pregnancy, the condition of the cervix, and the size and position of the uterus.
14. Measure the BP.
15. Obtain appropriate laboratory work.

BIBLIOGRAPHY

1. American College of Obstetricians and Gynecologists (ACOG). (2012). Noninvasive prenatal testing for fetal aneuploidy. Committee opinion No. 545. *Obstet Gynecol, 120*, 1532-1534.
2. Aruda, M. M., Waddicor, K., Frese, L., et al. (2010). Early pregnancy in adolescents: diagnosis, assessment, options counseling, and referral. *J Pediatr Health Care, 24*(1), 4-13.
3. Baby-Friendly USA. (2010). *Guidelines and evaluation criteria for facilities seeking baby-friendly designation.* Sandwich, MA: Baby-Friendly USA.
4. Benninger, C., & McCallister, J. (2010). Asthma in pregnancy: reading between the lines. *Nurse Pract, 35*(4), 10-20.
5. Bodurtha, J., & Strauss, J. F. III (2012). Genomics and perinatal care. *N Engl J Med, 366*(1), 64-73.
6. Cabbage, L. A., & Neal, J. L. (2011). Over-the-counter medications and pregnancy: an integrative review. *Nurse Pract, 36*(6), 22-28.
7. Carter, D. (2012). Elective early births put moms and infants at risk. *Am J Nurs, 112*(4), 19-20.
8. Creasy, R. K., Resnick, R., Iams, J. D., et al. (2014). *Creasy and Resnik's maternal-fetal medicine: principles and practice* (7th ed.). Philadelphia: Saunders.
9. Cunningham, F. G., Leveno, K., Bloom, S., et al. (2010). *Williams' obstetrics* (23rd ed.). Stamford, CT: Appleton & Lange.
10. Devine, K. S. (2012). The underutilization of emergency contraception. *Am J Nurs, 112*(4), 44-50.
11. Reference deleted in proofs.
12. Greene, M. F. (2012). Two hundred years of progress in the practice of midwifery. *N Engl J Med, 367*(18), 1732-1740.
13. Guttmacher Institute. (2013, June). *Facts on teens' sexual and reproductive health [Fact sheet].* http://www.guttmacher.org/pubs/FB-ATSRH.pdf.
14. Halloran, D. R., Marshall, N. E., Kunovich, R. M., et al. (2012). Obesity trends and perinatal outcomes in black and white teenagers. *Am J Obstet Gynecol, 207*(6), 492-e1-497.e7.
15. Hamilton, B. E., & Ventura, S. J. (2012). Birth rates for U.S. teenagers reach historic lows for all age and ethnic groups. *NCHS Data Brief 2012, 89,* 1-7.
16. Huang, H., Coleman, S., Bridge, J. A., et al. (2014). A meta-analysis of the relationship between antidepressant use in pregnancy and the risk of preterm birth and low birth weight. *Gen Hosp Psychiatry, 36*(1), 13-18.
17. Jansen, L., Gibson, M., Bowles, B. C., et al. (2013). First do no harm: interventions during childbirth. *J Perinat Educ, 22*(2), 83-92.
18. Keegan, J., Parva, M., Finnegan, M., et al. (2010). Addiction in pregnancy. *J Addictive Dis, 29*(2), 175-191.
19. Kelly-Weeder, S. (2012). Helping patients through the pain of infertility. *Nurse Pract, 37*(2), 47-52.
20. Kessenich, C. R., & Erigo-Backman, R. C. (2012). Using hCG testing in pregnancy and beyond. *Nurse Pract, 37*(5), 18-19.
21. King, T. L., Brucker, M. C., & Kriebs, J. M. (2013). *Varney's midwifery* (5th ed.). Sudbury, MA: Jones & Bartlett.
22. Krishna, I., & Lindsay, M. (2013). Breast cancer in pregnancy. *Obstet Gynecol Clin North Am, 40*(3), 559-571.
23. Lowe, N. K., & Ryan-Wenger, N. A. (2012). Uncomplicated UTIs in women. *Nurse Pract, 37*(5), 41-48.
24. Männistö, T., Mendola, P., Väaräsmäki, M., et al. (2013). Elevated blood pressure in pregnancy and subsequent chronic disease risk. *Circulation, 127*(6), 681-690.
25. March of Dimes. (2009). *Birth defects, Down syndrome.* White Plains, NY: March of Dimes Birth Defects Foundation.
26. Mateja, W. A., Nelson, D. B., Kroelinger, C. D., et al. (2012). The association between maternal alcohol use and smoking in early pregnancy and congenital cardiac defects. *J Women's Health, 21*(1), 26-34.
27. Nguyen, B. T., Cheng, Y. W., Snowden, J. M., et al. (2012). The effect of race/ethnicity on adverse perinatal outcomes among patients with gestational diabetes mellitus. *Am J Obstet Gynecol, 207*(4), 322-e1-322.e6.
28. O'Hara, M. W., Stuart, S., Watson, D., et al. (2012). Brief scales to detect postpartum depression and anxiety symptoms. *J Women's Health, 21*(12), 1237-1243.
29. Okoroh, E. M., Azonobi, I. C., Grosse, S. D., et al. (2012). Prevention of venous thromboembolism in pregnancy. *J Women's Health, 21*(6), 611-615.
30. Payne, R. J., Guinn, C., & Ponder, B. (2011). Supporting the couple with conception challenges. *Nurse Pract, 36*(8), 38-45.
31. Richardson, K. K., & Shannon, M. T. (2012). STI screening and treatment in pregnancy. *Nurse Pract, 37*(12), 30-37.

32. Reference deleted in proofs.
33. Sandall, J. (2013). Evidence supports midwife-led care models. *Am J Nurs, 113*(11), 15.
34. Reference deleted in proofs.
35. Urrutia, R. P., & Thorp, J. M. (2012). Vitamin D in pregnancy: current concepts. *Curr Opin Obstet Gynecol, 24*(2), 57-64.
36. Reference deleted in proofs.
37. Zhao, G., Ford, E. S., & Tsai, J., et al. (2012). Trends in health-related behavioral risk factors among pregnant women in the United States: 2001–2009. *J Women's Health, 21*(3), 255-263.

CHAPTER 31

Functional Assessment of the Older Adult

e http://evolve.elsevier.com/Jarvis/

31-1 © Diego Cervo, 2014/Shutterstock.

The United States has a large and expanding population of older adults. The implications of the graying of America are staggering for all health care systems (Fig. 31-1). In 2010 the U.S. population included 13.3% of people ≥65 years of age. This group accounted for 13.6 million short stay hospital discharges.[3] In 2011 older adults averaged more office visits than younger adults and had higher out-of-pocket health care expenditures than younger Americans.[3]

Many older Americans live with disabilities or have activity limitations, often because of multiple chronic conditions that may include sensory, physical, or mental impairments. Approximately 37% of older adults reported a severe disability requiring some type of assistance or personal caregiving, with only a small percentage (3.6%) residing in nursing homes.[3]

Personal caregiving can be formal (hired, paid caregivers) or informal (family, friends). Such services were valued at $450 billion per year in 2009.[2] In addition, *aging* or *older adult* cannot be defined only by the chronologic age of an individual as it is for Social Security (ages 65 years and older). Older adults are truly heterogeneous, and differences exist among biologic, social, physical, and emotional rates of aging.[26] Older age-groups are often categorized as young-old (65 to 74 years), middle-old (75 to 84 years), and old-old (85 years and older). Although the number of chronic diseases does increase with aging, remember that a substantial number of older adults both enjoy aging and report good-to-excellent health.[3]

The comprehensive assessment of an older adult requires knowledge of not only normal aging changes but also the consequences of chronic diseases, genetic makeup, and lifestyle. A comprehensive **geriatric assessment** is multidimensional and incorporates the physical examination and assessments of mental status, functional status, social and economic status, pain, and examination of the physical environment for safety concerns. Multiple disciplines may participate in this assessment, including physicians; nurses; physical, occupational, and speech therapists; social workers; case managers; nutritionists; and pharmacists. Early recognition of disabilities and treatable conditions is instrumental in preserving function and quality of life for older adults.

The normal changes of aging presented in previous chapters do not represent pathology; but with the imposition of acute and chronic illnesses, including hospitalization, an older adult may be predisposed to disability. Older adults may present to clinics or hospitals not only with an acute illness such as pneumonia, but also with ongoing chronic "geriatric syndromes" such as urinary incontinence, fragile skin, confusion, problems with eating or feeding, falls, or sleep disorders. If these syndromes are not identified early, an older adult may develop functional decline.

Normal aging changes and the development of disease may precipitate transition from home to a variety of settings where nursing-focused assessments are performed. Care may be provided in hospitals; skilled nursing, long-term care, assisted-living, and acute rehabilitation facilities; and hospice, senior centers, homes, and clinics (Fig. 31-2). The setting where care is provided usually determines the types of

31-2 © Alexander Raths, 2014/Shutterstock.

assessment and instruments used. However, the goal of the functional assessment remains the same: to identify an older adult's strengths and any limitations so appropriate interventions will promote independence and prevent functional decline.

FUNCTION

Functional ability refers to one's ability to perform activities necessary to live in modern society and includes driving, using the telephone, or performing personal tasks such as bathing and toileting. *Functional status* is one's actual performance of activities and tasks associated with his or her current life roles and depends on motivation, sensory capacity such as vision and hearing, degree of assistance needed to accomplish the tasks, and cognition.[34] For example, the effect that arthritis might have on a person's ability to exercise may affect physical function. A condition such as Alzheimer disease may affect problem solving, safety concerns, and motivation, which in turn affects function. Lack of social support or a safe physical setting is an environmental issue that affects functional status and possibly the ability to live independently. Functional status is not static; older adults may move continuously through varying stages of independence and disability.

The assessment of function is important to provide a baseline for continuing comparison, to predict prognosis, and to provide objective measures on the efficacy of treatments. Knowing only the person's medical diagnosis is not sufficient to predict functional abilities. Older adults may not experience the usual symptoms of an acute illness, and often a decline in functional status may herald the presence of another process such as an infection.

A functional assessment is the basis for care planning, goal setting, and discharge planning. It is needed for eligibility to obtain durable medical equipment, home modifications, and inpatient or outpatient rehabilitation services. For the older adult and family, a functional assessment can identify areas for current and future planning such as the most appropriate living situation.

A functional assessment includes three domains: **activities of daily living (ADLs), instrumental activities of daily living (IADLs),** and **mobility.**[32] A functional assessment is systematic, with attention to the particular needs of the person such as the presence of pain, fatigue, shortness of breath, or memory problems. There are two approaches to use for performing a functional assessment: (1) *asking individuals* about their abilities to perform the tasks (using self-reports), or (2) actually *observing* their ability to perform the tasks. For people with memory problems, the use of surrogate reporters (proxy reports) such as family members or caregivers may be necessary, keeping in mind that they may either overestimate or underestimate the actual abilities.

Activities of Daily Living

ADLs are tasks necessary for self-care. Typically, ADLs measure domains of eating/feeding, bathing, grooming (the individual tasks of washing face, combing hair, shaving, cleaning teeth), dressing (lower body and upper body), toileting (bowel and bladder), walking (including propelling a wheelchair), using stairs (ascending and descending), and transferring (e.g., bed to chair). The ADL instruments are designed as either self-report, observation of tasks, or proxy/surrogate report.

The Katz Index of Independence in ADL

The Katz Index of ADL[18] is based on the concept of physical disability and measures physical function in older adults and the chronically ill; it is the foundation for most of the newer functional assessment instruments.[32] It is widely used in both clinical practice and research to measure performance, evaluate treatment outcomes, and predict the need for continuing supervised care. Activities assessed are bathing, dressing, toileting, transferring from bed to chair, continence, and feeding. This instrument has been modified over the years since its development. A simplified method for scoring the instrument is to use a dichotomous rating of independence or dependence in the 6 activities (Fig. 31-3). One point is given for each independent item. Only activities that can be performed without help are rated as independent.

The Katz ADL scale is a useful instrument in many settings. The tool takes approximately 5 minutes to administer, but its use has limitations. In an outpatient setting or clinic visit, the provider cannot observe the older adult perform the activity and must rely on a self-report or surrogate report. In the hospital, nursing staff may be assisting with transferring or grooming activities and may underestimate ability for self-care. In addition, small changes in the ability to perform these activities may not be identified.

Remember that the instrument is measuring function at the current point in time and is valuable for planning specific types of assistance that the older person may need. For example, a person may be unable to bathe independently on hospital discharge but is independent in other ADLs. In this case, plan for a home health aide to go twice a week to the home to assist the older adult with bathing.

Additional Activity-of-Daily-Living Instruments

Additional tools used to assess ADL ability are the Barthel Index,[22] the Functional Independence Measure (FIM),[14] and the Rapid Disability Rating Scale-2 (RDS-2).[21] The Barthel Index includes definitions of each task to facilitate ease of scoring, has a comprehensive assessment of mobility, and is often used to follow progress in rehabilitation settings.[32] The FIM has been widely tested on older adults; it has a telephone, an in-person, and a proxy version of the instrument. It is more sensitive to change than the other ADL instruments but takes formal training and is more time consuming.[32] The RDS-2 is completed by a family member or professional caregiver familiar with the abilities of the older adult. It is designed to measure what the person can *actually do* versus what he or she could possibly do.

Katz Activities of Daily Living

Activities

Points (1 or 0)

Independence

(1 Point)

NO supervision, direction, or personal assistance

Dependence

(0 Points)

WITH supervision, direction, personal assistance, or total care

Bathing

Points _____

(1 Point) Bathes self completely or needs help in bathing only a single part of the body such as the back, genital area, or disabled extremity

(0 Point) Needs help with bathing more than one part of the body or with getting in or out of the tub or shower; requires total bathing

Dressing

Points _____

(1 Point) Gets clothes from closet and drawers and puts on clothes and outer garments complete with fasteners; may have help tying shoes

(0 Point) Needs help with dressing self or needs to be completely dressed

Toileting

Points _____

(1 Point) Gets to toilet, gets on and off, arranges clothes, cleans genital area without help

(0 Point) Needs help transferring to the toilet or cleaning self, or uses bedpan or commode

Transferring

Points _____

(1 Point) Moves into and out of bed or chair unassisted; mechanical transferring aides are acceptable

(0 Point) Needs help in moving from bed to chair or requires a complete transfer

Continence

Points _____

(1 Point) Exercises complete self-control over urination and defecation

(0 Point) Is partially or totally incontinent of bowel or bladder

Feeding

Points _____

(1 Point) Gets food from plate into mouth without help; preparation of food may be done by another person

(0 Point) Needs partial or total help with feeding or requires parenteral feeding

Total Points = _____

6 = High (patient independent)

0 = Low (patient very dependent)

Adapted from Gerontological Society of America. Katz, S., et al. (1970). Progress in the development of the index of ADL. *Gerontologist, 10, 20-30.*

31-3

Instrumental Activities of Daily Living

Many IADL instruments have been developed since the 1960s, with the goal of measuring functional abilities necessary for independent community living. Typically IADL tasks include shopping, meal preparation, housekeeping, laundry, managing finances, taking medications, and using transportation. Tasks such as yard work or home maintenance and leisure activities such as reading and other hobbies are included in some but not all IADL instruments. These instruments may have cultural and gender biases, especially in older cohorts.[32] IADL instruments measure tasks (doing laundry, cooking, housework) historically done by women, and many do not address activities done primarily by men such as home repairs and working in the yard.

Lawton Instrumental Activities of Daily Living

IADL measures address higher-order components of the Katz ADL scale and measure the more complex ADLs required for a person to adapt to the environment.[32] The instrument was originally developed to determine the most suitable living situation for an older adult. That is, determining competence and maintenance of life skills such as shopping, cooking, and managing finances is a meaningful way to assess function because these abilities are a prerequisite for independent living. The Lawton IADL scale contains 8 items (Fig. 31-4): use of telephone, shopping, meal preparation, housekeeping, laundry, transportation, self-medication, and management of finances.

The Lawton IADL instrument is designed as a self-report measure of performance rather than ability. Direct testing is

---

The Lawton Instrumental Activities of Daily Living Scale

A. Ability to Use Telephone
   1. Operates telephone on own initiative; looks up and dials numbers   1
   2. Dials a few well-known numbers   1
   3. Answers telephone, but does not dial   1
   4. Does not use telephone at all   0

B. Shopping
   1. Takes care of all shopping needs independently   1
   2. Shops independently for small purchases   0
   3. Needs to be accompanied on any shopping trip   0
   4. Completely unable to shop   0

C. Food Preparation
   1. Plans, prepares, and serves adequate meals independently   1
   2. Prepares adequate meals if supplied with ingredients   0
   3. Heats and serves prepared meals or prepares meals, but does not maintain adequate diet   0
   4. Needs to have meals prepared and served   0

D. Housekeeping
   1. Maintains house alone with occasional assistance (heavy work)   1
   2. Performs light daily tasks such as dishwashing, bed making   1
   3. Performs light daily tasks, but cannot maintain acceptable level of cleanliness   1
   4. Needs help with all home maintenance tasks   1
   5. Does not participate in any housekeeping tasks   0

E. Laundry
   1. Does personal laundry completely   1
   2. Launders small items, rinses socks, stockings, etc   1
   3. All laundry must be done by others   0

F. Mode of Transportation
   1. Travels independently on public transportation or drives own car   1
   2. Arranges own travel via taxi, but does not otherwise use public transportation   1
   3. Travels on public transportation when assisted or accompanied by another   1
   4. Travel limited to taxi or automobile with assistance of another   0
   5. Does not travel at all   0

G. Responsibility for Own Medications
   1. Is responsible for taking medication in correct dosages at correct time   1
   2. Takes responsibility if medication is prepared in advance in separate dosages   0
   3. Is not capable of dispensing own medication   0

H. Ability to Handle Finances
   1. Manages financial matters independently (budgets, writes checks, pays rent and bills, goes to bank); collects and keeps track of income   1
   2. Manages day-to-day purchases, but needs help with banking, major purchases, etc   1
   3. Incapable of handling money   0

Scoring: For each category, circle the item description that most closely resembles the client's highest functional level (either 0 or 1).

31-4

(Lawton, Brody, 1969.)

often not feasible (e.g., demonstrating the ability to prepare food while a hospital inpatient). Attention to the final score is less important than identifying a person's strengths and areas where assistance is needed. The instrument is useful in acute hospital settings for discharge planning and ongoing in outpatient settings. It would not be useful for those residing in institutional settings because many of these tasks are already being managed for the resident.

Additional IADL Instruments

Other IADL instruments available are the Older Americans Resources and Services Multidimensional Functional Assessment Questionnaire-IADL (OARS-IADL)[11] and the Direct Assessment of Functional Abilities (DAFA).[17] The OARS-IADL assesses 5 areas of personal function: social, economic, mental health, physical health, and self-care capacity; it is administered either as a self-report or trained observer instrument. The DAFA is a 10-item observational instrument for use with adults with dementia. It requires the person to demonstrate tasks of money management, shopping, hobbies, meal preparation, awareness, reading, and transportation.[32] The obvious strength of this instrument is the direct observation versus self-reporting or proxy reporting; however, it can take up to an hour and a half to complete; therefore it would not be feasible to use in an acute hospital setting.

Advanced Activities of Daily Living

Advanced activities of daily living (AADLs) are activities that an older adult performs as a member of a family, society, and community, including occupational and recreational activities.[13] Various AADL instruments commonly include self-care, mobility, work (either paid or volunteer), recreational activities/hobbies, and socialization. Occupational therapists often perform assessment of AADLs. The older adult sets priorities for these activities so interventions can be individualized.

Measuring Physical Performance

A disadvantage of many of the ADL and IADL instruments is the self-report or proxy report of functional activities. Incorporating an objective standardized measure of performance prevents overestimation or underestimation of abilities. Many of the physical performance measures also incorporate balance, gait, motor coordination, and endurance. Many of the tests are timed. Although there are clear advantages to directly observing the older adult perform the activities, there are some disadvantages. The instruments can be very time consuming, require training and special equipment, and have the possibility that the individual might fall or sustain an injury during the testing.

The Get Up and Go Test[25] is a reliable and valid test to quantify functional mobility. The test is quick; requires little training and no special equipment; and is appropriate to use in many settings, including hospitals and clinics. This instrument can predict a person's ability to go outside alone safely. As the practitioner observes, the person rises from a chair, walks 10 feet, turns, walks back to the chair, and sits down. Factors to note are sitting balance, transferring from sitting to standing (e.g., does the person need to push off the armrest to rise), pace and stability of walking, ability to turn without staggering, and sitting back down in the chair. Another instrument to assess gait and balance is the Tinetti Gait and Balance Evaluation,[39] a 28-point tool that is performed by trained observers and takes approximately 20 minutes to complete. Both of these instruments also provide useful information about falls risk.

Assessment of Risk for Functional Decline During Hospitalization

Losing the ability to perform ADLs and IADLs as a result of acute illness and hospitalization is common in older adults and can have significant negative consequences, including nursing home discharge and death.[7] This functional decline is attributable to the imposition of acute illness on an aging body with diminished physiologic reserve and to limited mobility commonly experienced during a hospital admission.[8] Because hospital-acquired functional decline has been noted to occur within 2 days of a hospital admission,[16] it is important to identify older adults who are at greatest risk for loss of ADLs or mobility at this critical time.

One easy-to-use assessment instrument is the Hospital Admission Risk Profile (HARP)[35] (Fig. 31-5). The HARP was developed based on three predictive variables for ADL loss during and after hospitalization for an acute medical illness: (1) older age, (2) impaired cognitive functioning, and (3) reduced IADL ability within 2 weeks before admission.[35] The HARP instrument assesses patients using age, an abbreviated 21-point Folstein Mini-Mental State Exam (MMSE), and IADL preadmission status.[35] The MMSE portion of the instrument consists of 10 orientation questions, registration (3 items), attention (5 items), and recall (previous 3 registration items). Depending on the score, patients are then identified as low, medium, or high risk for loss of ADLs and can be referred early for restorative interventions such as in-hospital rehabilitation, care on a geriatric unit, and multidisciplinary discharge planning.

Assessment of Cognition

Cognitive impairment resulting from disease may be attributed by patients, families, and health care providers to normal changes with aging and can delay diagnostic workup. In general, a gradual and mild-to-moderate decline in short-term memory may be attributable to aging; an older adult may need more time to learn new material or a new task or may need a system for reminders. Domains of cognition included in most mental status assessments are attention, memory, orientation, language, visuospatial skills, and higher cognitive functions such as the ability to plan and make decisions.

Altered cognition in older adults is commonly attributed to three disorders—**dementia, delirium,** or **depression**—although other disorders such as normal pressure hydrocephalus may contribute. Depressed persons often complain of memory impairment. Delirium presents as an acute change in cognition, affecting the domain of attention. It is usually

Hospital Admission Risk Profile (HARP)

1. Scoring range 0-5

A. Age

Age Category	Risk Score	Score =
<75	0	
75-84	1	
≥85	2	

B. Cognitive function (abbreviated MMSE*)

MMSE Score	Risk Score	Score =
15-21	0	
0-14	1	

C. IADL function prior to admission[†]

Independent IADLS	Risk Score	Score =
6-7	0	
0-5	2	

2. Risk categories

Total Score	Risk of Decline in ADL Function	TOTAL =
4 or 5	High risk	
2 or 3	Intermediate risk	
0 or 1	Low risk	

*Abbreviated MMSE includes only the following 21 components of the original 30-item test: orientation (10 items: year, season, month, date, day, city, county, state, hospital, floor), registration (3 unrelated items, such as hat, ball, tree), attention (5 items, such as spelling WORLD backwards), and recall (same 3 items as in registration). Each correct answer is scored one point.

[†] A person is judged independent in an activity if he or she is able to perform the activity without assistance. A person is scored dependent if he or she either does not perform an activity, requires the assistance of another person, or is unable to perform an activity. IADL activities include telephoning, shopping, cooking, doing housework, taking medications, using transportation, and managing finances.

31-5 (Sager, et. al., 1996.)

attributable to an acute illness such as an infection or a medication side effect, whereas people with Alzheimer dementia have alterations in word finding and naming objects in addition to memory problems (see Table 23-2, 10 Warning Signs of Alzheimer Disease, p. 677). These disorders commonly occur simultaneously with an acute illness and can complicate assessments. For example, people with dementia are at higher risk for delirium and, in the early stages of dementia, may also be depressed.

Cognitive assessments provide continuing comparisons with the individual's baseline to detect any acute changes such as with delirium. The assessments are not diagnostic but rather are for screening purposes and identify the need for a more

comprehensive workup. Cognitive assessments are important for discharge planning (e.g., will the person remember to take the prescribed medications) and to assess for readiness for learning. As with screening for ADLs and IADLs, assessment of cognition helps with determining the best discharge plan. Common assessment instruments are listed in Table 31-1.

Depression and Function

Depression is common in older adults, although it is not a normal part of aging or a natural reaction to acute illness or hospitalization. Although aging is often accompanied by loss and unwanted change, most older adults do not suffer from depression. Emotional experiences of sadness, grief, response

TABLE 31-1	**Common Cognitive Assessment Instruments**		
NAME OF INSTRUMENT	**TYPE OF TEST**	**DOMAINS COVERED**	**TIME**
Mini-Mental State Examination (Folstein et al., 1975)	Mental status	Orientation, immediate and delayed recall, working memory, language, visuospatial ability	10 minutes
Short Portable Mental Status Questionnaire (Pfeiffer, 1975)	Mental status	Orientation, general/personal information, working memory	5-10 minutes
Mini-Cog (Borson et al, 2003)	Mental status	Immediate and delayed recall, visuospatial ability	5-10 minutes
Blessed Orientation-Memory-Concentration Test (BOMC) (Katzman et al, 1983)	Mental status	Orientation, immediate and delayed recall, working memory	3-6 minutes
Geriatric Depression Scale, Short Form[41a]	Depression	Depression and changes in level of depression	5-10 minutes
Confusion Assessment Method[16a]	Delirium		
Neecham Confusion Scale (Neelon et al, 1996)	Delirium		

to loss, and temporary "blue" moods are considered normal. Persistent depression that interferes significantly with ability to function is not. Fortunately, mood disorders, including depression, are a commonly reversible psychiatric condition in later life.

Estimates of major depression in older people living in the community range from 8% to 15% but rise to up to 40% in hospitalized older patients.[6] Functional impairment in both ADLs and IADLs has been associated with higher levels of depressive symptoms.[6] Although older adults with physical impairments are at greater risk for depression, depression is not an inevitable consequence of functional impairment.

Prevention and treatment of depression are two effective targets for interventions aimed at reducing functional decline and increasing the time that an older adult maintains independence. It is vital to screen and identify those who have depressive symptoms. Several short screening instruments have been developed and validated for depression screening in the older adult. One example is the Geriatric Depression Scale, Short Form (Fig. 31-6).[36] Depression tends to be long lasting and can recur. Thus a wait-and-see approach to treatment is not desirable. Common treatment options are psychotherapy, antidepressant medications, and electroconvulsive therapy.

Geriatric Depression Scale (Short Form)

1. Are you basically satisfied with your life?	Yes	No
2. Have you dropped many of your activities and interests?	Yes	No
3. Do you feel that your life is empty?	Yes	No
4. Do you often get bored?	Yes	No
5. Are you in good spirits most of the time?	Yes	No
6. Are you afraid that something bad is going to happen to you?	Yes	No
7. Do you feel happy most of the time?	Yes	No
8. Do you often feel helpless?	Yes	No
9. Do you prefer to stay at home rather than go out and do new things?	Yes	No
10. Do you feel you have more problems with memory than most?	Yes	No
11. Do you think it is wonderful to be alive now?	Yes	No
12. Do you feel pretty worthless the way you are now?	Yes	No
13. Do you feel full of energy?	Yes	No
14. Do you feel that your situation is hopeless?	Yes	No
15. Do you think that most people are better off than you are?	Yes	No

*Score:*____/15. One point for "no" to questions 1, 5, 7, 11, 13; one point for "yes" to other questions. Normal: 3 ± 2; mildly depressed: 7 ± 3; very depressed: 12 ± 2.

31-6

(Sheikh, Yesavage, 1986.)

Social Domain

The quality of life that an older person experiences is closely linked to the success of social function. The social domain focuses on relationships within family, social groups, and the community and comprises multiple dimensions, including the sources of formal and informal assistance available from those relationships. Knowledge of the day-to-day routines can give you baseline information and a reference point to detect functional decline during future encounters.

A comprehensive social assessment is spread over several evaluation periods. Because approximately 80% of all care provided is by friends and family members, the social assessment also addresses assessment of caregivers.[27]

Social networks consist of informal supports that are accessed by the older adult.[40] Informal support is partly based on cultural beliefs regarding who should be providing care, prior relationships, and location and availability of the caregiver. Informal support includes family and friends and is usually provided free of charge. The total economic value of informal caregiving in the United States for all diseases is estimated to be at least $375 billion annually, almost twice as much as is spent on nursing home care.[28] Services provided include tasks such as ADLs, shopping, and paying bills.

Formal supports range from programs such as social welfare and other social service and health care delivery agencies such as home health care to church societies and senior centers.

The availability of assistance from family or friends frequently determines whether a functionally dependent older adult remains at home or is institutionalized. Several studies conclude that the presence of a caregiver is an important factor in the discharge plan of older adults from an acute care hospital.[5] Knowing who would be available to help the person if he or she becomes ill is important to document, even for healthy older adults.

Several standardized assessment instruments are available. The Norbeck Social Support Questionnaire[30, 31] was developed to measure the multiple components of social support.* It allows the individual to rate his or her own social network and perceived social support from the network and can also be used to measure social support with caregivers. Primary caregivers (especially spouse and adult children) often face high levels of demand and limitations on personal freedom that can result in increased stress, burden, and impaired physical health.

CAREGIVER ASSESSMENT

Most older adults with functional impairment live in the community with the help of informal support (commonly a spouse or other family member, often a daughter). Many spousal caregivers are as frail as the person for whom they are caring, or many adult children are themselves older than 65

years and may be having to cope with their own chronic illnesses. Although many caregivers experience satisfaction from providing care, great mental and physical stressors may also be linked with caregiving.[42] High levels of functional dependency place a burden on the caregiver and may result in caregiver burnout, sleep disturbances, depression, morbidity, and even increased mortality.[27]

An older person's need for institutionalization often is better predicted from assessment of the caregiver characteristics and stress than from the severity of the patient's illness. The health and well-being of the patient and caregiver are closely linked. For these reasons part of assessing an older adult involves paying attention to the well-being of the caregiver. A health care provider may help identify programs such as support groups, respite programs, adult daycare, or hired home health aides.

Assessment of Caregiver Burden

For individuals caring for a frail, frequently cognitively impaired older adult, the demands can be overwhelming. The level of care that the older adult requires may exceed caregiver ability. Caregiver burden is the perceived strain by the person who cares for an elderly, chronically ill, or disabled person. It is linked to the caregiver's ability to cope and handle stress. Signs of possible caregiver burnout include multiple somatic complaints, increased stress and anxiety, social isolation, depression, and weight loss.

Several formal screening tools are available that identify caregivers of any age who need a more comprehensive assessment; one example is the Modified Caregiver Strain Index.*[,38] Caregiver stress can potentially lead to elder mistreatment; a thorough assessment may identify opportunities to prevent and stop it (see Chapter 7).

CONTEXTS OF CARE

Older adults reside in and enter the health care system along multiple levels or contexts of care, including acute care hospitals, inpatient nursing facilities, in the community, and at home providing home health care.

The location of the care setting affects the ability to perform a comprehensive functional assessment. It may be more difficult in the acute care setting while the older adult is experiencing an acute illness; and the length of stay may be short versus that in a nursing facility, where an assessment may be achieved over time. In addition, if a resident resides in the home environment, the parameters of assessment will be broader than if he or she is in an inpatient long-term living situation.

Acute Care Setting

For older adults acute hospitalization offers the hope of relief of symptoms and treatment of illness and disease. But it also puts them at risk for adverse consequences of hospitalization,

---

*Norbeck Social Support Questionnaire is available online at http://evolve.elsevier.com/Jarvis.

*Activity for this Index is located in Jarvis, C., *Lab Manual for Physical Examination and Health Assessment*, 7th ed.

including functional decline, iatrogenic complications, and subsequent discharge to a nursing facility.[20] Researchers have found that older adults admitted to a hospital for acute illness will lose independent function in one or more ADLs.[20]

Hospitals appreciate the increased risk for functional decline and adverse outcomes, and targeted interventions to prevent decline have shown to be successful. One popular model of care is the Acute Care for Elders (ACE) unit, which is a dedicated unit within a hospital setting focused toward preventing functional decline in older adults through the design of the physical environment (e.g., bright lights, flooring to help prevent falls), collaboration among interdisciplinary teams, patient-centered care, and nursing protocols for clinical care (e.g., indwelling urinary catheter removal, reduction of restraint use, early mobilization). Acute care nurses equipped with specialized knowledge and skills have an impact on improving outcomes for the hospitalized older adult.

Community

The vast majority of older adults reside in the community, and misconceptions about nursing home statistics are common. Fewer than 5% of older adults live in nursing homes on any given day. The percentage increases from 1% of those ages 65 to 74 years to about 10% of those older than 85 years.[3] Since the mid-1980s the rate of nursing home residence for people older than 65 years has been declining, attributed partly to the increase in assisted-living facilities and the popularity and availability of home health care services.

One of the goals of community-based services is to help the older adult remain at home. Assessment of functional status helps to determine the type of services that an older adult needs to maintain independence and living at home. A low or negative result on a screening tool during assessment does not necessarily lead to the need for institutionalization. It may mean that the older adult requires increased services to maintain home living.

Home Care

Home care refers to a range of supportive social and health services provided in the home environment. Services include skilled nursing care, primary care, therapy (physical, occupational, and speech), social work, nutrition, case management, ADL assistance, and some durable medical equipment. The home care nurse is tending not only to the illness of the older adult but also to the home safety considerations, family dynamics, and functional ability. Because of advances in health care technology, equipment is smaller and more portable. As a result, people who once were limited to hospitalization can now be treated or managed at home. In addition to cost advantages with home care versus hospitalization, older adults have been shown to recover faster when at home in familiar settings than when placed in institutions and also can avoid the risk for infection exposure.

Assisted Living

Assisted-living facilities are a popular choice for older adults and typically are considered between home care and long-term care. There is great diversity in the services provided. Most facilities provide apartment-style living, although some single-family dwellings are licensed to provide care. Facilities offer homelike environments where residents have the opportunity for social interaction through group dining and activities. Some offer assistance with personal care and/or support with ADLs, transportation, and recreational activities as part of an overall package; others offer services that can be added separately.

Continuing-Care Retirement Communities

The unique feature of continuing-care retirement communities is that all care needs for the older adult can be met in one community, supporting the concept of aging in place. These facilities feature independent living arrangements, assisted-living care, and skilled nursing care that offer a variety of social and recreational activities. In these communities residents can progress through the continuum of care while residing in the same community. An older adult can enter at the independent level of living and then, as illness and/or functional limitations occur, can move to a higher level of support. Some older adults may never leave the independent living level, whereas others may progress to skilled nursing as the need for care arises.

MAINTAINING INDEPENDENCE

Exercise

Exercise and activity are essential for health promotion and maintenance in the older adult and to achieve an optimal level of functioning. A sedentary lifestyle is an important contributor to the loss in the ability to independently perform ADLs. Exercise does not prevent the process of aging, but it increases functional ability, helping to maximize the older adult's independence.

Exercise has positive health effects in older adults, including those with impairments.[41] These include improving cardiovascular function, postural stability, flexibility and range of motion, and strength and muscle mass; decreasing body fat; and possibly helping to reduce pain and discomfort. Because of these positive effects, falls risk and fractures may be decreased. In addition, participation in physical exercise has shown to reduce depressive symptoms and improve feelings of psychosocial well-being[41] (Table 31-2).

To help with compliance, physical activities should be readily available and have minimal cost associated with participation. Because pathology, both known and undiscovered, may be present in older adults (e.g., osteoporosis), the physical activity chosen should not put excessive stress on the skeletal system. Walking is a popular mode of exercise for cardiovascular endurance. Water activities or stationary cycling may be alternative modes for individuals when walking is not feasible. Developing an activity plan, particularly for older adults with chronic health conditions, may warrant clearance and input from a health care provider or referral to a specialty program (e.g., cardiac rehabilitation).

TABLE 31-2 WHO Recommended Levels of Physical Activity for Adults Ages 65 and Above
In adults ages 65 years and older, physical activity includes leisure-time physical activity (e.g., walking, dancing, gardening, hiking, swimming); transportation (e.g., walking or cycling); occupational (if the individual is still engaged in work); household chores; play, games, sports or planned exercise in the context of daily, family, and community activities.
To improve cardiorespiratory and muscular fitness and bone and functional health and reduce the risk of noncommunicable diseases, depression, and cognitive decline: • Older adults should do at least 150 minutes of moderate-intensity aerobic physical activity throughout the week, at least 75 minutes of vigorous-intensity aerobic physical activity throughout the week, or an equivalent combination of moderate- and vigorous-intensity activity. • Aerobic activity should be performed in bouts of at least 10 minutes' duration. • For additional health benefits, older adults should increase their moderate-intensity aerobic physical activity to 300 minutes per week or engage in 150 minutes of vigorous-intensity aerobic physical activity per week or an equivalent combination of moderate- and vigorous-intensity activity. • Older adults with poor mobility should perform physical activity to enhance balance and prevent falls on 3 or more days per week. • Muscle-strengthening activities involving major muscle groups should be done on 2 or more days a week. • When older adults cannot do the recommended amounts of physical activity because of health conditions, they should be as physically active as their abilities and conditions allow.[41]

31-7 © Monkey Business Images, 2014/Shutterstock.

Health Care Maintenance

Functional decline and a loss of independence are not inevitable consequences of aging. Although the prevalence of chronic disease increases with age, most older people remain functionally independent. However, given the presence of chronic disease among older adults, evidence-based interventions for screening and detection of health conditions and disease are important. The Agency for Healthcare Research and Quality (AHRQ) in partnership with AARP provides recommendations for daily steps to promote good health, screening tests, and medications to help in disease prevention in the publication *Staying Healthy at 50+*. It provides a guide for older adults to follow to ensure that they are receiving screening appropriate for their age and health status.

ENVIRONMENTAL ASSESSMENT

Common environmental hazards include inadequate lighting, loose throw rugs, curled carpet edges, obstructed hallways, cords in walkways, lack of grab bars in tub and shower,

and low and loose toilet seats. These hazards increase the risk for falls and fractures.[33] Environmental modification can promote mobility and reduce the likelihood of the older adult's falling.

Inquire about the safety of the neighborhood and ask whether older persons have transportation and/or services available in geographic proximity to where they live (Fig. 31-7). The community needs access to basic services such as food and clothing stores, pharmacists, financial institutions, health care facilities, and social service agencies. The community environment needs to provide safety conditions such as street lamps, sidewalks, and police and fire protection. These are especially important for older adults who need help in IADLs and who are still living within the community.

Older persons often have challenges not easily detected during an office visit. A home visit can reveal difficulties in the living situation such as household and bathing hazards, social isolation, family/caregiver stress, and nutrition issues. For example, a walk through the kitchen can assess the food preferences of the older adult. An empty refrigerator and/or kitchen cabinets may give clues to previously unrecognized functional impairment such as dementia, mobility challenges, or a decline in the ability to perform IADLs, which would warrant further assessment. Interventions such as home health assistance, transportation services, and shopping services may support the older adult to maintain community living.

Falls

Nearly 30% of older adults fall each year in the community; many of these falls result in serious physical injury such as fractures or head trauma and psychological injury such as fear of falling. Falls in older adults have multiple contributing factors such as gait and balance problems, poor vision, syncope, diabetic neuropathy, and dementia. Multifactorial assessments determine risk, home safety evaluations and interventions, and group and home-based exercise programs containing balance and strength training to reduce the rate and/or risk of falling. Tai Chi reduces the risk of falling, and exercise aimed to reduce falls also appears to reduce fractures. Reducing or gradually withdrawing psychotropic medications reduces falls; at this time vitamin D supplementation does not appear to reduce falls but may be effective for people with low vitamin D levels before treatment. Providing patient education as a single intervention to prevent falls is inconclusive.[12]

Older-Adult Drivers

Older-adult drivers account for 16% of all licensed drivers in the United States, 8% of all traffic crash injuries, and 18% of all pedestrian fatalities.[29] Safe driving requires intact cognitive functioning, sensory perception, good physical abilities (e.g., strength to turn the steering wheel and use pedals; enough range of motion to turn head and neck), alertness, and suitable reflexes. Early and routine attention to health care maintenance activities such as vision and hearing checks, exercise to maintain flexibility and range of motion, and workup of any cognitive abnormalities may allow the older adult to continue to drive safely for longer periods.

Driving represents independence, freedom, and control and is often a necessary part of functioning in daily life such as getting to work or shopping for groceries. It also facilitates remaining connected socially with family and friends. Driving cessation can be devastating to an older adult and lead to symptoms of depression[24] and steep declines in physical functioning.[10] If driving must be limited or cease altogether, it is important to establish a plan of action to enhance independence and maintain normal activity levels. This might mean accessing public transportation, carpooling, or increased involvement of family and friends for activities that require motor transportation. Many states, either by statute or regulation, have identified mandated physician reporting obligations for conditions such as sensory impairments or neurodegenerative illnesses.

Older adults often recognize that their driving abilities have changed and adjust their habits accordingly (e.g., limiting driving to daytime, good weather conditions, or only local driving). However, when this is not the case, family members, friends, or health care providers may be concerned enough about the safety of the older driver and others in the community that they need to intervene. One practical approach is a checklist of warning signs for when to stop driving (Table 31-3).[1] In addition, the American Automobile Association (AAA) and AARP provide online driver self-assessment tests, and local departments of motor vehicles and area agencies on aging can provide additional resources to help older adults and their families with ongoing assessment and planning.

Sleep

Sleep architecture changes with aging (e.g., more difficulty falling and staying asleep); however, significantly altered sleep patterns are not a normal part of aging, and the prevalence of insomnia is low in healthy older adults.[4] Most adults of all ages need about 8 hours of sleep per night to feel alert and

TABLE 31-3 **Warning Signs for When to Stop Driving**
1. Almost crashing, with frequent close calls
2. Finding dents and scrapes on the car, fences, mailboxes, garage doors, curbs, or the like
3. Getting lost
4. Having trouble seeing or following traffic signals, road signs, and pavement markings
5. Responding more slowly to unexpected situations; having trouble moving the foot from the gas to the brake pedal; confusing the two pedals
6. Misjudging gaps in traffic at intersections and on highway entrance and exit ramps
7. Experiencing road rage or having other drivers frequently honk at you
8. Easily becoming distracted or having difficulty concentrating while driving
9. Having a hard time turning around to check over your shoulder while backing up or changing lanes
10. Receiving traffic tickets or warnings from traffic or law enforcement officers in the last year or two

Adapted from AARP. (2010). *What are the warning signs that indicate someone should begin to limit driving or to stop altogether?* Available at www.aarp.org/home-garden/transportation/info-05-2010/Warning_Signs_Stopping.print.html.

rested. Medical and psychiatric illnesses such as cardiac and pulmonary disease, osteoarthritis, dementia, delirium, and depression, as well as side effects of the medications to treat these disorders (beta-blockers, corticosteroids, bronchodilators, decongestants, diuretics), are contributing factors to insomnia. Other causes of insomnia are intake of alcohol, nicotine, and caffeine; sleep apnea; restless legs syndrome; and circadian rhythm disturbances.[4] Detrimental consequences of poor sleep in older adults are poor health outcomes such as obesity, altered physical functioning, falls,[19] impaired cognition, and increased risk for death.[4]

Because medications such as sedatives and hypnotics, often used to treat insomnia, have many side effects for older adults such as falls and delirium, a nonpharmacologic approach to managing sleep in the hospital is recommended (Table 31-4). In the home, use of relaxing music; exposure to sunlight during the day; consistent bedtime routines; limiting food and drink after early evening; reduced light, noise, and room temperature; and whole-body relaxation may improve sleep. One instrument useful for measuring the quality and patterns of sleep in older adults is the Pittsburgh Sleep Quality Index (PSQI). The PSQI can be used across health care settings for initial and ongoing assessments.[37]

SPIRITUAL ASSESSMENT

Spirituality provides personal answers about the meaning and purpose of one's own life and how to interpret life events and regard them as "bigger than oneself." Spiritual health may improve with age, even as physical and mental health deteriorate. The aging process is a part of one's journey, with

TABLE 31-4 Nonpharmacologic Interventions to Promote Sleep

CATEGORY	INTERVENTION	RATIONALE
Dietary	Limit caffeine (coffee, tea, soft drinks, and chocolate) to 2 caffeinated drinks per day, none after lunch.	Caffeine promotes wakefulness by blocking adenosine receptors in the brain.
	Restrict alcohol to 1 drink per day, none after dinner.	Alcohol may shorten the time it takes to fall asleep; but it is metabolized quickly, and withdrawal occurs in the last half of the night, producing lighter sleep and aggravating obstructive sleep apnea, restless legs syndrome, sympathetic arousal, and sweating.
	Restrict fluid intake in the evening.	This reduces nighttime awakening resulting from a full bladder.
	Avoid heavy, spicy meals near bedtime.	This reduces nighttime awakening caused by heartburn.
	Have a light bedtime snack of milk or cheese and crackers.	This promotes sleep by reducing hypoglycemia.
Schedule	Adhere to a regular schedule for meals and sleep, using an alarm, if necessary, to ensure rising at a regular time. Limit naps to one 30-minute, early-afternoon nap.	Maintaining temporal patterns of rest and activity enhances synchrony with circadian rhythms. Excessive daytime napping weakens the homeostatic drive to sleep.
Environment	Maintain daytime light and nighttime dark. Open drapes and blinds; increase the wattage in lamps. Increase sunlight exposure to at least $\frac{1}{2}$ hour per day. Keep the sleep environment dark.	Circadian rhythms are established primarily by patterns of light and dark.
	Use the bed only for sleep or sex, not for work or watching television. Limit time spent in bed to the average time spent asleep. If not asleep after 30 minutes, get up and engage in a relaxing activity until the need to sleep is felt.	The bed becomes an environmental cue for sleep.
	Promote uninterrupted sleep (e.g., by controlling the noise level and limiting or consolidating nighttime interventions).	Limiting noise minimizes sleep disruption.
Activities	Maintain an active physical and social daytime schedule. Avoid passive activities such as watching television.	Vigorous activity promotes daytime arousal, prevents napping, and lessens depression, which can disrupt sleep.
	Keep to a relaxing bedtime ritual (e.g., using massage, reading, prayer, music, and warm baths).	Relaxing activities augment one's readiness for sleep. A warm bath enhances a drop in core temperature.
Delirium	Frequently reorient the patient by keeping a clock and calendar in the room and maintaining a regular schedule and associated light and dark patterns.	These measures decrease anxiety.

From Cole, C., & Richards, K. (2007). Sleep disruption in older adults. *Am J Nurs, 107*(5), 40-49.

capability for growth. Views on spirituality vary greatly from one adult to another and among people of the same faith or belief system. It is important to acknowledge spirituality as a powerful coping mechanism during stressful life events and during illness to the end of life.

Spiritual assessment is highly individual and may be delayed until a provider-client relationship has been developed. Open-ended questions provide a foundation for future dialogue. A sample question posed during the initial assessment may be, "Do you consider yourself to be a spiritual person?" If the person says "yes," a follow-up question could be, "How does that spirituality relate to your health or health care decisions?" Involving chaplains or clergy members when possible and appropriate can provide the older adult with support and serve as a resource to the clinician.

SPECIAL CONSIDERATIONS

Assessment of the functional status of an older adult can be more time consuming than for younger adults. For hospitalized or institutionalized older adults, consider assessing function during normal activities such as grooming, at mealtime, or during toileting.

Understand that a person with multiple medical problems may tire early and easily and that many medications have side effects that contribute to fatigue or affect attention span. Provide directions in written format if necessary. Have the older adult use sensory assistive devices (e.g., glasses, hearing aids) if necessary, and have hearing amplifiers and page magnifiers available (Fig. 31-8). Face the person as much as possible, speak slowly in a lower-pitched voice, and enunciate words clearly.

31-8 © tscaba, 2014/Shutterstock.

Be prepared to use interpreters rather than family members for non–English-speaking older adults.

Including the older adult in decision making about how the interview or testing is to be done establishes rapport and promotes self-esteem. Be aware of body language and behaviors, and be prepared to modify your approach. Touch can also help in establishing rapport and can reduce anxiety.

A functional assessment can be intimidating for older adults. Frustration or embarrassment may arise if some physical maneuvers cannot be performed or questions cannot be answered during cognitive testing. Older adults may also be tearful about the consequences of functional testing such as losing independent living or having a caregiver move into the home. Try to provide reassurance that not everyone can complete all of the tasks or answer all of the questions and that, to the extent possible, confidentiality will be honored.

Ensure adequate space if doing tests of mobility. An aging adult may need room to maneuver an assistive device. When testing mobility, stand close to him or her to prevent a fall. The environment should be well lighted with increased illumination; avoid high-gloss, shiny, slippery surfaces. Minimize

extraneous noise such as those from intercoms, televisions, or high-traffic areas. Warm rooms, access to fluids, proximity to a bathroom, and privacy are important.

Assessing Those in Pain

If the older adult is feeling pain or discomfort, the depth of knowledge gathered through the assessments will suffer. Alleviating pain should be a priority. It may be necessary to administer premedication before parts of the assessment, especially if the assessment requires movement. Another strategy is to use positioning to decrease pain. Ask which position is most comfortable. Providing comfort can help maximize the information gathered. It is paramount to remember that older adults with cognitive impairment do *not* experience less pain. This population suffers from conditions typically associated with pain (e.g., arthritis, osteoporosis, cancer, shingles) just as frequently as cognitively intact persons.

Several studies have demonstrated that those with cognitive impairment can provide self-report pain, which must be taken seriously.[15]

Assessing Older Adults with Altered Cognition

Cognitive impairment poses unique challenges. The older adult may not be able to actively participate in the evaluation and/or provide consistent answers. Gathering information from the older adult firsthand is always the best method but is not always feasible. To ensure the collection of reliable information, one strategy is to interview the caregiver and/or family to obtain subjective assessment data. Another is to arrange opportunities to assess the person during different times of the day when he or she may be more clearheaded.

Adults with cognitive impairment may need questions or directions broken down into single commands, with ongoing verbal cueing or a physical cue. For example, after getting the person's attention, the interviewer might say "sit here" and pat the chair. Never assume that he or she cannot respond to questions even when there is known cognitive impairment. Using *yes* or *no* questions may prevent frustration. Be relaxed and patient because a person with dementia may mirror your emotions. If a family member or caregiver needs to provide collateral information, avoid doing this in front of the older adult.

BIBLIOGRAPHY

1. AARP. (2010). *Know when to limit or stop driving.* www.aarp.org/home-garden/transportation/info-05-2010/ Warning_Signs_Stopping.print.html.
2. AARP Public Policy Institute. (2012). *Valuing the invaluable: 2011 update.* http://www.caregiver.org/caregiver/jsp/content _node.jsp?nodeid=439.
3. Administration on Aging. (2012). *A profile of older Americans.* http://www.aoa.gov/AoARoot/Aging_Statistics/Profile/ index.aspx.
4. Ancoli-Israel, S. (2009). Sleep and its disorders in aging populations. *Sleep Med, 10*(suppl. 1), S7-S11.

5. Bragstad, L. K., Kirevold, M., Hofoss, D., et al. (2012). Factors predicting a successful post-discharge outcome for individuals aged 80 years and over. *Int J Integr Care, 12*(10).
6. Chang-Quan, H., Xue, M., Bi-Rong, D., et al. (2010). Health status and risk for depression among the elderly. *Age Ageing, 39,* 23-30.
7. Covinsky, K. E., Justice, A. C., Rosenthal, G. E., et al. (1997). Measuring prognosis and case mix in hospitalized elders: the importance of functional status. *J Gen Intern Med, 12*(4), 203-208.

8. Creditor, M. C. (1993). Hazards of hospitalization of the elderly. *Ann Intern Med, 18*(3), 219-223.

9. Reference deleted in proofs.

10. Edwards J. D., Lunsman, M., Perkins, M., et al. (2009). Driving cessation and health trajectories in older adults. *J Gerontol Biol Sci, 64*(12), 1290-1295.

11. Fillenbaum, G. G., & Smyer, M. A. (1981). The development, validity, and reliability of the OARS multidimensional functional assessment questionnaire. *J Gerontol, 36*(4), 428-434.

11a. Folstein, M. F., Folstein, S. E., McHugh, P. R. (1975). Mini-mental state. *J Psychiatr Res, 12,* 189-198.

12. Gillespie, L. D., Robertson, M. C., Gillespie, W. J., et al. (2012). Interventions for preventing falls in older people living in the community. *Cochrane Database Syst Rev* 9, Art. No.: CD007146.

13. Guse, L. W. (2006). Assessment of the older adult. In K. L. Mauk (Ed.). *Gerontological nursing competencies for care* (pp. 265-292). Sudbury, MA: Jones & Bartlett.

14. Hamilton, B. B., Granger, C. V., Sherwin, F. S., et al. (1987). A uniform national data system for medical rehabilitation. In M. J. Fuher (Ed.). *Rehabilitation outcomes: analysis and measurement.* Baltimore: Brooks.

15. Herr, K. (2010). Pain in the older adult: an imperative across all health care settings. *Pain Manage Nurs, 11*(2), S1-S10.

16. Hirsch, C. H., Sommers, L., Olsen, A., et al. (1990). The natural history of functional morbidity in hospitalized patients. *J Am Geriatr Soc, 38*(12), 1296-1303.

16a. Inouye, S. K., van Dyck, C. H., Alessi, C. A., et al. (1990). Clarifying confusion: the confusion assessment method. *Ann Intern Med, 113,* 941-948.

17. Karagiozis, H., Gray, S., Sacco, J., et al. (1998). The direct assessment of functional abilities (DAFA). *Gerontologist, 38,* 113-121.

18. Katz, S., Ford, A. B., Moskowitz, R. W., et al. (1963). Studies of illness in the aged: the index of ADL, a standardized measure of biological and psychosocial functioning. *JAMA, 185,* 94-101.

19. Latimer Hill E., Cumming, R. G., Lewis, R., et al. (2007). Sleep disturbances and falls in older people. *J Gerontol Series A, Biol Sci Med Sci, 62*(1), 62-66.

20. Lee, S., Staffileno, B. A., Fogg, L. (2013). Influence of staff education on the function of hospitalized elders. *Nurs Outlook, 61*(1), E2-E8.

21. Linn, M., & Linn, B. (1982). The Rapid Disability Rating Scale-2. *J Am Geriatr Soc, 30,* 378-382.

22. Mahoney, F. I., & Barthel, D. W. (1965). Functional evaluation: the Barthel Index. *Maryland State Med J, 14,* 61-65.

23. Manning, L. K. (2013). Navigating hardships in old age: exploring the relationship between spirituality and resilience in later life. *Qual Health Res, 23*(4), 568–575.

24. Marottoli, R. A., Mendes de Leon, C. F., Glass, T. A., et al. (1997). Driving cessation and increased depressive symptoms. *J Am Geriatr Soc, 45,* 202-206.

25. Mathias, S., Nayak, U. S., & Isaacs, B. (1986). Balance in elderly patients: the "Get Up and Go" test. *Arch Phys Med Rehabil, 67,* 387-389.

26. Mauk, K. L. (2006). Introduction to gerontological nursing. In K. L. Mauk (Ed.), *Gerontological nursing: competencies for care* (pp. 5-28). Boston: Jones & Bartlett.

27. National Alliance for Caregiving; AARP. (2009). *Caregiving in the U.S.: executive summary.* Bethesda, Md.: National Alliance for Caregiving. http://www.caregiving.org/data/CaregivingUSAllAgesExecSum.pdf.

28. National Family Caregivers Association (NFCA). *Caregiving statistics.* www.caregiveraction.org/statistics/.

29. National Highway Traffic Safety Administration's National Center for Statistics and Analysis. (2007). *2007 data—traffic safety facts: older adults (DOT HS 810 992).* Washington, DC: National Highway Traffic Safety Administration.

29a. Neelon, V. J., Champagne, M. T., et al. (1996). The NEECHAM Confusion Scale. *Nurs Res, 45*(6), 324-330.

30. Norbeck, J. S., Lindsey, A. M., & Carrieri, V. L. (1980). The development of an instrument to measure social support. *Nurs Res, 30,* 264-269.

31. Norbeck, J. S., Lindsey, A. M., & Carrieri, V. L. (1983). Further development of the Norbeck Social Support Questionnaire: normative data and validity testing. *Nurs Res, 32,* 4-9.

32. Pearson, V. (2000). Assessment of function. In R. Kane & R. Kane (Eds.), *Assessing older persons: measures, meaning and practical applications* (pp. 17-48). New York: Oxford University Press.

33. Pighills, A.C., Torgerson, D.J., Sheldon, T.A., et al. (2011). Environmental assessment and modification to prevent falls in older people. *J Am Geriatr Soc, 59*(1), 26-33.

34. Richmond, T., Tang, S. T., Tulman, L., et al. (2004). Measuring function. In M. Frank-Stromberg, & S. J. Olsen (Eds.). *Instruments for clinical health-care research* (3rd ed.). Sudbury, MA: Jones & Bartlett.

35. Sager, M. A., Rudberg, M. A., Jalaluddin, M., et al. (1996). Hospital admission risk profile (HARP): identifying older patients at risk for functional decline following acute medical illness and hospitalization. *J Am Geriatr Soc, 44*(3), 251-257.

36. Sheikh, J. I., & Yesavage, J. A. (1986). Geriatric depression scale: recent evidence and development of a shorter version. *Clin Gerontol, 5,* 165-172.

37. Smyth, C. A. (2008). Evaluating sleep quality in older adults. *Am J Nurs, 108*(5), 42-51.

38. Onega, L. L. (2013). *The Modified Caregiver Strain Index (CSI).* Issue # 14. Accessed June 7, 2013, from http://consultgerirn.org/uploads/File/trythis/try_this_14.pdf.

39. Tinetti, M. E. (1986). Performance-oriented assessment of mobility problems on elderly patients. *J Am Geriatr Soc, 34,* 119-126.

40. Van Durme, T., Marq, J., Jeanmart, C., et al. (2012). Tools for measuring the impact of informal caregiving of the elderly. *Int J Nurs Stud, 49,* 490-504.

41. World Health Organization (2011). *Global recommendations on physical activity for health: 65 years and above.* http://www.who.int/dietphysicalactivity/factsheet_olderadults/en/.

41a. Yesavage, J. A., Brink, T. L., Rose, T. L., et al. (1983). Development and validation of a geriatric depression rating scale: a preliminary report. *J Psychiatr Res, 17,* 27.

42. Zarit., S. H., Femia, E. E., Kim, K., et al. (2010). The structure of risk factors and outcomes for family caregivers. *Aging Ment Health, 14* (2), 220-231.

ILLUSTRATION CREDITS

Acute Pain Management Guideline Panel, 1992.

Adams, G.L., Boies, L.R., Jr, & Hilger, P.A. (1989). *Boies fundamentals of otolaryngology: a textbook of ear, nose and throat diseases* (6th ed.). Philadelphia: Saunders.

Tables 5-6 (Retracted drum; Acute [purulent] otitis media [early stage]; Acute [purulent] otitis media [later stage]), 16-5 (Smooth, glossy tongue [atrophic glossitis])

Agricultural Research Service (ARS) (2012). Image Gallery. Beltsville, Maryland: United States Department of Agriculture.

AirStrip Technologies, © 2014. All rights reserved. Trademarks not belonging to AirStrip Technologies are the property of their respective companies. iPhone and is a registered trademark of Apple Inc. The information included about AirStrip products is intended for customers, partners, and healthcare professionals in the United States only. All information, including Prescribing Information for our products, abides by the laws, regulatory requirements, and medical practices for the United States only and may not be appropriate for use outside of the United States.

Albert, D.M., & Jakobiec, F.A. (1994). *Principles and practice of ophthalmology,* Philadelphia: Saunders.

Table 4-2 (Ectropion; Entropion)

Alfaro-LeFevre, R. (2009). *Critical thinking and clinical judgment: a practical appro*ach (4th ed.). Philadelphia: Saunders.

Ameerally, P.J., Colver. G.B. (2007). Cutaneous cryotherapy in maxillofacial surgery. *Journal of Oral and Maxillofacial Surgery, 65*(9), 1785-1792.

Table 5-2 (Carcinoma)

American Society of Human Genetics. (2004). www.ashg.org.

Anderson, R.C., Baker, E.J., Redington, A., Rigby, M.L., Penny, D., Wernovsky, G. (2010). *Paediatric cardiology* (ed. 3). Philadelphia: Churchill Livingstone.

Table 9-5 (Marfan syndrome)

Apgar, B.S., Brotzman, G.L., Spitzer, M. (2008). *Colposcopy: principles and practice* (ed. 2). Philadelphia, Saunders.

Atkinson, P., Kendall, R., Resnburg, L.V. (2011). *Emergency medicine: an illustrated color text* (1 ed.). Philadelphia: Churchill Livingstone.

Table 4-6 (Primary Angle-Closure Glaucoma)

Babu, M.S., Murthy, K.V.K.S.N., Sasidharan S. (2012). Burton's line. *The American Journal of Medicine 125*(10), 963-964.

Table 6-3 (Burton Line)

Black, M., Ambros-Rudolph, C.M., Edwards, L., Lynch, P.J. (2008). *Obstetric and gynecologic dermatology* (ed. 3). St. Louis: Mosby.

Bloom, A., Watkins, P.H., & Ireland, J. (1992). *Color atlas of diabetes* (2nd ed.). St. Louis: Mosby.

Bowden, V.R., Dickey, S.B., & Greenburg, C.S. (1998). *Children and their families: the continuum of care.* Philadelphia: Saunders.

Table 3-2 (Hydrocephalus)

Boyd-Monk, Heather, and Wills Eye Hospital, Philadelphia.

Tables 4-3 (Chalazion), 14-7 (Corneal abrasion)

Braddom, R.L. (2011). *Physical medicine and rehabilitation* (ed. 4). Philadelphia: Saunders.

Brady, Rick; Riva, Md.

Bunker, T., & Schranz, P.J. (1998). *Clinical challenges in orthopaedics: the shoulder.* London: Martin Dunitz, reproduced by permission of Taylor & Francis Books UK.

Table 2-2 (Atrophy; Dislocated shoulder; Joint effusion)

Busch, Niels.

Callen, J.P., et al. (1993). *Color atlas of dermatology.* Philadelphia: Saunders.

Tables 2-9 (Chickenpox [varicella]), 12-12 (Pediculosis capitis [head lice]; Trichotillomania), 12-13 (Beau's line; Splinter hemorrhages), 13-3 (Pilar cyst [wen], 16-2 (Herpes simplex 1; Angular cheilitis), 16-3 (Gingivitis), 16-4 (Candidiasis or monilial infe

Canale, S.T., Beaty, J.H. (2013). *Campbell's operative orthopaedics* (ed. 12). St. Louis: Mosby.

Table 2-4 (Dupuytren contracture)

Carroll, P. (2007). Health literacy: a critical patient safety tool. *RT: For decision makers in respiratory care 20*(7): 36.

Cavan Images.

Centers for Disease Control and Prevention (CDC) (2005, March 18). Public health image library (PHIL). Retrieved http://phil.cdc.gov.

Table 3-3 (Parotid gland enlargement)

Chudley, A.E., MD.

Table 2-8 (Talipes equinovarus)

Clark D.A. (2000). *Atlas of neonatology* (ed. 7). Philadelphia: Saunders.

Table 1-4 (Diastasis recti)

Clinical Slide Collection on the Rheumatic Diseases.1991, 1995, 1997. Used by permission of the American College of Rheumatology.

Tables 9-5 (Acromegaly [hyperpituitarism]), 12-13 (Late clubbing), 15-1 (Frostbite), 15-2 (Tophi), 22-4 (Carpal tunnel syndrome with atrophy of thenar eminence)

Comerci, George D., MD.

Table 9-5 (Anorexia nervosa)

Conroy K., Malata C.M. (2012). Epigastric hernia following DIEP flap breast reconstruction: complication or coincidence? *Journal of Plastic, Reconstructive & Aesthetic Surgery 65*(3), 387-391.

Table 1-4 (Epigastric hernia)

Cooper, Connie.

Dean, S., Garrett, N., Tyrrell, J. (2008). Management of enlarged cervical lymph nodes. *Paediatrics and Child Health, 118*(3), 118-122.

Dhillon, R.S., East, C.A. (2013). *Ear, nose and throat and head and neck surgery* (ed. 4). Philadelphia: Churchill Livingstone.

Table 5-6 (Perforation; Blue drum [hemotympanum])

Dieppe, P.A., Cooper, C., & McGill, N. (1991). *Arthritis and rheumatism in practice.* London: Gower Medical Publishing.

Tables 2-3 (Olecranon bursitis), 22-5 (Mild synovitis; Prepatellar bursitis), 22-6 (Achilles tenosynovitis; Acute gout)

Dockery, G.L. (1997). *Cutaneous disorders of the lower extremity.* Philadelphia: Saunders.

Tables 2-8 (Petechiae), 20-4 (Arterial-ischemic ulcer), 20-5 (Deep vein thrombophlebitis [DVT]), 22-6 (Tophi with chronic gout)

Douglas, G., Nicol, F., Robertson, C. (2013). *Macleod's clinical examination* (ed. 13). Philadelphia: Churchill Livingstone.

Table 6-6 (Acute tonsillitis and pharyngitis)

Edmond, R., Rowl, H.A.K., & Welsby, P. (1995). *Colour atlas of infectious diseases* (3rd ed., p. 161). London: Mosby.

Tables 4-3 (Urethritis [Urethral Discharge and Dysuria]), 24-4 (Syphilitic chancre), 26-2 (Syphilitic chancre; Abscess of Bartholin's gland)

Elshafieya, M.E., Zeeneldinb, A.A., Elsebaia, H.I., Moneerc, M., et al. (2011). Epidemiology and management of breast carcinoma in Egyptian males: experience of a single cancer institute. *Journal of the Egyptian National Cancer Institute 23*(3), 115-122.

Table 7-8 (Male breast cancer)

Evans, A.J., et al. 1998). *Atlas of breast disease management: 50 illustrative cases,* Philadelphia: Saunders.

Tables 7-3 (Dimpling), 17-6 (Carcinoma)

Feigin, R.D., & Cherry, J.D. (1998). *Textbook of pediatric infectious diseases* (4th ed.). Philadelphia: Saunders.

Tables 2-9 (Measles [rubeola] in dark skin), 16-4 (Koplik spots)

Feigin, R.D., et al. (2009). *Feigin and Cherry's textbook of pediatric infectious diseases* (6th ed.). Philadelphia: Saunders.

Ferguson, F. Department of Children's Dentistry, School of Dental Medicine, SUNY at Stony Brook, Stony Brook, NY.

Table 6-3 (Baby bottle tooth decay)

Fireman, P. (1996). *Atlas of allergies* (2nd ed.). London: Mosby.

Tables 2-4 (Wheal and urticaria [hives]), 15-6 (Insertion of tympanostomy tubes), 16-1 (Foreign body; Acute rhinitis, Allergic rhinitis; Nasal polyps)

Firestein, G.S., Budd, R.C., Gabriel, S.E., McInnes, I.B., O'Dell, J.R. (2013). *Kelley's textbook of rheumatology* (ed. 9). Philadelphia: Saunders.

Table 2-2 (Subacromial bursitis)

Flint, P.W., Haughey, B.H., Lund, V.J., Niparko, J.K., Richardson, M.A., Robbins, K.T., Thomas, J.R. (2010). *Cummings otolaryngology head & neck surgery* (ed. 5). Philadelphia: Saunders.

Table 6-6 (Oral Kaposi sarcoma)

Friedman, N., Pineda, R. (1998). *The Massachusetts Eye and Ear Infirmary illustrated manual of ophthalmology.* Philadelphia: Saunders.

Tables 4-3 (Blepharitis [inflammation of the eyelids]; Dacryocystitis [inflammation of the lacrimal sac]), 14-8 (Central gray opacity—nuclear cataract; Star-shaped opacity—cortical cataract), 14-9 (Excessive cup-disc ratio), 14-10 (Arteriovenous crossing [nicki]

Friedman, N., Kaiser, P.K., & Pineda, R. (2009). *The Massachusetts Eye and Ear Infirmary illustrated manual of ophthalmology* (3rd ed.). Philadelphia: Saunders.

Table 4-9 (Optic atrophy [disc pallor]; Papilledema [choked disc])

Friedman, N.J., Kaiser, P.K., Pineda R. (2014). *The Massachusetts Eye and Ear Infirmary Illustrated Manual of Ophthalmology* (ed. 4). Philadelphia: Saunders Elsevier.

Tables 4-3 (Basal cell carcinoma), 14-6 (Herpes Simplex), 14-10 (Moderate nonproliferative diabetic retinopathy; Severe nonproliferative diabetic retinopathy; Severe nonproliferative diabetic retinopathy; Proliferative diabetic retinopathy; Neovascularizations

Friedman-Kien, A.E. (1989). *Color atlas of AIDS.* Philadelphia: Saunders.

Table 2-12 (AIDS-related Kaposi sarcoma: Patch stage)

Gerontological Society of America. Katz S., et al. (1970). Progress in the development of the index of ADL. *Gerontologist 10*:20-30.

GlaxoSmithKline, 2013.

Glynn M. and Drake W.M. (2012). *Hutchison's clinical methods: an integrated approach to clinical practice* (23rd ed.). Philadelphia: Saunders/Elsevier Ltd.

Table 3-5 (Parkinson syndrome)

Goldenring, J.M., & Rosen, D.S. (2004). Getting into adolescent heads: an essential update. *Contemporary Pediatrics 21*(1), 64-68, 70, 73-74.

Gould, B.E., Dyer, R. (2011). *Pathophysiology for the health professions* (ed. 4). Philadelphia: Saunders.

Table 4-3 (Renal calculi)

Habif T.P., et al. (2005). *Skin disease: diagnosis and treatment* (2nd ed.). St Louis: Mosby.

Tables 2-8 (Strawberry mark [immature hemangioma]; Cavernous hemangioma [mature]; Venous lake), 15-2 (Chondrodermatitis nodularis helicus), 24-4 (Genital warts)

Habif, T.P., et al. (2001). *Skin disease: diagnosis and treatment.* St Louis: Mosby.

Tables 2-11 (Squamous cell carcinoma), 26-2 (Genital human papillomavirus [HPV] genital warts)

Hall, R., & Evered, D.C. (1990). *Color atlas of endocrinology* (2nd ed.). London: Mosby.

Tables 9-5 (Hypopituitary dwarfism; Gigantism) 11-3 (Marasmus), 13-4 (Myxedema [hypothyroidism])

Hawke, M. (1998). *Diagnostic handbook of otorhinolaryngology.* London: Martin Dunitz, reproduced by permission of Taylor & Francis Books UK.

Tables 6-1 (Perforated septum), 16-2 (Carcinoma; Retention "Cyst" [Mucocele]), 16-6 (Bifid Uvula)

Hicks, C.L., et al. (2001). Faces Pain Scale—Revised: toward a common metric in pediatric pain measurement. *Pain 93*, 173-183. 2001 the International Association for the Study of Pain (IASP).

Hockenberry, M.J. & Wilson, D.: *Wong's essentials of pediatric nursing* (9th ed.). St. Louis: Mosby.
  Tables 3-2 (Down syndrome), 14-2 (Upward palpebral slant)

Holgate, S.T., Church, M.K., Broide, D.H., Martinez, F.D. (2012). *Allergy* (ed. 4). Philadelphia: Saunders.
  Table 4-6 (Allergic conjunctivitis)

Hurwitz, S. (1993). *Clinical pediatric dermatology: a textbook of skin disorders of childhood and adolescence* (2nd ed.). Philadelphia: Saunders.
  Table 2-12 (Toxic alopecia; Alopecia areata; Traumatic alopecia: Traction alopecia; Seborrheic dermatitis [cradle cap])

Ibsen, O.A.C., & Phelan, J.A. (1992). *Oral pathology for the dental hygienist* (2nd ed.). Philadelphia: Saunders.
  Table 4-2 (Periorbital edema)

Ibsen, O.A.C., & Phelan, J.A. (1996). *Oral pathology for the dental hygienist* (2nd ed.). Philadelphia: Saunders.
  Tables 6-2 (Cleft lip), 16-3 (Epulis; Gingival hyperplasia), 16-5 (Ankyloglossia)

Jacquelyn C. Campbell, PhD, RN,1985, 1988, 2001.

Jones A., & Owen, R. (1995). *Color atlas of clinical orthopedics* (2nd ed.). London: Mosby.
  Tables 9-5 (Achondroplastic dwarfism), 22-5 (Swelling of menisci)

Kanski, J.J. (2009). *Clinical ophthalmology: a synopsis* (2nd ed.). Elsevier Ltd. 9780702031359.
  Table 3-5 (Cushing syndrome)

Keys, C., Lam, J.P.H. (2013). Foreskin and penile problems in childhood. *Surgery (Oxford) 31*(3), 130-134.
  Table 4-5 (Paraphimosis)

Krechel, S.W., & Bildner, J. (1995). CRIES—a new neonatal postoperative pain measurement score: initial testing of validity and reliability. *Pediatric Anesthesia, 5*, 53-61.

Kroenke, K., et al. (2007). Anxiety disorders in primary care: prevalence, impairment, comorbidity, and detection. *Annals of Internal Medicine, 146*(5), 317-325.

Lakatta, E.G. (1985). Cardiovascular function in later life, *Cardiovascular Medicine 10*, 37-40, 1985.

Latham, M.C., et al. (1980). *Scope manual on nutrition.* Kalamazoo: The Upjohn Company, Thomas Spies, MD.
  Table 1-4 (Pellagra; Rickets)

Lawton, M.P., & Brody, E.M. (1969). Assessment of older people: Self-maintaining and instrumental activities of daily living. *Gerontologist 9*:179-186.The Gerontological Society of America.

Leifer, B.P. (2009). Alzheimer's disease: seeing the signs early. *J Acad Nurse Pract*, 21(11), 588-595.

Lemmi and Lemmi, 2011.
  Tables 2-4 (Macule and patch; Papule and plaque; Nodule and tumor; Vesicle and bulla; Cyst; Pustule), 12-5 (Crust; Scale; Fissure; Erosion; Ulcer; Excoriation; Scar; Atrophic scar; Lichenification; Keloid), 12-8 (Telangiectasia; Spider or star angioma; Ecchymos

Liebert, P.S. (1996). *Color atlas of pediatric surgery* (2nd ed.). Philadelphia: Saunders.
  Table 5-1 (Branchial remnant and ear deformity), 15-2 (Sebaceous cyst), 22-4 (Polydactyly; Syndactyly), 24-5 (Phimosis; Hypospadias)

Lim, Eric Kian Saik. (2007). *Medicine & surgery: An integrated textbook* (ed. 1). Philadelphia: Churchill Livingstone.
  Table 5-6 (Scarred drum)

Liu,G.T.,Volpe,N.J.,Galetta S.L. (2010). *neuro-ophthalmology: diagnosis and management* (2nd ed.). Philadelphia: Saunders.
  Table 3-5 (Acromegaly)

Lookingbill D.P., & Marks, J.G. (1993). *Principles of dermatology* (2nd ed.). Philadelphia: Saunders.
  Tables 2-8 (Strawberry mark [immature hemangioma]), 12-10 (Primary contact dermatitis; Allergic drug reaction; Psoriasis), 12-11 (Basal cell carcinoma; Malignant melanoma), 12-12 (Tinea capitis [scalp ringworm]; Furuncle and abscess), 20-4 (Venous [stasis] ulcer

Lorenzo, G. D., Autorino, R., Perdonà, S., Placido, S.D. (2005). Management of gynaecomastia in patients with prostate cancer: a systematic review. *The Lancet 6*(12), 972-979.
  Table 7-8 (Gynecomastia)

Mansel, R. (1995). *Color atlas of breast diseases.* London: Mosby.
  Tables 7-3 (Edema [peau d'orange]; Fixation; Deviation in nipple pointing), 17-6 (Mammary duct ectasia; Intraductal papilloma; Paget's disease [intraductal carcinoma]), 17-7 (Mastitis; Breast abscess)

McCaffery, M., & Pasero, C. (1999). *Pain: clinical manual* (2nd ed.). St. Louis: Mosby.

McLaren, D.S. (1981). *Color atlas of nutritional disorders.* London: Wolfe Medical, C.E. Butterworth, Jr.
  Table 1-5 (Magenta tongue)

McWhorter, A., *Pediatric dentistry,* Baylor College of Dentistry, The Texas A & M University System, Dallas, TX.
  Table 6-3 (Dental caries)

Meningaud et al. (2007). Kimura's disease of the parotid region. *Journal of Oral and Maxillofacial Surgery 65*(1), 134-140.
  Table 3-3 (Parotid gland enlargement)

Meur, S., Mann, N. P. (2007). Infant outcomes following diabetic pregnancies. *Paediatrics and Child Health 17*(6), 217-222.
  Table 29-2 (Fetal macrosomia)

Mini Nutritional Assessment (MNA). ®Société des Produits Nestlé S.A., Vevey, Switzerland, Trademark Owners.

Moore, K.L., & Persaud, T.V.N. (1998). *Before we are born: essentials of embryology and birth defect* (5th ed.). Philadelphia: Saunders.
  Table 6-8 (Ambiguous genitalia)

Moore, K.L., & Persaud, T.V.N. (2008). *Before we are born: essentials of embryology and birth defects* (7th ed.). Philadelphia: Saunders.

Muram, D., Simmons, K.J. (2008). Pattern recognition in pediatric and adolescent gynecology—a case for formal education. *J Pediatr Adolesc Gynecol 21*(2), 103-108.
  Table 6-8 (Vulvovaginitis in child)

Murray, S.S., & McKinney, E.S. (2010). *Foundations of maternal-newborn and women's health nursing* (5th ed.). St. Louis: Saunders.

National Institute on Alcohol Abuse and Alcoholism (NIAAA). (Reprinted 2007).

Neville BW et al: *Oral and maxillofacial pathology* (3rd ed.). St. Louis, 2009, Saunders.
Table 6-3 (Meth mouth)

Nichols, F.H., & Zwelling, E. (1997). *Maternal-newborn nursing: theory and practice,* Philadelphia: Saunders.

Nolte, J., Sundsten, J. (2009). *The human brain: an introduction to its functional anatomy* (6th ed.). Philadelphia: Mosby/Elsevier.
Table 3-5 (Stroke or "Brain Attack")

Nursing Research Consortium on Violence and Abuse (NRCVA) (1988).

Paller, A.S., & Mancini, A.J. (2011). *Hurwitz clinical pediatric dermatology: a textbook of skin disorders of childhood and adolescence* (4th ed.). Philadelphia: Saunders.
Tables 2-8 (Port-wine stain [Nevus flammeus]; Purpura), 12-9 (Diaper dermatitis; Atopic dermatitis [eczema]; German measles [rubella]), 12-10 (Tinea corporis [ringworm of the body])

Pantagraph, The. (August 10, 1998). Bloomington, IL.

Patton, K.T., Thibodeau, G. A., Douglas, M.M. (2012). *Essentials of anatomy & physiology* (ed. 1). St. Louis: Mosby.

Peñas C.F., Cleland, J.A., Huijbregts, P.A. (2011). *Neck and arm pain syndromes: evidence-informed screening, diagnosis and management.* Philadelphia: Churchill Livingstone.
Table 2-2 (Frozen shoulder—adhesive capsulitis)

Peters and Pasvol (2009). *Atlas of tropical medicine and parasitology* (6th ed.). Philadelphia: Churchill Livingstone.
Table 6-4 (Candidiasis in Adult)

Pfenninger, J.L., Fowler, G. C. (2011). *Pfenninger and Fowler's procedures for primary care* (ed. 3). St. Louis: Mosby.
Table 6-6 (Peritonsillar Abscess)

Pfizer Laboratories Division, Pfizer Inc, New York. *A close look at VD: a slide presentation produced as a public service.*
Tables 4-4 (Genital herpes—HSV-2 infection), 26-2 (Red rash—contact dermatitis), 26-5 (Gonorrhea)

Polley, H.F., & Hunder, G.G. (1978). *Physical examination of the joints* (2nd ed.). Philadelphia: Saunders.
Table 2-3 (Gouty arthritis), 22-7 (Herniated nucleus pulposus)

Pomatto J.K., Calcaterra J., Kelly K.M., et al. (2006). A study of family head shape: environment alters cranial shape. *Clinical Pediatrics 45* (1), 55–64, 2006.
Table 3-2 (Plagiocephaly)

Potter, P.A., & Perry, A.G. (2009). *Fundamentals of nursing.* (7th ed.). St Louis: Mosby.
Table 2-6 (Decubitus Ulcer: Stages I-IV)

Potter, P.A., Perry, A.G., Stockert, P.,Hall, A. (2015). *Essentials for nursing practice* (ed. 8). St. Louis: Mosby.

Quiñones-Hinojosa A. (2012). *Schmidek and Sweets operative neurosurgical techniques: indications, methods and results* (6th ed.). Philadelphia: Saunders.
Table 3-2 (Craniosynostosis)

Rimsza, M.E. (1989). An illustrated guide to adolescent gynecology. *Pediatric Clinics of North America, 36*(3), 641.
Table 6-2 (Urethral caruncle)

Rossman, I. (1986). *Clinical geriatrics* (3rd ed.). Philadelphia: Lippincott.

Sager, M.A. et al (1996). Hospital admission risk profile (HARP): Identifying older patients at risk for functional decline following acute medical illness and hospitalization. *Journal of the American Geriatrics Society 44*(3), 251-257.

Scale Hickey, J.V. (1986). *Neurological and neurosurgical nursing* (2nd ed.). Philadelphia: Lippincott.

Scheie, H.G., & Albert, D.M. (1977). *Textbook of ophthalmology* (9th ed.). Philadelphia: Saunders.
Tables 4-6 (Iritis [circumcorneal redness]), 14-7 (Hypopyon)

Sheikh, J.I., & Yesavage, J.A. Geriatric Depression Scale (GDS): Recent evidence and development of a shorter version. In Brink, T.L. (1986). *Clinical gerontology: a guide to assessment and intervention.* Binghamton, NY: Haworth Press, pp. 165-173.

Sheridan, Daniel J., PhD, RN, FAAN. St. Louis, MO.

Skirven, T.M., Osterman, A.L., Fedorczyk, J.M., Amadio, P.C. (2011). *Rehabilitation of the hand and upper extremity* (ed. 6). St. Louis: Mosby.
Table 2-3 (Epicondylitis—Tennis elbow)

Sleisinger, M.H., & Fordtran, J.S. (1993). *Gastrointestinal diseases: pathophysiology, diagnosis, and management* (5th ed.). Vol 1, Philadelphia: Saunders.
Table 6-4 (Leukoplakia)

Slutsky D.J. (2010). *Principles and practice of wrist surgery.* Philadelphia: Saunders.
Table 2-4 (Ankylosis)

Spector, R.E. (2013). *Cultural diversity in health and illness* (8th ed.). Upper Saddle River, NJ: Pearson, pp. 376-378.

Spector, Rachel E., 2009.

Spitzer, Robert L., Williams, Janet B.W., Kroenke, Kurt, and colleagues, with an educational grant Pfizer Inc. No permission required to reproduce, translate, display, or distribute.

Streissguth, A.P. et al. (1980). Teratogenic effects of alcohol in humans and laboratory animals, *Science 209,* 353-361.
Table 3-2 (Fetal alcohol syndrome)

Stricker, Hans, Department of Urology, Henry Ford Hospital, Detroit MI.
Table 4-5 (Peyronie disease)

Studdiford J.S., Altschuler M. Salzman B., Tully A. (2009). *Images from the wards: diagnosis and treatment* (1st ed.). Philadelphia: Saunders.
Table 3-5 (Bell Palsy)

Swartz, M.H. (2005). *Textbook of physical diagnosis: history and examination* (5th ed.). Philadelphia: Saunders.
Tables 2-10 (Erythema migrans of Lyme disease), 13-3 (Thyroid—multiple nodules), 13-4 (Hyperthyroidism), 15-6 (Otitis media with effusion; Cholesteatoma; Bullous myringitis)

Symonds, E.M., MacPherson, M.B.A. (1997). *Color atlas of obstetrics and gynecology*, London: Mosby-Wolfe.
   Tables 6-3 (Uterine prolapse), 26-4 (Human papillomavirus [HPV, condylomata]; Carcinoma), 30-1 (Preeclampsia)
Tanner, J.M. (1962). *Growth at adolescence*. Oxford, England: Blackwell Scientific.
Taylor, K.B., & Anthony, L.E. (1983). *Clinical nutrition*. New York: McGraw-Hill.
   Table 1-5 (Follicular hyperkeratosis; Scorbutic gums; Bitot's spots)
Thomas, Pat, 2006.
   Tables 3-2 (Fetal alcohol syndrome [line drawing], 19-10 (Abnormal pulsations on the precordium), 19-11 (Congenital heart defects), 19-12 (Murmurs due to valvular defects), 21-3 (Liver, appendicitis, gallbladder, and others), 23-11 (Abnormal postures), 23-13 (Frontal release signs), 24-6 (Scrotum abnormalities), 24-7 (Inguinal anad femoral hernias)
Thomas, Pat, 2010.
   Tables 10-5 (Reflexive sympathetic dystrophy), 12-4 (Primary skin lesions [line drawings], 12-5 (Secondary skin lesions [line drawings], 15-4 (Ear canal abnormalities), 15-6 (Fungal infection [otomycosis]), 22-9 (Fibromyalgia syndrome), 23-9 (Patterns of motor)
Thomas, Pat, 2014.
   Tables 3-1 (Primary headaches), 13-4 (Hypothalamic-pituitary-thyroid axis), 15-3 (Hearing loss), 21-2 (Clinical portrait of intestinal obstruction), 23-6 (Ischemic and hemorrhagic stroke)
Thompson, D.N.P. (2010). Spinal dysraphic anomalies; classification, presentation and management. *Paediatrics and Child Health 20*(9), 397-403.
   Table 2-8 (Spina bifida)
Voepel-Lewis, T., Zanotti, J., Dammeyer, J.A., Merkel, S. (2010). Reliability and validity of the face, legs, activity, cry, consolability behavioral tool in assessing acute pain in critically ill patients. *American Journal of Critical Care, 19*(1),55-61. Printed with permission © The Regents of the University of Michigan.
Waldman, S.D. (2010). *Physical diagnosis of pain : an atlas of signs and symptoms* (ed. 2). Philadelphia: Saunders.
   Table 2-2 (Tear of rotator cuff)

Walker, J.M., & Helewa, A. (1996). *Physical therapy in arthritis*. Philadelphia: Saunders.
   Tables 2-4 (Ulnar deviation or drift; Degenerative joint disease, or osteoarthritis), 22-6 (Hallux valgus with bunion and hammertoes)
Walsh, T.D. et al. (2009). *Palliative medicine*. Philadelphia: Saunders.
   Table 20-2 (Lymphedema)
Warden, V., Hurley, A.C., & Voticer, L. (2003). Development and psychometric evaluation of the Pain Assessment in Advanced Dementia (PAINAD) Scale. *Journal of the American Medical Directors Association, 4*, 9-15.
Wenig B.M., Hefess C.S., & Adair, C.F. (1997). *Atlas of endocrine pathology*, Philadelphia: Saunders.
   Tables 9-5 (Endogenous obesity—Cushing syndrome), 16-5 (Carcinoma)
Yaffe, M.J., Lithwick, M., Wolfson, C., 2006.
Yeh, M.W., Duh, Q.Y. (2012). *Sabiston textbook of surgery: the biological basis of modern surgical practice* (19th ed.). Philadelphia: Saunders.
   Table 3-5 (Cushing syndrome)
Yoder-Wise P.S. (2014). *Leading and managing in nursing: revised reprint* (ed. 5). St. Louis: Mosby.
Zakus, S.M. (2001). *Mosby's clinical skills for medical assistants* (ed. 4). St. Louis: Mosby.
Zitelli, B.J., & Davis, H.W. (2002). *Atlas of pediatric physical diagnosis* (4th ed.). St Louis: Mosby.
   Tables 6-5 (Enlarged tongue [macroglossia]), 16-6 (Cleft palate), 22-5 (Osgood-Schlatter disease), 22-7 (Scoliosis [bending forward]), 22-8 (Congenital dislocated hip), 24-5 (Epispadias)
Zitelli, B.J., & Davis, H.W. (2007). *Atlas of pediatric physical diagnosis* (5th ed.). St Louis: Mosby.
   Tables 3-2 (Atopic [allergic] facies; Allergic salute and crease), 13-3 (Torticollis [wryneck]), 14-1 (Left esotropia; Exotropia), 21-4 (Umbilical hernia)
Zitelli, B.J., McIntire, S.C., Nowalk, A.J. (2012). *Atlas of pediatric physical diagnosis* (ed. 6). Philadelphia, Saunders.
   Table 5-2 (Battle sign)

b indicates boxed material, *f* indicates illustrations, and *t* indicates tables.

851